DIAGNOSIS AND TREATMENT
OF SKIN INFECTIONS

Diagnosis and Treatment of Skin Infections

EDITED BY
MARWALI HARAHAP
Professor of Dermatology
School of Medicine
University of North Sumatra
Medan, Indonesia

**Blackwell
Science**

© 1997 by
Blackwell Science Ltd
Editorial Offices:
Osney Mead, Oxford OX2 0EL
25 John Street, London WC1N 2BL
23 Ainslie Place, Edinburgh EH3 6AJ
350 Main Street, Malden
    MA 02148 5018, USA
54 University Street, Carlton
    Victoria 3053, Australia

Other Editorial Offices:
Blackwell Wissenschafts-Verlag GmbH
Kurfürstendamm 57
10707 Berlin, Germany

Blackwell Science KK
MG Kodenmacho Building
7-10 Kodenmacho Nihombashi
Chuo-ku, Tokyo 104, Japan

First published 1997

Set by Excel Typesetters Co., Hong Kong
Printed and bound in Italy by
G. Canale & C. SpA, Turin

The Blackwell Science logo is a
trade mark of Blackwell Science Ltd,
registered at the United Kingdom
Trade Marks Registry

DISTRIBUTORS

Marston Book Services Ltd
PO Box 269
Abingdon
Oxon OX14 4YN
(*Orders*: Tel: 01235 465500
       Fax: 01235 465555)

USA
Blackwell Science, Inc.
Commerce Place
350 Main Street
Malden, MA 02148 5018
(*Orders*: Tel: 800 759 6102
       617 388 8250
       Fax: 617 388 8255)

Canada
Copp Clark Professional
200 Adelaide St West, 3rd Floor
Toronto, Ontario M5H 1W7
(*Orders*: Tel: 416 597-1616
       800 815-9417
       Fax: 416 597-1617)

Australia
Blackwell Science Pty Ltd
54 University Street
Carlton, Victoria 3053
(*Orders*: Tel: 3 9347 0300
       Fax: 3 9347 5001)

A catalogue record for this title
is available from the British Library

ISBN 0-632-04757-7

Library of Congress
Cataloging-in-publication Data

Diagnosis and treatment of skin infections/
    edited by Marwali Harahap.
        p.   cm.
    Includes bibliographical references and
index.
    ISBN 0-632-04757-7
    1. Skin—Infections.   I. Harahap,
Marwali.
    [DNLM: 1. Skin Diseases, Infections—
diagnosis.
    2. Skin Diseases,
Infectious—therapy.   WR 220 D536
1997]
RL201.D53   1997
616.5—DC21
DNLM/DLC
for Library of Congress

Contents

List of Contributors

Gary L. Darmstadt MD, Division of Infectious Disease, Children's Hospital and Medical Center, University of Washington School of Medicine, Seattle, Washington, USA

Mervyn L. Elgart MD, Professor and Chairman, Department of Dermatology, George Washington University Medical Center, Washington, DC, USA

Sheila Fallon-Friedlander MD, Assistant Professor, Departments of Medicine and Pediatrics, Division of Dermatology, University of California, San Diego School of Medicine, and Division of Pediatric Dermatology, Children's Hospital, San Diego, California, USA

Ann F. Haas MD, Assistant Professor, Department of Dermatology, University of California, Davis, School of Medicine, Sacramento, California, USA

Eckart Haneke MD, Professor, Hautklinik, Academic Teaching Hospital, University of Düsseldorf, Wuppertal, Germany

Marwali Harahap MD, Professor of Dermatology, School of Medicine, University of North Sumatra, Rumah Sakit Umum H. Adam Malik, Medan, Indonesia

John A.D. Leake MD, M.F.H., Epidemic Intelligence Service, Division of Bacterial and Mycotic Diseases, Centers for Disease Control and Prevention, Atlanta, Georgia, USA

M. Reza P. Marwali MD, Department of Internal Medicine, Wayne State University, School of Medicine, Detroit, Michigan, USA

Monica L. McCrary MD, Department of Dermatology, Medical College of Georgia, Augusta, Georgia, USA

A. Colin McDougall MD, FRCP, FRCP (Edin), formerly Consultant in Clinical Research to the British Leprosy Relief Association (LEPRA), Department of Dermatology, The Slade Hospital, Headington, Oxford, UK

Lawrence Charles Parish MD, Clinical Professor, Department of Dermatology and Cutaneous Biology, Jefferson Medical College of Thomas Jefferson University, Philadelphia, Pennsylvania, USA

Martha S. Paterson MD, Department of Internal Medicine, University of Texas Medical Branch, Galveston, Texas, USA

David T. Roberts MB, ChB, FRCP (Glas), Consultant Dermatologist, Southern General Hospital and Victoria Infirmary, Clinical Director of Dermatology and Genitourinary Medicine, Southern General Hospital, Honorary Senior Lecturer, University of Glasgow, Glasgow, UK

Stephen K. Tyring MD, PhD, Professor, Departments of Dermatology, Microbiology, Immunology, and Internal Medicine, University of Texas Medical Branch, Galveston, Texas, USA

Anne E. Weilepp MD, Division of Dermatology, University of California, San Diego Medical Center, Children's Hospital, San Diego, California, USA

Warren J. Winkelman MD, Director, Immunodermatology Clinic, Montreal General Hospital, Assistant Professor of Medicine, McGill University, Faculty of Medicine, Montreal, Quebec, Canada

Joseph A. Witkowski MD, Clinical Professor, Department of Dermatology, University of Pennsylvania School of Medicine, Philadelphia, Pennsylvania, USA

Paul D. Wortman MD, Assistant Professor, Department of Dermatology, The Bowman Gray School of Medicine, Wake Forest University, Winston-Salem, North Carolina, USA

Preface

The intent of this book is to provide a practical approach to the recognition and therapy of skin infections. No attempt will be made to discuss the pathogeneses unless they are relevant to therapy.

Colour clinical photographs have been incorporated to aid diagnosis. The generous use of illustrative material is intended to highlight the seminal points of the chapter and render the text more accessible; readers will be aided in differentiating skin infections and selecting the proper therapeutic agent for a specific problem.

Skin infections in AIDS and HIV-immunocompromised patients are also discussed, because the field of infectious diseases is increasingly focused on the patient who is immunocompromised. Both the spectrum and the frequency of infections that occur with HIV or HIV immunosuppression continue to expand.

With the increase of international travel, tropical and 'exotic' illnesses are encountered with surprising frequency. Thus information about these infections and their therapy will be provided also in this volume.

This book will be of value for dermatologists, house officers, family practitioners and other physicians concerned with the diagnosis and treatment of skin infections.

The authors of various chapters have been chosen because of their special interest in the subjects they cover. They are outstanding authors, representing diverse institutions and subspecialties. I am most grateful to them for their contributions.

Marwali Harahap

Chapter 1
Principles of Anti-infective Therapy

Lawrence Charles Parish & Joseph A. Witkowski

The successful treatment of cutaneous infections is dependent upon an accurate diagnosis and the selection of appropriate anti-infective therapy. While some dermatological infections can be self-limiting and others may be eliminated coincidentally by the treatment of a concurrent dermatitis, many infections require rapid intervention if morbidity and even mortality are to be diminished [1].

Diagnosis

A major problem in establishing the diagnosis of infection is the determination of whether infection is causing the problem. Inflammation and infection can be very similar. Both may have the traditional elements of redness, swelling, tenderness and purulent discharge. The presence of pus usually indicates an infectious process, but sometimes so-called inflammatory pus can occur after electrosurgical procedures (Table 1.1) [2].

Several techniques are available to demonstrate the presence of an infectious process. While these are helpful, they cannot always be absolute and clinical correlation is necessary (Table 1.2).

An understanding of the variations resulting from anatomical location are extremely important. A topical antimicrobial agent will have difficulty in penetrating the thickened stratum corneum of the palm or sole. An oral antifungal agent may be unnecessary for the treatment of localized tinea pedis but is necessary for the control of nail and hair infections (Table 1.3).

The background of the infectious process must also be considered. A primary infection results from the organism attacking the skin, while a secondary infection is superimposed upon an underlying dermatitis. Appropriate therapy will cure the infection but it will not eliminate the underlying disease process. A tertiary infection reflects a systemic disease that has accompanying cutaneous manifestations.

Bacterial infections

Bacterial infections were sometimes treated successfully in the preantibiotic era. Judicious use of soap or antiseptics or localized débridement, including incision and drainage, could rid the skin of superficial pyoderma, an abscess or gangrene [3].

Table 1.1 Diagnostic considerations (adapted from reference [2]).

Clinical signs	Clinical symptoms	Laboratory findings	Microbiological findings
Redness	Pruritus	Leucocytosis	+ Gram stain (wbcs and stained bacterial components) + Culture
Swelling	Pain	Polymorphonucleocytosis	
Heat	Fever	Elevated erythrocyte sedimentation rate	
Induration	Chills		
Tenderness	Sweats	ASO titre	
Pustules	Malaise	DNase titre	
Purulent discharge	Headache		
Serous discharge			
Scaling			
Lymphangitis			
Lymphadenopathy			
Ulceration			

ASO, antistreptolysin O; DNase, deoxyribonuclease; wbcs, white blood cells.

Table 1.2 Diagnostic tools.

Bacterial	Viral	Fungal
Gram stain	Tzank smear	KOH scraping
Bacterial culture	Viral culture	Fungal culture
Other stains: Fite, Giemsa, Gomori, Warthin–Starry, Ziehl–Nielsen	Cutaneous biopsy Electron microscopy PCR	Cutaneous biopsy—stains with PAS, Gomori, hexamine silver Wood's rays
Polymerase chain reaction (PCR)		

PAS, periodic acid–Schiff.

Table 1.3 Primary pyogenic infections according to anatomical considerations.

Epidermal	Dermal	Circumscribed	Appendageal
Impetigo	Cellulitis	Abscess	Carbuncle
Ecthyma	Erysipelas	Paronychia	Folliculitis
	Lymphangitis		Furuncle
	Pyoderma		

A knowledge of whether a bacterium reported on culture is a pathogen (causative agent), colonizer (potential for being a pathogen but currently just present) or part of the normal flora is essential (Table 1.4).

Local treatment of a bacterial infection may include astringent compresses (aluminium subacetate (Burow's) 1:40, potassium permanganate 1:6000 or acetic acid 0.5%) for 20 minutes three times a day until the

Table 1.4 Pyogenic bacteria recovered from the skin.

Normal flora	Common pathogens	Uncommon pathogens
Aerobic		
Staphylococcus epidermidis	*Staphylococcus aureus*	*Actinetobacter* sp.
Staphylococcus saprophyticus	*Staphylococcus epidermidis*	*Enterobacter* sp.
Micrococcus	β-haemolytic *Streptococcus*, group A	*Streptococcus faecalis*
Corynebacterium	*Escherichia coli*	*Klebsiella* sp.
Brevibacterium	*Morganella morganii*	*Providencia stuartii*
	Proteus mirabilis	*Serratia marcescens*
	Proteus vulgaris	*Streptococcus agalactiae*
	Pseudomonas aeruginosa	β-haemolytic *Streptococcus*, groups B, C and G
Anaerobic		
Propionibacterium acnes		*Bacteroides fragilis*
Propionibacterium avidum		*Clostridium perfringens*

Table 1.5 Frequently used antimicrobial agents [3].

Agent	Amount	Time (days)
Oral		
Penicillins		
Penicillin V	250 mg qid	7–10
Amoxycillin with clavulanic acid	500 mg tid	7–10
Dicloxacillin	250 mg qid	7–10
Cephalosporins		
Cefaclor	250 mg tid	7–10
Cephalexin	250 mg qid	7–10
Cefadroxil	1 g qid	7–10
Cefuroxime axetil	250 mg bid	7–10
Cefprozil	500 mg qid	7–10
Cefpodoxime proxetil	400 mg bid	7–10
Macrolides		
Erythromycin	500 mg qid	7–10
Clarithromycin	500 mg bid	7–10
Azithromycin	500 mg qid	First day
	250 mg qid	Next 4
Tetracyclines		
Tetracycline	500 mg qid	7–10
Doxycycline	100 mg bid	First day
	50 mg bid	Next 6–9
Minocycline	200 mg initially	
	100 mg bid	Next 7–10
Quinolones		
Ciprofloxacin	500 mg bid	7–10
Ofloxacin	400 mg bid	7–10

Continued on page 4

Table 1.5 *Continued.*

Agent	Amount	Time (days)
Topical		
Bacitracin ointment	bid or tid	7–10
Betadine ointment	bid or tid	7–10
Fusidic acid ointment	bid or tid	7–10
Neomycin ointment	bid or tid	7–10
Mupirocin ointment	bid or tid	7–10
Silver sulphadiazine cream	bid or tid	7–10

bid, twice a day; tid, three times a day; qid, four times a day.

Table 1.6 Viral infections of the skin.

Human herpesvirus		Exanthemata of childhood		
Type	Associated disease	Number	Name	Aetiological agent
HHV-1, HSV-1	Herpes simplex infection, type I	First disease	Measles	Measles virus (morbillivirus)
HHV-2, HSV-2	Herpes simplex infection, type II	Second disease	Scarlet fever	β-haemolytic *Streptococcus*, group A
HHV-3, VZV	Varicella, herpes zoster infection	Third disease	Rubella	Rubella virus (togavirus)
HHV-4, EBV	Infectious mononucleosis (Epstein–Barr virus disease)	Fourth disease	Rubella scarlatinosa	Unknown
HHV-5, HCMV	Human cytomegalovirus disease	Fifth disease	Erythema infectiosum	Parvovirus, B19
HHV-6	Exanthema subitum (sixth disease)	Sixth disease	Exanthema subitum	Herpesvirus 6

HHV, human herpesvirus; HSV, herpes simplex virus; VZV, varicella zoster virus; EBV, Epstein–Barr virus; HCMV, human cytomegalovirus.

Table 1.7 Frequently used antiviral agents.

Acyclovir
Famciclovir
Ganciclovir
Valaciclovir

lesions are dry or antiseptic washes or soaks with chlorhexidine, hexa-chlorophane or pyrrolidone [4].

If the lesion is superficial and/or limited in extent, topical antimicrobial agents may be applied for 7–10 days. More extensive or deep infections require systemic therapy. Infections due to certain organisms, such as β-haemolytic *Streptococcus*, group A, mandate systemic treatment, as would

Table 1.8 Fungal infections of the skin.

Superficial	Subcutaneous	Deep
Candidiosis	Chromomycosis	Actinomycosis
Dermatophytosis	Lobo's disease	Coccidiomycosis
Tinea versicolor	Mycetoma	Cryptococcosis
	Rhinosporodiosis	Histoplasmosis
	Sporotrichosis	North American blastomycosis
		Paracoccidiomycosis

Table 1.9 Agents useful in treating fungal infections.

	Topical	Oral	Systemic
Historical agents			
Dyes			
Castellani's paint	×		
Gentian violet	×		
Keratolytic			
Whitfield's ointment	×		
Miscellaneous			
Potassium iodide		×	
Undecylenic acid	×		
Older agents			
8-Hydroxyquinoline			
Clioquinol	×		
Penicillium			
Griseofulvin		×	
Halogenated phenol			
Haloprogin	×		
Thiocarbamate			
Tolnaftate	×		
Newer agents			
Polyene antibiotics			
Nystatin	×	×*	
Amphotericin B	×		×
Pyrimidine			
Flucytosine	×		
Imidazoles			
Bifonazole	×		
Clotrimazole	×		
Econazole	×		
Ketoconazole	×	×	
Miconazole	×		×
Oxiconazole	×		
Sulconazole	×		
Tioconazole	×		
Triazoles			
Fluconazole		×	

Continued on page 6

Table 1.9 *Continued.*

Itraconazole		×
Terconazole	×	
Morpholine		
Amorolfine	×	
Hydroxypyridone		
Ciclopiroxolamine	×	
Allylamines		
Naftifine	×	
Terbinafine	×	×

* No systemic absorption.

certain locations — central face — and certain patients — diabetics, cardiac valve afflicted, mitral prolapse, rheumatic fever (Table 1.5) [5].

Viral infections

See Tables 1.6 and 1.7.

Fungal infections

See Tables 1.8 and 1.9.

References

1 Parish LC, Witkowski JA. Cutaneous bacterial skin infections: how to manage primary, secondary, and tertiary lesions. *Postgrad Med* 1992; **91**: 119–122, 125–126, 129–130.
2 Parish LC, Witkowski JA, Vassileva S. *Color Atlas of Cutaneous Infections*. Blackwell Science, Boston, 1995.
3 Witkowski JA, Parish LC. Wound cleansers. *Clin Dermatol* 1996; **14**: 89–94.
4 Parish LC, Witkowski JA. Aluminum acetate and chloride. In: Dollery C (ed.) *Therapeutic Drugs*, Vol. 1. Churchill Livingstone, Edinburgh, 1991, pp. A62–A63.
5 Parish LC, Witkowski JA. Systemic management of cutaneous bacterial infections. *Am J Med* 1991; **91**: 106S–110S.

Chapter 2
Staphylococcal and Streptococcal Skin Infections

Gary L. Darmstadt

Scope of skin infection

Staphylococcus aureus and *Streptococcus pyogenes* (group A β-haemolytic strep-tococci) are unsurpassed among human pathogens in their capability for infecting cutaneous and subcutaneous tissues (Tables 2.1–2.6) [1]. These organisms can infect each of the main layers of skin — the epidermis and dermis as well as subcutaneous tissues and fascia — and can cause a variety of skin lesions through several major pathogenetic mechanisms (Tables 2.3–2.6).

Primary infections develop in clinically normal skin, although minor breaks in the integrity of the skin may be required to initiate infection. These infections tend to be localized superficially in the epidermis and/or dermis, and develop due to local bacterial replication, leading to an inflammatory response within the skin. Superficial lesions are generally small; tenderness, if present, is localized; tissue necrosis, gangrene or abscess formation is minimal to absent; and few or no systemic manifestations develop. In many cases, these infections are self-limited, although antibiotic therapy may decrease the incidence of complications and hasten resolution. Some primary superficial infections, however, such as folliculitis, furunculosis, carbunculosis and paronychia, occasionally evolve into abscesses and/or extend from the epidermis and/or dermis to involve deeper subcutaneous tissues. Rarely, the infectious process progresses to tissue gangrene and necrosis and produces a range of systemic signs.

Secondary infections occur in previously diseased or wounded skin. Examples include infection of cysts (e.g. epidermal inclusion cyst), ulcers (e.g. decubitus ulcer), wounds (e.g. surgical wound; burn; arthropod bite or burrow) or dermatitis (e.g. atopic dermatitis, psoriasis).

From a site of primary or secondary skin infection, certain strains of *S. aureus* and *S. pyogenes* elaborate exotoxins, which cause disease directly (e.g. proteolytic activity of staphylococcal epidermolytic toxin on desmoglein I within desmosomes to cause scalded skin syndrome) or through release of other biologically active mediators, such as cytokines (e.g. toxic shock-like syndrome). These organisms are also capable of invading the bloodstream or lymphatics to cause disseminated skin lesions through bacterial replication at tertiary sites; coagulopathy; or vasculopathy. The tertiary skin

Table 2.1 Primary skin lesions due to *Staphylococcus aureus* or *Streptococcus pyogenes*.

Lesion	Definition	Disease example
Macule	Circumscribed, flat, unelevated discoloration. Results primarily from changes in epidermal melanin, producing hypopigmentation or hyperpigmentation; capillary dilatation, as in erythema; or purpura due to extravasation of red blood cells	Scarlet fever
Patch	Large macule >1 cm diameter	Perianal dermatitis
Papule	Circumscribed, solid elevation without visible fluid, <1 cm diameter. Major portion projects above the plane of the surrounding skin. May be located in the epidermis or dermis, around sebaceous glands, at the orifice of sweat ducts, or at hair follicles. Results from localized cellular hyperplasia or infiltration, metabolic deposits or oedema of the epidermis or dermis	Folliculitis
Plaque	Circumscribed, elevated, superficial, solid lesion >1 cm diameter. Generally flat, may be depressed centrally. Occupies a large area of skin in relation to its height above the skin surface. Often formed by confluence of papules. May involve the epidermis, dermis and/or subcutis	Erysipelas
Nodule	Palpable, circumscribed, elevated, solid lesion, extends more deeply than a papule, >0.5 cm diameter. Can be epidermal, epidermal–dermal, dermal, dermal–subdermal or subcutaneous	Furuncle
Pustule	Circumscribed elevation containing purulent exudate. Arises in the epidermis or upper dermis	Folliculitis
Vesicle	Circumscribed epidermal or subepidermal elevation containing clear fluid (serum, lymph, blood or extracellular fluid)	Impetigo
Bulla	Circumscribed collection of fluid >1 cm diameter. Located in the epidermis (flaccid, ruptures easily) or subepidermally (tense, ulceration and scarring often result)	Bullous impetigo
Wheal	Firm, evanescent, oedematous, elevated papule or plaque resulting from exudation of fluid into the upper dermis	Urticaria triggered by *S. pyogenes*

lesions can involve any of the deeper soft tissues, but spare direct involvement of the epidermis, due to its lack of vasculature. Finally, sterile skin lesions can form following postinfectious immunological or idiopathic mechanisms (Table 2.6).

Staphylococcus aureus and *S. pyogenes* are the most important bacterial agents of skin infections. *Staphylococcus aureus* was isolated from 71.9% of

Table 2.2 Secondary and special skin lesions due to *Staphylococcus aureus* or *Streptococcus pyogenes*.

Lesion	Definition	Disease example
Petechiae	Circumscribed macular deposit of red blood cells extravasated from dermal vessels, <0.5 cm diameter	Scarlet fever
Purpura	Circumscribed deposit of blood >0.5 cm diameter	Purpura fulminans
Ecchymosis	Macular area of haemorrhage >2 cm diameter	Purpura fulminans
Scale	Excess dead keratin and epidermal cells	Desquamation following scalded-skin syndrome
Crust	Collection of dried serum and cellular debris	Impetigo
Erosion	Focal loss of epidermis. Does not penetrate below the epidermal–dermal junction, heals without scarring	Bullous impetigo
Excoriation	Erosion caused mechanically, often linear, usually involving only the epidermis, rarely reaching the deep dermis	Secondarily infected eczema
Ulcer	Focal loss of epidermis and some portion of the dermis, tends to heal with scarring	Bacterial synergistic gangrene
Abscess	Localized collection of purulent material in a cavity formed by tissue disintegration or necrosis	Breast abscess
Necrosis	Death of tissue	Necrotizing fasciitis
Gangrene	Death of tissue due to loss of blood supply	Necrotizing fasciitis

Table 2.3 Classification of skin infections caused by *Staphylococcus aureus* or *Streptococcus pyogenes*.

Primary or secondary skin infection
Superficial
Subcutaneous
   Non-necrotizing
   Necrotizing

Bloodstream invasion
Disease due to coagulopathy
Tertiary skin infection: metastatic foci of bacterial replication
Invasion of blood-vessels: vasculopathy

Exotoxin-mediated disease

Immunologically mediated or idiopathic disease with sterile lesions

Table 2.4 Cutaneous and subcutaneous infections due to *Staphylococcus aureus* and *Streptococcus pyogenes*.

Disease entity	Infectious agent	Skin lesions
Superficial infections		
Impetigo	S. aureus	B, E, Pl, Pu, V
	S. pyogenes	Pl, Pu, V
Ecthyma	S. pyogenes	Pl, Pu, U
Blastomycosis-like pyoderma	S. aureus, S. pyogenes	A, Pl, U
Folliculitis	S. aureus, coagulase-negative staphylococci	A, P, Pu
Sycosis barbae	S. aureus	A, P, Pl, Pu
Blistering distal dactylitis	S. pyogenes, group B *Streptococcus*, S. aureus	B, V
Perianal dermatitis	S. pyogenes	Pa, Pl
Periocular infection		
Blepharitis	S. aureus	Pa, U
Internal hordeolum	S. aureus	A, Pa, Pu
External hordeolum	S. aureus	A, Pa, Pu
Dermatoblepharitis	S. aureus, S. pyogenes	Pl, Pu, V
Acute dacryocystitis	S. aureus, S. pyogenes	A
Dacryoadenitis	S. aureus, S. pyogenes	A
Abscesses		
Furuncle, carbuncle	S. aureus	A, N, P
Multiple sweat-gland abscesses	S. aureus	A, N, P, Pu
Paronychia	S. aureus, S. pyogenes	A, N, P
Breast abscess	S. aureus, group B *Streptococcus*	A, N
Perirectal abscess	S. aureus, S. pyogenes	A, N
Scalp abscess	S. aureus, S. pyogenes, group B or D streptococci	A, N, Pu
Suppurative sialadenitis	S. aureus, S. pyogenes	A, N
Botyromycosis	S. aureus, α-haemolytic streptococci	A, N, Pl
Non-necrotizing subcutaneous tissue infections		
Cellulitis	S. pyogenes, S. aureus, group B, C or G streptococci, Streptococcus pneumoniae	Pl
Erysipelas	S. pyogenes, group B, C, D or G streptococci, S. aureus, S. pneumoniae	B, Ec, Pe, Pl, V
Lymphangitis	S. pyogenes, group B or D streptococci, S. aureus	Pa

Continued

Table 2.4 *Continued.*

Disease entity	Infectious agent	Skin lesions
Necrotizing subcutaneous tissue infections		
Anaerobic cellulitis	Facultative streptococci, staphylococci	Pl, U
Bacterial synergistic gangrene (Meleney's ulcer)	Streptococci (anaerobic), *S. aureus*	Pl, U
Necrotizing fasciitis (Founier's gangrene)	Type I (mixed) infection: haemolytic or non-haemolytic non-group A streptococci, *S. aureus* Type II: *S. pyogenes* ± *S. aureus* Rare monomicrobial infections: group B, C, F or G streptococci, *S. aureus*, *S. pneumoniae*	B, Ec, Pe, Pl, Pur, U, V

A, abscess; B, bulla; E, erosion; Ec, ecchymosis; N, nodule; P, papule; Pa, patch; Pe, petechiae; Pl, plaque; Pu, pustule; Pur, purpura; U, ulcer; V, vesicle.

Table 2.5 Toxin-mediated diseases due to *Staphylococcus aureus* and *Streptococcus pyogenes*.

Disease entity	Infectious agent	Skin lesions
Scalded-skin syndrome	*S. aureus*	B, D, E, Er, P, Pa
Scarlet fever	*S. pyogenes*, *S. aureus*	D, Er, P, Pa, Pe
Toxic-shock syndrome	*S. aureus* *S. pyogenes**	B, D, Er, Ma-P, Pe, V B, D, Ma-P, Pa, Pe, V

* Commonly presents with localized swelling and erythema.
B, bulla; D, desquamation; E, erosion; Er, erythroderma; Ma-P, 'maculopapular'; P, papule ('scarlatiniform'); Pa, patch; Pe, petechiae; V, vesicle.

Table 2.6 Diseases with idiopathic or immunologically mediated skin lesions following infection with *Staphylococcus aureus* or *Streptococcus pyogenes*.

Disease entity	Infectious agent
Erythema elevatum diutinum	*S. pyogenes*
Erythema multiforme	*S. aureus*, *S. pyogenes*
Erythema nodosum	*S. pyogenes*
Guttate psoriasis	*S. pyogenes*
Henoch–Schoenlein purpura	*S. pyogenes*
Polyarteritis nodosa	*S. pyogenes*
Rheumatic fever	*S. pyogenes*
Sweet's syndrome	*S. aureus*, *S. pyogenes*
Scleroedema	*S. pyogenes*

all skin and skin-structure infections reported in children since 1980 and *S. pyogenes* was cultured from 30.4% (Table 2.7) [2–27]. The proportion of isolates that were either *S. aureus* or *S. pyogenes* was even higher (86.7% and 29.2%, respectively) when only lesions of impetigo were considered. Impetigo is the most common primary skin infection in children [28–31] and is caused almost exclusively by *S. aureus* and *S. pyogenes* (Table 2.4). The most common secondary skin infection, impetiginized atopic dermatitis, is also caused almost exclusively by *S. aureus*, although occasional isolates of *S. pyogenes* are found [32–35]. The next most common isolates from skin and skin-structure infections in children were *Staphylococcus epidermidis* (1.6%), *Escherichia coli* (1.0%) and group B *Streptococcus* (0.6%) (Table 2.7). When all Gram-negative enteric organisms were combined, they comprised only 2.0% of cases. This is significantly lower than the 16.7% (818 of 4907 isolates) and 15.4% (690 of 4473 isolates) prevalence of *S. epidermidis* or Gram-negative enteric bacilli, respectively, reported in clinical trials of skin infections in adults [36–54]. These data suggest that the focus when treating skin and skin-structure infections, particularly in children, must be on therapies that are effective against both *S. aureus* and *S. pyogenes*. Notable exceptions include complicated infections, such as infected decubitus ulcers, particularly those in the inguinal or perirectal

Table 2.7 Bacterial pathogens in skin and skin-structure infections in children. Compilation of data from 25 studies from 1980 to 1995 on impetigo and skin/skin-structure infections in children (references 3–27) which quantified the microorganisms isolated. (Adapted from reference [2].)

	Isolates (%)	
	Impetigo (*n* = 1155)	All (*n* = 2482)
COMMON		
Staphylococcus aureus	1001 (86.7)	2089 (71.9)
Streptococcus pyogenes	337 (29.2)	883 (30.4)
UNUSUAL		
Staphylococcus epidermidis	1 (0.1)	45 (1.6)
Escherichia coli	4 (0.3)	30 (1.0)
RARE		
Group B *Streptococcus*	8 (0.7)	17 (0.6)
α-Haemolytic streptococci	0	5 (0.2)
Enterococcus faecalis	2 (0.2)	8 (0.3)
Haemophilus influenzae type b	0	4 (0.1)
Gram-negative enteric bacilli		
Pseudomonas aeruginosa	0	8 (0.3)
Proteus vulgaris	0	8 (0.3)
Klebsiella spp.	6 (0.5)	9 (0.3)
Enterobacter spp.	1 (0.1)	2 (0.1)
All Gram-negative enteric bacilli	11 (1.0)	58 (2.0)

Table 2.8 Resident skin flora.

Characteristics
Attached to skin surface or in follicular canals
Stable, low numbers present
Low virulence

Flora
Micrococcaceae
  Coagulase-negative staphylococci
    Staphylococcus epidermidis (upper part of
      body)
    Staphylococcus hominis
    Staphylococcus saprophyticus (perineum)
    Staphylococcus capitis (sebum-rich areas)
    Staphylococcus auricularis (ear canal)
  Peptococcus spp.
  Micrococcus spp.
Diphtheroides
  Corynebacterium (moist intertriginous area)
    Corynebacterium jeikeium (multidrug-
      resistant)
  Brevibacterium (toe webs)
Propionibacterium (hair follicles, sebaceous glands)
Gram-negative rods
  Acinetobacter (moist intertriginous areas,
    perineum)
  Rarely *Klebsiella, Enterobacter, Proteus*

regions or on the buttocks, subcutaneous abscesses and burns, which are generally polymicrobial in origin and often include Gram-negative enteric and anaerobic organisms, enterococci and coagulase-negative staphylococci [55–60].

Mechanism of skin infection

Development of skin infection due to *S. aureus* or *S. pyogenes* involves a complex interaction among environmental and local ecological factors, such as the normal bacterial flora; predisposing tissue factors, such as local trauma; systemic and local tissue defence of the host; and bacterial virulence factors and synergism. The resident bacterial flora of the skin is low in virulence and stable in number and provides infrequent skin pathogens (Table 2.8). Normally, it appears to play a protective role, as alterations in the ecology of the resident flora through changes in temperature or humidity or by antibiotic administration may be associated with colonization and/or infection of the skin by *S. aureus* and *S. pyogenes*. Transient flora is introduced from the environment onto exposed skin or mucosal surfaces and appears to attach only in the presence of a disturbance in the integrity of the skin. *Staphylococcus aureus* and *S. pyogenes*, the most important of the transient bacteria, encounter a high degree of natural resistance to colonization and infection of the skin. Although most body sites are free from colonization with *S. aureus*, persistent nasal carriage is detected in 20–40% of immunocompetent adults, and up to 20% of people may be colonized on the perineum [61, 62]. This forms an important reservoir for infection of the skin, as staphylococci generally spread from the nose to normal skin prior to the initiation of lesions of impetigo [63]. Colonization of the skin with *S. pyogenes* occurs less frequently, but has been documented, particularly in areas with epidemics or a high endemic rate of impetigo. In these instances, in contrast to *S. aureus*, *S. pyogenes* colonizes the skin an average of 10 days before development of impetigo and appears in the nasopharynx only after the appearance of impetigo [63–65].

Initiation of infection appears to require a break in the integrity of the barrier function of the skin or mucous membrane, although the injury is often trivial or unapparent. The mechanism whereby injury facilitates infection of the skin may involve exposure or new synthesis of a receptor for adherence. The bacterial adhesins and cutaneous receptors for initial adherence of *S. aureus* or *S. pyogenes* to the skin, however, are largely unknown. Once this information is available, topical application of a purified bacterial adhesin or a cell-surface receptor might competively block pathogenic staphylococci and streptococci from adhering to the skin and provide novel approaches in the future to prevention or treatment of bacterial skin infections [66–68]. Competitive binding to cell-surface receptors by resident flora or transient flora of low virulence may also prevent pathogenic bacteria from colonizing skin. A non-virulent strain of *S. aureus* has been useful in neonates during nursery epidemics, to prevent colonization of the nasal mucosa with a pathogenic strain of *S. aureus*, and in adults, to prevent spread of recurrent staphylococcal abscesses within families [69, 70].

Once pathogenic bacteria have adhered to the skin, they must overcome several avenues of host defence before infection can develop. Intact, overlapping cells of the stratum corneum provide the first and foremost mechanism of defence. Breakdown products of the stratum corneum, including free fatty acids, polar lipids and glycosphingolipids, have antistaphylococcal and antistreptococcal activity [71]. Much of the resident flora, particularly the lipophilic corynebacteria, releases lipases and thus contributes to defence against *S. pyogenes* and *S. aureus* by liberating fatty acids from the triglycerides of sebum [72]. The acid mantle thus created favours growth of propionibacteria, which in turn produce propionic acid; this compound has relatively more antimicrobial activity against transient organisms than against resident flora. The skin's immune system, including antigen presentation by epidermal Langerhans cells and cytokine production by keratinocytes, plays a key role in defence from cutaneous infection [73]. On the other hand, compromise of immune defence is a primary predisposing factor for development of subcutaneous infections. This may occur locally, through trauma or surgery that compromises the barrier function of the skin, or involve systemic immune deficiency, particularly defects in neutrophil response (e.g. insufficient numbers of neutrophils; defects in neutrophil chemotaxis, phagocytosis or intracellular killing; or lack of opsonization) (Table 2.9). Humoral or cell-mediated immunity is relatively less important for combating skin infections due to *S. aureus* or *S. pyogenes*.

Following attachment, bacterial virulence factors may facilitate invasion of host cells and penetration to deeper levels within tissues, act to evade host defences and mediate clinical symptoms of the disease. Signs of the infection may develop as a direct result of bacterial factors (e.g. cytotoxicity), the immunological response to the presence of the bacteria, or both. Invasion of *S. pyogenes* may be facilitated by the M protein on its surface, possibly through the ability of M protein to impede phagocytosis by neutrophils by blocking deposition of complement component $C3_b$ opsonin on the organism [74]. Some strains of *S. pyogenes* produce a peptidase that cleaves the complement component $C5_a$, abrogating its function as a chemotactic factor for neutrophils and thus allowing the bacterium to avoid detection by phagocytes [75]. Streptococcal pyrogenic exotoxins A (SPE-A) and/or B (SPE-B), as well as certain M-protein fragments of *S. pyogenes* and the toxic-shock syndrome (TSS) toxin 1 (TSST-1) of *S. aureus*, appear to have the ability to interact simultaneously with the major histocompatibility complex class II antigen on antigen-presenting cells and specific Vβ regions of T-cell receptors, inducing massive synthesis and release of cytokines [76]. These cytokines may mediate systemic signs of toxicity seen in TSS, and tumour necrosis factor (TNF) may mediate, at least in part, the rapid, massive tissue destruction seen in streptococcal necrotizing fasciitis [77, 78]. Talkington *et al.* [79] found no relationship, however, between necrotizing soft-tissue involvement and production of pyrogenic exotoxin among patients with invasive *S. pyogenes* infections. Rather, tissue destruction was associated with protease activity. Protease activity is known to correlate with the ability of *S. aureus* to cause invasive disease [80]. A central feature of the pathology in necrotizing fasciitis, as in many other necrotizing soft-tissue infections, is vascular injury and thrombosis of arteries and veins passing through the fascia [81, 82]. Possible mechanisms for the vascular injury leading to tissue ischaemia and necrosis in streptococcal necrotizing fasciitis are direct cytolytic factors released from bacteria,

Table 2.9 Predisposing factors for skin infection with *Staphylococcus aureus* or *Streptococcus pyogenes*.

Alteration of normal skin flora
Chronic dermatoses
Corticosteroid therapy
Foreign body
Immunodeficiency disease (particularly involving neutrophils)
Malnutrition
Peripheral vascular disease
Skin trauma
Systemic disease (particularly diabetes mellitus)

immune-mediated vascular damage due to the inflammatory infiltrate surrounding the blood-vessels and/or non-inflammatory intravascular coagulation [83, 84].

Some skin infections appear to be caused by two or more organisms that act synergistically. Synergism occurs when a mixture of organisms causes a more severe infection than the sum of the damage caused by each of the organisms acting alone. In these instances, therapy is most effective when directed against all the pathogenic organisms present. Synergism does not appear to be a factor in most superficial skin infections, and, as a rule, superficial infections due to *S. aureus* and *S. pyogenes* can be treated with single antibiotics directed against them. In many instances, synergism is not necessary for abscess formation either, and *S. aureus* is commonly found alone in these lesions [57, 85–87]. In many necrotizing soft-tissue infections, however, synergism is operative [88]. Although *S. pyogenes* and occasionally *S. aureus* can act alone to cause necrotizing fasciitis, clinical evidence for potential synergy in some cases of streptococcal necrotizing fasciitis comes from the fact that *S. aureus* has also been cultured from the infected tissue of many patients [82, 89–91]. Proof of synergism requires that the infection be reproducible in an animal model. In the case of streptococcal necrotizing fasciitis, infection in an animal model was caused more often when *S. aureus* or crude staphylococcal α-lysin was coinjected with *S. pyogenes* [92]. A variety of anaerobic, aerobic and facultative bacteria also appear to be capable of acting synergistically as pathogens in necrotizing soft-tissue infections. Mechanisms of synergy are not well understood but may involve such factors as mutual protection from phagocytosis and intracellular killing; promotion of bacterial capsule formation; production of essential growth factors or energy sources; and utilization of oxygen by facultative bacteria, lowering host-tissue oxidation–reduction potential and facilitating growth of anaerobes [85, 93–95]. Until a necrotizing soft-tissue infection can be demonstrated to be due to a single organism, such as *S. pyogenes*, the antibiotic therapy given should be broadly effective against all possible pathogens.

Diagnosis of skin infection

Identification of the pathogen(s) causing a particular subcutaneous soft-tissue infection requires proper use and interpretation of diagnostic tests. If the surface of a wound or site of infection is swabbed and cultured, a number of organisms that are colonizing but not contributing directly to the disease process may be identified. If an organism is found on both Gram stain, or special stains in the case of fungi, and culture, it increases the likelihood that it is playing a pathogenic role. Chances of identifying the true pathogen(s) are increased further if cultures are obtained by swabbing the exudate directly from the source of suppuration, by fine-needle aspiration or by biopsy [96]. Cultures from abscesses and subcutaneous tissue infections should be obtained for both aerobic and anaerobic organisms. Standard recommendations include use of blood agar, chocolate agar and/or MacConkey's agar to identify the full range of pyogenic, fastidious and Gram-negative enteric organisms which may infect the skin and subcutaneous tissues. Isolation of anaerobic organisms can be accomplished by use of anaerobic media, such as *Brucella* agar supplemented with vitamin K_1 and haemin, and brain–heart infusion broth or thioglycolate broth. In the appropriate clinical setting, consideration should also be given to culture for saprophytic moulds. Once the pathogen(s) has been identified, antibiotic susceptibility testing may aid in adjusting the antibiotic regimen to optimally control the disease process.

Some skin diseases caused by infectious agents have characteristic histopathological findings (e.g. impetigo (Fig. 2.1)), which may aid in reaching a diagnosis. Additional studies on biopsy material, such as immunofluorescence testing and electron microscopy, may also be highly useful, particularly in excluding non-infectious diseases that may closely mimic a given skin infection.

In other cases, in order to formulate a diagnosis and treatment plan, it may be imperative to define the depth of infection. For example, in the case of soft-tissue infection, magnetic resonance imaging may be useful to distinguish cellulitis from necrotizing fasciitis or myositis. In the case of necrotizing soft-tissue infections, however, surgical exploration is necessary for definitive diagnosis and treatment.

Antigen detection or immunological tests have little utility in the managment of skin infections due to *S. aureus* or *S. pyogenes*. Antideoxyribonuclease (anti-DNase) B titres, however, may aid in confirming previous infection with *S. pyogenes* and may be useful in reaching a diagnosis of impetigo-associated poststreptococcal glomerulonephritis [97].

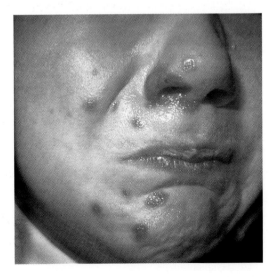

Fig. 2.1 Non-bullous impetigo. Honey-coloured, crusted papules and plaques due to *Staphylococcus aureus* on the face of a child.

Treatment of skin infection

Most superficial skin infections due to *S. aureus* or *S. pyogenes* can be treated effectively with local wound care and oral antibiotics. Depending on the age and health of the patient, the rapidity, severity and location of the infection and the presence of constitutional signs of illness, parenteral antibiotic therapy may be necessary. Surgical drainage and tissue débridement, particularly for treatment of abscesses and necrotizing infections, may also be required.

To devise an effective plan for antibiotic treatment of skin infections due to *S. aureus* or *S. pyogenes*, a number of factors must be taken into consideration (Table 2.10) [98, 99]. An increasingly important factor is the antibiotic resistance profile of the target microorganisms.

Antibiotic resistance of *Streptococcus pyogenes*

Erythromycin resistance

Oral erythromycin has been a gold-standard therapy for uncomplicated

Cost considerations
Basic treatment costs
  Per-dose cost
  Number of doses, i.e. duration and frequency of
    treatment
Indirect costs
  Compliance
    Frequency and length of therapy
    Palatability
  Incidence of treatment failure
  Incidence of adverse drug reaction, including
    drug interaction

Pharmacological considerations
Pharmacodynamic considerations
  Bactericidal
  Intrinsic activity against pathogens
  β-Lactamase stability
  Little potential for resistance development
  Little alteration of normal flora
Pharmaceutical considerations
  Available in concentrated suspension
  Palatable
  No direct gastrointestinal irritation
  Food does not interfere with absorption
Pharmacokinetic considerations
  High bioavailability
  Rapid intestinal absorption
  Good tissue penetration
  Long elimination half-life

Table 2.10 Considerations in selection of an oral antibiotic (adapted in part from references [2, 98 and 99]).

skin infection for the past several decades. Since the early 1970s, however, resistance of S. pyogenes to erythromycin has emerged as a potential problem. The first reports of widespread erythromycin resistance in S. pyogenes were from Japan in 1971, peaking in incidence at 60–70% during 1974–75 [100–102]. Emergence of erythromycin resistance was linked to increased macrolide use, and was associated with multidrug resistance to other macrolides, as well as chloramphenicol and tetracycline. Outbreaks of erythromycin-resistant S. pyogenes have also occurred periodically in various countries of Europe since 1984 [103, 104]. Of particular relevance to skin infections, the prevalence of erythromycin resistance among isolates from pus samples in Finland increased during 1990 from 11% to 31%, reaching a higher prevalence of resistance than pharyngeal isolates (20%) [105]. The resistant serotypes were associated with a 47% (nine of 19) rate of failure of erythromycin treatment of a small group of patients with pharyngitis, 10 times higher than the failure rate for treatment of erythromycin-sensitive strains. In North America, the prevalence of erythromycin resistance among isolates of S. pyogenes has remained below 5% [106, 107]. Although resistance of S. pyogenes to erythromycin is not currently of major clinical import, the threat of increased resistance exists, particularly if macrolide usage increases.

Inoculum effect

Classical resistance to penicillin has not been documented and the *in vitro* sensitivity of S. pyogenes to penicillin has not changed in four decades [106]. The apparent sensitivity of S. pyogenes to antibiotic therapy may, however, be affected by the inoculum (or Eagle) effect. An understanding of this phenomenon is important in the treatment of skin infections, particularly when faced with a severe, potentially life-threatening infection.

Eagle described the inoculum effect in an experimental mouse model of myositis [108]. By using a larger inoculum or longer time for proliferation and establishment of a fulminant infection with S. pyogenes before initiating treatment, the clinical efficacy of penicillin was reduced significantly [108–111]. Efficacy of the protein-synthesis inhibitor clindamycin, however, was not adversely altered by the inoculum effect [109]. Efficacy of erythromycin, also a protein-synthesis inhibitor, was altered to an intermediate degree. The inoculum effect on penicillin efficacy appears to be due to entry of bacteria into a slower or stationary phase of growth, rendering them less susceptible to the β-lactam antibiotics, such as penicillin, and the cephalosporins, which act by interupting cell-wall synthesis [108–111]. The inoculum effect may also be due to alterations in pencillin-binding proteins in slow-growing S. pyogenes, decreasing the target for the β-lactam antibiotics [110]. Considering the inoculum effect, along with the fact that clindamycin suppresses bacterial toxin synthesis, clindamycin is probably a better choice than penicillin for treatment of deep-seated, serious soft-tissue infections due to S. pyogenes [77].

Antibiotic resistance of *Staphylococcus aureus*

Penicillin resistance

The majority of skin isolates of *S. aureus* are resistant to penicillin, approaching rates of 100% in some areas [3, 12]. The *in vitro* resistance of *S. aureus* to penicillin has also been associated with penicillin treatment failure rates of 24–47% in studies conducted since 1980 [3, 10, 20, 25, 112]. Consequently, penicillin is an unacceptable empirical choice for treatment of uncomplicated skin and skin-structure infections, including impetigo. Given that amoxycillin and penicillin are both inactivated by the same mechanism of hydrolysis of the β-lactam ring by staphylococcal β-lactamase, amoxycillin is also an inappropriate choice.

Erythromycin resistance

The rate of erythromycin resistance among *S. aureus* strains isolated from sites of skin and soft-tissue infection in children in the continental USA was 10–20% between 1980 and 1992 [2], while the proportion of erythromycin-resistant *S. aureus* isolates from skin infections in Israel and Australia averaged 30–50% [12, 24]. It is not yet clear, however, whether *in vitro* erythromycin resistance is a clinically significant problem in the treatment of impetigo and other pyogenic skin infections [2].

Methicillin resistance

Emergence of methicillin resistance among isolates of *S. aureus* must also be considered in the design of a treatment plan. This form of resistance extends to the semisynthetic penicillins cloxacillin and dicloxacillin. Of primary concern is the observation that most isolates of methicillin-resistant *S. aureus* (MRSA) also produce β-lactamase and appear to serve as reservoirs of transmissible resistance elements for a variety of other antimicrobials, including erythromycin, clindamycin, tetracycline, sulphonamides, chloramphenicol, the cephalosporins and the quinolones [113]. Thus, the abbreviation MRSA should probably be used to indicate 'multiply resistant *S. aureus*'.

During the past decade, rates of methicillin resistance in *S. aureus* have risen dramatically. In 1991, an 11% incidence of methicillin resistance was found among the skin isolates of *S. aureus* from one series of patients in Texas [43]. In Japan, methicillin resistance among *S. aureus* isolates from dermatology patients rose from 24% in 1987–88 to 61% in 1988–89 [114]. In another site in Japan, MRSA increased from 34% of isolates in 1989 to 41.5% during 1991 [115].

Antibiotic susceptibility patterns of skin isolates of MRSA in Japan indicate that resistance to the quinolones is also increasing, further decreasing antibiotic options for control of these organisms. Currently, the only consistently reliable agent for treatment of MRSA is parenteral vancomycin.

Mupirocin resistance

High-level resistance (minimal inhibitory concentration (MIC) >500 µg/dl) to mupirocin has also emerged among isolates of MRSA, methicillin-sensitive *S. aureus* and coagulase-negative staphylococci [116–125]. Mupirocin resistance in staphylococci has been reported primarily in patients with severe skin disease who were admitted to dermatology wards, and appears to be associated with inappropriately long or intermittent mupirocin use [125]. *In vitro* high-level resistance has clinical significance, as it has been associated with failure to eradicate the organism from both colonized and infected adult patients [125]. Rates of high-level resistance in series of isolates of methicillin-sensitive *S. aureus* generally have been 0% [126–129], but rates of 0.3–0.4% and 3% have been reported in the larger series of isolates of MRSA and coagulase-negative staphylococci, respectively [123–130].

Antibiotic treatment

A number of oral antibiotics have been approved for treatment of skin and skin-structure infections due to *S. aureus* and *S. pyogenes* (Table 2.11) [2]. Primary considerations in choosing among them are outlined in Table 2.10. The gold-standard oral therapies for treatment of skin infections during the past two decades have been erythromycin, dicloxacillin, cloxacillin and cephalexin. Clindamycin has been used occasionally, particularly for treatment of recurrent, recalcitrant skin infections, such as furunculosis due to *S. aureus* [131]. Each of the gold-standard therapies has limitations to its use. The major limitation of erythromycin is gastrointestinal intolerance; dicloxacillin suffers from an unpalatable taste; and all of the agents, including cephalexin, must be given three to four times daily to optimize their effectiveness. The relative risk of *Clostridium difficile* toxin-associated diarrhoea is higher with clindamycin than with any other commonly used oral antibiotic, limiting its use as well.

Until this past decade, topical antibiotics for treatment of skin infections also had severe limitations. Although several studies demonstrated that topical (neomycin, bacitracin, polysporin, gentamicin or mixtures of these) treatment was superior to placebo or cleansing with 3% hexachlorophene soap [132], topical antibiotics were inferior to systemic antibiotics until the introduction of mupirocin (Bactroban) [133, 134].

Mupirocin

Mupirocin is produced during fermentation by *Pseudomonas fluorescens*. It was first introduced as an antibiotic in the UK in 1985, and has a unique

Table 2.11 Oral antibiotics approved for treatment of skin infections due to *Staphylococcus aureus* or *Streptococcus pyogenes* (adapted from reference [2]).

Antibiotic	Proprietary name	Paediatric dose (mg/kg/day)	Adult dose (mg/dose)	Dosing interval	Length of therapy
Amoxicillin/clav.	Augmentin	20–40	250–500	tid	10
Azithromycin*	Zithromax	10	†	qd	5
Cephalexin	Keflex	25–50	250–500	bid/qid	10
Cefaclor	Ceclor	20–40	250–500	tid	10
Cefadroxil	Duricef	30	500–1000	qd/bid	10
Cefpodoxime*	Vantin	10	400	bid	7–14
Cefprozil	Cefzil	20	250–500	qd/bid	10
Cefuroxime*	Ceftin	30	250–500	bid	10
Cephradine	Velocef	25–50	250–500	bid/qid	10
Clarithromycin	Biaxin	15	250–500	bid	10
Clindamycin	Generic	15	150–450	tid/qid	10
Cloxacillin	Generic	50	250–500	qid	10
Dicloxacillin	Generic	12.5–50	125–250	qid	10
Dirithromycin*‡	Dynabac	500 mg/day	500	qid	7
Erythromycin					
ethylsuccinate	Generic	40	400–800	tid/qid	10
estolate	Generic	30	250–1000	tid/qid	10
Loracarbef	Lorabid	15	200–400	bid	7

* Not approved for use in individuals less than 12 years of age.
† 500 mg qd day 1, 250 mg qd days 2–5.
‡ Dirithromycin paediatric dose in mg/day.
bid, twice a day; qd, every day; qid, four times a day; tid, three times a day.

chemical structure among antibiotics. Mupirocin is bactericidal at the concentration achieved following topical application, and is not absorbed systemically [135]. Therefore, side-effects from mupirocin, especially contact hypersensitivity, appear to be due to the polyethylene glycol vehicle rather than the active ingredient. Its mode of action is the reversible inhibition of bacterial isoleucyl-transfer ribonucleic acid (tRNA) synthetase; it has a relatively low affinity for mammalian isoleucyl-tRNA synthetase. *Micrococcus* spp., coryneforms and propionibacteria are less sensitive than *S. pyogenes* or *S. aureus* to mupirocin [118]; thus, the natural skin flora is left relatively undisturbed. Rare instances of bacterial resistance to mupirocin have been reported, as noted above. Several studies have shown that mupirocin is equal in efficacy to erythromycin for treatment of impetigo (see 'Impetigo', below).

Cephalosporins

The cephalosporins are bactericidal for most species through binding to penicillin-binding proteins and inhibition of mucopeptide synthesis in the bacterial cell wall. They have a relatively pleasing taste, are well tolerated, have little or no hepatic metabolism and cause few side-effects or drug interactions [136, 137]. The risk of an allergic reaction to a cephalosporin in a patient with a history of penicillin sensitivity is low, probably about 2% [138]. Consequently, these agents are generally safe to administer to penicillin-allergic patients, although caution and appropriate supervision is advisable. Differences among the cephalosporins in their side-effect profile are trivial, except that cefaclor appears to cause hypersensitivity reactions relatively more often (5.3%) than other cephalosporins or amoxycillin (3.7%) [138, 139]. Cephalosporins exhibit time-dependent or concentration-independent killing. Thus, the duration of time in which the drug concentration at its site of action (e.g. skin-blister fluid) is above the MIC or minimum bactericidal concentration of the pathogen is most closely correlated with ability to kill and with clinical outcome [140]. Oral cephalosporins that remain equal to or more than 50% but less than 90% of their dosing interval over the MIC for 90% of *S. aureus* isolates include cefuroxime axetil, cephalexin and cefadroxil [140]. This level of activity against *S. pyogenes* in skin and soft tissue is met by all cephalosporins tested (cephalexin, cefadroxil, cefaclor, cefprozil, cefuroxime axetil, loracarbef, cefpodoxime proxetil, cefixime). Although infrequent dosing intervals are convenient and associated with increased compliance, extending the dosing interval beyond that recommended for a given agent may increase the likelihood of clinical failure due to the time dependence for killing [141].

Cephalosporins can be subdivided into generations according to spectrum of activity against Gram-negative bacteria (Table 2.12). With increasing generation, Gram-negative coverage broadens, but Gram-positive activity, especially against *S. aureus*, may be sacrificed. Cephalosporins are not active against MRSA.

First-generation cephalosporins. First-generation cephalosporins have excellent activity against methicillin-sensitive *S. aureus* and *S. pyogenes*. Among the first-generation cephalosporins, cefadroxil has the advantages of ease of administration (i.e. twice a day (bid) without regard to meals) and excellent tissue penetration. It costs considerably more than cephalexin (Table 2.13), however. Cephalexin has also been shown to be effective for treatment of skin and skin-structure infections with bid dosing [142–144], but, considering its pharmacokinetics and time dependence for killing, there is theoretical cause for concern that bid dosing may not be adequate. Dosing three (tid) or four times a day (qid) is preferable.

Table 2.12 Oral cephalosporins available for treatment of skin infections.

First generation	Second generation	Third generation
Cefadroxil	Cefaclor	Cefpodoxime
Cephalexin	Cefuroxime	
Cephradine	Cefprozil	
	Loracarbef	

Table 2.13 Primary antibiotics for treatment of skin infections due to *Staphylococcus aureus* or *Streptococcus pyogenes* (adapted from reference [2]).

Antibiotic	Dosing	Tissue penetration	Activity*	Cost†
Erythromycin	tid/qid	+++	++	2.60
Cephalexin	bid/qid	++	+++	3.26
Cloxacillin	qid	+++	+++	
Dicloxacillin	qid	+++	+++	14.40
Amoxycillin/clav.	tid	++	++++	31.04
Cefadroxil	qd/bid	+++	+++	24.20
Cefprozil	qd/bid	+++	$+++\frac{1}{2}$	33.40
Loracarbef	bid	++	++	15.48
Clarithromycin	bid	+++	++	22.20

* Activity against *S. aureus* and *S. pyogenes*.
† Wholesale cost in US dollars to Children's Hospital and Medical Center, Seattle, Washington, USA, for a course of therapy for a 20-kg child at the mid-dose range.
bid, twice a day; qd, every day; qid, four times a day; tid, three times a day.

Second-generation cephalosporins. Cefprozil is a second-generation cephalosporin that has superior activity against methicillin-sensitive *S. aureus* compared with cephalexin, cefaclor and cefuroxime, but has slightly less activity than amoxycillin/clavulanate [145, 146]. Cefprozil is the second-generation agent of choice for treatment of skin and skin-structure infections. Its major advantage over first-generation cephalosporins, erythromycin, dicloxacillin and amoxycillin/clavulanate for treatment of skin infections is the convenience and thus increased compliance associated with qd dosing. Its side-effect profile is also more favourable than these agents. Otherwise, it is not distinctly better and is significantly more expensive than cephalexin, erythromycin and dicloxacillin (Table 2.13).

Cefuroxime axetil is a prodrug that is de-esterified to the active cefuroxime moiety in the intestinal mucosa. It has greater stability than cefaclor to β-lactamases and is similar in activity to amoxycillin/clavulanate. It does not offer any distinct advantages over other cephalosporins for empirical treatment of uncomplicated skin and skin-structure infections and is relatively expensive (Table 2.13). Therefore, its use for treatment of skin and skin-structure infections should be limited.

Cefaclor has several disadvantages compared with its second-generation counterparts. These include its more frequent dosing (tid), decreased absorption in the presence of food, decreased activity against Gram-negative bacilli, decreased β-lactamase stability relative to cephalexin and higher propensity for hypersensitivity reactions, including the highest rate of serum sickness among the commonly used antimicrobial agents [139, 147–149]. Cefaclor is currently overused for treatment of skin infections.

Loracarbef is a carbacepham, a new class of β-lactamase antibiotics that resemble the cephalosporins in structure, but differ by replacement of the sulphur atom in position 1 of the cepham nucleus with a methylene group. It has equivalent to slightly increased β-lactamase stability relative to cefaclor, but less stability compared with cephalexin, cefadroxil or cefuroxime [150]. Its spectrum of antimicrobial activity is similar to that of the second-generation cephalosporins and amoxycillin/clavulanate [151]. Loracarbef has excellent activity against *S. pyogenes* and most isolates of methicillin-sensitive *S. aureus*. Loracarbef has no distinctive advantages over similar agents [152].

Third-generation cephalosporins. Third-generation cephalosporins are active against most Gram-negative enteric organisms, but are variable in their activity against Gram-positive cocci, particularly methicillin-sensitive *S. aureus*. Cefixime, for example, has the best Gram-negative activity of the oral cephalosporins and has excellent activity against *S. pyogenes* [145, 153]. It has essentially no activity against methicillin-sensitive *S. aureus*, however, due to low affinity for its β-lactam-binding proteins. Cefixime should not be used for treatment of primary skin and skin-structure infections. Cefdinir is similar to cefixime in its spectrum of activity, but has improved staphylococcal coverage. Nevertheless, serum bactericidal titres are only 1:2 or 1:4 for methicillin-sensitive *S. aureus*, below the desirable level of 1:8 or greater [153]. Likewise, ceftibuten, cefetamet and cefteram lack sufficient activity against *S. aureus*. Cefpodoxime axetil is the only third-generation cephalosporin that can be considered for treatment of uncomplicated skin infections. There is no inherent advantage, however, in the broader spectrum of activity of the third-generation cephalosporins. On the contrary, the broad spectrum of activity tends to exert increased selective pressure for the emergence of antibiotic resistance.

Macrolides

The macrolides are bacteriostatic, but may be bactericidal in high concentrations or against susceptible organisms. They inhibit bacterial RNA-dependent protein synthesis by binding to the 50S subunit of the 70S ribosome in the organism. Although erythromycin has been a front-line therapy for treatment of skin and skin-structure infections, its use is limited by gastrointestinal side-effects, erratic bioavailability, the need for tid or qid dosing and increasing resistance among isolates of *S. aureus*. Two macrolides (e.g. clarithromycin, azithromycin) with a lower incidence of gastrointestinal side-effects, improved pharmacokinetic properties and broader *in vitro* antimicrobial activity have appeared on the market in suspension form since 1994 [154, 155]. Like erythromycin, the new macrolides are also safe for use in patients with penicillin or sulpha allergies. The 14-hydroxy metabolite of clarithromycin enhances activity against susceptible isolates of *S. pyogenes*; thus, activity against *S. pyogenes* is excellent [156]. Activity of the new macrolides against methicillin-sensitive *S. aureus*, however, is no better than that of erythromycin, although the new macrolides are concentrated more than 30-fold in neutrophils that have phagocytized *S. aureus* [157]. Thus, the same concerns regarding erythromycin-resistant *S. aureus* apply to the new macrolides and, like erythromycin, the new macrolides should not be used to treat severe staphylococcal infections. Activity against MRSA remains poor.

Clarithromycin. Clarithromycin is better and more consistently absorbed than erythromycin. Like erythromycin, clarithromycin is metabolized by the cytochrome P450 system in liver hepatocytes and can affect the clearance of drugs metabolized by that system, such as theophylline, carbamazepine, phenytoin, digoxin and cyclosporin. In a comparative trial, although the rate of *S. aureus* resistance was 18% to clarithromycin compared with 1% for cefadroxil, they were equal in rate of clinical cure and pathogen eradication [26]. For treatment of uncomplicated skin and skin-structure infections, the primary advantages of clarithromycin compared with erythromycin are less frequent dosing and fewer gastrointestinal side-effects [158]. Compared with cephalexin and cefadroxil, both of which are well tolerated and can be dosed bid, there is little advantage to the use of clarithromycin except less selective pressure for emergence of β-lactamase resistance. Of lesser consequence is the threat of increased resistance of *S. pyogenes* to erythromycin with increased macrolide use.

Azithromycin. Azithromycin has a nitrogen molecule inserted into the lactone ring, and is thus a member of the macrolide subgroup called the azalides. It is highly concentrated in tissues (10–100-fold, compared with 5–10-fold for erythromycin) and within macrophages and neutrophils (up to 26-fold greater than erythromycin) [154, 155, 159] and may be transported within phagocytes to areas of inflammation [160]. Drug concentration in tissue reaches approximately 3 µg/ml, which is above the MIC_{90} of *S. pyogenes* and most isolates of methicillin-sensitive *S. aureus* [162]. Due to its slow release from tissues, the elimination half-life from serum (approximately 2 days) and tissue (2–3 days) is extremely long [159]. Consequently, azithromycin can be dosed once daily for a relatively short period of time (5 days) for treatment of skin and skin-structure infections. Although it interacts with the cytochrome P450 system, no clinically significant drug interactions have been observed [155, 161]. Furthermore, it has an excellent safety profile [155, 161–164].

The macrolide which was approved most recently (August 1995) for treatment of skin and skin-structure infections is dirithromycin. Dirithromycin is less active, however, than other macrolides against *S. pyogenes* [165]. Currently, it is approved only for use in adults with uncomplicated skin and skin-structure infections which are known to be due to *S. aureus*. As a result, it is not appropriate for empirical treatment of skin and skin-structure infections.

Quinolones

Several quinolones have shown excellent efficacy for treatment of skin and skin-structure infections in adults [36–41, 43, 48, 50]. Their use, however, has been complicated by superinfection and the rapid development of resistance, particularly among isolates of *S. aureus* [166]. Quinolones also have limited activity against *S. pyogenes*, and are not appropriate for treatment of skin infections known to be due to *S. aureus* or *S. pyogenes*.

Systemic antibiotic therapy

The β-lactamase-resistant penicillins nafcillin, oxacillin and methicillin are generally considered to be the first-line agents for treatment of serious skin and soft-tissue infections due to *S. aureus* or *S. pyogenes*. Treatment of *S. pyogenes* may be achieved with penicillin. A first-generation cephalosporin (e.g. cefazolin) is a suitable alternative to the penicillins. For more serious, deep-seated infections, however, particularly those due to exotoxin-producing isolates, clindamycin may be advantageous. In all serious infections, the susceptibility profile of the isolate(s) should be determined and the results used to optimize antibiotic selection.

Superficial skin infections

Superficial skin infections occur in the epidermis and/or dermis and tend to be localized and associated with few constitutional symptoms or signs. Primary superficial infections tend to have a characteristic clinical presentation. This section will focus on a description of these entities. Secondary superficial infections may be more difficult to recognize, as they involve further alteration of previously diseased or damaged skin by a superimposed skin infection.

Impetigo

Definition, epidemiology, aetiology

Impetigo is a superficial infection localized in the subcorneal portion of the epidermis. It accounts for 1–2% of all visits to pediatricians [29] and comprises approximately 10% of all skin problems in children and 50–60% of all bacterial skin infections [30, 31] making it the most common bacterial skin infection in children. There are two classic forms of impetigo: non-bullous and bullous.

Non-bullous impetigo. Non-bullous impetigo (impetigo contagiosa) accounts for more than 70% of cases of impetigo [3, 17, 20, 167–168]. It is most common in regions with a warm, humid climate. Among indigent schoolchildren in the southern USA in the summer, the prevalence of impetigo reaches 40–50%, with 85% of children becoming infected over the course of a summer [169]. From the 1940s to the mid-1960s, non-bullous impetigo in the USA was primarily of staphylococcal origin [3, 170]. During the later 1960s and the 1970s, S. pyogenes became the predominant pathogenic organism. At that time, the clinical response of non-bullous impetigo to penicillin was found to be excellent, regardless of whether culture of the lesion grew pure S. pyogenes, mixed S. pyogenes and penicillin-resistant S. aureus or pure penicillin-resistant S. aureus [171, 172]. These findings, which may have occurred due to interference with growth of S. pyogenes in culture by a bacteriocin produced by S. aureus [173], appeared to confirm the relative importance of S. pyogenes in the pathogenesis of the lesions. Studies during epidemics in the 1960s showed that clinically normal skin became colonized with S. pyogenes an average of 10 days before development of impetigo. In approximately 74% of episodes, the same serotype was recovered from clinically normal skin and the subsequent lesion of impetigo [64], suggesting that colonized skin served as the primary source and probably the initial step for development of skin infection. It was not until 15–20 days after the appearance of impetigo that S. pyogenes colonized the nasopharynx. Since the early 1980s, S. aureus has again become the predominant organism of non-bullous impetigo [10]. In contrast to streptococci, staphylococci generally spread from the nose to normal skin, and thence are able to infect the skin [63, 168]. Staphylococci can now be cultured from approximately 85% of lesions of impetigo of most populations and are the sole pathogen in approximately 50–60% of cases [2, 3, 13, 17, 19, 24], whereas S. pyogenes can be cultured from approximately 30–40% of lesions and is the sole pathogen in only about 5% of cases; occasionally, group B, C, G or F streptococci are present. Recent studies have demonstrated that treatment regimens which utilize antistaphylococcal agents now produce superior cure rates compared with regimens which employ β-lactamase-sensitive antibiotics. Several serotypes of S. pyogenes, termed 'impetigo strains', are found most frequently in lesions of non-bullous impetigo [65], and are different from those which cause pharyngitis. The S. aureus types which cause non-bullous impetigo are variable, but are generally not from phage group 2, the group associated with toxin production and bullous impetigo [168]. Whereas S. aureus can be cultured from lesions of impetigo on individuals of all ages, S. pyogenes is most common in children of preschool age and is unusual before 2 years of age except in highly endemic areas [170, 174].

Lesions of endemic non-bullous impetigo form most commonly on skin which has been traumatized, such as at varicella lesions, insect bites, abrasions, lacerations and burns. It appears that either colonization of normal-appearing skin, followed by a break in its barrier function, or direct inoculation of pathogens, concurrently with or following a skin wound, can lead to the infection [175]. Non-bullous impetigo also develops secondarily on previously diseased skin. Virtually any skin disease that violates the integrity of the barrier function of the skin may become infected in this manner. Impetiginization of atopic dermatitis, the most common form of secondary impetigo, almost uniformly involves *S. aureus*, although *S. pyogenes* can be cultured occasionally [32, 33]. Modes of transmission of the organisms responsible for impetigo are not clear but in most cases appear to involve direct contact with infected lesions. Fomites and the non-biting *Hippelates* fly can also contribute to spread of the infection. There is no sex or racial predilection.

Bullous impetigo. Bullous impetigo usually occurs sporadically, most often in infants and young children. A warm, humid climate favours its development and, consequently, like non-bullous impetigo, it is most common in the summer months in temperate climates. Unlike non-bullous impetigo, it is always caused by coagulase-positive *S. aureus*; approximately 80% are from phage group 2, 60% are type 71 and most of the remainder are types 3A, 3B, 3C and 55 [168, 176]. Lesions of bullous impetigo appear to develop on intact skin as a manifestation of localized toxin production (exfoliatin or epidermolytic toxins A or B) [177, 178].

Clinical characteristics

Non-bullous impetigo. Non-bullous impetigo begins as a tiny vesicle or pustule and rapidly develops into a honey-coloured crusted plaque, which is generally less than 2 cm in diameter (Figs 2.1 and 2.2). Lesions are associated with little to no pain or surrounding erythema, and constitutional symp-

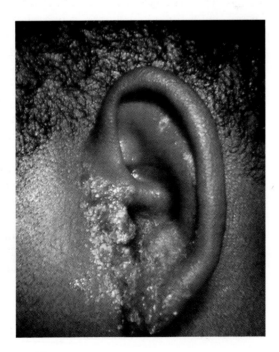

Fig. 2.2 Non-bullous impetigo. Crusted plaque of non-bullous impetigo.

toms are generally absent. Pruritus occurs occasionally, and regional adenopathy is found in up to 90% of cases [97, 168]. Leucocytosis is present in approximately 50% of patients [179].

In most studies of impetigo since 1980, the clinical appearance of lesions of non-bullous impetigo which yielded only *S. aureus* could not be distinguished from those that yielded only *S. pyogenes* or those that yielded both [10, 17, 20, 168]. It was claimed in the past that impetigo lesions due to *S. pyogenes* were deeper, more apt to ulcerate and more often associated with regional lymphadenopathy, tissue oedema and erythema, while infection with *S. aureus* was associated with early suppuration and possibly tissue necrosis [29, 32, 180]. It was also suggested that impetigo on the face was more commonly due to *S. aureus*, while lesions on the extremities tended to be caused by *S. pyogenes*. These clinical distinctions appear to have blurred.

When impetigo develops secondarily on previously diseased skin, it may be more difficult to recognize, as clinical signs of the infection are intermingled with those of the primary disease process. In atopic dermatitis, for example, impetiginization may present with little more than a mild exacerbation of the dermatitis, manifested as increased pruritus, erythema and superficial crusted erosions (Fig. 2.3). As the infection worsens, fissures develop and the dermatitis may become frankly exudative. Development of an odour may also indicate secondary impetiginization. While impetigo tends to be localized in primary infections, it may generalize rapidly when superimposed on skin affected with a primary disease, such as atopic dermatitis or chickenpox, or on skin that has been traumatized, such as with insect bites.

Bullous impetigo. Bullous impetigo presents with flaccid, transparent bullae, most commonly on skin of moist, intertriginous areas and occasionally on the face or extremities. Bullae may occur singly or several may be clustered

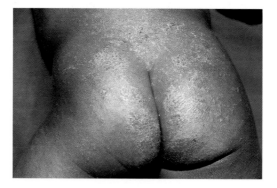

Fig. 2.3 Secondary non-bullous impetigo. Multiple excoriated, lichenified, erythematous plaques of atopic dermatitis on the buttocks of a child. Impetiginized, focal, crusted erosions and excoriations are present within the plaques. Secondary infection in this setting is nearly always due to *Staphylococcus aureus*.

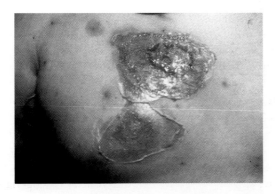

Fig. 2.4 Bullous varicella. Crusted, flaky, erythematous erosions with a rim of scale extending from chickenpox lesions on the chest of a child. Damage to the integrity of the epidermal barrier by the chickenpox lesions facilitates secondary infection with *Staphylococcus aureus*. Epidermolytic toxin produced locally by *S. aureus* damages desmosomes, forming subcorneal bullae. An erosion is apparent following rupture of the bullae.

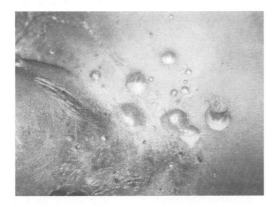

Fig. 2.5 Bullous impetigo. Multiple bullae in the inguinal region of an infant. Pus has formed a layer in the dependent portion of the bullae.

regionally. In bullous varicella, generalized bullae may develop when an exotoxin-producing strain of *S. aureus* infects lesions of chickenpox, producing moist, mildly tender, denuded areas that extend from the chickenpox vesicles (Fig. 2.4) [134]. Influx of leucocytes may lead to turbidity of bullae fluid; if the patient is stationary, pus may form a layer on the dependent portion of the bullae (Fig. 2.5). Due to the superficial location of the subcorneal bullae, they rupture easily, leaving a narrow rim of scale at the edge of a shallow, moist, erythematous erosion (Fig. 2.6). The erosion does not penetrate below the epidermal–dermal junction and thus it heals without scarring. Postinflammatory pigmental changes, however, may be present for weeks to months. Surrounding erythema, regional adenopathy and constitutional symptoms are generally absent.

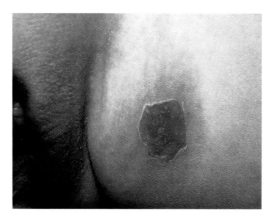

Fig. 2.6 Bullous impetigo. Shallow, erythematous erosion with a rim of scale in the inguinal region of an infant.

Without treatment, individual lesions of impetigo may progress slowly for several weeks, but in most cases will resolve spontaneously without scarring or complications within approximately 2 weeks [63]. The disease often lasts several weeks, however, with new lesions developing, probably following autoinoculation, as older lesions resolve. Cellulitis has been reported in approximately 10% of patients, but this figure may be an overestimation [168]. Lymphangitis, suppurative lymphadenitis, guttate psoriasis and scarlet fever may be associated with streptococcal disease. There is no correlation, however, between number of lesions and clinical involvement of the lymphatics or development of cellulitis in association with streptococcal impetigo [168]. Possible complications of impetigo due to haematogenous spread include osteomyelitis, septic arthritis, pneumonia and septicaemia. Positive blood cultures are rarely found.

Infection with nephritogenic strains of *S. pyogenes* can result in acute poststreptococcal glomerulonephritis. The clinical character of impetigo lesions is not different between those that lead to poststreptococcal glomerulonephritis and those that do not. The most commonly affected age-group is school-aged children of 3–7 years old. The latent period, from onset of impetigo to development of poststreptococcal glomerulonephritis, averages 18–21 days, which is longer than the 10-day latency period following pharyngitis [65, 181]. Acute poststreptococcal glomerulonephritis occurs sporadically, due primarily to M type 12 infection of the pharynx, and epidemically, following either pharyngeal or skin infection. Impetigo-associated epidemics are caused by M groups 2, 49, 53, 55, 56, 57 and 60 [65, 181], whereas M groups 1 and 12 are most often associated with glomerulonephritis following pharyngitis. The most common site of *S. pyogenes* infection that results in acute poststreptococcal glomerulonephritis varies according to geographical location. Whereas 76% of symptomatic acute poststreptococcal glomerulonephritis in children in Chicago was associated with upper respiratory-tract infection [182], 40–80% of episodes of the disease in children in the south-eastern USA followed impetigo [65, 183, 184]. In general, since the 1960s, acute poststreptococcal glomerulonephritis in the USA has appeared more frequently following pharyngitis than after impetigo [185]. The true incidence of acute poststreptococcal glomerulonephritis is difficult to determine, as many mild or subclinical cases go undetected. A prospective study of 248 children with streptococcal infection demonstrated that 22% developed asymptomatic urinary abnormalities or a low-serum C3 concentration or both [186]. The risk of nephritis after impetigo varies widely with the strain of S. pyogenes. During an epidemic of acute nephritis due to S. pyogenes of M group 49, 24% of children with streptococcal impetigo developed acute nephritis or unexplained haematuria; the risk was highest in children less than $6\frac{1}{2}$ years of age (43%) [187]. Multiple subclinical and clinical cases of nephritis often occur within a family [65]. Strains of S. pyogenes which are associated with endemic impetigo in the USA have little or no nephritogenic potential [187]. For example, there have been no cases of glomerulonephritis among the more than 500 patients from trials which compared the efficacy of treatment with erythromycin to that with mupirocin [13, 15–17, 19, 24, 167]. Acute rheumatic fever does not occur following impetigo.

Diagnosis

Although the number of infectious agents capable of causing a vesiculobullous rash is lengthy, the number of common infectious agents besides S. aureus and S. pyogenes is limited, consisting of the enteroviruses, varicella zoster and herpes simplex viruses (HSV). Bullous impetigo, occurring independently or as a superinfection of varicella lesions, is probably the most common cause of bullae in children. Other bullous eruptions, such as staphylococcal scalded-skin syndrome (SSSS), erythema multiforme (with HSV or *Mycoplasma pneumoniae* infection) and the haemorrhagic bullae which can accompany sepsis with Gram-negative organisms, particularly *Pseudomonas aeruginosa* (ecthyma gangraenosum) and *Neisseria meningitidis*, fortunately are relatively infrequent. The number of non-infectious conditions that closely mimic the eruption caused by these organisms, however is disproportionately large, often leading to confusion or delay in diagnosis. The appearance of bullae caused by thermal injury or a hypersensitivity response to insect bites is virtually identical to that of bullous impetigo. Similarly, nummular eczema may closely mimic non-bullous impetigo. Nevertheless, consideration of the season; the patient's age; a history of exposure to infectious agents or recent ingestion of medications, prior disease and concurrent symptoms; and the morphology, distribution and evolution of the eruption will routinely allow one to make a diagnosis of impetigo on an empirical basis. Swabbing the blister fluid or beneath the lifted edge of a crusted plaque generally yields reliable culture results. If S. aureus is acting as a pathogen of impetigo rather than a colonizer of a primary vesiculobullous process, the organism will generally be identifiable on Gram stain as well as in culture. In cases where aetiology remains in doubt, a biopsy, utilizing histopathological evaluation, immunofluorescence staining and occasionally electron microscopy, may be helpful, particularly in excluding non-infectious bullous disorders.

Histopathological examination of an early lesion of impetigo shows vesicopustule formation in the subcorneal or granular region of the epidermis (Fig. 2.7). The blister cavity is larger in the bullous form. Neutrophils are generally visible within the cavity of the blister, and often in the underlying epidermis as they migrate from dermal blood-vessels. Acantholytic cells may be present at the base of the vesicle or bulla. The underlying stratum malpighii and/or papillary dermis is spongiotic, and a mixed infiltrate of lymphocytes and neutrophils surrounds the blood-vessels of the superficial dermal plexus. Biopsy of lesions in later stages may reveal serous crust and neutrophilic debris overlying a superficially eroded epidermis. Unless Gram-positive cocci can be cultured from the vesicle, it may be impossible to differentiate impetigo from pemphigus foliaceus histopathologically. Pemphigus foliaceus tends to have more acantholysis and fewer neutrophils within the subcorneal blister, and may have dyskeratotic changes in cells of the granular layer [188]. Clinically, pemphigus folliaceus differs from impetigo in its presentation, with multiple, small, flaccid blisters which easily rupture, leaving erythematous, crusted erosions. Subcorneal pustular dermatosis may also be indistinguishable histopathologically from impetigo, but its clinical presentation is that of crops of grouped pustules in a serpiginous outline, generally on the abdomen or in the axillary and inguinal folds, sparing the face.

Although immunological tests have little place in the diagnosis of impetigo, they may occasionally be useful retrospectively for confirmation of disease. Anti-DNase B is the test of choice for detecting preceding streptococcal impetigo. After an episode of non-bullous impetigo caused by *S. pyogenes*, the antistreptolysin O (ASO) response is slight or absent, perhaps due to binding of streptolysin O by lipids, including cholesterol, in the skin [189]. Of patients with uncomplicated impetigo, 67% had elevated anti-DNase B titres, while 43% developed an elevated ASO titre [97]. The anti-hyaluronidase test also is thought to be superior to the ASO test in documenting a preceding streptococcal skin infection [190]. The strep-

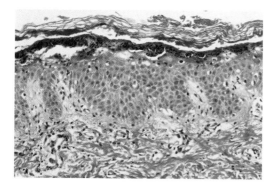

Fig. 2.7 Bullous impetigo. Haematoxylin–eosin-stained skin-biopsy specimen taken from a lesion of bullous impetigo. A subcorneal bulla contains an acute inflammatory infiltrate.

tozyme test measures more than five antibodies to streptococcal antigens, including anti-DNase B ASO, and antihyaluronidase. When only one of the antibodies is minimally elevated, however, false-negative results may be obtained [191]. In addition, the combination of individual anti-DNase B and ASO tests is more effective than the streptozyme test in detecting preceding *S. pyogenes* infection [192].

Treatment

In areas with a high prevalence of erythromycin-resistant strains of *S. aureus*, superficial, localized, non-bullous impetigo located away from the mouth might be best treated topically with mupirocin. Several studies have demonstrated that mupirocin applied three times daily for 7–10 days is equal to or greater in effectiveness than oral erythromycin ethylsuccinate 30–50 mg/kg/day for 7–10 days for treatment of impetigo in children [13, 15–17, 19, 24]. Treatment success rate with mupirocin was greater than 90%, regardless of whether the length of treatment was 7, 8 or 10 days. There were fewer side-effects of treatment [13, 15, 17, 24], in some cases lesions cleared more rapidly and the rate of eradication of pyogenic bacteria was equivalent [167], or greater [16, 17] in those treated with topical mupirocin compared with systemic erythromycin. A cost-effectiveness analysis evaluated the total cost, including physician fees, transportation expenses and cost of the medication for a 10-day course of treatment with mupirocin compared with erythromycin ethylsuccinate. Although the cost of treatment was significantly greater for mupirocin ($62.30) than for erythromycin ($56.85), this extra cost was offset by increased side-effects (43% vs. 22%) and number of schooldays (3.0 vs. 1.2) and workdays (0.5 vs. 0.2) missed in the group treated with erythromycin [167].

Studies that have compared the effectiveness of mupirocin with that of erythromycin have generally restricted their patient population to those with superficial, localized, primary pyoderma. Low-grade fever [15, 24], and regional adenopathy [24], however, are not absolute contraindications to treatment with mupirocin. Lesions around the mouth in children should probably not be treated with mupirocin, as the medication may be licked off [17].

A patient with recurrent impetigo should be evaluated for carriage of *S. aureus* in the nares, although approximately 25% of carriers will harbour *S. aureus* at sites other than the nares, such as the perineum or axillae [193]. Nasal carriage of both methicillin-susceptible strains of *S. aureus* and MRSA has been eliminated in greater than 90% of individuals within 2–4 days through use of topical mupirocin [129, 194], thereby reducing rates of staphylococcal infection in patients with atopic dermatitis or on haemodialysis [33]. Coagulase-negative staphylococci and coryneforms subsequently became the dominant nasal flora and may have contributed to prevention of reacquisition of *S. aureus* by bacterial interference [195]. In time, however, measured in weeks to months, the nares become recolonized. In order to prevent the emergence of resistant strains, use of mupirocin to eliminate nasal carriage should be reserved for outbreaks, particularly when MRSA is involved, or for patients with recurrent staphyloccocal impetigo, particularly if the phage types that are cultured from the nares and from impetiginous lesions are identical [129, 196].

For impetigo that is more widespread or has become complicated by involvement of deeper tissues, including cellulitis, suppurative lymphadenitis, furunculosis, abscess formation or suppurative lymphadenitis, or if significant constitutional symptoms are present, an oral antibiotic active against β-lactamase-producing strains of *S. aureus* should be prescribed. Although, dicloxacillin is a first-line oral agent for treatment of staphylococcal infections, its usefulness, particularly in infants and young children who cannot swallow a pill, is limited by poor taste and gastrointestinal complaints [147]. Erythromycin and cephalexin also remain first-line agents for treatment of skin and skin-structure infections in children. The clinical significance of *in vitro* erythromycin resistance in the treatment of skin infections in children is unclear and must be assessed on a local basis. Cephalexin, primarily due to its lower cost, is still the cephalosporin of choice. The superior taste and adverse-events profile, uniform efficacy and potential for twice-daily dosing, however, make cephalexin a more attractive option in many cases. If bid dosing of cephalexin proves to be ineffective and tid or qid dosing around meals is unmanageable, either cefadroxil (qd or bid dosing) or cefprozil (qid dosing) may be preferred. The ease of administration of cefprozil must be weighed against its slightly higher cost compared with cefadroxil (Table 2.13).

If the local rate of resistance to erythromycin is low among isolates of *S. aureus*, erythromycin is preferred, provided that dosing tid to qid and its gastrointestinal side-effects are manageable. Either erythromycin or cephalexin is suitable for penicillin-allergic patients. Cefadroxil, cefprozil, loracarbef, claithromycin and amoxycillin/clavulanate are second-line agents for treatment of uncomplicated impetigo. Choice among these agents may be guided primarily by issues of cost, compliance, local availability, patient/parent acceptability and physician preference, since each is clinically effective in more than 90% of patients studied [2, 22, 23, 25, 26, 132, 153]. Cefuroxime may be useful in the uncommon instance of a moderately severe skin infection due to a β-lactamase-producing Gram-negative organism with proved susceptibility to cefuroxime. Clindamycin remains of value primarily in infections with strains of *S. aureus* that are known to produce toxins, as well as in treating patients with recurrent staphylococcal infections, such as furunculosis/carbunculosis, or infections with anaerobic organisms, such as many abscesses, burns and ulcers. Bullous impetigo in a neonate must be treated parenterally; first-line agents include β-lactamase-resistant antistaphylococcal penicillins, such as methicillin, oxacillin or nafcillin. Culture and antibiotic susceptibility testing of the pathogens should be utilized to guide therapy. Aggressive treatment may prevent development of complications, such as septicaemia, pneumonia, septic arthritis and osteomyelitis.

There is little evidence to suggest that a 10-day course of therapy is superior to a 7-day course. Because studies, except those with loracarbef and azithromycin, have utilized 10 days of therapy, drug manufacturers have recommended this length of treatment. In general, if a satisfactory clinical response has not been achieved after 7 days of therapy, it is advisable to swab beneath the lifted edge of a crusted lesion to obtain a Gram stain, culture and antibiotic-susceptibility profile of the pathogen(s).

Treatment, whether systemic or topical, in cases of impetigo-associated acute poststreptococcal glomerulonephritis does not prevent the development of glomerulonephritis in the index case [170, 197], but may prevent spread of impetigo to others and thus reduce the incidence of acute poststreptococcal glomerulonephritis in the community.

Ecthyma

Definition, epidemiology, aetiology

Ecthyma resembles non-bullous impetigo in onset and appearance but gradually evolves into a deeper, more chronic infection. Lesions occur most frequently on the legs, particularly in the setting of poor hygiene and malnutrition, and at sites of pruritis, such as insect bites, scabies or pediculosis, which are subject to frequent scratching [198]. The causative agent is usually *S. pyogenes*; *S. aureus* is also cultured from most lesions but is probably a secondary invader. Alternatively, the infection may involve synergism between the two organisms.

Clinical characteristics

The initial lesion is a vesicle or vesicopustule with an erythematous base that erodes through the epidermis into the dermis to form a well-defined, thickly crusted ulcer with elevated margins up to 4 cm in diameter, surrounded by a rim of erythema (Fig. 2.8). Because the lesion extends into the dermis, healing is frequently accompanied by scar formation. Complications include lymphadentitis, lymphangitis, cellulitis and, rarely, poststreptococcal glomerulonephritis.

Diagnosis

Diagnosis of ecthyma can generally be made by visual inspection, although clinical distinction from impetigo may not be possible. Treatment for these two entities is the same, however, so biopsy, which reveals a prominent acute inflammatory infiltrate surrounding an ulcer that extends into the superficial dermis, is not needed to confirm the diagnosis in most cases.

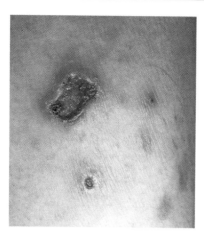

Fig. 2.8 Ecthyma. Well-defined, crusted ulcer due to *Streptococcus pyogenes* on the thigh.

Other unusual infections, such as anthrax, cutaneous diphtheria and ecthyma gangraenosum can closely mimic ecthyma. Primary cutaneous anthrax infection develops approximately 2–5 days after inoculation of *Bacillus anthracis* organisms on to exposed skin. A painless papule evolves into a serosanguinous vesicle or bulla, which is surrounded by brawny, non-pitting oedema. The site becomes progressively discoloured, haemor-rhagic and necrotic, with central eschar formation. Satellite vesicles and regional adenitis may be present, but lymphangitis is absent. Constitutional symptoms are common. Anthrax is usually characterized by a more rapid course and greater degree of haemorrhage, gelatinous oedema and consti-tutional symptoms than ecthyma. Diagnosis of anthrax can be confirmed by culture of the Gram-positive bacillus.

Primary cutaneous infection with *Corynebacterium diphtheriae* occurs predominantly in malnourished, unimmunized children in crowded, unsanitary conditions. Secondary infection of skin affected by pre-existing trauma, dermatitis or pyoderma with *S. pyogenes* is the most common form of cutaneous diphtheria in the USA. The infected site is erythematous, oedematous and purulent and is usually covered partially with a greyish, adherent membrane. Primary cutaneous diphtheria, a disease mainly of tropical environments, begins as a tender papulopustule, which breaks down to form a punched-out ulcer with a membranous base and oedema-tous, rolled, bluish margins [199–201]. Regional lymphadenopathy is common, but systemic signs, except in infants, are absent to mild. Differen-tiation from ecthyma may require culture of the organism.

Ecthyma gangraenosum is a necrotic ulcer covered with a grey-black eschar. It is generally a sign of *P. aeruginosa* bacteraemia in neutropenic patients with leukaemia or aplastic anaemia. It can also occur, however, as a primary cutaneous infection by inoculation. Similar lesions may also develop as a result of infection with other agents, such as *Aeromonas hydrophila, Enterobacter* spp., *E. coli, Proteus* spp., *Pseudomonas cepacia, Serratia marcescens, Stenotrophomonas maltophilia, Aspergillus* spp., *Fusarium* spp., and

Candida albicans [202]. The lesion begins as a red or purpuric macule, which vesiculates and then ulcerates; there is a surrounding rim of pink to violaceous skin. The punched-out ulcer develops raised edges, with a dense, black, depressed, crusted centre. Lesions may be single or multiple; patients with bacteraemia commonly have lesions in apocrine areas. Histopathological examination allows distinction of this entity from ecthyma. One sees bacterial invasion of the adventitia and media of dermal veins but not arteries; the intima and lumina are spared.

Treatment

Systemic antibiotic therapy to cover *S. pyogenes* and *S. aureus*, as for impetigo, is recommended. Local wound care, including removal of eschar, cleansing and application of occlusive ointment, may aid healing.

Blastomycosis-like pyoderma (dermatitis vegetans)

Definition, epidemiology, aetiology

Blastomycosis-like pyoderma appears to be an exuberant cutaneous reaction to bacterial infection in a host with defective immunity [203]. It has been described in individuals with a variety of underlying conditions, including malnutrition, ulcerative colitis, alcoholism, lymphoma and immunodeficiency [204–206]. *Staphylococcus aureus* and *S. pyogenes* are the organisms isolated most commonly, but several other organisms have been associated with these lesions, including *P. aeruginosa*, *Proteus mirabilis*, diphtheroids, *Bacillus* spp. and *Clostridium perfringens*.

Clinical characteristics

Hyperplastic, crusted plaques in the flexures or on the extremities are characteristic (Fig. 2.9), sometimes forming from the coalescence of multiple, pinpoint, purulent, crusted abscesses. Central clearing may occur. Alternatively, ulceration and sinus-tract formation may develop, and additional lesions may appear at sites distant from the site of inoculation. Regional lymphadenopathy is common, but fever is not.

Diagnosis

Diagnosis depends largely on the exclusion of other conditions. The differential diagnosis includes deep fungal infection, particularly blastomycosis, tuberculous, atypical mycobacterial infection, iododerma, pyoderma gangraenosum and pemphigus vegetans. Histopathological examination reveals pseudoepitheliomatous hyperplasia and abscesses composed of neutrophils and/or eosinophils; giant cells are usually lacking. Underlying immunodeficiency should be ruled out.

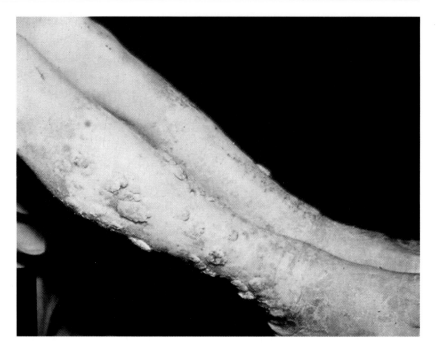

Fig. 2.9 Blastomycosis-like pyoderma. Hyperplastic, crusted nodules and plaques on the legs.

Treatment

Malnutritional and other underlying conditions should be addressed. Selection of antibiotics should be guided by susceptibility testing, as the response to antibiotics is often poor. Antibiotic efficacy appears to be enhanced when combined with curettage of lesions to a clean base [205]. Application of caustic substances, such as silver nitrate, to hyperplastic granulation tissue may also be helpful [205].

Folliculitis

Definition, epidemiology, aetiology

This superficial infection of the hair follicle is predominantly due to *S. aureus*, although coagulase-negative staphylococci are occasionally involved. A moist environment, maceration, poor hygiene, application of an occlusive emollient and drainage from adjacent wounds and abscesses can be provocative factors.

Clinical characteristics

Folliculitis presents as discrete, dome-shaped pustules with an erythematous base, located at the ostium of the pilosebaceous canals, usually on the scalp, buttocks or extremities. The lesions are asymptomatic to mildly tender. Occasionally, a lesion may extend to involve deeper tissues and form an abscess. Human immunodeficiency virus (HIV)-infected patients may develop confluent erythematous patches, with satellite pustules in intertriginous areas, and violaceous plaques composed of superficial follicular pustules in the scalp, axillae or groin [207].

Diagnosis

The causative organism of folliculitis can be identified by Gram stain and culture of purulent material from the follicular orifice.

Sycosis barbae is a deeper, more severe, recurrent, inflammatory form of folliculitis due to *S. aureus*, involving the entire depth of the follicle. Erythematous, follicular papules and pustules develop on the chin, upper lip and angle of the jaw, primarily in young black males. Papules may coalesce into plaques, and healing may occur with scarring. Affected individuals are frequently found to be *S. aureus* nasal carriers.

Candida is prone to cause satellite follicular papules and/or pustules surrounding patches of candidal intertrigo, particularly in patients on long-term corticosteroid or antibiotic therapy. *Malassezia furfur* can also produce pruritic, 2- to 3-mm, erythematous, perifollicular papules and papulopustules on the back, chest and extremities, particularly in patients with diabetes mellitus, or on long-term systemic corticosteroids or antibiotics. Diagnosis is made by potassium hydroxide examination of scrapings from a lesion. A skin biopsy is often necessary to identify grape-like clusters of yeast, and short, septate branching hyphal fragments ('spaghetti and meatballs') in widened follicular ostia, mixed with keratinous debris.

Gram-negative folliculitis occurs primarily in patients with acne vulgaris who have received long-term therapy with broad-spectrum systemic antibiotics. A superficial pustular form, due to *Klebsiella* spp., *Enterobacter* spp., *E. coli*, or *P. aeruginosa*, occurs around the nose and spreads to the cheeks and chin. A deeper, nodular form on the face and trunk is caused by *Proteus* spp. Culture of infected follicles is necessary to establish the diagnosis.

Hot-tub folliculitis is attributable to *P. aeruginosa*, predominantly serotype O-11. The lesions are pruritic papules and pustules or deeply erythematous to violaceous nodules, which develop 8–48 hours after exposure and are most dense in areas covered by a bathing-suit. Patients occasionally develop fever, malaise and lymphadenopathy. The organism is cultured from pus.

Treatment

An attempt should be made to identify and eliminate predisposing factors. Topical antibiotic cleansers, such as chlorhexidine or hexachlorophene, are usually effective for mild cases, but more severe cases may require use of a penicillinase-resistant systemic antibiotic, such as cephalexin, dicloxacillin or cloxacillin. In chronic recurrent folliculitis, daily application of a benzoyl peroxide lotion or gel can facilitate resolution.

Treatment of sycosis barbae with warm saline compresses and topical antibiotics, such as mupirocin, will generally clear the infection. More extensive, recalcitrant cases may require therapy with systemic β-lactamase-resistant antibiotics, as well as elimination of *S. aureus* from sites of carriage, using mupirocin or rifampicin.

Blistering dactylitis

Definition, epidemiology, aetiology

Blistering dactylitis is a superficial blistering infection, most commonly of the distal volar fat pad on the phalanges of school-aged children [208]. It can also occur, however, in infants and adults. There is usually no preceding history of trauma. The causal organism is nearly always *S. pyogenes*, but blistering dactylitis has also occurred as a result of infection with *S. aureus* or group B streptococci [209, 210]. *Streptococcus pyogenes* is occasionally isolated concurrently from the oropharynx.

Clinical characteristics

Bullae up to approximately 2 cm in diameter develop on an erythematous base (Fig. 2.10). More than one digit may be involved, as may the volar surfaces of the proximal phalanges, the toes and the palm. Lesions are asymptomatic to mildly tender; systemic symptoms are generally absent. If left untreated, blisters may continue to enlarge and extend to the paronychial area. Poststreptococcal glomerulonephritis has not occurred following blistering distal dactylitis.

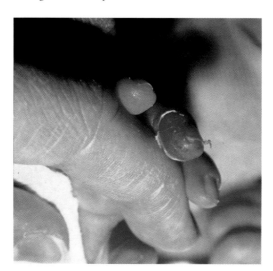

Fig. 2.10 Blistering dactylitis. Erythematous erosion with a rim of scale following rupture of a bulla on the distal finger of an infant infected locally with *Streptococcus pyogenes* (photograph courtesy of Alfred T. Lane, MD).

Diagnosis

Blisters are filled with a purulent fluid, which contains polymorphonuclear leucocytes and infecting organisms. The reason for blister formation is unclear, but location of the infection in areas of skin with a thickened stratum corneum appears to be a factor. Diagnosis can be confirmed by Gram stain and culture.

Treatment

The infection responds to incision and drainage and a 10-day course of systemic therapy with a β-lactamase-resistant penicillin or cephalosporin, such as cephalexin, dicloxacillin or cloxacillin. Penicillin-allergic patients can be treated with erythromycin or clindamycin.

Perianal dermatitis

Definition, epidemiology, aetiology

Perianal dermatitis is a superficial, perianally localized form of *S. pyogenes* infection; the infection has also been caused by *S. aureus* [211]. Although it was termed perianal cellulitis in the past, subcutaneous tissue is not typically involved, and it is more properly referred to as a dermatitis. It presents most commonly in boys (70% of cases) between the ages of 6 months and 10 years, but has been reported in adults. Asymptomatic adults may also serve as carriers [212, 213]. The anal carrier rate in children with positive pharyngeal cultures for *S. pyogenes* was 6% in one study of 100 children [214] and 0% in a group of 25 children [215]. Among a control group of 119 children who presented for well-child care, only one was culture-positive for *S. pyogenes*, suggesting that the rate of perianal colonization may be higher in those with *S. pyogenes*-associated pharyngitis than in the general population [215]. On the other hand, among children with perianal dermatitis, more than 50% (16 of 25 patients in one study) [215] have concurrent positive perianal and pharyngeal cultures with an identical *S. pyogenes* type [215, 216], and approximately 10% have symptomatic pharyngitis [215]. The mechanism for concurrent pharyngeal and anal involvement with *S. pyogenes* may involve passage of live organisms from the colonized or infected pharynx through the gastrointestinal tract or, alternatively, digital contamination from the infected anus to the oropharynx or vice versa. Rarely, perianal dermatitis has been associated with impetigo caused by *S. pyogenes*; in each case, impetigo preceded the dermatitis, suggesting that *S. pyogenes* spread from the impetigo lesion to the perianal skin [215, 217]. It is not currently known whether anal or pharyngeal colonization tends to occur first. Familial spread of perianal dermatitis is common, particularly when family members share the same bath water.

The incidence of perianal dermatitis is not known precisely. In their original description of this condition, Amren *et al.* [216] reported an incidence of one in 2000 patient visits over a 15-month period. More recently, in one paediatric practice, 31 patients—or one in 218 patient visits —were diagnosed with perianal dermatitis during a 9-month period of time [215].

Clinical characteristics

Presentation most commonly includes perianal dermatitis (90% of cases) and pruritis (80% of cases) [216, 218]. Approximately half of patients have rectal pain, most commonly described as burning inside the anus during defecation, and one-third have blood-streaked stools. Faecal hoarding is a frequent behavioural response to the infection. The rash is superficial, erythematous, well marginated, non-indurated and confluent from the anus outward (Fig. 2.11). Acutely (<6 weeks' duration), the rash tends to be bright red, moist and tender. Local induration or oedema may occur. With time, painful fissures, a dried mucoid discharge or psoriasiform plaques with yellow, peripheral crusts become more prominent and the erythema subsides. In girls, the perianal rash may be associated with vulvovaginitis, manifested as vaginal discharge and vulvar redness [215]. Overall, approximately 10% of cases of vulvovaginitis in girls are due to *S. pyogenes* [219]. Patients may also present with guttate psoriasis, emphasizing that the anus should be examined in all such cases [220].

Diagnosis

Duration of symptoms before diagnosis ranges from a few days to several months (mean 6 months) [218], and in one case 13 months elapsed from onset of symptoms to diagnosis [215]. The differential diagnosis of perianal dermatitis includes psoriasis, seborrhoeic dermatitis, candidiasis, pinworm infestation, sexual abuse and inflammatory bowel disease. Differentiation from these other conditions can be accomplished by culturing a moderate

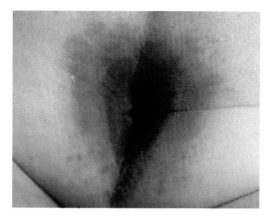

Fig. 2.11 Perianal dermatitis. Bright red plaque due to *Streptococcus pyogenes* on the anus of a child (photograph courtesy of Alfred T. Lane, MD).

to heavy growth of *S. pyogenes* from perianal swabs. Individuals with asymptomatic perianal colonization have light growth of *S. pyogenes* on blood agar. Direct antigen studies for *S. pyogenes* are also very sensitive (89%), but may be falsely negative early in the course of the disease [215, 216]. Antistreptolysin O and antiDNase B titres do not rise [216]. The index case and family members should be cultured initially, and follow-up cultures to document bacteriological cure after a course of treatment are recommended.

Treatment

A single 10-day course of oral penicillin will resolve the condition in the majority of patients; however, recurrence rates of 40–50% have been reported, emphasizing the need for close follow-up, including repeat culture. Erythromycin estolate or ethylsuccinate are alternative treatments for persons who are allergic to penicillin, who have failed a course of penicillin or who are infected with *S. aureus*. Clindamycin has also been used successfully to treat persons with recurrent perianal dermatitis. Mupirocin has been used in conjunction with oral antibiotics to treat recurrences, but has not been evaluated as a single-drug therapy.

Periocular infection

The skin over the eyelids is the thinnest in the body and the subcutaneous tissue is loose and lacks fat. Consequently, signs of inflammation in this site are readily apparent, and superficial infections may be complicated by abscess formation or cellulitis of adjacent tissues. Inflammation of the eyelid margin, known as blepharitis, is most commonly due to *S. aureus* [221]. The infection can also be caused by *S. epidermidis* and, rarely, by *Moraxella* in children. Other Gram-negative bacilli, such as *Pseudomonas* spp. or *P. mirabilis*, or fungi, such as *Candida*, may cause blepharitis, primarily in immunosuppressed patients. Viral agents, particularly herpes simplex virus (HSV), varicella zoster virus (VZV) and molluscum contagiosum, and parasitic infestations with scabies and pubic or head lice can affect the eyelids as well. Application of contaminated make-up or contact-lens solution, poor hygiene, tear deficiency and the presence of seborrhoeic dermatitis, acne rosacea, atopy and immunosuppression are predisposing conditions [222]. Staphylococcal blepharitis involves the skin of the anterior portion of the eyelids, and may extend to involve the ciliofollicles or accessory glandular structures. Blepharitis due to *S. aureus* is typically chronic and bilateral, but may also present acutely. The anterior lid margin is erythematous, with hard scales around the base of the lashes. Removal of the crust may leave a superficial ulceration at hair-follicle ostia. Lashes may be lost, and conjunctivitis is common, particularly when the *S. aureus* isolate is a producer of exotoxins. Keratitis may also develop, presumably due to hypersensitivity reactions to staphylococcal exotoxins or other bacterial antigens [223]. Fluorescein examination may reveal punctate erosions of the cornea. The differential diagnosis includes contact dermatitis and allergic conjunctivitis. Both of these conditions are associated with pruritus, which may induce the patient to rub the lids, producing secondary erythema and swelling. Treatment of staphylococcal blepharitis includes warm compresses, careful débridement of scales and topical application of antibiotics, such as bacitracin, erythromycin or sulphacetamide. Topical corticosteroid drops, given briefly, may decrease inflammation.

Staphylococcal blepharitis is often associated with infection of the glands of the eyelids. When the infection involves the meibomian glands, which are long sebaceous glands that extend through the tarsal plate, it is called an internal hordeolum, as the abscess is within the tarsal plate. This presents with diffuse lid swelling, erythema, tenderness and pointing toward the skin or conjunctival surface, since the orifices of these glands are located along the posterior eyelid border. When the glands of Zeis, which are small sebaceous glands attached directly to the hair follicles, become infected, the term external hordeolum or sty is used. This lesion is smaller and more superficial than an internal hordeolum. An external hordeolum presents as a well-defined, pinpoint, erythematous pustule on the lid margin that points toward the skin surface. Both forms of hordeolum generally respond to application of warm compresses and topical antibiotics. Systemic antibiotics or surgical drainage are generally not required.

Dermatoblepharitis results from either *S. aureus* or *S. pyogenes*, and is a form of impetigo that extends from the adjacent skin to the eyelid. A potential complication of *S. pyogenes* infection is necrotizing erysipelas of the eyelid [224]. When VZV or HSV affects the eyelids, it typically also involves the adjacent skin in a dermatoblepharitis. Varicella zoster virus presents with a painful, dermatomal eruption, usually involving all three branches (frontal, lacrimal and nasociliary) of the ophthalmic division of the trigeminal nerve, although involvement of an isolated branch may occur. Herpes simplex virus infection is usually accompanied by typical skin lesions, follicular conjunctivitis and pleomorphic epithelial keratitis, and may be associated with ipsilateral preauricular adenopathy.

Staphylococcus aureus is the most common pathogen in acute dacryocystitis, which is inflammation of the lacrimal sac [225]. Various streptococci, including *S. pyogenes*, are involved in some cases. Predisposing conditions include obstruction of the nasolacrimal duct (often due in neonates to an imperforate membrane at the distal end of the duct), nasal polyps or dacryolithiasis. It presents with pain, swelling and redness in the area of the tear sac along the nose, just inferior and medial to the medial canthus. Purulent material can be expressed by rubbing toward the lacrimal puncta. Culture of this material and antibiotic-susceptibility testing of the isolate may aid in antibiotic selection. Localized cellulitis, including orbital cellulitis, may ensue. Treatment should include warm compresses, lacrimal-sac massage to express purulent material, topical antibiotics and systemic (usually oral) penicillinase-resistant or β-lactamase-resistant antistaphylococcal antibiotics. If *S. pyogenes* alone is identified, penicillin is used. Dacryoadenitis is inflammation of the main lacrimal gland. Common bacterial causes of acute infection are *S. aureus* and *S. pyogenes*. Infection may develop from local inoculation, often following trauma, or in the course of bacteraemia. Dacryoadenitis presents with localized pain, erythema and swelling, often producing an S-shaped deformity of the lid margin. Occasionally, ocular mobility is restricted. Surrounding cellulitis may develop, and distinction from preseptal or orbital cellulitis must be made. Treatment includes systemic antibiotics and surgical drainage of the abscess cavity.

Abscesses

An abscess is a localized collection of pus in a cavity formed by disintegration or necrosis of tissue. It is recognized clinically by the presence of a firm, tender, erythematous nodule that becomes fluctuant. Constitutional symptoms in association with an abscess are generally absent, unless the process has extended into deeper tissues or the bloodstream. Histopathologically, a cutaneous abscess is covered by normal epidermis but the dermis contains a dense aggregate of acute inflammatory cells surrounded by a fibrinoid wall. Cutaneous and subcutaneous abscesses most commonly evolve by local extension of a primary infectious process in the epidermis and/or dermis, such as a cutaneous abscess originating from a skin appendage (e.g. furuncle, carbuncle, infundibular cyst, periporitis) or from a secondarily infected skin tumour or site of skin disease or injury. An abscess can also arise by direct traumatic implantation or invasion of pathogens into subcutaneous tissue or, occasionally, by haematogenous spread. Often no predisposing factor can be identified, although a number of processes that disrupt the integrity of the barrier function of the skin or the integrity of local immunological processes, particularly neutrophil function, are associated with abscess formation (see Table 2.9). Despite the extensive list of immunodeficiency diseases associated with abscess formation, most individuals with recurrent abscess formation (e.g. furunculosis) lack evidence of immunodeficiency.

Staphylococcus aureus is the single most common pathogen of cutaneous and subcutaneous abscesses [57]. It is particularly prevalent, frequently as the sole pathogen, in abscesses of the neck, trunk and extremities, although it can be found in all areas where abscesses originate on skin surfaces. For abscesses from which only one organism is isolated, *S. aureus* is responsible in the vast majority of cases [57, 86, 87]. The principal pathogens, however, vary with location of the lesion on the body. Most abscesses of the perineal region (inguinal, buttocks, perirectal, vulvovaginal) contain multiple anaerobic stool organisms, particularly *Bacteroides* spp., although occasionally anaerobes appear to be capable of acting alone to cause the abscess. In general, cultures from perineal or perioral abscesses and ulcers of both children and adults contain organisms that originated from adjacent mucous membranes rather than skin, whereas lesions remote from the rectum or mouth contain primarily organisms which reside normally on skin at that site [56, 58, 59, 86, 87, 226, 227].

Furuncle and carbuncle

Definition, epidemiology, aetiology

These follicular cutaneous abscesses may originate from a preceding folliculitis or arise initially as a nodular abscess. Sites of predilection are hair-bearing areas on the face, neck, axillae, buttocks and groin. The causative agent is almost always *S. aureus*, which has a predilection for binding to abraded perifollicular skin. Certain strains of *S. aureus*, such as phage type 80/81, appear to have particular propensity for causing furuncles. Conditions that predispose to furuncle formation include a warm, humid environment, obesity, hyperhidrosis, maceration, friction and pre-existing dermatitis. They are more common in males than in females. Furunculosis is also more common in individuals with low serum iron, diabetes mellitus, malnutrition, HIV infection or other immunodeficiency states, particularly those involving defects in neutrophil function. Most individuals with furunculosis, including recurrent disease, however, do not have an identifiable immune deficiency. Recurrent furunculosis is frequently associated with carriage of *S. aureus* in the nares, axillae or perineum, or sustained close contact with someone who is a carrier.

Clinical characteristics

A furuncle presents as a deep-seated, tender, erythematous, perifollicular papule, which evolves into a nodule. Influx of neutrophils, followed by vessel thrombosis, suppuration and central tissue necrosis, leads to rupture and discharge of a central core of necrotic tissue, destruction of the follicle and scarring. Surrounding cellulitis may develop. Pain may be intense if the lesion is situated in an area where the skin is relatively fixed, such as in the external auditory canal or over nasal cartilage. Patients with furuncles usually have no constitutional symptoms, although bacteraemia may occur, particularly in association with malnutrition or manipulation of the lesion [228]. Rarely, severe lesions on the upper lip or cheek may lead to cavernous sinus thrombosis [229].

A carbuncle is an infection of a group of contiguous follicles, with multiple drainage points and inflammatory changes in surrounding connective tissue. Carbuncles may be accompanied by fever, leucocytosis and bacteraemia.

Diagnosis

Other bacteria or fungi may occasionally cause furuncles or carbuncles; therefore, Gram stain and culture of the pus are indicated.

Treatment

Treatment includes frequent application of a hot, moist compress to facilitate drainage of lesions. Large lesions may require surgical drainage. Carbuncles and large or multiple furuncles, particularly those located on the central face, should be treated with oral penicillinase-resistant systemic antibiotics, such as cephalexin, dicloxacillin or cloxacillin. The penicillin-allergic patient can be treated with clindamycin or erythromycin, although emergence of erythromycin resistance among isolates of *S. aureus* has limited the utility of the latter agent. Successful treatment of recurrent cases has been achieved by colonization of the individual with a non-virulent strain of *S. aureus*, such as 502A, following a course of systemic therapy to eradicate the carrier state; however, this form of treatment is no longer in common practice [230].

The carriage state may be eliminated temporarily by application of mupirocin ointment for 5 days to the anterior nares. Attention to personal hygiene, use of an antibacterial soap and prophylactic low-dose oral anti-staphylococcal penicillin or clindamycin may also be beneficial.

Hidradenitis suppurativa. Hidradenitis suppurativa is a chronic, inflammatory, suppurative disorder of the apocrine glands. The disease is probably initiated by plugging of apocrine gland ducts with keratinous debris. Bacterial infection, particularly with *S. aureus, Streptococcus milleri, E. coli* and possibly anaerobic streptococci, appears to be important in the progressive dilatation below the obstruction. The underlying mechanism of hidradenitis suppurativa is controversial, but it appears to be an androgen-dependent condition [231]. Onset usually occurs during puberty or early adulthood. Solitary or multiple painful, erythematous nodules, deep abscesses and contracted scars are sharply confined to areas of skin containing apocrine glands in the axillae, anogenital region and, occasionally, the scalp, posterior aspect of the ears, female breasts and around the umbilicus. When the disease is severe and chronic, sinus tracts, ulcers and thick, linear fibrotic bands develop. Hidradenitis suppurativa tends to persist for many years, punctuated by relapses and partial remissions. Complications include cellulitis, ulceration or burrowing abscesses, which may perforate adjacent structures in the anogenital region, forming fistulas to the urethra, bladder, rectum or peritoneum. Episodic inflammatory arthritis develops in some patients. A minority of patients have the follicular occlusion triad, which includes acne conglobata and perifolliculitis capitis (dissecting cellulitis of the scalp); a tetrad with pilonidal sinus has also been described. Each of these conditions, which share similarities in pathogenesis, may also occur singly in a given patient. Early lesions are often mistaken for infected epidermal cysts, furuncles, scrofuloderma, actinomycosis, cat-scratch disease, granuloma inguinale or lymphogranuloma venereum. Sharp localization to areas of the body which bear apocrine glands, however, should suggest hidradenitis. When involvement is limited to the anogenital region, the condition may be difficult to distinguish from, and may coexist with, Crohn's disease. Patients should be counselled to avoid tight-fitting clothes, as occlusion may exacerbate the condition. The effectiveness of topical antibiotics is limited. Systemic antibiotics, chosen on the basis of bacterial culture and susceptibility tests, should be administered in the acute phase. Empirical therapy may be initiated with tetracycline, doxycycline or minocycline (provided the patient is older than 8 years); clindamycin or cephalosporins may also be effective. Some patients require long-term treatment with tetracycline or erythromycin. Intralesional triamcinolone acetonide (5–10 mg/ml) is often helpful in early disease. The addition of prednisone 40–60 mg/day for 7–10 days, tapering gradually as inflammation subsides, to the regimen of patients who respond poorly to antibiotics may decrease fibrosis and scarring. Ultimately, surgical measures may be required for control or cure.

Multiple sweat-gland abscesses (periporitis)

Definition, epidemiology, aetiology

Sweat-gland abscesses develop rarely in neonates, most often in association with malnutrition or debilitation, although healthy infants may also be affected [232]. Due to the almost uniform presence of *S. aureus* in the lesions, the infection has also been referred to as 'periporitis staphylogenes'. It appears that, in most cases, lesions of miliaria become infected secondarily, followed by extension into the sweat-gland apparatus and occasionally into the adjacent subcutaneous tissue. Miliaria-like lesions, however, are not a constant feature [232].

Clinical characteristics

The 2- to 20-mm dome-shaped, well-defined, nodular abscesses present most commonly on the neck, occiput, back, buttocks and thighs. Multiple lesions usually occur. Superficial vesicles and/or pustules (periporitis) are sometimes found before or in association with the nodules. Unlike furuncles and carbuncles of follicular origin, they are non-tender, non-pointing and cold. Constitutional signs are usually absent but may accompany numerous large abscesses. Lymphangitis or cellulitis occurs rarely. Healing generally occurs over several weeks without scarring.

Diagnosis

Gram stain of pus expressed from lesions generally reveals Gram-positive cocci in clusters, and cultures grow *S. aureus*. The condition can be differentiated from furunculosis by the absence of pointing, tenderness, local heat and relation to hair follicles.

Treatment

Therapy includes control of factors that predispose to miliaria, such as fever or skin occlusion; correction of malnutrition; local care of abscesses, including saline-solution compresses; and β-lactamase-stable antistaphylococcal antibiotics.

Paronychia

Definition, epidemiology, aetiology

Acute paronychia involves localized inflammation and infection of the nail fold, usually following local injury. The primary disorder is separation of the eponychium from the nail plate, followed by secondary invasion of the space by pathogens. It occurs most commonly in children who suck their fingers or in individuals who bite their nails, have poor hygiene or engage in activities that cause maceration and/or trauma to the nail fold. In the majority of cases, mixed oropharyngeal flora are found; *S. aureus* and *S. pyogenes* are the most common aerobic organisms, while anaerobic pathogens include *Bacteroides* spp., *Fusobacterium nucleatum* and Gram-positive cocci, particularly *Peptostreptococcus* spp. [233, 234]. Occasionally, Gram-negative organisms, such as *Pseudomonas* spp., *Proteus* spp. and *E. coli*, are involved. *Candida albicans* is implicated in chronic infection.

Clinical characteristics

The lateral nail fold becomes warm, erythematous, oedematous and painful. A purulent exudate may develop. Dermatitis often occurs around the affected area and may contribute to initiation and/or perpetuation of the problem.

Diagnosis

Acute paronychia can usually be diagnosed by clinical inspection. Both aerobic and anaerobic cultures of purulent material are recommended.

Herpes simplex virus infection may also occur in the paronychial area (i.e. herpetic whitlow). It is typically preceded by a prodrome of pain and presents with vesicles on an erythematous base. The lesion may become purulent or necrotic. Due to the thickness of the stratum corneum on the fingers, the vesicles may appear to be more deeply set than is generally observed with HSV infections. Occasionally, it may be necessary to perform a Tzanck smear, direct fluorescent-antibody test and/or culture to identify the virus.

Treatment

Attention must be directed toward eliminating or reducing predisposing factors of nail-fold maceration and trauma. Warm compresses are generally curative for superficial lesions. Drainage of the abscess may be facilitated by gently pushing the nail fold away from the nail plate. Antibiotics, in addition to incision and drainage, are needed for treatment of deeper lesions. Dicloxacillin, cloxacillin or cephalexin is the antibiotic of choice for treatment of infections caused by *S. aureus*, while amoxycillin plus clavulanic acid is preferred for empirical treatment, due to the emergence of β-lactamase-producing anaerobes [234]. Chronic paronychia sometimes precedes an episode of acute infection and may require management after the acute infection has been cleared.

Breast abscess

Definition, epidemiology, aetiology

Breast abscess is an uncommon infection of neonates, usually due to *S. aureus*. Infection is occasionally due to group B *Streptococcus, E. coli, Salmonella* spp., *P. mirabilis* or *P. aeruginosa*. Although anaerobic organisms can be isolated from up to 40% of infections, their pathogenic role in neonates is questionable and therapy directed specifically against them is unnecessary [235, 236].

Breast abscess develops in full-term neonates during the first 1–6 weeks of life, most commonly during the second to third weeks of life [235–239]. Incidence of breast abscess is approximately equal in males and females during the first 2 weeks of life, but thereafter the incidence in girls is approximately twice that of boys [237]. The fact that physiological breast enlargement is more common in infant girls than in boys after, but not before 2 weeks of age suggests that this may be a factor in the pathogenesis of breast abscess [237, 240]. Breast manipulation has also been suggested as a predisposing factor [237]. Infants with *S. aureus* breast abscess are also, as a rule, colonized with the same organism on nasal or pharyngeal mucous membranes [235]. It seems likely that *S. aureus* may spread from the nasopharynx to colonize the skin of the nipple, and may move from there up the ducts of the physiologically enlarged, predisposed breast in a retrograde fashion, perhaps facilitated by breast manipulation, to infect deeper tissues [235].

Clinical characteristics

Breast abscess presents initially with breast enlargement, accompanied by varying degrees of erythema, induration and tenderness. Progression to fluctuance may or may not occur, depending in part on how early antibiotic therapy is initiated. Bilateral infection occurs in less than 5% of cases [235]. Affected infants usually lack fever (present in approximately one-third) or constitutional symptoms, such as irritability or toxicity; leucocytosis (>15 000/mm³) is found in approximately half to two-thirds of patients [235]. Breast abscess due to *S. aureus* is accompanied by cutaneous pustules or bullae on the trunk, particularly in the perineal region, in 25–50% of patients [235, 237]. The symptoms, age of presentation and clinical findings of infants with breast abscess due to Gram-negative bacilli or those that harbour anaerobes are similar to those of infants infected with *S. aureus*, except that infants infected with *Salmonella* spp. generally also have gastrointestinal illness [235, 239]. The most common complication of breast abscess is cellulitis, which develops in approximately 5–10% of affected infants [235, 237]. Cellulitis is generally localized, but can extend rapidly to involve the shoulder and/or abdomen. Other complications, such as bacteraemia, pneumonia, osteomyelitis or sepsis, are unusual. Scar formation, leading to decreased breast size following puberty, can occur as a late complication [237].

Diagnosis

Gram stain of material expressed from the nipple or obtained by needle aspiration or incision and drainage can help to guide initial antibiotic therapy. The presence of cutaneous vesicles or bullae may help to identify the presence of *S. aureus*. Blood cultures should be obtained, but, unless the infant is febrile or ill-appearing, cultures of urine and cerebrospinal fluid are unnecessary.

Treatment

If fluctuance is present, the abscess must be drained surgically; antibiotic therapy is adjunctive. If fluctuance is absent, early antibiotic therapy alone may be curative and prevent abscess development. A β-lactamase-resistant antistaphylococcal antibiotic should be given parenterally. If Gram-negative bacilli are seen on Gram stain or the infant appears ill, initial therapy should include an aminoglycoside or cefotaxime. If no organisms are seen on Gram stain, antibiotics for control of both *S. aureus* and Gram-negative bacilli should be started while awaiting culture results. Once infection has begun to subside and constitutional signs are absent, therapy may be completed orally with cloxacillin, dicloxacillin or cephalexin if the infection was due to *S. aureus* alone. In most instances, a total of 5–7 days of therapy is sufficient, although many experts continue treatment for 10–14 days [235].

Perirectal abscess

Definition, epidemiology, aetiology

Perirectal abscess tends to occur in healthy neonates and infants, more often boys than girls. There may be no apparent predisposing factor, or the abscess may develop following minor abrasions or fissures, particularly in association with diarrhoea or constipation. Children who develop peri-rectal abscess, however, usually have a predisposing condition, such as: neutropenia in association with neoplastic disease, autoimmunity or chemotherapy administration; neutrophil dysfunction due to immunodefi-ciency disease, such as chronic granulomatous disease; acquired immune deficiency syndrome (AIDS); diabetes mellitus; corticosteroid therapy; ulcerative colitis or Crohn's disease; hidradenitis suppurativa; or rectal surgery. Initiation of perirectal abscess appears to involve a break in the mucosal barrier or occlusion of anal crypts; thus, in those with granulocy-topenia, the risk for development of an abscess or perirectal cellulitis increases with perirectal mucositis, haemorrhoids, rectal fissure or manipulation.

The organisms in perirectal abscesses are predominantly mixed anaero-bic and aerobic flora of the intestine and skin of the anal verge, including *S. aureus* and *S. pyogenes*, as well as *Bacteroides* spp., *Peptococcus* spp., *Peptostrep-tococcus* spp., *Porphyromonas* spp., *Fusobacterium* spp., *Clostridium* spp., *E. coli*, *P. aeruginosa*, *Klebsiella* spp. and *Proteus* spp. [241–245]. Perirectal abscess is rarely due to *Entamoeba histolytica*, *Mycobacterium* spp., *Nocardia* spp. and *Actinomyces* spp.

Clinical characteristics

Superficial abscess in the infant usually presents with signs of pain on defe-cation, sitting or walking and the presence of redness, swelling and tender-ness in the perianal region. Such abscesses can potentially extend in several directions: inferiorly along the anal sphincter to exit next to the anus on the buttock (fistula in ano); laterally through the external sphincter to the ischiorectal fossa to form a deep abscess; or superiorly to the deep space between the internal sphincter and the levator ani muscles [246–248]. An abscess in deeper tissues may be accompanied by poorly localized, deep pain and constitutional signs. An anorectal abscess may not be apparent externally, but pain is generally elicited upon rectal examination. Compli-cations, which occur more commonly in children with underlying disease, include anorectal fistula, abscess recurrence, bacteraemia and necrotizing fasciitis.

Treatment

In immunocompetent infants, a superficial perianal abscess can drain spontaneously and be self-limiting. Recommended management, however, includes prompt drainage and exploration of the abscess and fistulae and Sitz baths. Administration of antibiotics, such as clindamycin and an aminoglycoside to cover *S. aureus*, β-lactamase-resistant anaerobic bacteria and aerobic Gram-negative bacilli, may prevent regional spread of the infection and decrease the incidence of complications [242]. In the absence of fluctuance, extensive soft-tissue disease or evidence of sepsis, a trial of parenteral antimicrobial therapy may be initiated alone. A 7–10-day course of antibiotics is recommended. If fluctuance or progression of disease becomes apparent, surgery should be undertaken. Children with granulocytopenia may have absence or delayed development of erythema, induration and fluctuance. A chronic fistula may require a fistulotomy [247].

Scalp abscess

Definition, epidemiology, aetiology

Scalp abscess develops at the insertion site of a fetal-scalp monitoring electrode. The reported incidence of scalp abscess following placement of a spiral fetal-scalp electrode, the type used since the early 1970s, ranges from 0.1 to 1.0% in retrospective studies [249]. Prospective studies have reported the incidence to be 0.56% [250] and 4.5% [251].

Predisposing factors for abscess development have not been clearly identified. The most plausible hypothesis for the pathogenesis of scalp abscess is that the infection occurs through ascension of normal cervical flora into the uterus following rupture of membranes, aided by procedures which gain access to the uterine cavity. Placement of the electrode then serves to break the cutaneous barrier and provide a foreign-body nidus for infection in the subcutaneous tissue. Okada *et al.* [251] found significant risk factors to be longer duration of ruptured membranes; longer duration of monitoring; monitoring for high-risk indications, particularly prematurity; and nulliparous birth, possibly due to increased risk of infection of oedematous, hypoxic caput succedaneum. Plavidal and Werch [252] also found an association between prolonged rupture of membranes and development of scalp abscess, while Wagener *et al.* [250] reported that duration of ruptured membranes or duration of monitoring were not significant risk factors. Risk factors in their study included a number of vaginal examinations, concurrent monitoring with an intrauterine-pressure catheter, use of more than one spiral electrode, fetal-scalp blood sampling, maternal diabetes and endomyometritis. They speculated that procedures which serve to provide increased access of vaginal flora to the infant or more trauma to the scalp may increase the risk of abscess development. Scalp trauma and compression *per se*, however, are questionable factors in the pathogenesis of scalp abscess, as most authors have not noted abscess formation at sites of scalp trauma and abrasion due to forceps or vacuum extraction, at sites of fetal blood sampling or in association with haematomas [249–253]. Exceptions exist, however, as cephalohaematomas may become infected, and similar rates of scalp abscess have been reported among infants monitored with scalp electrodes and those who were not monitored but were delivered by forceps or vacuum extraction [254]. A threefold greater, but statistically insignificant, rate of scalp abscess has also been noted among infants delivered by vacuum extraction compared with spontaneous vaginal delivery [251].

Scalp abscess is typically a polymicrobial infection. Cultures from approximately one-third of abscesses reveal aerobic or facultative organisms alone, 10–25% grow anaerobes alone and 40–60% grow a mixture of aerobic, facultative and anaerobic bacteria [249, 251, 255]. The most common aerobic isolates are *S. aureus*, group A, B or D streptococci, *S. epidermidis* and, occasionally, *Haemophilus influenzae* type b, *E. coli*, *Klebsiella pneumoniae*, *Enterobacter* spp., *P. aeruginosa* and *Neisseria gonorrhoeae*. The role of *S. epidermidis* as a pathogen is questionable. Common anaerobic isolates are *Peptococcus* spp., *Peptostreptococcus* spp., *Bacteroides* spp., *Propionibacterium acnes* and *Clostridium* spp. The anaerobic flora in the abscesses reflects that found in the normal cervix during labour [256].

Clinical characteristics

Presentation occurs most commonly on the third or fourth day of life, but may be as early as the first day and as late as 3 weeks of life [249]. The lesion appears initially as a localized, erythematous area of induration 0.5 to approximately 2 cm in diameter. The site may become fluctuant or pustular. Regional lymphadenopathy may be present, but other more serious complications, such as cranial osteomyelitis, subgaleal abscess, necrotizing fasciitis of the scalp, bacteraemia and sepsis, are rare. Death associated with a complication of fetal-scalp electrode placement has been described in a premature infant who developed *E. coli* scalp abscess and septicaemia [257].

Diagnosis

Infants who are subjected to scalp-electrode monitoring *in utero* should be followed closely during the first weeks of life for evidence of infection. Parents should be instructed in surveillance and, if an abscess is noted, it is advisable to remove the hair directly around the lesion to allow for closer observation. Culture for both aerobic and anaerobic organisms can be obtained by needle aspiration or swabbing the exudate from the puncture site.

The primary differential diagnostic concern is HSV infection [249]. The time of appearance of these lesions (peak incidence 4–10 days) overlaps with that for scalp abscess, and they may be indistinguishable clinically. Dissemination may also occur [258]. Consequently, if suspicion of HSV exists, therapy with acyclovir should be initiated while awaiting diagnostic test results.

Treatment

Many lesions resolve spontaneously, but, if fluctuance develops without spontaneous suppuration, incision and drainage are necessary, although extensive débridement should not be performed. If surrounding cellulitis is present, a 5–7-day course of parenteral antibiotic therapy is usually sufficient, with culture results guiding antibiotic choice.

Suppurative sialadenitis (salivary-gland abscess)

Definition, epidemiology, aetiology

Acute suppurative sialadenitis occurs in neonates, particularly those born prematurely, and in children and adults with salivary stasis from ductal obstruction or decreased production of saliva [259]. Predisposing factors include calculi; stricture of a salivary duct; local trauma; a septic focus in the oral cavity, such as a dental infection; neoplasm of the oral cavity; dehydration; malnutrition; medications that diminish salivary flow, such as antihistamines, diuretics and tranquillizers; autoimmune disorders; or immunosuppression [260–262]. In adults, the most common cause is a previous surgical procedure [263]. Most cases involve the parotid gland, although obstruction due to stones occurs more commonly in Wharton's duct of the submandibular salivary gland than in Stensen's duct of the parotid gland [261].

   Staphylococcus aureus is the most common pathogen [264]. The infection is often polymicrobial, however, involving a variety of streptococci, including *S. pyogenes, Streptococcus viridans* and *Streptococcus pneumoniae*; enteric Gram-negative bacilli, such as *E. coli*; and anaerobes, particularly *Bacteroides* spp., *Peptostreptococcus* spp. and pigmented *Prevotella* spp. [260, 265]. Rarely, *H. influenzae, Bartonella henslae, Eikenella corrodens, Treponema pallidum, Actinomyces* spp., *Mycobacterium tuberculosis* and atypical mycobacteria cause salivary-gland suppuration [260, 265]. In neonates, *P. aeruginosa* and *Moraxella catarrhalis* have been identified [262].

   Some children have recurrent episodes of acute parotitis. Recurrence of parotid-gland infection is uncommon in neonates relative to children or adults, while recurrence of submaxillary sialadenitis is the rule [261, 262]. Alpha-haemolytic streptococci are most consistently identified during acute recurrences of infection [264]. Spontaneous resolution usually occurs around the time of puberty.

Clinical characteristics

The infection presents with acute, unilateral onset of erythema, tenderness and oedema of the soft tissue overlying the affected gland. Parotitis presents with swelling of the preauricular area, extending to the angle of the mandible. The papilla of Stensen's duct may be erythematous, oedematous and exuding pus. Constitutional signs of fever and chills and leucocytosis are usually present. Abscess formation is uncommon in the paediatric population; when it occurs, the submandibular gland is likely to be the affected gland [262]. Suppuration is seen most commonly in debilitated elderly patients. Complications include spread of infection to the face or external auditory canal; to the neck, causing respiratory obstruction; to local facial bones, causing temporomandibular-joint arthritis or mandibular osteomyelitis; or to the bloodstream. It may take several months for enlargement of the affected gland to resolve.

Diagnosis

Diagnosis and management can be aided by Gram stain and culture of exudate from the duct of the affected salivary gland. Massage of the gland may be necessary to express pus through the duct. Culture of material obtained from the duct may become contaminated with oral flora, however, making identification of anaerobes unreliable by this means [260]. Needle aspiration of a suppurative gland allows for recovery of the full range of pathogens, but suppuration is generally not present early in the course of the infection. In this instance, aspiration of sterile saline solution following its introduction into the gland may allow recovery of the pathogens.

The most common cause of parotid swelling in children is mumps caused by paramyxovirus. A number of other viral agents can also cause parotitis. Unlike bacterial infection, however, viral parotitis is not suppurative.

Treatment

Blood cultures should be obtained from all affected patients, and neonates should undergo a full sepsis work-up, including cultures of blood, urine and cerebrospinal fluid. Patients should be hospitalized and given intravenous fluids to maintain adequate hydration; salivary-gland massage to empty pus from the ducts; sialogogues, such as lemon juice or acid sweets, to increase flow of saliva; and parenteral antibiotic therapy. Until culture results are available, a penicillinase-resistant antistaphylococcal antibiotic, such as methicillin, nafcillin or oxacillin, is recommended empirically, particularly if *S. aureus* was the predominant organism seen on Gram stain of secretions expressed from the duct. Clindamycin may become necessary to cover anaerobes. If Gram-negative bacilli are present, ceftazadime or gentamicin should be included. When no organisms can be seen on Gram stain, empirical therapy with a combination of clindamycin and gentamicin is appropriate while awaiting culture results [266]. If no improvement is noted within 4–5 days, surgery should be considered to identify and drain an abscess. Out-patient therapy can be completed orally, using dicloxacillin, cloxacillin or cephalexin for *S. aureus* or clindamycin if anaerobes were present. Treatment of Gram-negative pathogens must be guided by susceptibility-test results. Infection of the submandibular gland is usually due to sialolithiasis and is subject to recurrence; consequently, surgical excision of the gland is the treatment of choice [261, 262].

Acute episodes of recurrent suppurative parotitis can be treated in most cases with oral penicillin. Gram stain and culture of ductal exudate may aid in identifying unusual pathogens. In between episodes, gentle probing of the duct may help to ensure its patency [262]. A search should be made for causes of obstruction. Occasionally, recurrent parotitis is unresponsive to antibiotics and is associated with altered glandular architecture on sialography. In this instance, total parotidectomy is the treatment of choice [262]. Nearly all cases, however, respond to conservative management.

Botryomycosis

Definition, epidemiology, aetiology

Cutaneous botryomycosis is an unusual, chronic, suppurative disease characterized by the presence of granules formed by clusters of bacteria within a suppurative focus. It is most commonly associated with *S. aureus* infection, but can also result from infection with other bacteria, including α-haemolytic streptococci, *P. aeruginosa*, *E. coli*, *Proteus* spp., *Bacillus* spp., *S. marcescens*, *Neisseria* spp., *P. acnes* and *Peptostreptococcus* spp. [267, 268]. Although most patients are otherwise healthy, predisposing conditions appear to include cutaneous trauma, presence of a foreign body, malnutrition, systemic corticosteroid therapy, diabetes mellitus, alcoholism, HIV infection and cell-mediated immunodeficiency [269–271]. Pathogenesis of this condition is unclear, but it is most widely regarded as a symbiotic balance between a pathogen of relatively low virulence and the tissue resistance of the host, which may be attenuated [268, 271, 272]. It presents in cutaneous and visceral forms.

Clinical characteristics

Cutaneous infection presents with firm, non-tender subcutaneous nodules, sometimes associated with purulent sinus tracts, or with verrucous plaques associated with purulent exudate. Occasionally, the exudate appears granular to the naked eye. Exposed surfaces, particularly on the extremities, are affected most commonly, although intertriginous and gluteal areas are also frequently involved [269, 271]. Most patients present with a solitary lesion but multiple lesions may occur. Occasionally, the infection extends to underlying muscle and bone [273, 274]. A patient with immunodeficiency due to HIV infection presented with papulonodular lesions resembling prurigo nodularis [270].

Diagnosis

Histopathological examination of biopsy specimens reveals either acute inflammation or mixed acute, chronic and granulomatous inflammation and central suppuration or microabscesses, which contain granules similar to those seen in actinomycosis and the mycetomas. The characteristic granules consist of clusters of swollen basophilic-staining bacterial cells, surrounded by an eosinophilic matrix. With use of special stains, the cocci of *S. aureus* can be distinguished from the filaments of *Actinomyces* [268]. Size of the granules varies from several micrometres up to 2 mm in diameter. The amorphous matrix of the granules contains immunoglobulin G (IgG) and is apparently produced by the host in response to bacterial antigens [270].

Treatment

The lesions of botryomycosis are indolent and are often refractory to antibacterial therapy. Antibacterial therapy must be tailored according to the susceptibility profile of the pathogen. The treatment of choice in refractory cases is often excision. Carbon dioxide (CO_2) laser therapy has also been shown to be effective [275, 276].

Secondary infection of cutaneous tumours

Epidermal inclusion cyst

Epidermal inclusion cyst (epidermoid or infundibular cyst) is a sharply circumscribed, dome-shaped, firm, freely movable, skin-coloured nodule, often with a central dimple or punctum, which is a plugged, dilated pore of a pilosebaceous follicle. A mass of layered keratinized material, which may have a cheesy consistency, fills the cavity. Epidermoid cysts form most frequently on the face, neck, chest or upper back and may periodically become inflamed and infected secondarily, particularly in association with acne vulgaris. The causative organism is most commonly *S. aureus*. The cyst wall may also rupture and induce an inflammatory reaction in the dermis. The wall of the cyst is derived from the follicular infundibulum and consists of stratified epithelium; a granular layer is present. A fluctuant, infected cyst should first be excised, drained and packed, and the patient should be placed on an antibiotic that covers against *S. aureus*. After inflammation subsides, the cyst should be removed.

Pilar cyst

Pilar cyst is clinically indistinguishable from an epidermal inclusion cyst. It presents as a smooth, firm, mobile nodule, predominantly on the scalp but occasionally on the face, neck or trunk. The cyst may become infected with *S. aureus*, inducing inflammation and occasionally suppuration and ulceration. The cyst wall is composed of epithelial cells with indistinct intercellular bridges. The peripheral cell layer of the wall shows a pallisade arrangement, which is not seen in an epidermoid cyst. There is no granular layer present, the cyst cavity contains homogeneous eosinophilic keratinous material, and foci of calcification are seen in one-quarter of cases. The propensity to develop pilar cysts is inherited in an autosomal dominant manner; more than one cyst generally develops. Multiple pilar and epidermoid cysts, desmoid tumours, fibromas, lipomas or osteomas may be associated with colonic polyposis or adenocarcinoma in Gardner's syndrome. Patients with an infected pilar cyst should be treated with antistaphylococcal, β-lactamase-stable oral antibiotics, such as dicloxacillin, cloxacillin or cephalexin. Once the inflammation has subsided, the cyst can be shelled out easily from the dermis.

Pilomatricoma

Pilomatricoma is a benign tumour which presents as a 3–30-mm, firm, solitary, deep dermal or subcutaneous tumour on the head, neck or upper extremities. The overlying epidermis is usually normal; the tumour may occasionally be located more superficially, however, imparting a blue-red coloration to the overlying skin. Pilomatricomas may enlarge rapidly due to infection and inflammation, or haemorrhage, and occasionally may perforate the epidermis. Histopathologically, irregularly shaped islands of epithelial cells are embedded in a cellular stroma. Two types of cells make up the islands: basophilic cells and shadow cells. Calcium deposits are found in 75% of tumours. Infected lesions can be treated in the same manner as for pilar cysts.

Subcutaneous tissue infections

The subcutaneous tissue compartment is continuous over the entire body and consists of loose connective tissue containing blood- and lymphatic vessels and fat. The fascia is subdivided into superficial and deep components. The superficial fascia, located between the dermis and the deep fascia, is further subdivided into two layers. The outer layer, of variable thickness, contains loose collagenous tissue and fat. The inner layer of the superficial fascia is a thin membrane that has relatively little fat but is rich in elastic tissue. Superficial arteries, veins, nerves and lymphatics lie within the superficial fascia. The deep fascia is a membranous sheet surrounding and separating muscles into functioning units and forming the deepest boundary of the subcutaneous tissue compartment.

The most basic determination to be made when confronted with a soft-tissue infection is whether it is non-necrotizing or necrotizing; the former responds to antibiotic therapy alone, while the latter requires prompt surgical removal of all devitalized tissue in addition to antimicrobial therapy. Necrotizing soft-tissue infections are potentially life-threatening conditions, characterized by rapidly advancing, local tissue destruction and systemic toxicity. Tissue necrosis distinguishes them from cellulitis, in which an inflammatory infectious process involves, but does not destroy, subcutaneous tissue. Unlike an abscess, necrotizing soft-tissue infections involve relatively diffuse tissue necrosis and lack localized purulence.

Non-necrotizing subcutaneous infections

Cellulitis

Definition, epidemiology, aetiology

Cellulitis is characterized by infection and inflammation of loose connective tissue, with limited involvment of the dermis and relative sparing of the epidermis. A break in the skin due to previous trauma, surgery or an underlying skin lesion predisposes to cellulitis. Cellulitis is also more common in individuals with lymphatic stasis, diabetes mellitus or immunosuppression.

Streptococcus pyogenes and *S. aureus* are the most common aetiological agents. Occasionally, *S. pneumoniae*, group G or C streptococci and, in neonates, group B streptococci or rarely *E. coli* are the causal organism. In patients who are immunocompromised or have diabetes mellitus, a number of other bacterial or fungal agents may be involved, notably *P. aeruginosa*; *A. hydrophila* and occasionally other Enterobacteriaceae; *Legionella* spp.; the Mucorales, particularly *Rhizopus* spp., *Mucor* spp. and *Absidia* spp.; and *Cryptococcus neoformans*. Children with relapsed nephrotic syndrome may develop cellulitis due to *E. coli* [277]. In children aged 3 months to 3–5 years, *H. influenzae* type b has been an important cause of facial cellulitis, but its incidence has declined significantly since institution of immunization against this organism [278].

Clinical characterisitics

Cellulitis presents clinically as an area of oedema, warmth, erythema and tenderness. The lateral margins tend to be indistinct because the process is deep in the skin. Application of pressure may produce pitting. Although distinction cannot be made with certainty in any particular patient, cellulitis due to *S. aureus* tends to be more localized and may suppurate, while infections due to *S. pyogenes* tend to spread more rapidly and may be associated with lymphangitis. Regional adenopathy and constitutional signs and symptoms of fever, chills and malaise are common. Complications of cellulitis include subcutaneous abscess, osteomyelitis, septic arthritis, thrombophlebitis, bacteraemia and necrotizing fasciitis. Lymphangitis or glomerulonephritis can also follow infection with *S. pyogenes*.

Cellulitis due to *H. influenzae* type b generally develops rapidly, is often accompanied by bacteraemia, tends to have a bluish-red coloration, lacks an apparent portal of entry and, when located on the cheek (i.e. facial cellulitis), is often associated with ipsilateral otitis media and occasionally meningitis. Cellulitis due to *S. pneumoniae* may closely resemble that due to *H. influenzae* type b [279, 280]. Facial cellulitis associated with a portal of entry, such as a tooth abscess or cutaneous trauma, is generally due, respectively, to mouth anaerobes or to either *S. pyogenes* or *S. aureus* [281].

Periorbital or preseptal cellulitis. Periorbital (i.e. preseptal) cellulitis develops anterior (i.e. superficial) to an intact orbital septum. The orbital septum is composed of fascia that extends from the periostium of the bones which form the orbit to the margins of the upper and lower eyelids. When the infection is associated with trauma to the periorbital skin or extension of infection from adjacent skin (e.g. dermatoblepharitis) or eyelid structures (e.g. hordeolum, dacryocystitis, dacryoadenitis), the most common pathogens are *S. aureus* or *S. pyogenes*. Additional potential agents include *H. influenzae* type b or *S. pneumoniae*, particularly in infants and young children less than 5 years of age. These latter agents generally cause the infection following bacteraemic spread. Periorbital cellulitis presents with erythema and swelling of the eyelid. Systemic signs of toxicity are variable in degree. Rapidly progressive, non-suppurative cellulitis of the eyelid, which may progress to eyelid gangrene, can be caused by *S. pyogenes* [224]. Extension to the orbit may occur, presumably due to secondary inflammation. Preseptal cellulitis due to *H. influenzae* type b may have a bluish-purple hue.

Orbital cellulitis. Cellulitis that extends to involve structures behind (i.e. posterior to) the septum in the orbital space is called orbital cellulitis. It is usually associated with sinusitis or direct penetrating trauma to the orbital septum. *Staphylococcus aureus* is the most common cause, particularly following trauma. *Streptococcus pyogenes*, nontypeable *H. influenzae* and *S. pneumoniae* may cause the disease in association with contiguous infection of the sinuses or oral cavity. Orbital cellulitis presents with eyelid erythema and oedema, conjunctival hyperaemia, chemosis, proptosis, decreased and painful extraocular movements, decreased visual acuity, fever and constitutional signs. As the infection progresses, an abscess of the orbital tissue and subperiosteum develops [282]. Computed tomography is necessary to define the extent of infection. Nausea and vomiting may herald the development of cavernous sinus thrombosis.

Saphenous-vein cellulitis. Saphenous-vein cellulitis may occur in individuals who have had the vein removed for use in coronary-artery bypass surgery [283]. Non-group A β-haemolytic streptococci (groups B, C, F) have been implicated, but the causal organisms have not been identified in most cases. Marked oedema, erythema and tenderness are present along the venectomy path, sometimes mimicking erysipelas or acute thrombophlebitis. Lymphangitis is occasionally present, and fever, chills and toxicity are common. Most patients have had an associated tinea pedis, which may provide a portal of entry.

Diagnosis

Aspirates from the leading edge of inflammation, skin biopsy and blood cultures collectively allow identification of the causal organism in approximately 25% of cases of cellulitis [284]. Yield of the causative organism is approximately one-third when the site of origin of the cellulitis is apparent, such as an abrasion or ulcer. An aspirate taken from the point of maximum inflammation yields the causal organism more often than does a leading-edge aspirate [285]. Lack of success in isolating an organism stems primarily from the low number of organisms present within the lesion.

Treatment

Empirical therapy for cellulitis should be directed by the history. The location and character of the cellulitis and the age and immune status of the patient. Cellulitis in the neonate should prompt a full sepsis work-up, followed by initiation of empirical therapy intravenously with a β-lactamase-stable antistaphylococcal antibiotic, such as methicillin, and an aminoglycoside, such as gentamicin, or a cephalosporin, such as cefotaxime. Treatment of cellulitis in the infant or child younger than about 5 years of age should provide coverage for *S. pyogenes* and *S. aureus* as well as *H. influenzae* type b and *S. pneumoniae*. The work-up should include a blood culture and, if the infant is younger than 1 year of age, signs of systemic toxicity are present or an adequate examination cannot be obtained, a lumbar puncture should also be performed. In most cases of cellulitis on an extremity, regardless of age, *S. aureus* and *S. pyogenes* are the cause and bacteraemia is unlikely. Nevertheless, blood cultures should be obtained. If fever, lymphadenopathy and other constitutional signs are absent (e.g. white blood cell count <15 000), treatment of cellulitis on an extremity may be initiated orally on an out-patient basis with a penicillinase-resistant penicillin, such as dicloxacillin or cloxacillin, or a first-generation cephalosporin, such as cephalexin. If improvement is not noted or the disease progresses significantly within the first 24–48 hours of therapy, parenteral therapy becomes necessary. If fever, lymphadenopathy and/or constitutional signs are present, therapy should be initiated parenterally. Penicillinase-resistant penicillin such as oxacillin or nafcillin is effective in most cases. Once the erythema, warmth, oedema and fever have decreased significantly, a 10-day course of treatment may be completed on an out-patient basis. Immobilization and elevation of an affected limb, particularly early in the course of therapy, may help to reduce swelling and pain.

Children younger than 1 year of age who develop facial or periorbital cellulitis should receive antibiotics intravenously, regardless of the severity of the infection. A lumbar puncture should be included to rule out meningitis. Therapy to cover *S. aureus* and *S. pyogenes* as well as *H. influenzae* type b and *S. pneumoniae* can be initiated with a third-generation cephalosporin, such as ceftriaxone or cefotaxime; the second-generation agent cefuroxime, provided that meningitis has been ruled out; or nafcillin and chloramphenicol. Individuals older than 1 year of age with mild localized signs of infection and a lack of all signs of systemic disease can be considered for out-patient management with an agent such as amoxycillin/clavulanate or possibly cefuroxime axetil. If a purulent wound was present adjacent to the inflamed eyelid, an antistaphylococcal agent, such as dicloxacillin, cephalexin or clindamycin, should suffice. In most cases, however, therapy in patients with facial or periorbital cellulitis should be initiated parenterally. If an adequate response is achieved within 2–5 days of parenteral therapy, a 7–10-day course of therapy can be completed with an oral agent. Culture and antibiotic-susceptibility results, when available, should be used to guide the choice of oral antibiotic.

Orbital cellulitis is a medical emergency. If the response to parenteral antibiotic therapy is not prompt or signs of optic-nerve compression, such as decreased vision or colour perception, are present, surgical decompression of the orbital space and infected sinuses must be undertaken. Cultures for both aerobic and anaerobic organisms should be obtained and the results used to guide antibiotic therapy. A penicillinase-resistant penicillin or clindamycin, plus ceftriaxone or cefotaxime, will provide adequate empirical coverage, as will vancomycin plus chloramphenicol in the penicillin-allergic patient. It is recommended that intravenous antibiotic therapy continue for at least 5 days following abscess drainage and for a total of 14–21 days.

Erysipelas

Definition, epidemiology, aetiology

Erysipelas is a superficial form of cellulitis, involving the dermis and upper subcutaneous tissue, with prominent lymphatic involvement. It occurs sporadically, and usually begins at a break in the skin. Common portals of entry include leg ulcers; sites of local trauma; dermatoses, particularly intertrigo or tinea pedis; insect bites; and heel fissures [290]. In neonates, infection may originate in the umbilical stump and spread to the abdominal wall, or on the external genitalia at an infected circumcision site. Predisposing host factors include a history of venous or lymphatic obstruction, nephrotic syndrome and diabetes mellitus. Approximately one-third of patients have a history of preceding upper respiratory-tract infection, presumably viral in origin. At the time that erysipelas develops, throat swabs are generally negative for *S. pyogenes*. The most common site of erysipelas is the lower extremities; in the past, the face was the favoured site [286, 287].

The bacteriological cause of erysipelas is *S. pyogenes* in the majority of cases. Group G as well as group B, C or D streptococci are involved occasionally, particularly in hosts who have been compromised by surgery or other illness. *Staphylococcus aureus, S. pneumoniae, K. pneumoniae, Yersinia enterocolitica* and *H. influenzae* type b are rarely implicated.

Clinical characteristics

Onset of erysipelas is abrupt, with fever, chills and malaise, followed within a day or two by cutaneous signs. A small area of burning and redness develops into a warm, shiny, bright red, confluent, indurated, tender plaque with a brawny, *peau d'orange* appearance and elevated, sharply demarcated margins, particularly on the face (Fig. 2.12). Vesicles, haemorrhagic bullae, petechiae and ecchymoses may develop in the plaque, and regional adenopathy may be present. Complications include bacteraemia (5%), abscess, gangrene, thrombophlebitis and glomerulonephritis. Fine desquamation and sometimes residual pigmentation accompany resolution of the plaque.

Diagnosis

Diagnosis of erysipelas is made primarily on clinical grounds. Skin culture from the portal of entry may be helpful in identifying the causal organism [287]. Latex-particle agglutination tests for streptococcal antigens in skin-

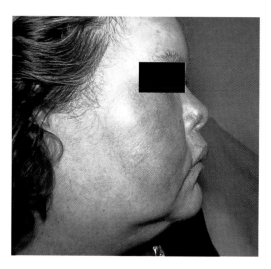

Fig. 2.12 Erysipelas. Well-defined, erythematous plaque due to *Streptococcus pyogenes*.

biopsy specimens can be more sensitive than skin culture [288]. Injecting sterile saline into the advancing edge of the plaque, followed by culture of aspirated fluid, is usually futile due to the low number of organisms present. Serological tests for ASO and anti-DNase B titres can be conclusive in approximately 40% of cases, but are only helpful in retrospect [289]. Skin biopsy shows oedema and vascular dilatation in the dermis and upper subcutis; occasionally, organisms can be seen within lymphatic vessels, particularly early in the course of infection. Neutrophils are often seen infiltrating the tissues and lymphatic channels.

Treatment

Prompt institution of parenteral penicillin is the mainstay of treatment. In most cases, parenteral penicillin for 10 days is effective. A switch can be made in immunocompetent hosts to oral antibiotics after a clinical response is noted, of within 1–2 days. In more indolent cases, oral therapy alone may be sufficient. Local wound care and attention to predisposing factors are also important. If the presence of staphylococci is a concern, a β-lactamase-resistant antibiotic should be used. Patients with recurrent disease may need to remain on prophylactic therapy for prolonged periods with penicillin, erythromycin or an alternative antistreptococcal drug [286]. Use of support stockings and maintenance of good skin hygiene may also aid in the prevention of recurrences.

Lymphangitis

Definition, epidemiology, aetiology

Lymphatic vessels in the skin begin as a blind loop in the subpapillary dermis and the dermal papillae. They comprise a rich network of vessels throughout the dermis and subcutaneous tissues, forming a superficial plexus below the subpapillary venous plexus and a deeper collecting system at the junction of the reticular dermis and the subcutis, which, in turn, drains into larger subcutaneous channels. In the extremities, the lymphatics that run superficial to the deep fascia connect with the deeper subfascial lymphatics, primarily at the antecubital, axillary, popliteal and inguinal lymph nodes.

Lymphangitis occurs when a local skin infection is not fully contained and spreads to cause inflammation in the walls and soft tissue surrounding dilated lymphatic vessels. Primary predisposing factors are local trauma to skin on an extremity with lymphatic stasis due to malfunction of the lymphatic vessels. The aetiology of lymphatic dysfunction includes congenital malformation, trauma or surgery, previous infection, chronic inflammation, associated venous disease and tumour infiltration.

Acute inflammation of lymphatic channels is usually due to infection with *S. pyogenes. Staphylococcus aureus* and groups B and D streptococci cause lymphangitis on occasion. Other rare infectious agents of acute lymphangitis include *Pasteurella multocida* and *Spirillium minus* (rat-bite fever). Following the bite of a mosquito in an area endemic for filariasis, such as Africa, South-East Asia and South America, acute lymphangitis and/or lymphadenitis may be caused by *Wuchereria bancrofti* or *Brugia malayi*.

Clinical characteristics

Acute lymphangitis presents most commonly on an extremity with an erythematous, tender, linear streak measuring millimetres to a few centimetres in width (Fig. 2.13). The streak extends proximally from the portal of entry, which may or may not be visible as a site of local infection. Typical infectious sites of origin include impetigo, ecthyma, cellulitis and paronychia. The regional lymph nodes are enlarged and tender, and the distal extremity may become oedematous. Systemic manifestations of infection, including fever, chills, malaise and headache, tend to develop quickly and are often out of proportion to the degree of local signs. Leucocytosis is often present, and bacteraemia may ensue. Following infection, some individuals develop chronic distal-extremity lymphoedema, which worsens with subsequent infections and progressive lymphatic fibrosis. Ultimately, the epidermis may become hyperkeratotic, warty and studded with vesicles and bullae containing lymphatic fluid. Lymphangitis originating at the interdigital web of the thumb can present particular problems, as the lymphatic drainage from this site may bypass the epitrochlear and axillary nodes and enter the subpectoral nodes. Complications can include subpectoral abscess, chest-wall cellulitis and pleural effusion [290].

Diagnosis

Gram stain and culture of the initial skin lesion or culture of the blood may reveal the causative organism. Thrombophlebitis on the leg may also

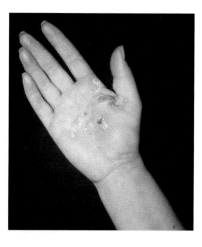

Fig. 2.13 Lymphangitis. Erythematous streak of lymphangitis on the volar forearm emanating from plaques of impetigo on the palm.

present with a tender, swollen, red streak, but tender lymphadenopathy and a focal, distal skin infection are absent. Nodular lymphangitis, due most commonly to *Sporothrix schenckii* or *Mycobacterium marinum*, is generally not associated with significant tenderness, regional lymphadenopathy or systemic signs of illness.

Treatment

The affected limb should be elevated and a search made for the portal of entry of the causative organism. In some instances, a treatable process, such as tinea pedis, may create the minor breaks in the skin.

Penicillin is the empirical treatment of choice for lymphangitis, although suspicion of infection due to *S. aureus* should prompt use of a penicillinase-resistant antistaphylococcal penicillin. Patients with systemic signs of illness should be hospitalized and treated parenterally. Occasionally, early, mild disease can be managed initially with procaine penicillin G, followed by oral penicillin V. As in the management of erysipelas, patients with recurrent disease and predisposing factors, such as chronic lymphoedema, may need to remain on prophylactic therapy for prolonged periods with penicillin, erythromycin or an alternative antistreptococcal drug [286]. In those with recurrent disease, attention should be given to conservative measures, such as exercise, local skin care and pressure-gradient bandages or hosiery.

Necrotizing subcutaneous infections

Necrotizing soft-tissue infections form a continuum of diseases, some of which develop primarily in the more superficial layer(s) of the subcutaneous tissues, while others typically extend to the deep fascia and muscle. Although the rapidity and extent of tissue destruction and the aetiological agent(s) vary, they characteristically present with a paucity of early cutaneous signs relative to the rapidity and degree of destruction of the subcutaneous tissues. Early clinical findings include ill-defined cutaneous erythema and oedema that extends beyond the area of erythema. In distinction from cellulitis, pain, tenderness and constitutional signs tend to be out of proportion to the cutaneous findings. This is particularly true with involvement of the fascia and muscle. In general, patients with involvement of the superficial or deep fascia and muscle tend to be more acutely and systemically ill and have more rapidly advancing disease than those with infection confined solely to subcutaneous tissues above the fascia. Cutaneous signs, such as vesiculation or bulla formation, ecchymoses, crepitus, anaesthesia or necrosis, are ominous and indicative of advanced disease [78].

Classification of necrotizing soft-tissue infections has undergone multiple revisions over the years, resulting in a multitude of confusing names in the literature, often with more than one name for the same condition.

Adding to the confusion is the fact that different organisms may produce similar clinical manifestations, and the same organism may be capable of causing a variety of clinical signs in different hosts or in the same host over time (e.g. streptococcal cellulitis, necrotizing fasciitis, myositis). Current classification schemes for necrotizing soft-tissue infections focus on the depth of soft-tissue destruction and the aetiological agent(s) [291]. Anaerobic cellulitis, bacterial synergistic gangrene and Meleney's ulcer involve primarily subcutaneous tissues, sparing fascia and muscle. When infection involves the deep layer of superficial fascia but largely spares adjacent skin, deep fascia and muscle, it is termed necrotizing fasciitis. Synergistic necrotizing cellulitis is clinically indistinguishable from necrotizing fasciitis in most cases, but frequently extends to involve the deep fascia and muscle. This section describes staphylococcal and streptococcal infections that lead to inflammation and/or destruction of subcutaneous tissues as deep as the inner layer of the superficial fascia. Conditions with principal involvement of muscle, such as myositis and pyomyositis, are not considered.

Tertiary or haematogenous infections of the subcutaneous tissues occur most commonly in immunocompromised hosts, and may lead to an abscess or necrotizing soft-tissue infection. Although a wide range of organisms, including bacteria and fungi, can be involved, the most common are *S. aureus* or *P. aeruginosa*.

Anaerobic cellulitis

Definition, epidemiology, aetiology

Anaerobic cellulitis primarily involves subcutaneous tissue, sparing fascia and muscle. It develops in devitalized subcutaneous tissues following spread of a local primary infection or introduction of the pathogen(s) into subcutaneous tissue by trauma or during surgery. The infection is most prevalent on areas of the body subject to faecal soiling, such as the perineum, abdominal wall, buttocks and lower extremities. Rarely, it occurs as a tertiary infection following bacteraemia with *Clostridium septicum* in an immunocompromised patient with a solid tumour or haematological malignancy and neutropenia [292]. In this setting, however, progression to myonecrosis usually occurs rapidly.

The condition is indistinguishable whether it is caused by a mixture of non-clostridial pathogens or by *Clostridium* spp., usually *C. perfringens*, acting alone. Non-clostridial anaerobic cellulitis is due to a variety of facultative streptococci and staphylococci and facultative or aerobic Gram-negative bacilli, such as *E. coli*, *K. pneumoniae* or *Aeromonas* spp., generally acting synergistically with anaerobes, such as *Bacteroides* spp., *Peptostreptococcus* spp. or *Peptococcus* spp.

Clinical characteristics

Onset of anaerobic cellulitis follows an incubation period of several days, with development of localized, ill-defined erythema, oedema and tenderness. Once established, destruction of subcutaneous tissue can spread rapidly, but the usual course is indolent relative to clostridial myonecrosis, with little tissue oedema, necrosis or pain and few constitutional symptoms. Generally, there is minimal cutaneous discoloration, even late in the infection. In contrast, as clostridial myonecrosis advances, the skin becomes bronze-coloured, with dark-coloured bullae and patches of necrosis. Gas formation, with tissue crepitus, is extensive in anaerobic cellulitis, however, extending well beyond that expected based on the clinical appearance of the skin and beyond that seen with myonecrosis. The gas in tissue is usually visible on radiographs. A thin, dark, foul-smelling exudate may drain from the wound.

Diagnosis

Gram-stained smears of tissue or exudate demonstrating the blunt-ended, thick, Gram-positive bacilli of *C. perfringens* may help to distinguish clostridial infection. The inflammatory infiltrate is often more substantial with non-clostridial anaerobic cellulitis, particularly early in the course of the disease, as tissue damage with *Clostridium* spp. infection appears to be due in large part to histotoxic exotoxins. Identification of *Clostridium* bacilli in a patient without acute, severe illness is reassuring that myonecrosis is not involved. Surgical exploration is necessary, however, to definitively distinguish anaerobic cellulitis from clostridial myonecrosis; muscle appears pink in anaerobic cellulitis but not in myonecrosis. Other facultative organisms may be present in association with *Clostridium*, so definitive identification of the pathogen(s) involved should await culture of aspirates or tissue specimens obtained during surgery.

Treatment

At the time of surgery, all areas of necrotic tissue must be exposed and débrided, but fascia and muscle may be spared. Broad-spectrum antibiotics must be initiated that will control all possible pathogens. Recommended initial antibiotic therapy includes intravenous ampicillin, clindamycin or metronidazole, and an aminoglycoside. Some favour use of ampicillin and chloramphenicol or ampicillin-sulbactam. Final antibiotic selection can be tailored according to results of cultures and antibiotic-susceptibility testing.

Bacterial synergistic gangrene

Definition, epidemiology, aetiology

This rare, chronic gangrenous infection of the skin and subcutaneous tissue presents almost uniformly on the trunk following abdominal surgery. The most common sites are at the exit of a fistulous tract, particularly following appendectomy or drainage of empyema, or in association with an ileostomy or colostomy [293]. Occasionally it develops in close proximity to chronic ulceration on an extremity. A related lesion, chronic undermining ulcer of Meleney, occurs most commonly following lymph-node surgery in the neck, axillae or groin, or occasionally after colonic or gynaecological surgery.

Bacterial synergistic gangrene is thought to be due to microaerophilic or anaerobic streptococci, in combination with *S. aureus* or occasionally *Proteus* spp. or other Gram-negative bacilli [294]. In classic animal experiments reported in the 1920s, Brewer and Meleney [88] reproduced the clinical lesions by injecting a combination of microaerophilic non-haemolytic streptococci and *S. aureus* into the skin, and proposed that the infection was due to synergism between these organisms. Other investigators have demonstrated that *Proteus* could be substituted for *S. aureus* [295] and that identical lesions, on both a clinical and a histopathological basis, can be caused by cutaneous amoebiasis due to *E. histolytica* [293]; in steroid-dependent patients, atypical mycobacteria, particularly *Mycobacterium kansasii* and *Mycobacterium chelonei*, can cause an identical clinical syndrome [296].

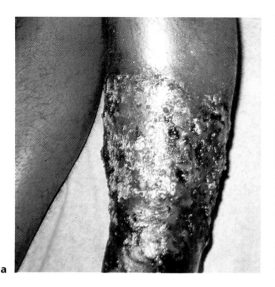 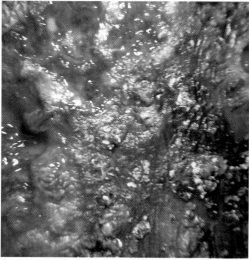

a

b

Fig. 2.14 Bacterial synergistic gangrene. (a) Thickly crusted, gangrenous ulceration on the forearm. (b) Red, exudative granulation tissue forms the base of the ulcer.

Clinical characteristics

Bacterial synergistic gangrene begins with localized tenderness, erythema and oedema, followed by severe pain and slow but inexorable gangrenous ulceration. The ulcer characteristically has a base of red granulation tissue, with grey to yellow exudate and a sharply demarcated gangrenous serpiginous border (Fig. 2.14a,b). Surrounding the ulcer is a raised dusky to purple margin and a peripheral ring of erythema and oedema. Meleney's ulcer is characterized by burrowing necrotic sinus tracts, which emerge at distant sites to form additional ulcers. Systemic signs are minimal in both conditions. Without treatment, these lesions have little to no tendency to heal and ultimately destroy large areas of skin and subcutaneous tissue.

Treatment

Although antimicrobial therapy alone has been curative in some cases, both wide surgical débridement of all necrotic tissue, extending into normal tissue, and antibiotic therapy (e.g. penicillin or clindamycin and gentamicin) are recommended [294]. Treatment, however, should be based on culture and susceptibility testing of organisms recovered from surgical material.

Necrotizing fasciitis

Definition, epidemiology, aetiology

Necrotizing fasciitis is a subcutaneous tissue infection that involves the deep layer of superficial fascia but largely spares adjacent epidermis, deep fascia and muscle. Relatively few organisms possess sufficient virulence to cause necrotizing fasciitis when acting alone. The most fulminant infections, associated with toxic-shock syndrome (TSS) and a high case-fatality rate, are caused by *S. pyogenes* [89, 297]. When due to *S. pyogenes*, the disease has been termed type II necrotizing fasciitis [90]. Streptococcal necrotizing fasciitis in the absence of TSS may occur and is seldom fatal, but may be associated with substantial morbidity. A subacute form of streptococcal necrotizing fasciitis, with slowly advancing tissue necrosis and eschar formation and a lesser degree of blood-vessel thrombosis in histopathological sections, has also been described [82]. Necrotizing fasciitis can occasionally be caused by *S. aureus*, *C. perfringens*, *C. septicum*, *P. aeruginosa*, *Vibrio* spp., particularly *Vibrio vulnificus*, and fungi of the order Mucorales, particularly *Rhizopus* spp., *Mucor* spp. and *Absidia* spp. [89, 298–302]. Necrotizing fasciitis has also been reported to occur on rare occasions due to non-group A streptococci, such as group B, C, F or G streptococci, *S. pneumoniae* or *H. influenzae* type b. Necrotizing fasciitis may be a polymicrobial infection. In this instance, it is termed type I disease [90]. In most of these cases, a mixture of anaerobic bacteria and aerobic and/or facultative bacteria appear to act together to cause tissue necrosis [90]. The most common aerobic or facultative bacteria are several species of haemolytic or non-haemolytic non-group A streptococci, *S. aureus*, *E. coli*, *Enterobacter* spp. and a variety of other Enterobacteriaceae and *Pseudomonas* spp. The anaerobes present are similar to those found in subcutaneous abscesses: *Bacteroides* spp., *Peptostreptococcus* spp., *Peptococcus* spp., *Prevotella* spp., *Porphyromonas* spp., *Clostridium* spp. and *Fusobacterium* spp. [90, 91]. Infections due to any one organism or combination of organisms cannot be distinguished clinically from one another, although development of crepitus signals the presence of *Clostridium* spp. or Gram-negative bacilli, such as *E. coli*, *Klebsiella*, *Proteus* and *Aeromonas*.

Necrotizing fasciitis may occur anywhere on the body; the most common locations, however, are the extremities, abdomen and perineal region. Common predisposing conditions in neonates are omphalitis and balanitis after circumcision [303, 304]. The incidence of necrotizing fasciitis is highest in hosts with systemic or local tissue immunocompromise, such as those with diabetes mellitus, neoplasia, peripheral vascular disease, recent surgery or intravenous drug abuse or on immunosuppressive treatment, particularly corticosteroids. The infection can also occur in healthy individuals following minor puncture wounds, abrasions or lacerations; blunt trauma; surgical procedures, particularly of the abdomen, gastrointestinal or genitourinary tracts or the perineum; or hypodermic-needle injection. Since the mid-1980s, there has been a resurgence of fulminant necrotizing soft-tissue infections due to *S. pyogenes*, which may occur in previously healthy individuals with little or no apparent compromise of immunological or skin integrity [89]. Recent cases in children have highlighted the occurrence of necrotizing fasciitis due to *S. pyogenes* following superinfection of varicella lesions [305–308]. Children with varicella and invasive *S. pyogenes* infection have tended to display onset, recrudescence or persistence of high fever and signs of toxicity after the third to fourth day of varicella [305, 309].

Clinical characteristics

Necrotizing fasciitis begins with acute onset of local swelling, erythema, tenderness and heat (Fig. 2.15). Fever is usually present, and pain is out of proportion to cutaneous signs [305–307]. Lymphangitis and lymphadenitis are usually absent. The infection advances along the superficial fascial plane, and initially there are few cutaneous signs to herald the serious nature and extent of subcutaneous tissue necrosis that is occurring. Skin changes may appear over 24–48 hours, as nutrient vessels are thrombosed and cutaneous ischaemia develops. Cutaneous signs include formation of bullae, filled initially with straw-coloured and later bluish to haemorrhagic fluid, and darkening of affected tissues from red to purple to blue. Skin anaesthesia and finally frank tissue gangrene and slough develop, due to the ischaemia and necrosis. Children with varicella lesions may initially

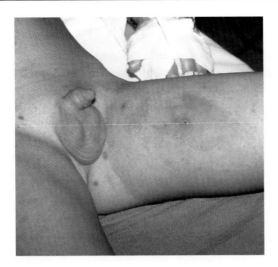

Fig. 2.15 Necrotizing fasciitis. Acute onset of swelling, erythema and exquisite tenderness heralds development of necrotizing fasciitis of the thigh due to *Streptococcus pyogenes*. A chickenpox lesion provided the portal of entry for the bacteria.

show no cutaneous signs of superinfection with invasive *S. pyogenes*, such as erythema or swelling [305]. Significant systemic toxicity may accompany necrotizing fasciitis, including shock, organ failure and death. Advance of the infection in this setting can be rapid, progressing to death within hours. The combined case-fatality rate among children and adults with streptococcal TSS (STSS) and necrotizing fasciitis has been approximately 60% [78]. Death is less common, however, in children and in cases not complicated by STSS. In fact, there were no deaths reported among a series of 10 children seen at Seattle Children's Hospital over a 15-month period [305].

Fournier's gangrene is a form of necrotizing fasciitis that occurs in the male genital area, sometimes confined to the scrotum, but involving the perineum, penis and/or abdominal wall in other cases. It is caused by a synergistic type I infection or, occasionally, spread of streptococcal balanitis.

Diagnosis

Histopathologically, necrotizing fasciitis involves necrosis and suppuration of the superficial fascia; oedema and an acute inflammatory infiltrate in the deep dermis, subcutaneous fat and fascia; microorganisms present within destroyed tissue; and thrombosis of arteries and veins at all levels of tissue [81–83]. Some thrombosed vessels are surrounded by an inflammatory infiltrate and/or microorganisms, others may be vasculitic, while non-inflammatory intravascular coagulation may be present in others [81, 83]. Early in infections due to *S. pyogenes* or *Clostridium* spp., inflammatory cells may be lacking at sites of tissue damage [310].

Definitive diagnosis is made by surgical exploration, which must be undertaken as soon as the diagnosis is suspected. Necrotic fascia and subcutaneous tissue are grey and offer little resistance to blunt probing. Although magnetic-resonance imaging may aid in delineating the extent and tissue planes of involvement, this procedure should not delay surgical intervention [311]. Frozen-section incisional biopsy taken early in the course of the infection can aid management by decreasing the time to diagnosis and helping to establish margins of involvement [81]. Gram stain of tissue can be particularly useful if chains of Gram-positive cocci, indicative of infection with *S. pyogenes*, are seen.

Treatment

Early supportive care, surgical débridement and parenteral antibiotic administration are mandatory. All devitalized tissue must be removed to freely bleeding edges, and repeat exploration is generally indicated within 24–36 hours to confirm that no necrotic tissue remains. This may need to be repeated on several occasions until devitalized tissue has ceased to form. Daily, meticulous wound care is also paramount. The testes can generally be saved in Fournier's gangrene, because they have a separate blood supply from the adjacent fascia and skin.

Antibiotic therapy must be initiated parenterally as soon as possible with broad-spectrum agents against all potential pathogens. Most experts recommend initial empirical therapy with penicillin, ampicillin or nafcillin; clindamycin; and an aminoglycoside for coverage against *S. pyogenes* and the broad spectrum of potential anaerobic and Gram-negative pathogens [77, 310, 312]. Due to the presence of large numbers of *S. pyogenes* in type II infections and their entry into a slower or stationary phase of growth, *S. pyogenes* may become less susceptible to the β-lactam antibiotics, such as penicillin and the cephalosporins, which act by interrupting cell-wall synthesis [108, 109, 111]. Since efficacy of the protein-synthesis inhibitor clindamycin is not adversely altered by the inoculum effect, it may be preferable to penicillin for treatment of deep-seated, serious soft-tissue infections due to *S. pyogenes* [109]. Additional theoretical reasons for the superiority of clindamycin include its suppression of bacterial toxin synthesis and monocyte synthesis of TNF-α, and facilitation of phagocytosis by inhibiting synthesis of M protein [313–315]. Adjunctive therapies under investigation include hyperbaric oxygen and intravenous administration of pooled γ-globulin [77, 297, 303, 316–318].

Diseases mediated by exotoxins

Exotoxin-mediated diseases caused by *S. aureus* or *S. pyogenes* are due to the effects of extracellular toxin(s) produced at a focus of infection or colonization. The site of bacterial replication is typically inconspicuous in relation to the clinical effects of the toxin(s). Toxins can act locally, as in bullous impetigo, or, as with the diseases discussed in this section, can cause widespread clinical signs of disease due to haematogenous spread. To exert their effects, toxins may act directly, as when staphylococcal epidermolytic toxin binds to and disrupts desmosomes to cause bullous impetigo or staphylococcal scalded skin syndrome (SSSS). Alternatively, toxins may act indirectly, as when staphylococcal TSST-1 activates T lymphocytes to secrete massive amounts of cytokines; the cytokines, in turn, trigger the multisystem dysfunction that constitutes staphylococcal TSS. In most instances, however, both direct toxicity and indirect toxicity are responsible for the disease manifestations, as in scarlet fever, where cytotoxicity and Arthus and delayed hypersensitivity skin reactions cause the rash.

Scarlet fever (scarlatina)

Definition, epidemiology, aetiology

Scarlet fever is characterized by fever, oral mucous membrane changes and an exanthem associated with elaboration of SPE(s) from a focus of infection or colonization. Scarlet fever was more common and was frequently more severe during the mid- to late nineteenth century than it is has been in the past several decades; at that time, it was the most common infectious cause of death among children, and epidemics with mortality rates as high as 30% were reported [319–322]. Scarlet fever encompasses a spectrum of illness, but the vast majority of cases now fall into the mild or moderate groups [323]; the deadly toxic and septic forms seen during the scarlet-fever pandemic of the 1800s are now rare [322, 324–326]. Since the mid-1980s, however, there has been an increase in the incidence of severe, invasive, group A streptococcal infections, including STSS, in association with SPE production, particularly SPE-A [77, 79, 297, 324, 325, 327]. The clinical features of surgical, toxic or septic scarlet fever and STSS overlap, and some cases classified as severe forms of scarlet fever during the pandemic might now be considered cases of STSS [320, 327, 328].

Approximately 90% of isolates of *S. pyogenes* produce one or more of the antigenically distinct SPEs A, B or C [329]. Most cases of scarlet fever reported around the turn of the century are thought to have been due primarily to strains of *S. pyogenes* that produced SPE-A [321, 327, 329–332], although this has not been clearly substantiated [322]. Decline in the prevalence of SPE-A-producing strains of *S. pyogenes* appears to have been associated with the decreased incidence and severity of scarlet fever in recent decades [321, 329, 330]. Nevertheless, isolates of *S. pyogenes* from patients with scarlet fever in the 1980s were much more likely (45%) to possess the gene for SPE-A (called *spe*A) than were clinical isolates from patients with a variety of other streptococcal diseases (15%) [333]. Furthermore, presence of the gene for either SPE-B or SPE-C did not correlate with the ability of a strain to cause scarlet fever [334], suggesting that scarlet fever may still be caused predominantly by SPE-A-producing strains. All three of the SPEs are capable of causing the clinical features of scarlet fever, however, and isolates from recently affected patients have expressed various combinations of the SPEs [320, 328, 330]. Strains that produced SPE-B or SPE-C, but not SPE-A, were associated with scarlet fever in England in the early 1980s [330], but approximately half of children with scarlet fever in Czechoslovakia in the mid-1980s harboured isolates that produced SPE-A [320]. Greater intensity and duration of the exanthem was associated with strains that produced two or three SPEs [320]. Scarlet fever is occasionally caused by strains of group C or G streptococci, which produce exotoxins that are antigenically distinct from the SPEs of group A streptococci [331, 335].

During the course of scarlet fever, protective antibody is generated against SPE. Antibody to exotoxin does not provide protection against future infection with *S. pyogenes*, but, by the age of 10 years, 80% of children have developed lifelong protective antibodies against the toxins. Consequently, the disease primarily affects children between 4 and 8 years old. Recurrent attacks are exceptional, due to protective cross-reactivity of antibody against all three streptococcal exotoxins. Disease is also rare in children younger than 2 years of age, apparently due to the presence of maternal antiexotoxin antibodies and the lack of prior hypersensitization to the exotoxins, which is necessary for development of the exanthem [336]. In temperate climates, scarlet fever occurs more commonly during the late autumn, winter and early spring. It appears to be less common in tropical environments, perhaps due to immunity to exotoxins acquired during frequent subclinical infections [337].

The most common infection that leads to scarlet fever is tonsillopharyngitis due to *S. pyogenes*. Rash develops, however, in less than 10% of individuals with streptococcal tonsillopharyngitis [338]. Scarlet fever also occurs following streptococcal skin and soft-tissue infection and infection of surgical wounds (surgical scarlet fever) or the uterus (puerperal scarlet fever). The incubation period is generally 1–4 days. Spread of infection occurs primarily via airborne droplets produced by sneezing and coughing or by direct contact with an infected skin lesion. Transmission can occur from clinically infected as well as asymptomatically colonized individuals. Foodborne outbreaks have occurred in association with improper preparation or refrigeration of food or pasteurization of milk [339].

Clinical characteristics

Mild to moderate scarlet fever associated with tonsillopharyngitis typically presents abruptly with fever and sore throat, followed within 1–2 days by the appearance of rash. The illness may be accompanied by headache, nausea, vomiting, abdominal pain, myalgias and malaise. Exudative tonsillopharyngitis is accompanied by erythematous oral mucous membranes and petechiae and punctate erythematous macules on the hard and soft palate and uvula (Forschheimer's spots). The tongue is covered initially by a yellowish-white coat; protruding red papillae give the appearance of a 'white strawberry tongue'. Within approximately 2–4 days, disappearance of the white coating reveals a beefy red tongue with engorged papillae, known as a 'red strawberry tongue' (Fig. 2.16).

Rash generally appears first on the base of the neck, the face and the upper trunk and generalizes over the next 1–2 days. The lower legs are involved last and least, and the palms and soles are usually spared. Generalized, blanchable erythroderma is punctuated by numerous pinpoint, erythematous, blanchable papules, which impart a sandpaper-like texture. Occlusion of sweat glands is apparently responsible for producing the papular rash. Erythema tends to be accentuated in the skin folds of the neck, axillae, antecubital fossae and inguinal and popliteal creases and may develop into linear arrays of petechiae, called Pastia's lines, due to capillary

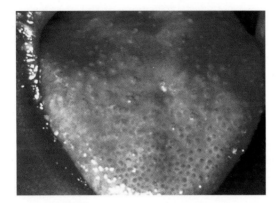

Fig. 2.16 Scarlet fever. Enlarged papillae on the tongue of an individual with scarlet fever due to *Streptococcus pyogenes*.

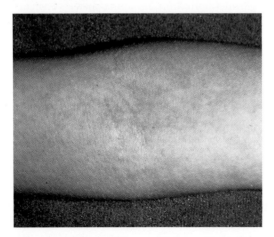

Fig. 2.17 Scarlet fever. Multiple pinpoint erythematous papules on the diffusely erythematous arm of an individual with scarlet fever due to *Streptococcus pyogenes*. Linear arrays of petechiae in the antecubital fossa form Pastia's lines. (Photograph courtesy of Alfred T. Lane, MD.)

fragility (Fig. 2.17). Circumoral pallor may be prominent against the background erythema of the face, although the face is occasionally spared. Generalized lymphadenopathy and/or splenomegaly occurs occasionally. Leucocytosis (e.g. 12000–16000/mm^3) with a left shift is common; eosinophilia (e.g. 10–20%) can also occur after a few days of illness.

The rash fades over approximately 5–7 days, followed approximately 7–10 days later by fine superficial desquamation on the face and trunk, particularly in the axillae and groin. Sheets of scale peel off the hands and feet; this may be most marked on the distal digits and at the base of the nails. Desquamation and peeling may continue for weeks. Months after the acute illness, transverse grooves (Beau's lines) may become apparent on the nails and telogen effluvium can develop. Toxin-mediated complications of the acute illness, such as myocarditis, may occur, but most complications are the result of direct bacterial invasion of tissues and are no more common than with other streptococcal infections of the pharynx or skin. Possible complications include peritonsillar abscess or cellulitis; cervical lymphadenitis; retropharyngeal abscess; otitis media; bronchopneumonia; meningitis; brain abscess; intracranial venous sinus thrombosis; bacteraemia with metastatic foci of infection, such as osteomyelitis, suppurative arthritis, endocarditis or liver abscess; and septicaemia. Late complications include rheumatic fever and acute poststreptococcal glomerulonephritis (see 'Impetigo').

Toxic cases of scarlet fever begin with severe sore throat and painful cervical lymphadenopathy; high fever, greater than 40°C; delirium; and rash. Severe cases, akin to those described by Osler as malignant scarlet fever [340], may progress to convulsions, coma and death within approximately 24 hours. Septic cases involve bacterial invasion of local soft tissues of the neck with suppuration, leading to otitis media with perforation, mucopurulent sinusitis, bronchopneumonia, upper-airway obstruction, sepsis and death. Necrotizing fasciitis or myositis is not present in even the most severe forms of scarlet fever.

Diagnosis

Diagnosis is generally made on clinical grounds and can be confirmed by culture of *S. pyogenes* from a focal site of infection, such as the throat or skin. When a throat culture is obtained properly from a symptomatic individual, false-negative results are obtained in less than 10% of cases. Highly specific, rapid antigen-detection technology is available for detection of tonsillopharyngeal infection and some cases of skin infection [341]; thus, a positive antigen-detection test result is sufficient for confirmation of infection due to *S. pyogenes*. False-negative results can occur, however, particularly with low-level infection. Furthermore, antigen-detection tests fail to identify infection due to non-group A streptococci. Consequently, a negative antigen-detection test result should be followed up with a confirmatory throat culture. A rise in the ASO titre, particularly following tonsillopharyngeal infection, or the anti-DNase B titre following skin infection (see 'Impetigo') provides retrospective evidence of streptococcal infection.

Histopathogically, dermal blood and lymphatic vessels show diffuse vasodilatation, which is most prominent around hair follicles. Perivascular oedema, mononuclear-cell infiltrates and occasional haemorrhage are also noted, but there is no evidence of vasculitis. The epidermis may appear spongiotic in the acute phase; parakeratosis is prominent during the desquamative stage.

An eruption virtually identical to that of streptococcal scarlet fever is caused by toxin-producing strains of *S. aureus*. Exudative tonsillopharyngitis is lacking in staphylococcal scarlet fever, however, and this entity is typically associated with focal infection, such as an abscess, septic arthritis, osteomyelitis or wound infection [342–345]. Staphylococcal scarlet fever may be an abortive form of SSSS, particularly when mucous membrane changes are lacking or minor in degree [346]. These cases are presumably mediated by the effects of epidermolytic toxin. Other cases share features with TSS and may be mediated by other staphylococcal toxins, such as TSST-1, enterotoxin B or enterotoxin C.

Exudative pharyngitis and a rash similar to that of scarlet fever have also been associated with infection caused by *Arcanobacterium haemolyticum* [347–356]. The infection is commonly accompanied by pruritus, anterior cervical or submandibular lymphadenopathy, low-grade fever and a non-productive cough. Most patients are between 10 and 25 years of age, and in this age-group pharyngitis with scarlatina is as likely to be due to *A. haemolyticum* as to *S. pyogenes* [350]. The scarlatiniform eruption appears 1–4 days after onset of pharyngitis, developing first on the distal extremities and spreading centrally over the next 2–3 days. Rash may also involve the neck, chest and back, but the face, palms and soles are spared. Desquamation frequently occurs as the rash resolves, often on the hands and feet, but it is generally less prominent than that seen following scarlet fever. Rash does not appear to be a feature of *A. haemolyticum* infection in the tropics, and rash has not been reported in association with *A. haemolyticum* infection at sites other than the pharynx [353, 357, 358]. The organism grows more slowly than *S. pyogenes* on sheep-blood agar, and does not produce significant β-haemolysis before 24–36 hours, when throat cultures for *S. pyogenes* are typically read for the final time. Growth and β-haemolysis are enhanced when the organism is cultured on rabbit- or human-blood agar. Within 48 hours on these media, haemolysis is prominent and a black opaque dot at the centre of each colony is visible and remains if the colony is scraped aside. As with scarlet fever, the exanthem is presumably due to an extracellular toxin. Kawasaki disease can also present with oral mucous membrane changes and a scarlatiniform rash virtually indistinguishable clinically from scarlet fever. Features that may be helpful in diagnosing Kawasaki disease, however, include prominent conjunctivitis, occasionally sparing the limbus; uveitis on slit-lamp examination; marked elevation of the erythrocyte sedimentation rate and C-reactive protein; sterile pyuria;

and prolonged fever. Fever tends to resolve within 5–6 days in scarlet fever, whereas fever for more than 5 days is a diagnostic criterion for Kawasaki disease. Additional infectious diseases that must be considered in the differential diagnosis of scarlet fever include SSSS and TSS (see below), rubella, measles, infectious mononucleosis and parvovirus B19 or echovirus 14 infection. The cutaneous eruption caused by drug-hypersensitivity reaction can also closely mimic scarlet fever [359, 360].

Treatment

Early treatment of scarlet fever is associated with reduced infectivity, more rapid resolution of disease and prevention of acute complications and of rheumatic fever [361]. The drug of choice for treatment of scarlet fever is penicillin, due to its narrow spectrum of activity, low cost and proved efficacy for preventing rheumatic fever. Since eradication of *S. pyogenes* from the pharynx is necessary to prevent rheumatic fever, a prolonged treatment course of 10 days is necessary. Patients who are acutely ill may benefit from an intramuscular injection of benzathine penicillin G, 1.2 million units in adults or 600 000 units for children who weigh less than 27 kg. Intramuscular injection is associated with less discomfort if the formulation is warmed to room temperature prior to administration. The dose of orally administered penicillin V is 250 mg tid for 10 days. In penicillin-allergic patients, erythromycin estolate 20–40 mg/kg/day in two to four divided doses or erythromycin ethylsuccinate 40–50 mg/kg/day in three to four divided doses, up to a maximum of 1 g/day, should be administered for 10 days. Twice-daily dosing is probably sufficient for children, but data supporting this dosing interval in adults are lacking. The newer macrolides azithromycin and clarithromycin appear to be effective, and may be useful in instances of gastrointestinal intolerance to erythromycin. Narrow-spectrum oral cephalosporins are also effective, acceptable alternatives [362, 363], but should not be administered to patients with immediate anaphylactic hypersensitivity to penicillin [138].

Staphylococcal scalded-skin syndrome

Definition, epidemiology, aetiology

Staphyloccocal scalded-skin syndrome is a staphylococcal epidermolytic toxin-mediated disease characterized by cutaneous tenderness and superficial, widespread blistering and/or desquamation [364]. It occurs predominantly in infants and children under 5 years of age. Decreased renal clearance and decreased immunity to the toxins may account for the fact that the disease is most common in infants and young children. Disease in adults occurs predominantly in those with immunocompromise and/or renal failure [365]. Staphylococcal scalded-skin syndrome is caused predominantly by phage-group II staphylococci, particularly strains 71 and 55, which are present at localized sites of infection [177, 366, 367]. Occasionally, a group I or III isolate is involved. Foci of infection include the nasopharynx or, less commonly, the umbilicus, urinary tract, a cutaneous wound, conjunctivae or the blood. Severity of the disease is related to the toxin load, rather than the nature of the focal infection, since the clinical manifestations are mediated by haematogenous spread, in the absence of specific antitoxin antibody to, of staphylococcal epidermolytic (or exfoliative or exfoliatin) toxins A or B [177, 366]. Investigators have utilized the toxins to reproduce the disease in both animal models and human volunteers [366, 368, 369].

Clinical characteristics

Onset of the rash may be preceded by malaise, fever, irritability and exquisite tenderness of the skin. Generalized macular erythema evolves rapidly into a scarlatiniform eruption, which is accentuated in flexural and periorificial areas. There may be pharyngitis, conjunctivitis and superficial erosions of the lips, but intraoral mucosal surfaces are spared. Characteristically, circumoral erythema is prominent. The brightly erythematous skin may acquire a wrinkled appearance, leading to thick flaky desquamation, particularly in the flexures, over approximately 2–5 days. In severe cases, the erythrodermic phase is followed by the development of diffuse, sterile, flaccid blisters and erosions. Bullous desquamation of large sheets of skin in the neonate is known as Ritter's disease (Fig. 2.18). At this stage, areas of

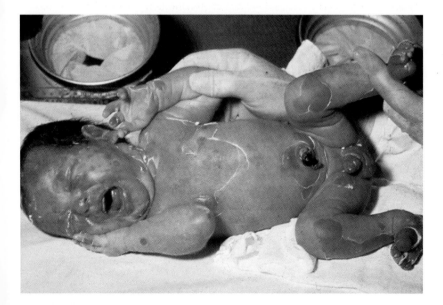

Fig. 2.18 Staphylococcal scalded-skin syndrome. Diffuse, superficial desquamation in a neonate with Ritter's disease. As with bullous impetigo, separation of the skin occurs at the subcorneal layer due to the action of epidermolytic toxin on desmosomes.

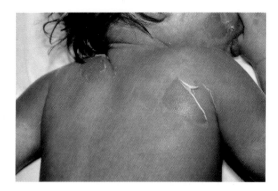

Fig. 2.19 Staphylococcal scalded-skin syndrome. Lateral shear force produced the superficial erosion (Nikolsky sign) on the right upper back of a toddler with staphylococcal scalded-skin syndrome. Diffuse, scarlatiniform erythroderma is present on the face, back and proximal arms. (Photograph courtesy of Alfred T. Lane, MD.)

epidermis may separate in response to gentle shear force (Nikolsky sign) (Fig. 2.19). As large sheets of epidermis peel away, moist, glistening, denuded areas become apparent, initially in the flexures and subsequently over much of the body surface. As the exposed denuded skin dries, it develops a crusted, flaky appearance. Distinctive radial crusting and fissuring around the eyes, mouth and nose develop approximately 2–5 days after the onset of erythroderma in all forms of the disease. Healing occurs without scarring in 10–14 days. Although some patients appear ill, many are reasonably comfortable except for the marked skin tenderness. Recovery is usually rapid, but complications, such as excessive fluid loss, electrolyte imbalance, faulty temperature regulation, secondary cutaneous infection, pneumonia, septicaemia and cellulitis, may cause increased morbidity. Mortality, due predominantly to sepsis, is rare but is higher in infants with Ritter's disease. Omphalitis, endocarditis and severe surgical-wound infections have also been described.

A presumed abortive form of the disease presents with diffuse, scarlatiniform, tender erythroderma, which is accentuated in the flexural areas, but does not progress to blister formation. In these patients, the Nikolsky sign may be absent. While the exanthem is similar to that of streptococcal scarlet fever, strawberry tongue and palatal petechiae are absent. Presence of cutaneous tenderness and early desquamation also help to distinguish SSSS from scarlet fever.

Diagnosis

Intact bullae are consistently sterile, unlike those of bullous impetigo, but cultures should be obtained from all suspected sites of localized infection and from the blood in an attempt to identify the source for elaboration of the epidermolytic toxins. Histopathologically, the site of blister cleavage is subcorneal, through the granular layer. Absence of an inflammatory infiltrate is characteristic. In cases that demand a rapid diagnosis, the exfoliated corneal layer can be seen on a frozen biopsy specimen of the desquamating epidermis. Scattered acantholytic cells, which are evident histopathologically in the cleft-like bullae, can also be seen in a Tzanck preparation. The epidermolytic toxins appear to produce the granular-layer split by binding to desmoglein I within desmosomes [370–372]. There is evidence that the toxins are members of the trypsin-like serine protease family, and may exert their action through proteolysis [373]. Ultrastructural studies have consistently demonstrated separation of the two halves of the desmosome without preceding cytolysis.

Staphylococcal scalded-skin syndrome may be mistaken for a number of other blistering and exfoliating disorders, including scarlet fever, bullous impetigo, epidermolysis bullosa, epidermolytic hyperkeratosis, pemphigus, drug eruption, erythema multiforme and (Lyell's disease) drug-induced toxic epidermal necrolysis (TEN). Toxic epidermal necrolysis can often be distinguished by a history of drug ingestion, presence of the Nikolsky sign only at sites of erythema and absence of perioral crusting. Distinction between the skin lesions of TEN and SSSS may require histopathological examination of a skin-biopsy specimen; TEN results in full-thickness epidermal necrosis, with a blister cleavage plane in the lowermost epidermis, while the cleavage plane in SSSS is subcorneal. Distinguishing between these conditions is particularly important, since mortality rates as high as 30% have been reported with TEN and avoidance of the offending drug is crucial to preventing a recurrence.

Treatment

Systemic therapy, either orally, in cases of localized involvement, or parenterally, with a semisynthetic penicillinase-resistant penicillin should be administered promptly. The skin should be gently moistened and cleansed with Burow's solution, Dakin's solution or isotonic saline. Handling of the patient should be minimized, particularly early in the course of the disease. Application of an emollient will provide lubrication and may decrease discomfort in the resolution phase. Topical antibiotics are unnecessary, and corticosteroids are detrimental and should be avoided [374].

Staphylococcal toxic-shock syndrome

Definition, epidemiology, aetiology

Staphyloccocal TSS is characterized by acute onset of high fever; erythrodermic, scarlatiniform rash, followed by desquamation, particularly on the hands and feet; hyperaemic mucous membranes; hypotension; and multiorgan compromise. It is due to infection or colonization with a toxin-producing strain of S. aureus in a susceptible host with low to absent levels of specific antitoxin antibody [375–377]. Toxic-shock syndrome was first described in 1978 in children who were colonized or infected on a mucosal surface (vaginal, nasopharyngeal, tracheal) or in a focal, sequestered site (empyema, cutaneous abscess) with phage-group I *S. aureus* [378]. In the late 1970s to early 1980s, however, the most prevalent form of the syndrome occurred in the USA in young, healthy women using hyperabsorbent tampons during menstruation [379–381]. Recognition of the association of menstrual TSS with use of hyperabsorbent tampons and removal of those tampons from the market in the early 1980s resulted in a decrease in the incidence of TSS [379, 381, 382]. Since 1986, half or more of cases worldwide have continued to occur in women who are vaginally colonized or infected during menstruation; this continues to be the group at highest risk [383]. A significant proportion of cases are associated with a wide variety of focal *S. aureus* infections [383–387]. The most common non-menstrual settings for TSS are upper-airway infections, such as sinusitis or tracheitis, burns and minor skin infections [388]. Non-menstrual TSS has occurred as a complication of a myriad of surgical procedures; nasal packing appears to pose an especially high risk [388]. It occurs more often in females than in males (approximately 2:1) [383], at a mean age of approximately 30 years in females, similar to that for menses-associated TSS, and approximately age 40 years in males [383, 389]. Toxic-shock syndrome has been reported in individuals from infancy to the ninth decade of life, but it occurs rarely in children [378, 383, 384, 390–400].

Toxic-shock syndrome is caused by toxin-producing strains of *S. aureus*, particularly phage types 29, 52 and 29/52 of phage-group 1 [401]. A significant proportion of isolates (30–40%) are non-typable [402]. Strains that cause TSS are not new, but appear to have increased in prevalence among clinical isolates and acquired the capability to produce exotoxin [401, 402]. Many of the isolates appear to have developed from a single clone [403]. Manifestations of disease are mediated by one or more staphylococcal toxins acting alone or in concert [402]. Approximately 90–95% of menstrual cases of TSS are due to strains of *S. aureus* that are capable of producing TSST-1, while approximately 60% of non-menstrual cases are associated with strains that produce this toxin [401, 404, 405]. In contrast, only 5–25% of all clinical isolates of *S. aureus* produce TSST-1 [402]. Other staphylococcal toxins, particularly enterotoxin B, mediate TSS under some circumstances; in other cases, enterotoxins, such as A or C1, are coproduced with TSST-1 and appear to worsen disease due primarily to TSST-1 [405–412]. Colonization or infection with a toxigenic strain of *S. aureus* is not sufficient for production of TSS, however, even in a host lacking protective antitoxin antibody. It appears that the conditions present locally (e.g. neutral pH, aerobic environment, slightly elevated CO_2 level, high protein level) must favour expression of toxin [413]. Not surprisingly, the unique environment at foci of infection in patients with non-menstrual TSS is similar to that in the vagina with tampon use during menstruation [413]. The nasopharynx, on the other hand, appears to allow for colonization and the development of antibody against TSST-1 in the absence of clinical disease [414, 415]. The importance of local conditions at the site of infection is also highlighted in children, who rarely develop TSS, despite the fact that they are frequently, more often than adults, infected or colonized with strains of *S. aureus* that are toxigenic [390, 415]. Neonates receive protective antibody from the mother. Approximately 80% of infants under 1 years of age have levels of anti-TSST-1 antibody that are considered protective. Half or less of children aged 1–4 years, however, have protective levels of antibody [390]; nevertheless, their incidence of TSS is exceedingly low. The prevalence of protective antibody levels rises to 80–90% or more in the general population over age 20 years [377, 390, 416], and yet this is the age-group most frequently affected. Women who develop menstrual TSS, however, lack protective levels of antibody and tend to develop antibody slowly, if at all, often only after several episodes over 1–2 years.

Once staphylococcal exotoxins have been produced and released into the circulation, they mediate manifestations of TSS, predominantly through superantigen stimulation of massive cytokine release, primarily TNF-α and interleukin 1 (IL-1) from monocytes and IL-2 and TNF-β from lymphocytes [407, 417, 418]. Direct cytotoxic action of the staphylococcal enterotoxins may also play a role in pathogenesis, as may enhancement by TSST-1 of susceptibility to endotoxin or synergistic action of staphylococcal enterotoxins with streptococcal exotoxins [388, 403, 407, 419, 420]. It has also been proposed that *E. coli* may facilitate multiplication of *S. aureus* in the vagina [402].

Toxic-shock syndrome has occurred in individuals from whom only coagulase-negative staphylococci have been isolated, suggesting that these bacteria can rarely cause the syndrome [411, 421, 422]. Some investigators, however, have been unable to detect production of TSST-1 or the presence of the gene for toxic-shock toxin in isolates of coagulase-negative staphylococci [402, 423, 424].

Clinical characteristics

Toxic-shock syndrome encompasses a range of relatively mild to rapidly fatal disease. Characteristically, however, patients develop a well-defined constellation of signs over a brief period of time (Table 2.14). Some patients experience a prodrome of malaise, myalgias, low-grade fever or vomiting during the week before acute onset of illness [380]. Short incubation periods of approximately 48 hours are typical for postoperative TSS, and may be particularly abbreviated following nasal surgery [425]. On average, the interval from antecedent injury or precipating event to onset of symptoms of TSS is longer for cases unrelated to menstruation (e.g. 7 days) than for mentrually associated cases (e.g. 3 days) [389]. Local signs of inflammation and infection are typically trivial to absent [381, 386, 389]. Women with menstrual TSS may have vaginal discharge, hyperaemia and ulceration of the vaginal mucosa, perineal tenderness, labial oedema and occasionally vaginal cellulitis [380]. Onset of disease is marked by abrupt

Table 2.14 Case definition of toxic-shock syndrome due to *Staphylococcus aureus*.

Major criteria (all four must be present)
Fever: temperature ≥38.9°C (102°F)
Rash: scarlatiniform erythroderma
Hypotension: systolic blood pressure < fifth percentile by age for children <16 years
old, ≤90 mmHg for adults; orthostatic syncope, dizziness or drop in diastolic blood
pressure ≥15 mmHg from lying to sitting position
Desquamation: 1–2 weeks after onset of illness, particularly the palms, soles and
distal digits

Multisystem involvement (three or more present)
Gastrointestinal: emesis and/or diarrhoea present at onset of illness
Musculoskeletal: myalgias; creatine phosphokinase level twofold or more above the
upper limit of normal
Mucous membranes: conjunctival, oropharyngeal and/or vaginal hyperaemia
Renal: BUN or serum creatinine level twofold or more above the upper limit of
normal; pyuria (≥ five leucocytes/high-power field) in the absence of urinary-tract
infection
Hepatic: total bilirubin, aspartate aminotransferase and/or alanine aminotransferase
level twofold or more above the upper limit of normal
Haematological: platelets ≤100 000/mm³
Central nervous system: disorientation or alteration of consciousness without focal
neurological signs and while fever is absent

Negative
Serological tests for Rocky Mountain spotted fever, leptospirosis or measles

BUN, blood urea nitrogen.

development of high fever, associated with chills, abdominal pain, headache, nausea, emesis, diarrhoea, myalgias and weakness. Hypotension ensues rapidly, leading to tissue ischaemia and multiorgan injury [425]. Hypotension appears to be due to both decreased vasomotor tone, resulting in peripheral vascular congestion, and hydrostatic leakage of fluid into the interstitium. These physiological alterations lead to decreased intravascular volume and marked reduction in venous return, particularly when coupled with large fluid losses through diarrhoea. Multiorgan-system involvement follows, due to poor tissue perfusion as well as the action of toxin or toxin-induced mediators on cells throughout the body [425]. Capillary leak and loss of vascular tone may not improve for days, requiring massive fluid administration and resulting in diffuse, non-pitting peripheral oedema. Patients present without focal neurological or meningeal signs, but confusion and disorientation may become significant, presumably due to development of cerebral oedema, and may progress to seizures and coma [425, 426]. Renal failure, adult respiratory distress syndrome, myocardial dysfunction and disseminated intravascular coagulation may be life-threatening. Laboratory abnormalities are protean, reflecting the multisystem injury. Serum protein and albumin are uniformly low. Haematological disturbances include leucocytosis, with a predominance of immature forms, thrombocytopenia and evidence of disseminated intravascular coagulation; renal abnormalities include reduced urine output, pyuria, proteinuria and elevated blood urea nitrogen (BUN) and creatinine; electrolyte abnormalities include hypocalcaemia, hypophosphataemia and hypomagnesaemia; and hepatic enzymes and bilirubin and muscle creatine phosphokinase are elevated [380].

Rash is typically a presenting feature, developing in virtually all patients within 1–3 days of onset of disease [389]. A diffuse, macular, erythrodermic, scarlatiniform eruption is most common, sometimes developing first on the trunk and spreading to the extremities. Scattered erythematous papules may also be present [427]. The eruption is often accentuated in flexural areas and may be patchy [392, 428]. Typically, the rash fades over a few days; on occasion, it becomes petechial during the first week. In the setting of thrombocytopenia, purpura can develop, and, on rare occasions, vesicles and bullae form. Pharyngitis and hyperaemia of conjunctival and mucosal membranes may be prominent and may progress to oral, oesophageal, vaginal and/or bladder mucosal ulcerations or subconjuctival haemorrhage. Strawberry tongue is present in more than half of patients and palatal petechiae may be present occasionally [429]. Oedema of the hands and feet is characteristic. One to two weeks after onset of illness, approximately half of patients develop a pruritic, diffuse, maculopapular, sometime urticarial eruption, typically involving the palms and soles but sparing the face [430, 431]. This secondary eruption generally lasts 2–7 days, and may be accompanied by oedema of the face and extremities [431]. Full-thickness desquamation of the skin, particularly of the subungual areas of the digits, the palms and soles, occurs as a rule 10–21 days after onset of the disease.

Toxic-shock syndrome presents in a similar manner, regardless of age, sex and association with menses. Children, however, are more apt to suffer respiratory embarrassment [396]. Non-menstrual cases are more frequently acquired nosocomially, associated with prior antibiotic use, and more commonly involve central nervous system (CNS) manifestations or anaemia than menstrual cases, but have less prominent musculoskeletal signs of tenderness or weakness [389]. A variant of TSS has presented in individuals with AIDS, with prolonged, diffuse, cutaneous erythema, desquamation, conjunctival injection, hypotension and multiorgan involvement [395, 432]. Mean duration of the recalcitrant illness was 50 days. Enterotoxin-producing strains of *S. aureus* were isolated from the blood, cutaneous lesions or sinuses.

Most patients with TSS improve after approximately 3–5 days of therapy. Mortality is now low, approximately 3%, and approaches zero among menstrual cases at major medical centres [385]. Overall, the severity of non-menstrual cases may be greater than those associated with menses [389]. Recurrence is rare following non-menstrual TSS, but can occur in up to one-quarter of women with menstrual TSS, particularly if antibiotic therapy is inadequate during the acute illness or tampon use continues [379, 389]. Delayed or absent development of protective antibody probably contributes to the risk of recurrence. Potential sequelae are numerous, involving the major organ systems affected during acute disease. More common sequelae include prolonged fatigue, weakness or myalgia; reversible hair loss, consistent with telogen effluvium or possibly toxin-induced anagen effluvium; shedding of nails or appearance of Beau's lines; vocal-cord paralysis; limb paraesthesia; amenorrhoea; prolonged renal failue; carpal-tunnel syndrome; difficulties with recent memory, computation and concentration; abnormal electroencephalogram; and impaired capillary refilling, leading to cyanotic extremities [380, 388, 425].

Diagnosis

Diagnosis is based on clinical recognition of the syndrome (Table 2.14) and requires the presence of high fever, rash followed by desquamation, hypotension and involvement of three or more organ systems. Supportive evidence is provided by negative results of diagnostic tests for other diseases in the differential diagnosis. While recovery of *S. aureus* from a normally sterile site provides supportive evidence for a diagnosis of TSS, the initial focus of infection may occur at a site that is frequently colonized, such as the upper-respiratory or genital tracts, making culture results difficult to interpret. Demonstration of toxin production by the isolate also supports its role in pathogenesis of the disease. Suspicion of TSS should be aroused whenever systemic toxicity develops rapidly, out of proportion to local signs of infection [433].

Histopathological examination shows a superficial, perivascular infiltrate of neutrophils, lymphocytes and a few eosinophils; epidermal spongiosis; individually necrotic keratinocytes; and papillary oedema [427, 428]. Although nuclear dust may be seen within the infiltrate on occasion, fibrin deposition in the walls of venules, and thus vasculitis, is lacking. When blisters form, they are located subepidermally, and ulcerations involve the full thickness of the epidermis. Biopsy generally permits differentiation from TEN or other drug eruptions [427, 428].

The differential diagnosis of TSS is broad, due to its wide variety and spectrum of presentation. Initially, based on cutaneous and mucosal signs, it may be most easily confused with streptococcal scarlet fever, Kawasaki disease, SSSS, atypical measles, leptospirosis, Rocky Mountain spotted fever, viral exanthematous diseases and drug-induced syndromes, including Stevens–Johnson syndrome and TEN. Development of shock and multiorgan involvement are not characteristic of these entities, except perhaps in severe cases of Kawasaki disease/infantile polyarteritis nodosa or TEN. Toxic epidermal necrolysis develops following medication ingestion and can generally be distinguished from TSS on the basis of its histopathological findings of interface dermatitis and subepidermal vesiculation [427, 428]. Furthermore, development of exquisite skin tenderness, bullae and full-thickness epidermal erosions characterize TEN but are unusual in TSS. Toxic-shock syndrome may be particularly difficult to distinguish from Kawasaki disease. Kawasaki disease, however, including the severe systemic form that resembles and probably can be equated with infantile polyarteritis nodosa, presents almost uniformly in children under age 10. Prominent crusting and fissuring of the lips, morbilliform or erythema multiforme-like rash, lymphadenopathy, coronary aneurysm, thrombocytosis and marked elevation of C-reactive protein and the erythrocyte sedimentation rate favour a diagnosis of Kawasaki diasease [346].

Treatment

Treatment of TSS centres around intensive supportive management of shock and multiorgan failure, identification and drainage of infection and prompt institution of antibacterial therapy. Initial evaluation must include a chest radiograph and culture of all potential focal sites of infection, including the blood, urine and vagina. Vaginal tampons or contraceptive devices must be removed. Vaginal irrigation to remove preformed toxin is recommended if suspicion of vaginal infection exists, although efficacy of this measure has not been proved [431]. If illness develops following surgery, the surgical wound must be explored and cultured, even in the absence of overt signs of inflammation, particularly if no other source of infection can be found. Any accessible focal site of infection must be drained. Initial screening laboratory studies for organ dysfunction should include a complete blood count with differential; electrolytes, including calcium and magnesium; hepatic transaminases and bilirubin; BUN, creatinine and urinalysis; and creatine phophokinase. Vital signs, blood pressure, weight, urine output, peripheral perfusion and respiratory and mental status must be monitored frequently.

Hypotension is due largely to venous pooling of blood and capillary leak into the interstitium, creating a state of high cardiac output and low venous return. Consequently, large volumes of crystalloid (i.e. electrolyte solution) and colloid (i.e. albumin) are typically needed to maintain tissue perfusion and reverse organ failure [431, 434]. Measurement of blood pressure, heart rate, urine output and central venous pressure facilitate assessment of intravascular volume. Invasive monitoring with a Swan–Ganz catheter may be necessary. After fluid resuscitation is initiated, signs of adult respiratory distress syndrome may become apparent. While intubation and administration of continuous airway pressure may be necessary to manage this complication, fluid resuscitation should not be curtailed, as recurrence of shock may ensue [434]. Myocardial failure may require use of inotropic and antiarrhythmic agents, along with maintenance of adequate venous return and atrial filling pressure through carefully monitored fluid administration [435].

Antibiotic therapy is necessary to eliminate bacterial toxin production, but is unlikely to alter the acute course of the disease unless given early, before significant amounts of toxin reach the circulation. A penicillinase-resistant antistaphylococcal antibiotic, such as oxacillin or nafcillin, or a first- or possibly second-generation cephalosporin should be administered intravenously at the maximal recommended dose for weight and age. In the event that the patient may have acquired a methicillin-resistant isolate nosocomially or has an indwelling catheter, therapy may be initiated with vancomycin. Antibiotic choice can be tailored once the susceptibility profile of the isolate is known. A 10-day course of therapy may be completed with an oral agent (e.g. dicloxacillin, cephalexin) once the patient has defervesced, has stabilized and is taking fluids by mouth. Inadequate therapy is a risk factor for recurrence of disease. If recurrence of menstrual TSS occurs despite adequate antibiotic therapy during the acute episode and discontinuation of tampon use, eradication of the carrier state may be attempted with rifampicin (20 mg/kg/day for 5 days) in conjunction with a β-lactam antibiotic; or with clindamycin (300 mg every 6 hours for 7 days), following the acute course of antibacterial therapy [434]. Rifampicin should not be given alone, due to the propensity to select for resistant isolates. Administration of an oral contraceptive pill or an oral β-lactamase antibiotic during menses may also be effective for treatment of recurrent disease [425, 436]. Patients with severe shock, particularly those unresponsive to initial antibiotic therapy may benefit from early administration of methylprednisolone 10 mg/kg every 8–12 hours [437]. Use of corticosteroids is controversial, however, and benefit has not been demonstrated prospectively. In addition, administration of IVIG 400 mg/kg may be considered for treatment of TSS with unrelenting shock and organ failure despite optimal management [400, 425, 434], since high levels of antibody to TSST-1 have been found in intramuscular immunoglobulin and IVIG preparations [431]. Decreased mortality following administration of IVIG has been demonstrated using a rabbit model of TSS [438] and IVIG has been used in burn-associated TSS in children in the UK [400].

Streptococcal toxic-shock syndrome

Definition, epidemiology, aetiology

Streptococcal toxic-shock syndrome is characterized by acute onset of shock and multisystem organ failure, due to *S. pyogenes* infection at a normally sterile site [439]. Attention was focused on this entity in the late 1980s, when adults in the USA were described with fulminant manifestations of invasive streptococcal disease [77, 324, 327]. Since then, STSS has occurred in persons of all ages, primarily in North America and Europe, at an estimated incidence of 10–20 cases per 100 000 population, with no sex predilection [440, 441]. Children appear to be less apt than adults to develop STSS in the setting of invasive group A streptococcal disease [442]. Unlike staphylococcal TSS, STSS is associated with invasion of *S. pyogenes*; consequently most patients are bacteraemic and/or have focal tissue infection at the time of presentation [77, 89, 440]. Streptococcal toxic-shock syndrome develops most often in the setting of a minor, focal skin and/or soft-tissue infection [76–78, 89, 325, 327, 443, 444], which presumably provides a portal of entry [89, 325, 440]. The integrity of the skin need not be grossly damaged for invasion to occur, as cases of STSS have developed following minor, non-penetrating trauma that resulted in ecchymosis, haematoma or muscle strain [89, 440]. The mucous membranes can also be penetrated, as invasive infection may follow pharyngeal carriage [445, 446], pharyngitis [447], postpartum vaginal infection [77], or puerperal sepsis [448–451] or may develop in the setting of influenza. Recent cases of STSS in children with varicella have highlighted the role of these lesions as a potential portal for *S. pyogenes* invasion [305, 307, 309, 452–454]. The reason invasive disease is found in children with varicella but is exceedingly rare in adults [455] is not known, but may be related to the fact that children have higher skin and pharyngeal carriage rates for *S. pyogenes* than adults [456]. Anecdotal reports suggest an association between use of non-steroidal anti-inflammatory agents and progression of infection to STSS [457]. Most cases of STSS involve patients who were previously healthy, although underlying conditions, such as intravenous drug abuse and diabetes mellitus, are present in some patients [77]. Lack of antibody against exotoxin appears to be a risk factor for severe, invasive disease and STSS [458, 459].

Most isolates of *S. pyogenes* that cause STSS are M-protein types 1, 3, 12 and 28 that produce SPE-A or SPE-B [77, 79, 89, 325, 327, 460–463]. Streptococcal pyrogenic exotoxins can cause shock and multiorgan damage in animal models and can stimulate cytokine release from monocytes in a manner similar to TSST-1, suggesting parallels in pathogenesis of STSS and staphylococcal TSS [463–467]. Streptococcal pyrogenic exotoxin B has protease activity and may be capable of damaging tissue directly [468]. Additional virulence factors, such as streptococcal M protein, streptolysin O, cell-wall components and synergistic action with other toxins (e.g. TSST-1), appear to contribute to the pathogenesis of invasive streptococcal infections, including STSS [78, 79, 84, 419, 440].

Clinical characteristics

Streptococcal toxic-shock syndrome is characterized by acute onset and early, frequently fulminant progression to shock and multiorgan compromise or failure. An influenza-like prodromal illness of fever, chills, myalgia and diarrhoea heralds STSS in approximately 20% of patients [77]. The most common presenting sign of STSS is fever, generally accompanied by tachycardia, confusion and hypotension. One-tenth of patients present with profound shock and hypothermia. All patients rapidly develop hypotensive shock, accompanied in most by early renal impairment and onset of adult respiratory distress syndrome. Renal impairment tends to progress for the first few days regardless of therapy, often necessitating dialysis, but function is regained within 4–6 weeks in nearly all patients. Toxic cardiomyopathy is a life-threatening complication that is characterized by decreased contractility and cardiac output and refractory shock [461].

A cardinal distinguishing feature — the most common (85%) initial symptom of STSS—is abrupt onset of severe, localized pain out of proportion to physical findings, which may even be absent [77]. Pain most commonly involves an extremity, but may originate from the abdomen, chest or pelvis. Most patients have localized swelling and erythema at the site of pain. Soft-tissue infection becomes apparent in 80% of patients and evolves in the majority of cases (70%) into severe subcutaneous infections (e.g. necrotizing fasciitis, myositis) that require surgical débridement. Development of vesicles and bullae (5%) is a late, ominous sign of tissue devitalization [77, 469]. Patients without soft-tissue infection have a variety of focal infections, including endophthalmitis, osteomyelitis, myositis, pneumonia, perihepatitis, peritonitis, myocarditis and sepsis [77, 309, 443, 461].

Early in the course of STSS, conjunctival and/or oropharyngeal mucous membrane hyperaemia may be present, but strawberry tongue is uncommon [327, 443, 454]. Other cutaneous signs in a minority of patients include a petechial, maculopapular or diffuse scarlatiniform eruption [324, 443, 446, 452]. Rarely, eruptions may appear several days into the course of the illness [324], and may even develop concurrently with the desquamation that develops in some patients (20–30%) 1–2 weeks after onset of illness [440, 443, 469].

Laboratory abnormalities reflect the multiorgan-system dysfunction. Haemoglobinuria, elevation of serum creatinine and leucocytosis with a marked left shift develop early. As the disease progresses, the majority of patients display hypoalbuminaemia, hypocalcaemia, anaemia and thrombocytopenia. Soft-tissue infection, particularly development of necrotizing fasciitis and myositis, is reflected in an elevation of creatine phosphokinase [77, 89].

Mortality rates of 30% or more have been reported in small series made up primarily of adults. The mortality rate in children, however, may be somewhat lower [442].

Diagnosis

Definitive diagnosis of STSS requires isolation of *S. pyogenes* from a normally sterile site on a patient with hypotension and multiorgan failure (Table 2.15). Features of STSS overlap with staphylococcal TSS, possibly due to similarities in their molecular pathogenesis, and with streptococcal necrotizing fasciitis, because most cases of STSS originate from a focus of infection involving skin and/or soft tissue. In general, however, STSS is a more fulminant disease, which is associated more often with bacteraemia, an identifiable focal site of infection, bulla formation, extensive soft-tissue devitalization, disfiguring morbidity and a lethal outcome than staphylo-

Table 2.15 Case definition of toxic-shock syndrome due to *Streptococcus pyogenes* (for definitive diagnosis; modified from [439]).

Major criteria (both must be present)

Isolation of *Streptococcus pyogenes* from a normally sterile site, such as blood, cerebrospinal, pleural or peritoneal fluid, tissue or surgical wound (isolation from a non-sterile site, such as throat, sputum, vagina or skin, permits classification as a probable case)

Hypotension: systolic blood pressure < fifth percentile by age for children <16 years old, ≤90 mmHg for adults

Multisystem involvement (two or more present)

Renal: serum creatinine level twofold or more above the upper limit of normal (≥177 μmol/l or 2 mg/dl for adults) or twofold above baseline if impairment pre-existed

Hepatic: total bilirubin, aspartate aminotransferase and/or alanine aminotransferase level twofold or more above the upper limit of normal or twofold above baseline if impairment pre-existed

Haematological: platelets ≤100 000/mm^3 and/or presence of DIC

Endovascular: presence of adult respiratory distress syndrome, diffuse capillary leak manifested by generalized oedema or pleural or peritoneal effusions with hypoalbuminaemia

Dermatological: generalized erythematous macular eruption ± desquamation

Dermatological: soft-tissue necrosis (e.g. necrotizing fasciitis, myositis, gangrene)

DIC, disseminated intravascular coagulation.

coccal TSS. Scarlatiniform eruption, conjunctival or mucous membrane hyperaemia, strawberry tongue and late desquamation are present less frequently in STSS than in staphylococcal TSS.

Treatment

Patients suspected of having STSS should be managed in an intensive-care setting, due to the rapidly progressive, fulminant nature of the syndrome. Early management consists of aggressive intravenous fluid resuscitation, culture of potential sites of infection, early surgical exploration of suspected deep-seated infections, débridement of devitalized tissue (see 'Necrotizing fasciitis') and prompt administration of antibiotics. Inotropic agents may be necessary to manage refractory shock due to toxic cardiomyopathy [435, 461]. Use of adrenaline in patients with intractable hypotension may be complicated by gangrene of digits [440].

While ruling out septic shock from Gram-negative bacilli or *S. aureus* or polymicrobial necrotizing fasciitis, broad-spectrum antimicrobial therapy should be initiated, as discussed for necrotizing fasciitis. Once a diagnosis of STSS is made, therapy can be tailored. Clindamycin has advantages over penicillin (see 'Necrotizing Fasciitis'), although many experts recommend use of both agents concurrently for treatment of STSS [76, 297, 440]. Neutralization of circulating exotoxin is appealing theoretically, but directed antibody therapy is not yet available. Simulation of this effect has been attempted with use of IVIG [318, 470], but its efficacy for treatment of STSS has not been determined.

References

1 Darmstadt GL, Marcy SM. Skin and soft tissue infections. In: Long SS, Prober CG, Pickering LK (eds) *Principles and Practice of Pediatric Infectious Disease*. Churchill Livingstone, New York, 1996: 476–517.

2 Darmstadt GL. Oral antibiotic therapy for uncomplicated bacterial skin infections in children. *Pediatr Infect Dis J* 1997; **16**:227–240.

3 Schachner L, Taplin D, Scott GB, Morrison M. A therapeutic update of superficial skin infections. *Pediatr Clin North Am* 1983; **30**: 397–404.

4 Aronoff SC, Murdell D, O'Brien CA, Klinger JD, Reed MD, Blumer JL. Efficacy and safety of ceftriaxone in serious pediatric infections. *Antimicrob Agents Chemother* 1983; **24**: 663–666.

5 Fleisher GR, Wilmott CM, Campos JM. Amoxicillin combined with clavulanic acid for the treatment of soft tissue infections in children. *Antimicrob Agents Chemother* 1983; **24**: 679–681.

6 Steele RW. Ceftriaxone therapy of meningitis and serious infections. *Am J Med* 1984; **77** (Suppl 4C): 50–53.

7 Jaffe AC, O'Brien CA, Reed MD, Blumer JL. Randomized comparative evaluation of Augmentin and cefaclor in pediatric skin and soft tissue infections. *Curr Ther Res* 1985; **38**: 160–168.

8 Ells LD, Mertz PM, Piovanetti Y, Pekoe GM, Eaglstein WH. Topical antibiotic treatment of impetigo with mupirocin. *Arch Dermatol* 1986; **122**: 1273–1276.

9 Arredondo JL. Efficacy and tolerance of topical mupirocin compared with oral dicloxacillin in the treatment of primary skin infections. *Curr Ther Res* 1987; **41**: 121–127.

10 Barton LL, Friedman AD. Impetigo: a reassessment of etiology and therapy. *Pediatr Dermatol* 1987; **4**: 185–188.

11 Coskey RJ, Coskey LA. Diagnosis and treatment of impetigo. *J Am Acad Dermatol* 1987; **17**: 62–63.

12 Rogers M, Dorman DC, Gapes M, Ly J. A three-year study of impetigo in Sydney. *Med J Aust* 1987; **147**: 63–65.

13 Goldfarb J, Crenshaw D, O'Horo J, Lemon E, Blumer JL. Randomized clinical trial of topical mupirocin versus oral erythromycin for impetigo. *Antimicrob Agents Chemother* 1988; **32**: 1780–1783.

14 Barton LL, Friedman AD, Portilla MG. Impetigo contagiosa: a comparison of erythromycin and dicloxacillin therapy. *Pediatr Dermatol* 1988; **5**: 88–91.

15 McLinn S. Topical mupirocin vs systemic erythromycin treatment for pyoderma. *Pediatr Infect Dis J* 1988; **7**: 785–790.

16 Mertz PM, Marshall DA, Eagelstein WH, Piovanetti Y, Montalvo J. Topical mupirocin treatment of impetigo is equal to oral erythromycin. *Arch Dermatol* 1989; **125**: 1069–1073.

17 Barton LL, Friedman AD, Sharkey AM, Schneller DJ, Swierkosz EM. Impetigo contagiosa III: comparative efficacy of oral erythromycin and topical mupirocin. *Pediatr Dermatol* 1989; **6**: 134–138.

18 Dagan R, Bar-David Y. Comparison of amoxicillin and clavulanic acid (Augmentin) for the treatment of nonbullous impetigo. *Am J Dis Child* 1989; **143**: 916–918.

19 Britton JW, Fajardo JE, Krafte-Jacobs B. Comparison of mupirocin and erythromycin in the treatment of impetigo. *J Pediatr* 1990; **117**: 827–829.

20 Demidovich CW, Wittler RR, Ruff ME, Bass JW, Browning WC. Impetigo: current etiology and comparison of penicillin, erythromycin, and cephalexin therapies. *Am J*

Dis Child 1990; **144**: 1313–1315.

21 Esterly NB, Nelson DB, Dunne WM. Impetigo. *Am J Dis Child* 1991; **145**: 125–126.

22 Jacobs RF, Brown WD, Chartrand S *et al.* Evaluation of cefuroxime axetil and cefadroxil suspensions for treatment of pediatric skin infections. *Antimicrob Agents Chemother* 1992; **36**: 1614–1618.

23 Hanfling MJ, Hausinger SA, Squires J. Loracarbef vs cefaclor in pediatric skin and skin structure infections. *Pediatr Infect Dis J* 1992; **11**: S27–S30.

24 Dagan R, Bar-David Y. Double-blind study comparing erythromycin and mupirocin for treatment of impetigo in children: implications of a high prevalence of erythromycin resistant *Staphylococcus* strains. *Antimicrob Agents Chemother* 1992; **36**: 287–290.

25 Rodriguez-Solares A, Perez-Gutierrez F, Prosperi J, Milgram E, Martin A. A comparative study of the efficacy, safety and tolerance of azithromycin, dicloxacillin and flucloxacillin in the treatment of children with acute skin and skin-structure infections. *J Antimicrob Chemother* 1993; **31** (Suppl E): 103–109.

26 Hebert AA, Still JG, Rueman PD. Comparative safety and efficacy of clarithromycin suspensions in the treatment of mild to moderate skin and skin structure infections in children. *Pediatr Infect Dis J* 1993; **12**: S112–S117.

27 Linder CW, Nelson K, Paryani S, Stallworth JR, Blumer JL. Comparative evaluation of cefadroxil and cephalexin in children and adolescents with pyodermas. *Clin Ther* 1993; **15**: 46–56.

28 Darmstadt GL, Lane AT. Impetigo: an overview. *Pediatr Dermatol* 1994; **11**: 293–303.

29 Lookingbill DP. Impetigo. *Pediatr Rev* 1985; **7**: 177–181.

30 Hayden GF. Skin diseases encountered in a pediatric clinic. *Am J Dis Child* 1985; **139**: 36–38.

31 Tunnessen WW. A survey of skin disorders seen in pediatric general and dermatology clinics. *Pediatr Dermatol* 1984; **1**: 219–222.

32 Leyden JJ, Kligman AM. Rationale for topical antibiotics. *Cutis* 1978; **22**: 515–528.

33 Dhar S, Kanwar AJ, Kaur S, Sharma P, Ganguly NK. Role of bacterial flora in the pathogenesis and management of atopic dermatitis. *Ind J Med Res* 1992; **95**: 234–238.

34 Leyden JJ, Marples RR, Kligman AM. *Staphylococcus aureus* in the lesions of atopic dermatitis. *Br J Dermatol* 1974; **90**: 525–530.

35 Aly R, Maibach HI, Shinefield HR. Microbial flora of atopic dermatitis. *Arch Dermatol* 1977; **113**: 780–782.

36 Powers RD, Schwartz R, Snow RM, Yarbrough DR. Ofloxacin versus cephalexin in the treatment of skin, skin structure, and soft-tissue infections in adults. *Clin Ther* 1991; **13**: 727–736.

37 Gentry LO, Ramirez-Ronda CH, Rodriguez-Noriega E, Thadepalli H, del Rosal PL, Ramirez C. Oral ciprofloxacin vs parenteral cefotaxime in the treatment of difficult skin and skin structure infections: a multicenter trial. *Arch Intern Med* 1989; **149**: 2579–2583.

38 Dominguez J, Palma F, Vega ME *et al.* Prospective, controlled, randomized non-blind comparison of intravenous/oral ciprofloxacin with intravenous ceftazidime in the treatment of skin or soft-tissue infections. *Am J Med* 1989; **87** (Suppl 5A): 136S–137S.

39 Parish LC, Jungkind DL. Systemic antimicrobial therapy in skin and skin structure infections: comparison of texafloxacin and ciprofloxacin. *Am J Med* 1991; **91** (Suppl 6A): 115S–119S.

40 Fass RJ, Plouffe JF, Russell JA. Intravenous/oral ciprofloxacin versus ceftazidime in the treatment of serious infections. *Am J Med* 1989; **87** (Suppl 5A): 164S–168S.

41 Gentry LO, Rodriguez-Gomez G, Zeluff BJ, Khoshdel A, Price M. A comparative evaluation of oral ofloxacin versus intravenous cefotaxime therapy for serious skin and skin structure infections. *Am J Med* 1989; **87** (Suppl 6C): 57S–60S.

42 Powers RD. Soft tissue infections in the emergency department: the case for the use of 'simple' antibiotics. *South Med J* 1991; **84**: 1313–1315.

43 Neldner KH. Double-blind randomized study of oral temafloxacin and cefadroxil in patients with mild to moderately severe bacterial skin infections. *Am J Med* 1991; **91** (Suppl 6A): 111S–114S.

44 Parish LC, Doyle CA, Durham SJ, Wilber RB. Cefprozil versus cefaclor in the treatment of mild to moderate skin and skin structure infections. *Clin Ther* 1992; **14**: 458–469.

45 Tack KJ, Wilks NE, Semerdijian G *et al.* Cefpodoxime proxetil in the treatment of skin and soft tissue infections. *Drugs* 1991; **42** (Suppl 3): 51–56.

46 Ballantyne F. Cefadroxil in the treatment of skin and soft tissue infections. *J Antimicrob Chemother* 1982; **10** (Suppl B): 143–147.

47 Welsh O, Saenz C. Topical mupirocin compared with oral ampicillin in the treatment of primary and secondary skin infections. *Curr Ther Res* 1987; **41**: 114–120.

48 Lipsky BA, Yarbrough DR, Walker FB, Powers RD, Morman MR. Ofloxacin versus cephalexin for treating skin and soft tissue infections. *Int J Dermatol* 1992; **311**: 443–445.

49 Schupbach CW, Olovich KG, Dere WH. Efficacy of cefaclor AF in the treatment of skin and skin-structure infections. *Clin Ther* 1992; **14**: 470–479.

50 Lentino JR, Augustinsky JB, Weber TM, Pachucki CT. Therapy of serious skin and soft tissue infections with ofloxacin administered by intravenous and oral route. *Chemotherapy* 1991; **37**: 70–76.

51 Parish LC, Aten EM. Treatment of skin and skin structure infections: a comparative study of Augmentin and cefaclor. *Cutis* 1984; **34**: 567–570.

52 Solomon E, McCarty JM, Mormon MR *et al.* Comparison of cefprozil and amoxycillin–clavulanate potassium in the treatment of skin and skin structure infections in adults. *Adv Ther* 1992; **9**: 156–165.

53 Nolen T, Conetta BJ, Durham SJ, Wilber RB. Safety and efficacy of cefprozil vs cefaclor in the treatment of mild to moderate skin and skin structure infections. *Infect Med* 1992; **9** (Suppl E): 56–67.

54 Parish LC, Witkowski JA. Ceforanide compared with cefazolin in skin and soft tissue infections. *Cutis* 1984; **33**: 313–319.

55 Brook I. Anaerobic and aerobic bacteriology of decubitus ulcers in children. *Am Surg* 1980; **46**: 624–626.

56 Brook I. Microbiological studies of decubitus ulcers in children. *J Pediatr Surg* 1991; **26**: 207–209.

57 Brook I, Finegold SM. Aerobic and anaerobic bacteriology of cutaneous abscesses in children. *Pediatrics* 1981; **67**: 891–895.

58 Brook I, Frazier EH. Aerobic and anaerobic bacteriology of wounds and cutaneous abscesses. *Arch Surg* 1990; **125**: 1445–1451.

59 Brook I. Antimicrobial therapy of skin and soft tissue infection in children. *J Am Podiatr Med Assoc* 1993; **83**: 398–405.

60 Brook I, Randolph JG. Aerobic and anaerobic bacterial flora of burns in children. *J Trauma* 1981; **21**: 313–318.

61 Martin RR, Buttram V, Besch P, Kirkland JJ, Petty GP. Nasal and vaginal *Staphylococcus aureus* in young women: quantitative studies. *Ann Intern Med* 1982; **96**: 951–953.

62 Barth JH. Nasal carriage of staphylococci and streptococci. *Int J Dermatol* 1987; **26**: 24–26.

63 Dajani AS, Ferrieri P, Wannamaker LW. Natural history of impetigo. II. Etiologic agents and bacterial interactions. *J Clin Invest* 1972; **51**: 2863–2871.

64 Ferrieri P, Dajani AS, Wannamaker LW, Chapman SS. Natural history of impetigo. I. Site sequence of acquisition and familial patterns of spread of cutaneous streptococci. *J Clin Invest* 1972; **51**: 2851–2862.

65 Dillon HC Jr. Streptococcal infections of the skin and its complications: impetigo and nephritis. In: Wannamaker LW, Masten P (eds) *Streptococci and Sreptococcal Diseases.* Academic Press, New York, 1972, pp. 571–587.

66 Roth RR, James WD. Microbiology of the skin: resident flora, ecology, infection. *J Am Acad Dermatol* 1989; **20**: 367–390.

67 Aly R, Shinefield HR, Maibach HI. *Staphylococcus aureus* adherence to nasal epithelial cells: studies of some parameters. In: Maibach H, Aly R (eds) *Skin Microbiology: Relevance to Clinical Infection.* Springer-Verlag, New York, 1981, pp. 171–179.

68 Feingold DS. Bacterial adherence, colonization and pathogenicity. *Arch Dermatol* 1986; **122**: 161–163.

69 Shinefield HR, Ribble JC, Boris M *et al.* Bacterial interference: its effect on nursery acquired infection with *Staphylococcus aureus*. Preliminary observations on artificial colonization of newborns. *Am J Dis Child* 1963; **105**: 646–654.

70 Steele RW. Recurrent staphylococcal infection in families. *Arch Dermatol* 1980; **116**: 189–190.

71 Miller SJ, Aly R, Shinefield HR, Elias PM. *In vitro* and *in vivo* antistaphylococcal activity of human stratum corneum lipids. *Arch Dermatol* 1988; **124**: 209–215.

72 Ushijima T, Takahashi M, Ozaki Y. Acetic, propionic, and oleic acid as the possible factors influencing the predominant residence of some species of *Propionibacterium* and coagulase negative *Staphylococcus* on normal human skin. *Can J Microbiol* 1984; **30**: 647–652.

73 Nickoloff BJ, Griffiths CEM, Barker JNMN. The role of adhesion molecules, chemotactic factors and cytokines in inflammatory and neoplastic skin disease— 1990 update. *J Invest Dermatol* 1990; **94**: 151S–157S.

74 Jacks-Weis J, Kim Y, Cleary P. Restricted deposition of C3 on M+ group A streptococci: correlation with resistance to phagocytosis. *J Immunol* 1982; **128**: 1897–1902.

75 Cleary P, Prabu U, Dale J, Wexler D, Handley J. Streptococcal C5a peptidase is a highly specific endopeptidase. *Infect Immun* 1992; **60**: 5219–5223.

76 Bisno AL, Stevens DL. Streptococcal infections of skin and soft tissues. *N Engl J Med* 1996; **334**: 240–245.

77 Stevens DL, Tanner MH, Winship J *et al.* Severe group A streptococcal infections associated with a toxic shock-like syndrome and scarlet fever toxin. *N Engl J Med* 1989; **321**: 1–8.

78 Stevens DL. Invasive group A streptococcal infections: the past, present and future. *Pediatr Infect Dis J* 1994; **13**: 561–566.

79 Talkington DF, Schwartz B, Black CM *et al.* Association of phenotypic and genotypic characteristics of invasive *Streptococcus pyogenes* isolates with clinical components of streptococcal toxic shock syndrome. *Infect Immun* 1993; **61**: 3369–3374.

80 Todd J, Roberson S, Roe M. Relationship of protease production to invasiveness of *Staphylococcus aureus* strains, abstr 275, 1991. In: *Program Abstract 31st Interscience Conference Antimicrobial Agents Chemotherapy.* American Socitey of Microbiology, Washington, DC.

81 Stamenkovic I, Lew PD. Early recognition of potentially fatal necrotizing fasciitis. *N Engl J Med* 1972; **310**: 1689–1693.

82 Barker FG, Leppard BJ, Seal DV. Streptococcal necrotizing fasciitis: comparison between histological and clinical features. *J Clin Pathol* 1987; **40**: 335–341.

83 Umbert IJ, Winkelmann RK, Oliver GF, Peters MS. Necrotizing fasciitis: a clinical, microbiologic, and histopathologic study of 14 patients. *J Am Acad Dermatol* 1989; **20**: 774–781.

84 Bryant AE, Kehoe MA, Stevens DL. Streptococcal pyrogenic exotoxin A and streptolysin O enhance PMNL binding to protein matrixes. *J Infect Dis* 1992; **166**: 165–169.

85 Brook I. The role of encapsulated anaerobic bacteria in synergistic infections. *FEMS*

Microbiol Rev 1994; **13**: 65–74.

86 Meislin HW, Lerner SA, Graves MH *et al*. Cutaneous abscesses: anaerobic and aerobic bacteriology and outpatient management. *Ann Intern Med* 1977; **87**: 145–149.

87 Ghoneim ATM, McGoldrick J, Blick PWH, Flowers MW, Marsden AK, Wilson DH. Aerobic and anaerobic bacteriology of subcutaneous abscesses. *Br J Surg* 1981; **68**: 498–500.

88 Brewer GE, Meleney FL. Progressive gangrenous infection of the skin and subcutaneous tissues, following operation for acute perforative appendicitis: a study of symbiosis. *Ann Surg* 1926; **84**: 438–450.

89 Stevens DL. Invasive group A streptococcus infections. *Clin Infect Dis* 1992; **14**: 2–13.

90 Giuliano A, Lewis F, Hadley K, Blaisdell FW. Bacteriology of necrotizing fasciitis. *Am J Surg* 1977; **134**: 52–56.

91 Brook I, Frazier EH. Clinical and microbiological features of necrotizing fasciitis. *J Clin Microbiol* 1995; **33**: 2382–2387.

92 Seal DV, Kingston D. Streptococcal necrotizing fasciits: development of an animal model to study its pathogenesis. *Br J Exp Pathol* 1988; **69**: 813–831.

93 Kingston D, Seal DV. Current hypotheses on synergistic microbial gangrene. *Br J Surg* 1990; **77**: 260–264.

94 Brook I. Encapsulated anaerobic bacteria in synergistic infections. *Microbiol Rev* 1986; **50**: 452–457.

95 Roberts DS. Synergistic mechanisms in certain mixed infections. *J Infect Dis* 1969; **120**: 720–724.

96 Lee PC, Turnidge J, McDonald PJ. Fine-needle aspiration biopsy in diagnosis of soft tissue infections. *J Clin Microbiol* 1985; **22**: 80–83.

97 Dillon HC, Reeves MSA. Streptococcal immune responses in nephritis after skin infection. *Am J Med* 1974; **56**: 333–346.

98 Blumer JL, O'Brien CA, Lemon E, Capretta TM. Skin and soft tissue infections: pharmacologic approaches. *Pediatr Infect Dis J* 1985; **4**: 336–341.

99 Blumer JL, Lemon E, O'Horo J, Snodgrass DJ. Changing therapy for skin and soft tissue infections in children: have we come full circle? *Pediatr Infect Dis J* 1987; **6**: 117–122.

100 Nakae M, Murai T, Kaneko Y, Mitsuhashi S. Drug resistance in *Streptococcus pyogenes* isolated in Japan (1974–1975). *Antimicrob Agents Chemother* 1977; **12**: 427–428.

101 Maruyama S, Yoshioka H, Fujita K, Takimoto M, Satake Y. Sensitivity of group A streptococci to antibiotics. *Am J Dis Child* 1979; **133**: 1143–1145.

102 Miyamoto Y, Takizawa K, Matsushima A, Asai Y, Nakatsuka S. Stepwise acquisition of multiple drug resistance by beta-hemolytic streptococci and difference in resistance patterns by type. *Antimicrob Agents Chemother* 1978; **31**: 399–404.

103 Holmstrom L, Nyman B, Rosengren M *et al*. Outbreaks of infections with erythromycin-resistant group A streptococci in child care centers. *Scand J Infect Dis* 1990; **22**: 179–185.

104 Warren RE, Haines D, Walpole E *et al*. Erythromycin-resistant *Streptococcus pneumoniae. Lancet* 1988; **ii**: 1432–1433.

105 Seppala H, Nissinen A, Jarvinen H *et al*. Resistance to erythromycin in group A streptococci. *N Engl J Med* 1992; **326**: 292–297.

106 Gerber MA. Antibiotic resistance in group A streptococci. *Pediatr Clin North Am* 1995; **42**: 539–551.

107 Coonan KM, Kaplan EL. *In vitro* susceptibility of recent North American group A streptococcal isolates to eleven oral antibiotics. *Pediatr Infect Dis J* 1994; **13**: 630–635.

108 Eagle H. Experimental approach to the problem of treatment failure with penicillin. 1. Group A streptococcal infection in mice. *Am J Med* 1952; **13**: 389–399.

109 Stevens DL, Gibbons AE, Bergstrom R, Winn V. The Eagle effect revisited: efficacy of clindamycin, erythromycin, and penicillin in the treatment of streptococcal myositis. *J Infect Dis* 1988; **158**: 23–28.

110 Stevens DL, Yan S, Bryant AE. Penicillin-binding protein expression at different growth stages determines penicillin efficacy *in vitro* and *in vivo*: an explanation for the inoculum effect. *J Infect Dis* 1993; **167**: 1401–1405.

111 Brook I. Inoculum effect. *Rev Infect Dis* 1989; **11**: 361–368.

112 Dillon HC. Topical and systemic therapy for pyodermas. *Int J Dermatol* 1980; **19**: 443–451.

113 Moreira BM, Daum RS. Antimicrobial resistance in staphylococci. *Pediatr Clin North Am* 1995; **42**: 619–648.

114 Akiyama H, Yamada T, Simoe K, Kanzaki H, Arata J. Characteristic and susceptibilities to antimicrobial agents of *Staphylococcus aureus* isolates isolated in dermatology. *Chemotherapy (Japan)* 1990; **38**: 9–20.

115 Nishijima S, Namura S, Mitsuya K, Asada Y. The incidence of isolation of methicillin-resistant *Staphylococcus aureus* (MRSA) strains from skin infections during the past three years (1989–1991). *J Dermatol* 1993; **20**: 193–197.

116 Rahman M, Noble WC, Cookson B. Mupirocin-resistant *Staphylococcus aureus*. Lancet 1987; **ii**: 387.

117 Baird D, Coia J. Mupirocin-resistant *Staphylococcus aureus*. Lancet 1987; **ii**: 387–388.

118 Cookson BD. Mupirocin resistance in staphylococci. *J Antimicrob Chemother* 1990; **25**: 497–503.

119 Smith GE, Kennedy CTC. *Staphylococcus aureus* resistant to mupirocin. *J Antimicrob Chemother* 1988; **21**: 141–142.

120 Rahman M, Noble WC, Cookson B. Transmissible mupirocin resistance in *Staphylococcus aureus*. *Epidemiol Infect* 1989; **102**: 261–270.

121 Moy JA, Caldwell-Brown D, Lin AN, Pappa KA, Carter DM. Mupirocin-resistant *Staphylococcus aureus* after long term treatments of patients with epidermolysis bullosa. *J Am Acad Dermatol* 1990; **22**: 893–895.

122 Connolly S, Noble WC, Phillips I. Mupirocin resistance in coagulase-negative staphylococci. *J Med Microbiol* 1993; **39**: 450–453.

123 Naguib MH, Naguib MT, Flournoy DJ. Mupirocin resistance in methicillin-resistant *Staphylococcus aureus* from a veterans hospital. *Chemotherapy* 1993; **39**: 400–404.

124 Eady EA, Cove JH. Topical antibiotic therapy: current status and future prospects. *Drugs Exp Clin Res* 1990; **26**: 423–433.

125 Bradley SF, Ramsey MA, Morton TM, Kauffman CA. Mupirocin resistance: clinical and molecular epidemiology. *Infect Control Hosp Epidemiol* 1995; **16**: 354–358.

126 Redhead RJ, Lamb YJ, Rowsell RB. The efficacy of calcium mupirocin in the eradication of nasal *Staphylococcus aureus* carriage. *Br J Clin Pract* 1991; **45**: 252–254.

127 Hill RL, Duckworth GJ, Casewell MW. Elimination of nasal carriage of methicillin-resistant *Staphylococcus aureus* with mupirocin during an outbreak. *J Antimicrob Chemother* 1988; **22**: 377–384.

128 Maple PA, Hamilton-Miller JM, Brumfitt W. Comparison of the *in vitro* activities of the topical antimicrobials azelaic acid, nitrofurazone, silver sulphadiazine, and mupirocin against methicillin-resistant *Staphylococcus aureus*. *J Antimicrob Chemother* 1992; **29**: 661–668.

129 Kauffman CA, Terpenning MS, Xiaogong H *et al*. Attempt to eradicate methicillin-resistant *Staphylococcus aureus* from a long-term-care facility with the use of mupirocin ointment. *Am J Med* 1993; **94**: 371–378.

130 Cookson BD, Lacey RW, Noble WC, Reeves DS, Wise R, Redhead RJ. Mupirocin-resistant *Staphylococcus aureus*. Lancet 1990; **335**: 1095–1096.

131 Klempner MS, Styrt B. Prevention of recurrent staphylococcal skin infections with low-dose oral clindamycin therapy. *JAMA* 1988; **260**: 2682–2685.

132 Ruby RJ, Nelson JD. The influence of hexachlorophene scrubs on the response to placebo or penicillin therapy in impetigo. *Pediatrics* 1973; **52**: 854–859.

133 Derrick CW, Dillon HC Jr. Further studies on the treatment of streptococcal skin infection. *J Pediatr* 1970; **77**: 696–700.

134 Tunnessen WW Jr. Practical aspects of bacterial skin infections in children. *Pediatr Dermatol* 1985; **2**: 255–265.

135 Ward A, Campoli-Richards DM. Mupirocin: a review of its antibacterial activity, pharmacokinetic properties, and therapeutic use. *Drugs* 1986; **32**: 425–444.

136 Ruff ME, Schotik DA, Bass JW, Vincent JM. Antimicrobial drug suspensions: a blind comparison of taste of fourteen common pediatric drugs. *Pediatr Infect Dis J* 1991; **10**: 30–33.

137 Rodriguez WJ, Wiedermann BL. The role of newer oral cephalosporins, fluoroquinolones, and macrolides in the treatment of pediatric infections. *Adv Pediatr Infect Dis* 1994; **9**: 125–159.

138 Anderson JA. Cross-sensitivity to cephalosporins in patients allergic to penicillin. *Pediatr Infect Dis J* 1986; **5**: 557–561.

139 Levine LR. Quantitative comparison of adverse reactions to cefaclor vs amoxycillin in a surveillance study. *Pediatr Infect Dis J* 1985; **4**: 358–361.

140 Quintiliani R, Nightingale CH, Freeman CD. Pharmacokinetic and pharmacodynamic considerations in antibiotic selection, with particular attention to oral cephalosporins. *Infect Dis Clin Pract* 1995; **4** (Suppl 2): S58–S63.

141 Gerber AU. Impact of the antibiotic dosage schedule on efficacy in experimental soft tissue infections. *Scand J Infect Dis Suppl* 1991; **74**: 147–154.

142 Derrick CW, Reilly K. The role of cephalexin in the treatment of skin and soft tissue infections. *Postgrad Med J* 1983; **59** (Suppl 5): 43–46.

143 DiMattia AF, Sexton MJ, Smialowicz CR *et al.* Efficacy of two dosage schedules of cephalexin in dermatologic infections. *J Fam Pract* 1981; **12**: 649–652.

144 Dillon HC Jr. Treatment of staphylococcal skin infections: a comparison of cephalexin and dicloxacillin. *J Am Acad Dermatol* 1983; **8**: 177–181.

145 Jones RN, Barry AL. BMY-28100, a new oral cephalosporin: antimicrobial activity against nearly 7000 recent clinical isolates, comparative potency with other oral agents, and activity against beta-lactamase producing isolates. *Diagn Microbiol Infect Dis* 1988; **9**: 11–26.

146 Ritchie DJ, Hopefl AW, Milligan TW, Bryne JE, Maddux MS. *In vitro* activity of clarithromycin, cefprozil, and other common oral antimicrobial agents against Gram-positive and Gram-negative pathogens. *Clin Ther* 1993; **15**: 107–113.

147 Goldfarb J. New antimicrobial agents. *Pediatr Clin North Am* 1995; **42**: 717–735.

148 Heckert SR, Stryker WS, Collin KL, Manson JE, Platt R. Serum sickness in children after antibiotic exposure: estimates of occurrence and morbidity in a health maintenance organization population. *Am J Epidemiol* 1990; **132**: 336–342.

149 Wise R. The pharmacokinetics of the oral cephalosporins—a review. *J Antimicrob Chemother* 1990; **26** (Suppl E): 13–20.

150 Brogden RN, McTavish D. Loracarbef: a review of its antimicrobial activity, pharmacokinetic properties and therapeutic efficacy. *Drugs* 1993; **45**: 716–736.

151 Doern G. *In vitro* activity of loracarbef and effects of susceptibility test methods. *Am J Med* 1992; **92** (Suppl 6A): 7S–15S.

152 Stamos JK, Yogev R. Oral cephalosporins: the newest of the new. *Contemp Pediatr* 1993; 10(5): 28–51.

153 Neu HC. Oral β-lactam antibiotics from 1960 to 1994. *Infect Dis Clin Pract* 1995; **4** (Suppl 2): S39–S49.

154 Rodvold KA, Piscitelli SC. New oral macrolides and fluoroquinolone antibiotics: an overview of pharmacokinetics, interactions and safety. *Clin Infect Dis* 1993; **17** (Suppl 1): S192–S199.

155 Williams JD, Sefton AM. Comparison of macrolide antibiotics. *J Antimicrob Chemother* 1993; **31** (Suppl C): 11–26.

156 Hoover WW, Barrett MS, Jones RN. Clarithromycin *in vitro* activity enhanced by its major metabolite, 14-hydroxyclarithromycin. *Diagn Microbiol Infect Dis* 1992; **15** 259–266.

157 Ishiguro M, Koga H, Kohno S *et al.* Penetration of macrolides into human polymorphonuclear leucocytes. *J Antimicrob Chemother* 1989; **24**: 719–729.

158 Craft JC, Siepman N. Overview of the safety profile of clarithromycin suspension in

pediatric patients. *Pediatr Infect Dis J* 1993; **12**: S142–S147.

159 Foulds G, Shepard RM, Johnson RB. The pharmacokinetics of azithromycin in human serum and tissues. *J Antimicrob Chemother* 1990; **25** (Suppl A): 73–82.

160 McDonald PJ, Pruul H. Phagocyte uptake and transport of azithromycin. *Eur J Clin Microbiol Infect Dis* 1991; **10**: 828–833.

161 Hopkins SJ. Clinical toleration and safety of azithromycin. *Am J Med* 1991; **91** (Suppl 3A): 40S–55S.

162 Hopkins SJ. Clinical toleration and safety of azithromycin in adults and children. *Rev Contemp Pharmacother* 1994; **5**: 383–389.

163 Hopkins SJ, Williams D. Clinical tolerability and safety of azithromycin in children. *Pediatr Infect Dis J* 1995; **14**: S67–S71.

164 Hopkins S. Clinical safety and tolerance of azithromycin in children. *J Antimicrob Chemother* 1993; **31** (Suppl E): 111–117.

165 Bauernfeind A. *In-vitro* activity of dirithromycin in comparison with other new and established macrolides. *J Antimicrob Chemother* 1993; **31** (Suppl C): 39–49.

166 Lieberman JM. Bacterial resistance in the '90s. *Contemp Pediatr* 1994; **11**: 72–99.

167 Rice TD, Duggan AK, DeAngelis C. Cost effectiveness of erythromycin versus mupirocin for the treatment of impetigo in children. *Pediatrics* 1992; **89**: 210–214.

168 Dillon HC. Impetigo contagiosa: suppurative and non-suppurative complications. *Am J Dis Child* 1968; **115**: 530–541.

169 Nelson KE, Bisno AL, Waytz P *et al*. The epidemiology and natural history of streptococcal pyoderma: an endemic disease of rural southern United States. *Am J Epidemiol* 1976; **103**; 270–283.

170 Dagan R. Impetigo in childhood: changing epidemiology and new treatments. *Pediatr Ann* 1993; **22**: 235–240.

171 Dajani AS, Hill PL, Wannamaker LW. Experimental infection of the skin in the hamster simulating human impetigo. II. Assessment of various therapeutic regimens. *Pediatrics* 1971; **48**: 83–90.

172 Dillon HC Jr. The treatment of streptococcal skin infections. *J Pediatr* 1970; **76**: 676–684.

173 Dajani AS, Wannamaker LW. Demonstration of a bactericidal substance against beta-hemolytic streptococci in supernatant fluids of streptococcal cultures. *J Bacteriol* 1969; **97**: 985–991.

174 Blumberg RW, Feldman DB. Observations on acute glomerulonephritis associated with impetigo. *J Pediatr* 1962; **60**: 677–685.

175 Maddox JS, Ware JC, Dillon HC Jr. The natural history of streptococcal skin infection: prevention with topical antibiotics. *J Am Acad Dermatol* 1985; **13**: 207–212.

176 Wannamaker LW. Differences between streptococcal infections of the throat and of the skin. *N Engl J Med* 1970; **282**: 23–30.

177 Melish ME, Glasgow LA. Staphylococcal scalded skin syndrome: the expanded clinical syndrome. *J Pediatr* 1971; **78**: 958–967.

178 Elias PM, Levy W. Bullous impetigo: occurrence of localized scalded skin syndrome in an adult. *Arch Dermatol* 1976; **112**: 856–858.

179 Burnett JW. Management of pyogenic cutaneous infections. *N Engl J Med* 1962; **266**: 164–169.

180 Maibach H. Soft tissue infections. In *Oral Antibiotics in Dermatology. Proceedings of the 17th Hawaii Dermatology Seminar*, 1993, pp. 3–6.

181 Baraff LJ, Fine RN, Knutson DW. Poststreptococcal acute glomerulonephritis: fact and controversy. *Ann Intern Med* 1979; **91**: 76–86.

182 Lewy JE, Salinas-Madrigal L, Herdson PB, Perani CL, Metcoff J. Clinico-pathologic correlations in acute poststreptococcal glomerulonephritis. *Medicine* 1971; **50**: 453–501.

183 Travis LB, Dodge WG, Beathard GA *et al*. Acute glomerulonephritis in children: a review of the natural history with emphasis on prognosis. *Clin Nephrol* 1973; **1**: 169–181.

184 Sanjad S, Tolaymat A, Whitworth J, Levin S. Acute glomerulonephritis in children: a review of 153 cases. *South Med J* 1977; **70**: 1202–1206.

185 Tejani A, Ingulli E. Poststreptococcal glomerulonephritis: current clinical and pathologic concepts. *Nephron* 1990; **55**: 1–5.

186 Sagel , Treser G, Ty A, Yoshizawa N *et al.* Occurrence and nature of glomerular lesions after group A streptococci infections in children. *Ann Intern Med* 1973; **79**: 492–499.

187 Anthony BF, Kaplan EL, Wannamaker LW, Briese FW, Chapman SS. Attack rates of acute nephritis after type 49 streptococcal infection of the skin and of the respiratory tract. *J Clin Invest* 1969; **48**: 1697–1704.

188 Lever WF, Schaumburg-Lever G. Bacterial disease. In: Lever WF, Schaumburg-Lever G (eds) *Histopathology of the Skin*, 7th edn. JB Lippincott, Philadelphia, 1990, pp. 318–351.

189 Kaplan EL, Wannamaker LW. Suppression of the antistreptolysin O response by cholesterol and by lipid extracts of rabbit skin. *J Exp Med* 1976; **144**: 754–767.

190 Ortiz JS, Finklea JF, Potter EV, Poon-King T, Ali D, Earle DP. Endemic nephritis and streptococcal infections in South Trinidad: surveillance studies during the first year following a major epidemic. *Arch Intern Med* 1970; **126**: 640–646.

191 El-Kholy A, Hafez K, Krause RM. Specificity and sensitivity of the streptozyme test for the detection of streptococcal antibodies. *Appl Microbiol* 1974; **27**: 748–752.

192 Klein GC, Jones WL. Comparison of the streptozyme test with the antistreptolysin O, antideoxyribonuclease B, and antihyaluronidase tests. *Appl Microbiol* 1971; **21**: 257–259.

193 Dancer SJ, Noble WC. Nasal, axillary, and perineal carriage of *Staphylococcus aureus* among women: identification of strains producing epidermolytic toxin. *J Clin Pathol* 1991; **44**: 681–684.

194 Doebbeling BN, Breneman DL, Neu HC *et al.* Elimination of *Staphylococcus aureus* nasal carriage in health care workers: analysis of six clinical trials with calcium mupirocin ointment. *Clin Infect Dis* 1993; **17**: 466–474.

195 Martin RR, White A. The reacquisition of staphylococci by treated carriers: a demonstration of bacterial interference. *J Lab Clin Med* 1968; **71**: 791–797.

196 Mulligan ME, Murray-Leisure KA, Ribner BS *et al.* Methicillin-resistant *Staphylococcus aureus*: a consensus review of the microbiology, pathogenesis, and epidemiology with implications for prevention and management. *Am J Med* 1993; **94**: 313–328.

197 Hall WD, Blumberg RW, Moody MD. Studies in children with impetigo: bacteriology, serology, and incidence of glomerulonephritis. *Am J Dis Child* 1973; **125**: 800–806.

198 Kelly C, Taplin D, Allen AM. Streptococcal ecthyma. *Arch Dermatol* 1971; **103**: 306.

199 Livingood CS, Perry OJ, Forrester JS. Cutaneous diphtheria: a report of 140 cases. *J Invest Dermatol* 1946; **7**: 341–364.

200 Riddell GS. Cutaneous diphtheria: epidemiological and dermatological aspects of 365 cases amongst British prisoners of war in the Far East. *J Roy Army Med Corps* 1950; **95**: 64–87.

201 Harnish JP, Tronca E, Nolan CM, Turck M, Holmes KK. Diphtheria among alcoholic urban adults: a decade of experience in Seattle. *Ann Intern Med* 1989; **111**: 71–82.

202 Bodey GP. Dermatologic manifestations of infections in neutropenic patients. *Infect Dis Clin North Am* 1994; **8**: 655–675.

203 Brown CS, Kligman AM. Mycosis-like pyoderma. *Arch Dermatol* 1957; **75**: 123–125.

204 Brunsting LA, Underwood LJ. Pyoderma vegetans in association with chronic ulcerative colitis. *Arch Dermatol* 1979; **60**: 161–172.

205 Stone OJ. Hyperinflammatory proliferative (blastomycosis-like) pyodermas: review, mechanisms and therapy. *J Dermatol Surg Oncol* 1986; **12**: 271–273.

206 Welch KJ, Burke WA, Park HK. Pyoderma vegetans: association with diffuse T-cell

lymphoma (large cell type). *J Am Acad Dermatol* 1989; **20**: 691–693.

207 Becker BA, Frieden IJ, Odom RB, Berger TG. Atypical plaquelike staphylococcal folliculitis in human immunodeficiency virus-infected persons. *J Am Acad Dermatol* 1989; **21**: 1024–1026.

208 Hays GC, Mullard JE. Blistering distal dactylitis: a clinically recognizable streptococcal infection. *Pediatrics* 1975; **56**: 129–131.

209 Schneider JA, Parlette HL. Blistering distal dactylitis: a manifestation of group A β-hemolytic streptococcal infection. *Arch Dermatol* 1983; **118**: 879–880.

210 Norcross MC, Mitchell DF. Blistering distal dactylitis caused by *Staphylococcus aureus*. *Cutis* 1993; **51**: 353–354.

211 Montemarano AD, James WD. *Staphylococcus aureus* as a cause of perianal dermatitis. *Pediatr Dermatol* 1993; **10**: 259–262.

212 Richman DD, Breton SJ, Goldmann DA. Scarlet fever and group A streptococcal surgical wound infection traced to an anal carrier. *J Pediatr* 1977; **90**: 387–390.

213 Schaffner W, Lefkowitz LB, Goodman JS *et al.* Hospital outbreak of infections with group A streptococci traced to an asymptomatic anal carrier. *N Engl J Med* 1969; **280**: 1224–1225.

214 Asnes RS, Vail D, Grebin B, Sprunt K. Anal carrier rate of group A beta-hemolytic streptococci pharyngitis. *Pediatrics* 1973; **52**: 438–441.

215 Kokx NP, Comstock JA, Facklam RR. Streptococcal perianal disease in children. *Pediatrics* 1987; **80**: 659–663.

216 Amren DP, Anderson AS, Wannamaker LW. Perianal cellulitis associated with group A streptococci. *Am J Dis Child* 1966; **112**: 546–552.

217 Krol AL. Perianal streptococcal dermatitis. *Pediatr Dermatol* 1990; **7**: 97–100.

218 Spear RM, Rothbaum RJ, Keating JP, Blaufuss MC, Rosenblum JL. Perianal streptococcal cellulitis. *J Pediatr* 1985; **107**: 557–559.

219 Schwartz RH, Wientzen RL, Barsanti RG. Vulvovaginitis in prepubertal girls: the importance of Group A streptococcus. *South Med J* 1982; **75**: 446–447.

220 Rehder PA, Eliezer ET, Lane AT. Perianal cellulitis: cutaneous group A streptococcal disease. *Arch Dermatol* 1988; **124**: 702–704.

221 Smolin G, Okumoto M. Staphylococcal blepharitis. *Arch Ophthalmol* 1977; **95**: 812.

222 Friedlander MH, Masi RJ, Osumoto M. Ocular microbial microflora in immunodeficient patients. *Arch Ophthalmol* 1980; **98**: 1211–1213.

223 Valenton MJ, Okumoto M. Toxin-producing strains of *Staphylococcus epidermidis* (albus): isolates from patients with staphylococcal blepharoconjuctivitis. *Arch Ophthalmol* 1973; **89**: 186–189.

224 Stone L, Codere F, Ma SA. Streptococcal lid necrosis in previously healthy children. *Can J Ophthalmol* 1991; **26**: 386–390.

225 Hurwitz JJ, Rodgers KJA. Managment of acquired dacryocystitis. *Can J Ophthalmol* 1983; **18**: 213–216.

226 Kontiainen S, Rinne E. Bacteria isolated from skin and soft tissue lesions. *Eur J Clin Microbiol* 1987; **6**: 420–422.

227 Brook I. Bacteriologic study of paronychia in children. *Am J Surg* 1981; **141**: 703–705.

228 Dyk T, Kuriata D. Lethal septic shock in a 20-year-old girl following extrusion of a furuncle of the nape. *Wiad Lek* 1976; **29**: 1571–1574.

229 Alekseev VN, Leshchenko AP, Bytotov AA. Furuncle of the upper lip complicated by thrombosis of the cavernous sinus and septic pneumonia. *Vestn Khir* 1979; **122**: 43–44.

230 Strauss WB, Maibach HI, Shinefield HR. Bacterial interference treatment of recurrent furunculosis. *JAMA* 1969; **208**: 861–863.

231 Ebling FJG. Hidradenitis suppurativa: an androgen-dependent disorder. *Br J Dermatol* 1986; **115**: 259–262.

232 Maibach H, Kligman A. Multiple sweat gland abscesses of infants. *JAMA* 1960; **174**: 140–142.

233 Brook I. Aerobic and anaerobic microbiology of paronychia. *Ann Emerg Med* 1990; **19**: 994–996.

234 Brook I, Calhoun L, Yocum P. Beta-lactamase-producing isolates of *Bacteroides* species from children. *Antimicrob Agents Chemother* 1980; **18**: 164–166.

235 Walsh M, McIntosh K. Neonatal mastitis. *Clin Pediatr* 1986; **25**: 395–399.

236 Bailey LA. *Pseudomonas aeruginosa* mastitis in a neonate. *Pediatr Infect Dis J* 1993; **12**: 104.

237 Rodoy RC, Nelson JD. Breast abscess during the neonatal period. *Am J Dis Child* 1975; **129**: 1031–1034.

238 Nelson JD. Suppurative mastitis in infants. *Am J Dis Child* 1973; **125**: 458–459.

239 Brook I. The aerobic and anaerobic microbiology of neonatal breast abscess. *Pediatr Infect Dis J* 1991; **10**: 785–786.

240 Parmelee AH. *Management of the Newborn*. Year Book Medical Publishers, Chicago, 1952, p. 247.

241 Enberg RN, Cox RH, Burry VF. Perirectal abscess in children. *Am J Dis Child* 1974; **128**: 360–361.

242 Kreiger RW, Chusid MJ. Perirectal abscess in childhood: review of 29 cases. *Am J Dis Child* 1979; **133**: 411–412.

243 Brook I, Martin WJ. Aerobic and anaerobic bacteriology of perirectal abscess in children. *Pediatrics* 1980; **66**: 282–284.

244 Arditi M, Yoger R. Perirectal abscess in infants and children: report of 52 cases and review of the literature. *Rev Infect Dis* 1990; **9**: 411–415.

245 Glenn J, Cotton D, Westley R, Pizzo P. Anorectal infections in patients with malignant disease. *Rev Infect Dis* 1988; **10**: 42–52

246 Grant CS, Al-Salem AH, Anim JT *et al.* Childhood fistula-in-ano: a clincopathological study. *Pediatr Surg Int* 1991; **6**: 207–209

247 Longo WE, Touloukian RJ, Seashore JN. Fistula in ano in infants and children: implications and management. *Pediatrics* 1991; **87**: 737–739.

248 Piazza DJ, Radhakrishnan J. Perianal abscess and fistula-in-ano in children. *Dis Colon Rectum* 1990; **33**: 1014–1016.

249 Cordero L, Anderson CW, Zuspan FP. Scalp abscess: a benign and infrequent complication of fetal monitoring. *Am J Obstetr Gynecol* 1983; **146**: 126–130.

250 Wagener MM, Rycheck RR, Yee RB, McVay JF, Buffenmyer CL, Harger JH. Septic dermatitis of the neonatal scalp and maternal endomyometritis with intrapartum internal fetal monitoring. *Pediatrics* 1984; **74**: 81–85.

251 Okada DM, Chow AW, Bruce VT. Neonatal scalp abscess and fetal monitoring: factors associated with infection. *Am J Obstetr Gynecol* 1977; **129**: 185–189.

252 Plavidal FJ, Werch A. Fetal scalp abscess secondary to intrauterine monitoring. *Am J Obstetr Gynecol* 1976; **125**: 65–70.

253 Cordero L, Hon EH. Scalp abscess: a rare complication of fetal monitoring. *J Pediatr* 1971; **78**: 533–537.

254 Hutchins CJ. Scalp infection after fetal monitoring in labour. *NZ Med J* 1978; **87**: 390–392.

255 Brook I, Frazier EH. Microbiology of scalp abscess in newborns. *Pediatr Infect Dis J* 1992; **11**: 766–768.

256 Thadepalli H, Chan WH, Maidman JE *et al.* Microflora of the cervix during normal labor and the puerperium. *J Infect Dis* 1978; **137**: 468–472.

257 Turbeville DF, Heath RE Jr, Bowen FW Jr, Killiam AP. Complications of fetal scalp electrodes: a case report. *Am J Obstetr Gynecol* 1975; **122**: 530–531.

258 Golden SM, Merenstein GB, Todd WA *et al.* Disseminated herpes simplex neonatorum: a complication of fetal monitoring. *Am J Obstetr Gynecol* 1977; **123**: 917–918.

259 Leake D, Leake R. Neonatal suppurative parotitis. *Pediatrics* 1970; **46**: 203–207.

260 Brook I. Diagnosis and management of parotitis. *Arch Otolaryngol Head Neck Surg* 1992; **118**: 469–471.

261 Kaban LB, Mulliken JB, Murray JE. Sialadenitis in childhood. *Am J Surg* 1978; **135**: 570–576.

262 Myer C, Cotton RT. Salivary gland disease in children: a review. *Clin Pediatr* 1986; **25**: 314–322.

263 Carlson RG, Glas WW. Acute suppurative parotitis: twenty-eight cases in a county hospital. *Arch Surg* 1963; **86**: 659–663.

264 David RB, O'Connell EJ. Suppurative parotitis in childhood. *Am J Dis Child* 1970; **119**: 332–335.

265 Brook I, Frazier EH, Thompson DH. Aerobic and anaerobic microbiology of acute suppurative parotitis. *Laryngoscope* 1991; **101**: 170–172.

266 Marcy SM. Infection of the salivary glands (sialadenitis). In: Kaplan SL (ed.) *Current Therapy in Pediatric Infectious Disease*, 3rd edn. Mosby Year Book, St Louis, 1993, pp. 28–29.

267 Mehregan DA, Su WPD, Anhalt JP. Cutaneous botryomycosis. *J Am Acad Dermatol* 1991; **24**: 393–396.

268 Winslow DJ. Botryomycosis. *Am J Pathol* 1959; **35**: 153–167.

269 Buescher ES, Hebert A, Rapini RP. Staphylococcal botryomycosis in a patient with hyperimmunoglobulin-E-recurrent infection (Job's) syndrome. *Pediatr Infect Dis J* 1988; **7**: 431–433.

270 Patterson JW, Kitces EN, Neafie RC. Cutaneous botryomycosis in a patient with acquired immunodeficiency syndrome. *J Am Acad Dermatol* 1987; **16**: 238–242.

271 Brunken RC, Lichon-Chao N, Van den Broek H. Immunologic abnormalities in botryomycosis. *J Am Acad Dermatol* 1983; **9**: 428–434.

272 Magrou J. Les formes actinomycotiques du staphylocoque. *Ann Inst Pasteur* 1919; **33**: 344–374.

273 Picou K, Batres E, Jarratt M. Botryomycosis: a bacterial cause of mycetoma. *Arch Dermatol* 1979; **115**: 609–610.

274 Hacker P. Botryomycosis. *Int J Dermatol* 1983; **22**: 455–458.

275 Brown MD, Headington JT. Solitary plaque on the foot (botryomycosis). *Arch Dermatol* 1990; **126**: 815–818.

276 Leffell DJ, Brown MD, Swanson NA. Laser vaporization: a novel treatment of botryomycosis. *J Dermatol Surg Oncol* 1989; **15**: 703–705.

277 Asmar BI, Bashour BN, Fleischmann LE. *Escherichia coli* cellulitis in children with idiopathic nephrotic syndrome. *Clin Pediatr* 1987; **26**: 592–594.

278 Vadheim CM, Greengerg DP, March SM, Froeschle J, Ward JI. Safety evaluation of PRP-D *Haemophilus influenzae* type b conjugate vaccine in children immunized at 18 months of age and older: follow-up study of 30 000 children. *Pediatr Infect Dis J* 1990; **9**: 555–561.

279 Dagan R, Englehard D, Piccard E, Israeli Pediatric Bacteremia and Meningitis Group. Epidemiology of invasive childhood pneumococcal infections in Israel. *JAMA* 1992; **268**: 3328–3332.

280 Baker RC, Bausher JC. Meningitis complicating acute bacteremic facial cellulitis. *Pediatr Infect Dis J* 1986; **5**: 421–423.

281 Carter S, Feldman WE. Etiology and treatment of facial cellulitis in pediatric patients. *Pediatr Infect Dis J* 1983; **2**: 222–224.

282 Chandler JR, Langenbrunner DJ, Stevens ER. The pathogenesis of orbital complications in acute sinusitis. *Laryngoscope* 1970; **80**: 1414–1428.

283 Baddour LM, Bisno AL. Recurrent cellulitis after saphenous venectomy for coronary artery bypass surgery. *Ann Intern Med* 1982; **97**: 493–496.

284 Hook EW III, Hooton TM, Horton CA *et al*. Microbiologic evaluation of cutaneous cellulitis in adults. *Arch Intern Med* 1986; **146**: 295–297.

285 Howe PM, Fajardo JE, Orcutt MA. Etiologic diagnosis of cellulitis: comparison of aspirates obtained from the leading edge and the point of maximal inflammation. *Pediatr Infec Dis J* 1987; **6**: 685–686.

286 Chartier C, Grosshans E. Erysipelas. *Int J Dermatol* 1990; **29**: 459–467.

287 Jorup-Ronstrom C. Epidemiologic, bacteriological and complicating features of erysipelas. *Scand J Infect Dis* 1986; **18**: 519–524.

288 Bernard P, Toty L, Mounier M, Denis F, Bonnetblanc JM. Early detection of streptococcal group antigens in skin samples by latex particle agglutination. *Arch Dermatol* 1987; **123**: 468–470.

289 Leppard BJ, Seal DV, Colman G *et al.* The value of bacteriology and serology in the diagnosis of cellulitis and erysipelas. *Br J Dermatol* 1985; **112**: 559–567.

290 Amren DP. Lymphangitis. In: Wannamaker LW, Nelson JM (eds) *Streptococci and Streptococcal Diseases.* Academic Press, New York, 1972, p. 545.

291 Sapico FL. Commentary: necrotizing soft tissue infections. *Infect Dis Clin Pract* 1993; **2**: 330–331.

292 Moses AE, Hardan I, Simhon A *et al. Clostridium septicum* bactermia and diffuse spreading cellulitis of the head and neck in a leukemic patient. *Rev Infect Dis* 1991; **13**: 525–527.

293 Davon J, Jones DM, Turner L. Diagnosis of Meleney's synergistic gangrene. *Br J Surg* 1988; **75**: 267–271.

294 Mbonu OB, Nwako FA. Synergistic bacterial gangrene and allied lesions: a unified etiological theory. *Int Surg* 1983; **68**: 323–324.

295 Lyall A, Stuart RD. Progressive postoperative gangrene of the skin: observations on aetiology and treatment in 2 cases. *Glasgow Med J* 1948; **29**: 1–18.

296 Lewis RT. Necrotizing soft-tissue infections. *Infect Dis Clin North Am* 1992; **6**: 693–703.

297 Finegold DS, Weinberg AN. Group A streptococcal infections: an old adversary reemerging with new tricks? *Arch Dermatol* 1996; **132**: 67–70.

298 Weitzman I. Saprophytic molds as agents of cutaneous and subcutaneous infection in the immunocompromised host. *Arch Dermatol* 1986; **122**: 1161–1168.

299 Wilson CB, Siber GR, O'Brien TF, Morgan AP. Phycomycotic gangrenous cellulitis. *Arch Surg* 1976; **111**: 532–538.

300 Newton WD, Cramer FS, Norwood SH. Necrotizing fasciitis from invasive phycomycetes. *Crit Care Med* 1987; **15**: 331–332.

301 Howard RJ, Pessa ME, Brennaman BH, Ramphal R. Necrotizing soft-tissue infections caused by marine vibrios. *Surgery* 1985; **98**: 126–130.

302 Murphy JJ, Granger R, Blair GK, Miller GC, Fraser GC, Magee JF. Necrotizing fasciitis in childhood. *J Pediatr Surg* 1995; **30**: 1131–1134.

303 Sawin RS, Schaller RT, Tapper D, Morgan A, Cahill J. Early recognition of neonatal abdominal wall necrotizing fasciitis. *Am J Surg* 1994; **167**: 481–484.

304 Goldberg GN, Hansen RC, Lynch PJ. Necrotizing fasciitis in infancy: report of three cases and review of the literature. *Pediatr Dermatol* 1984; **2**: 55–63.

305 Brogan TV, Nizet V, Waldhausen JHT, Rubens CE, Clarke WR. Group A streptococcal necrotizing fasciitis complicating varicella: a series of ten patients. *Pediatr Infect Dis J* 1995; **14**: 588–594.

306 Falcone PA, Pricolo YE, Edstrom LE. Necrotizing fasciitis as a complication of chickenpox. *Clin Pediatr* 1988; **27**: 339–343.

307 Vugia DJ, Peterson CL, Meyers HB *et al.* Invasive group A streptococcal infections in children with varicella in Southern California. *Pediatr Infect Dis J* 1996; **15**: 146–150.

308 Peterson CL, Vugia DJ, Meyers HB *et al.* Risk factors for invasive group A streptococcal infections in children with varicella: case–control study. *Pediatr Infect Dis J* 1996; **15**: 151–156.

309 Doctor A, Harper MB, Fleisher GR. Group A β-hemolytic streptococcal bacteremia: historical overview, changing incidence, and recent association with varicella. *Pediatrics* 1995; **96**: 428–433.

310 Dellinger EP. Severe necrotizing soft-tissue infections: multiple disease entities requiring a common approach. *JAMA* 1981; **246**: 1717–1721.

311 Zittergruen M, Grose C. Magnetic resonance imaging for early detection of

necrotizing fasciitis. *Pediatr Emerg Care* 1993; **9**: 26–28.

312 Patino JF, Castro D. Necrotizing lesions of soft tissues: a review. *World J Surg* 1991; **15**: 235–239.

313 Stevens DL, Maier KA, Mitten JE. Effect of antibiotics on toxin production and viability of *Clostridium perfringens*. *Antimicrob Agents Chemother* 1987; **31**: 213–218.

314 Gemmell CG, Peterson PK, Schmeling D *et al.* Potentiation of opsonization and phagocytosis of *Streptococcus pyogenes* following growth in the presence of clindamycin. *J Clin Invest* 1981; **67**: 1249–1256.

315 Stevens DL, Bryant AE, Hackett SP. Antibiotic effects on bacterial viability, toxin production, and host response. *Clin Infect Dis* 1995; **120** (Suppl 2): S154–S157.

316 Riseman JA, Zamboni WA, Curtis A, Graham DR, Konrad HR, Ross DS. Hyperbaric oxygen therapy for necrotizing fasciitis reduces mortality and the need for débridements. *Surgery* 1990; **108**: 847–850.

317 Shupak A, Shoshani O, Goldenberg I, Barzilai A, Moskuna R, Bursztein S. Necrotizing fasciitis: an indication for hyperbaric oxygen therapy? *Surgery* 1995; **118**: 873–878.

318 Barry W, Hudgins L, Donta ST, Pesanti EL. Intravenous immunoglobulin therapy for toxic shock syndrome. *JAMA* 1992; **267**: 3315–3316.

319 Quinn RW. Epidemiology of group A streptococcal infections: their changing frequency and severity. *Yale J Biol Med* 1982; **55**: 265–270.

320 Knoll H, Sramek J, Vrbova K *et al.* Scarlet fever and the types of erythrogenic toxins produced by the infecting streptococcal strains. *Int J Med Microbiol* 1991; **276**: 94–106.

321 Stollerman GH. Changing group A streptococci: the reappearance of streptococcal 'toxic shock'. *Arch Intern Med* 1988; **148**: 1268–1270.

322 Katz AR, Morens DM. Severe streptococcal infections in historical perspective. *Clin Infect Dis* 1992; **14**: 298–307.

323 Weaver GH. Scarlet fever. In: Abt IA (ed.) *Pediatrics*. WB Saunders, Philadelphia, 1925, pp. 298–362.

324 Bartter T, Dascal A, Carroll K, Curley FJ. Toxic strep syndrome: a manifestation of group A streptococcal infection. *Arch Intern Med* 1988; **148**: 1421–1424.

325 Belani K, Schlievert PM, Kaplan EL, Ferrieri P. Association of exotoxin-producing group A streptococci and severe disease in children. *Pediatr Infect Dis J* 1991; **10**: 351–354.

326 Shaunak S, Wendon J, Monteil M, Gordon AM. Septic scarlet fever due to *Streptococcus pyogenes* cellulitis. *Quart J Med* 1988; **258**: 921–925.

327 Cone LA, Woodland DR, Schlievert PM *et al.* Clinical and bacteriologic observations of a toxic shock-like syndrome due to *Streptococcus pyogenes*. *N Engl J Med* 1987; **317**: 146–149.

328 Kohler WD, Gerlach D, Knoll H. Streptococcal outbreaks and erythrogenic toxin type A. *Zbl Bakt Hyg A* 1987; **266**: 104–115.

329 Schlievert PM, Bettin KM, Watson DW. Production of pyrogenic exotoxin by groups of streptococci: association with group A. *J Infect Dis* 1979; **140**: 676–681.

330 Hallas G. The production of pyogenic exotoxins by group A streptococci. *J Hyg* 1985; **95**: 47–57.

331 Dick GF, Dick GH. A skin test for susceptibility to scarlet fever. *JAMA* 1924; **82**: 265–266.

332 Dick GF, Dick GH. Etiology of scarlet fever. *JAMA* 1924; **82**: 301–302.

333 Yu C, Ferretti JJ. Molecular epidemiologic analysis of the type A streptococcal exotoxin (erythrogenic toxin) gene (speA) in clinical *Streptococcus pyogenes* strains. *Infect Immun* 1989; **57**: 3715–3719.

334 Yu C, Ferretti JJ. Frequency of the erythrogenic toxin B and C genes (speB and speC) among clinical isolates of group A streptococci. *Infect Immun* 1991; **59**: 211–215.

335 Corson AP, Garagusi VF, Chretien JH. Group C β-hemolytic streptococci causing

pharyngitis and scarlet fever. *South Med J* 1989; **82**: 1119–1120.

336 Schlievert PM, Bettin KM, Watson DW. Reinterpretation of the Dick test: the role of group A streptococcal pyrogenic exotoxin. *Infect Immun* 1979; **26**: 467–472.

337 Murray JF. Bantu immunity to scarlet fever toxin. *J Hyg* 1943; **43**: 170–172.

338 Breese BB. Beta hemolytic streptococcal infections in children. *Pediatr Clin North Am* 1960; **7**: 843–867.

339 Duca E, Teodorovici G, Radu C *et al.* A new nephritogenic *Streptococcus. J Hyg* 1969; **67**: 691–698.

340 Osler W. *The Principles and Practice of Medicine*, 2nd edn. Appleton, New York, 1895, pp. 71–80.

341 Kaplan EL, Reid HF, Johnson DR *et al.* Rapid antigen detection in the diagnosis of group A streptococcal pyoderma: influence of a 'learning curve effect' on sensitivity and specificity. *Pediatr Infect Dis J* 1989; **8**: 591–593.

342 Stevens FA. The occurrence of *Staphylococcus aureus* infection with a scarlatiniform rash. *JAMA* 1927; **88**: 1957–1958.

343 Aranow H, Wood WB. Staphylococcic infection simulating scarlet fever. *JAMA* 1942; **119**: 1491–1495.

344 Dunnet WN, Schallibaum EM. Scarlet-fever-like illness due to staphylococcal infection. *Lancet* 1960; **ii**: 1227–1229.

345 Feldman CA. Staphylococcal scarlet fever. *N Engl J Med* 1962; **267**: 877–888.

346 Hansen RC. Staphylococcal scalded skin syndrome, toxic shock syndrome, and Kawasaki disease. *Pediatr Clin North Am* 1983; **30**: 533–544.

347 Fell HWK, Nagington J, Naylor GRE. *Corynebacterium haemolyticum* infections in Cambridgeshire. *J Hyg* 1977; **79**: 269–274.

348 Banck G, Nyman M. Tonsillitis and rash associated with *Corynebacterium haemolyticum. J Infect Dis* 1986; **154**: 1037–1040.

349 Selander B, Ljungh A. *Corynebacterium haemolyticum* as a cause of nonstreptococcal pharyngitis. *J Infect Dis* 1986; **154**: 1041.

350 Miller RA, Brancato F, Holmes KK. *Corynebacterium haemolyticum* as a cause of pharyngitis and scarlatiniform rash in young adults. *Ann Int Med* 1986; **105**: 867–872.

351 Nyman M, Banck G, Thore M. Penicillin tolerance in *Arcanobacterium haemolyticum. J Infect Dis* 1990; **161**: 261–265.

352 Kain KC, Noble MA, Barteluk RL, Tubbesing RH. *Arcanobacterium haemolyticum* infection: confused with scarlet fever and diphtheria. *J Emerg Med* 1991; **9**: 33–35.

353 Waagner DC. *Arcanobacterium haemolyticum*: biology of the organism and diseases in man. *Pediatr Infect Dis J* 1991; **10**: 933–939.

354 Karpathios T, Drakonaki S, Zervoudaki A *et al. Arcanobacterium haemolyticum* in children with presumed streptococcal pharygotonsillitis or scarlet fever. *J Pediatr* 1992; **121**: 735–737.

355 Carlson P, Renkonen O, Kontiainen S. *Arcanobacterium haemolyticum* and streptococcal pharyngitis. *Scand J Infect Dis* 1994; **26**: 283–287.

356 Gaston DA, Zurowski SM. *Arcanobacterium haemolyticum* pharyngitis and exanthem. *Arch Dermatol* 1996; **132**: 61–64.

357 MacLean PD, Lieboe AA, Rosenberg AA. A hemolytic corynebacterium resembling *Corynebacterium ovis* and *Corynebacterium pyogenes* in man. *J Infect Dis* 1946; **79**: 69–90.

358 Wickremesinghe RSB. *Corynebacterium haemolyticum* infections in Sri Lanka. *J Hyg* 1981; **87**: 271–276.

359 Boguniewicz M, Leung DYM. Hypersensitivity reactions to antibiotics commonly used in children. *Pediatr Infect Dis J* 1995; **14**: 221–231.

360 Roujeau JC, Stern RS. Severe adverse cutaneous reactions to drugs. *N Engl J Med* 1994; **331**: 1272–1285.

361 Randolph MF, Gerber MA, DeMeo KK *et al.* Effect of antibiotic therapy on the clinical course of streptococcal pharyngitis. *J Pediatr* 1985; **106**: 870–875.

362 Pichichero ME, Margolis PA. A comparison of cephalosporins and penicillins in the

treatment of group A beta-hemolytic streptococcal pharyngitis: a meta-analysis supporting the concept of microbial copathogenicity. *Pediatr Infect Dis J* 1991; **10**: 275–281.

363 Pichichero ME. Cephalosporins are superior to penicillin for treatment of streptococcal tonsillopharyngitis: is the difference worth it? *Pediatr Infect Dis J* 1993; **12**: 268–274.

364 Elias PM, Fritsch P, Epstein EH. Staphylococcal scalded skin syndrome: clinical features, pathogenesis, and recent microbiological and biochemical developments. *Arch Dermatol* 1977; **113**: 207–219.

365 Norden CW, Mendelow H. Staphylococcal scalded skin syndrome in adults. *N Engl J Med* 1974; **290**: 577.

366 Melish ME, Glasgow LA. The staphylococcal scalded skin syndrome—development of an experimental model. *N Engl J Med* 1970; **282**: 1114–1119.

367 Parker MT, Tomlinson AJH, Williams REO. Impetigo contagiosa: the association of certain types of *Staphylococcus aureus* and *Streptococcus pyogenes* in superficial skin infections. *J Hyg* 1955; **53**: 458.

368 Elias PM, Fritsch P, Tappeiner G, Mittermayer H, Wolff K. Experimental staphylococcal toxic epidermal necrolysis (TEN) in adult humans and mice. *J Lab Clin Med* 1974; **84**: 414–424.

369 Elias PM, Mittermayer H, Fritsch P, Tappeiner G, Wolff K. Staphylococcal toxic epidermal necrolysis (TEN): the expanded mouse model. *J Invest Dermatol* 1974; **63**: 467–475.

370 Lillibridge CB, Melish ME, Glasgow LA. Site of action of exfoliative toxin on the staphylococcal scalded skin syndrome. *Pediatrics* 1972; **50**: 723–738.

371 Elias PM, Fritsch P, Dahl MV, Wolff K. Staphylococcal exfoliative toxin: pathogenesis and subcellular site of action. *J Invest Dermatol* 1975; **65**: 501–512.

372 Takagi Y, Futamura S, Asada Y. Action site of exfoliative toxin on keratinocytes. *J Invest Dermatol* 1990; **94**: 52A.

373 Dancer SJ, Garratt R, Saldanha J *et al*. The epidermolytic toxins are serine proteases. *FEBS Lett* 1990; **268**: 129–132.

374 Rudolph RI, Schwartz W, Leyden JJ. Treatment of staphylococcal toxic epidermal necrolysis. *Arch Dermatol* 1974; **110**: 559–562.

375 Bonventre PF, Linnemann C, Weckbach LS *et al*. Antibody responses to toxic-shock-syndrome (TSS) toxin by patients with TSS and by healthy staphylococcal carriers. *J Infect Dis* 1984; **150**: 662–666.

376 Notermans S, VanLeeuwen WJ, Dufrenne J, Tips PD. Serum antibodies to enterotoxins produced by *Staphylococcus aureus* with special reference to enterotoxin F and toxic shock syndrome. *J Clin Microbiol* 1983; **18**: 1055–1060.

377 Vergeront JM, Stolz SJ, Crass BA, Nelson DB, Davis JB, Bergdoll MS. Prevalence of serum antibody to staphylococcal enterotoxin F among Wisconsin residents: implications for toxic shock syndrome. *J Infect Dis* 1983; **148**: 692–698.

378 Todd J, Fishaut M, Kapral F, Welch T. Toxic-shock syndrome associated with phage-group-I staphylococci. *Lancet* 1978; **ii**: 1116–1118.

379 Davis JP, Chesney PJ, Wand PJ, LaVentre M. Toxic-shock syndrome: epidemiologic features, recurrence, risk factors, and prevention. *N Engl J Med* 1980; **303**: 1429–1435.

380 Chesney PJ, Davis JP, Purdy WK, Wand PJ, Chesney RW. Clinical manifestations of toxic shock syndrome. *JAMA* 1981; **246**: 741–748.

381 Shands KN, Schmid GP, Dan BB *et al*. Toxic-shock syndrome in menstruating women: association with tampon use and *Staphylococcus aureus* and clinical features in 52 cases. *N Engl J Med* 1980; **303**: 1436–1442.

382 Broome CV. Epidemiology of toxic shock syndrome in the United States: overview. *Rev Infect Dis* 1989; **11** (Suppl 1): S14–S21.

383 Gaventa S, Reingold AL, Hightower AW *et al*. Active surveillance for toxic shock syndrome in the United States: 1986. *Rev Infect Dis* 1989; **11** (Suppl 1): S28–S34.

384 Reingold AL, Shands KN, Dan BB, Broome CV. Toxic-shock syndrome not associated with menstruation. *Lancet* 1982; **i**: 1–4.

385 Reingold AL. Epidemiology of toxic shock syndrome, United States, 1960–1984. *MMWR* 1985; **33**: 19SS–22SS.

386 Reingold AL, Hagrett NT, Dan BB *et al*. Non-menstrual toxic shock syndrome: a review of 130 cases. *Ann Intern Med* 1982; **96**: 871–874.

387 Reingold AL. Non-menstrual toxic shock syndrome: the growing picture. *JAMA* 1983; **249**: 932.

388 Resnick SD. Toxic shock syndrome: recent developments in pathogenesis. *J Pediatr* 1990; **116**: 321–328.

389 Kain KC, Schulzer M, Chow AW. Clinical spectrum of nonmenstrual toxic shock syndrome (TSS): comparison with menstrual TSS by multivariate discriminant analyses. *Clin Infect Dis* 1993; **16**: 100–106.

390 Jacobson JA, Kasworm EM, Reiser RF, Bergdoll MS. Low incidence of toxic shock syndrome in children with staphylococcal infection. *Am J Med Sci* 1987; **294**: 403–407.

391 Wiesenthal AM, Todd JK. Toxic shock syndrome in children aged 10 years or less. *Pediatrics* 1984; **74**: 112–117.

392 Buchdahl R, Levin M, Wilkins B *et al*. Toxic shock syndrome. *Arch Dis Child* 1985; **60**: 563–567.

393 Spearman PW, Barson WJ. Toxic shock syndrome occurring in children with abrasive injuries beneath casts. *J Pediatr Orthop* 1992; **12**: 169–172.

394 McCarthy VP, Peoples WM. Toxic shock syndrome after ear piercing. *Pediatr Infect Dis J* 1988; **7**: 741–742.

395 Kline MW, Dunkle LM. Toxic shock syndrome and the acquired immunodeficiency syndrome. *Pediatr Infect Dis J* 1988; **7**: 736–738.

396 Solomon R, Truman T, Murray DL. Toxic shock syndrome as a complication of bacterial tracheitis. *Pediatr Infect Dis J* 1983; **4**: 298–299.

397 Surh L, Read SE. Staphylococcal tracheitis and toxic shock syndrome in a young child. *J Pediatr* 1984; **105**: 585–587.

398 Cheneaud M, Leclerc F, Martinot A. Bacterial croup and toxic shock syndrome. *Eur J Pediatr* 1986; **145**: 306–307.

399 Donaldson JD, Maltby CC. Bacterial tracheitis in children. *J Otolaryngol* 1989; **18**: 101–104.

400 Cole RP, Shakespeare PG. Toxic shock syndrome in scalded children. *Burns* 1990; **16**: 221–224.

401 Ejlertsen T, Jensen A, Lester A, Rosdahl VT. Epidemiology of toxic shock syndrome toxin-1 production in *Staphylococcus aureus* strains isolated in Denmark between 1959–1990. *Scand J Infect Dis* 1994; **26**: 599–604.

402 See RH, Chow AW. Microbiology of toxic shock syndrome: overview. *Rev Infect Dis* 1989; **11** (Suppl 1): S55–S60.

403 Musser JM, Schlievert PM, Chow AW *et al*. A single clone of *Staphylococcus aureus* causes the majority of cases of toxic shock syndrome. *Proc Nat Acad Sci* 1990; **87**: 225–229.

404 Schlievert PM, Shands KN, Schmid GP, Nishimura RD. Identification and characterization of an exotoxin from *Staphylococcus aureus* associated with toxic shock syndrome. *J Infect Dis* 1981; **143**: 509–516.

405 Garbe PL, Arko RJ, Reingold AL *et al*. *Staphylococcus aureus* isolates from patients with nonmenstrual toxic shock syndrome. *JAMA* 1985; **253**: 2538–2542.

406 Schlievert PM. Staphylococcal enterotoxin B and toxic-shock syndrome toxin-1 are significantly associated with non-menstrual TSS. *Lancet* 1986; **i**: 1149–1150.

407 Parsonnet J. Mediators in the pathogenesis of toxic shock syndrome: overview. *Rev Infect Dis* 1989; **11** (Suppl 1): S263–S269.

408 Lee VTP, Chang AH, Chow AW. Detection of staphylococcal enterotoxin B among toxic shock syndrome (TSS)- and non-TSS-associated *Staphylococcus aureus* isolates.

J Infect Dis 1992; **166**: 911–915.

409 Bohach GA, Kreiswirth BN, Novick RP, Schlievert PM. Analysis of TSS isolates producing staphylococcal enterotoxins B and C1 with use of Southern hybridization and immunologic assays. *Rev Infect Dis* 1989; **11** (Suppl 1): S75–S81.

410 Chang AH, Musser JM, Chow AW. A single clone which produces both TSST-1 and SEA causes the majority of menstrual TSS (abstract). *Clin Res* 1989; **39**: 36A.

411 Crass BA, Bergdoll MS. Toxin involvement in toxic shock syndrome. *J Infect Dis* 1986; **153**: 918–926.

412 Milner LS, de Jager J, Thomson PD, Doehring RO. Toxic shock syndrome caused by staphylococcal enterotoxin B. *South Afr Med J* 1983; **63**: 822–824.

413 Todd JK, Todd BH, Franco-Buff A, Smith CM, Lawellin DW. Influence of focal growth conditions on the pathogenesis of toxic shock syndrome. *J Infect Dis* 1987; **155**: 673–681.

414 Ritz HL, Kirkland JJ, Bond GG, Warner EK, Petty GP. Association of high levels of serum antibody to staphylococcal toxic shock antigen with nasal carriage of toxic shock antigen-producing strains of *Staphylococcus aureus*. *Infect Immun* 1984; **43**: 954–958.

415 Jacobson JA, Kasworm EM, Crass BA, Bergdoll MS. Nasal carriage of toxigenic *Staphylococcus aureus* and prevalence of serum antibody to toxic-shock-syndrome toxin 1 in Utah children. *J Infect Dis* 1986; **153**: 356–359.

416 Bergdoll MS, Crass BA, Reiser RF, Robbins RN, Davis JP. A new staphylococcal enterotoxin F, associated with toxic-shock syndrome *Staphylococcus aureus* isolates. *Lancet* 1981; **1**: 1017–1021.

417 Miethke T, Wahl C, Heeg K, Echtenacher B, Krammer PH, Wagner H. T cell-mediated lethal shock triggered in mice by the superantigen staphylococcal enterotoxin B: critical role of tumor necrosis factor. *J Exp Med* 1992; **175**: 91–98.

418 Miethke T, Duschek K, Wahl C, Heeg K, Wagner H. Pathogenesis of the toxic shock syndrome: T cell mediated lethal shock caused by the superantigen TSST-1. *Eur J Immunol* 1993; **23**: 1494–1500.

419 Smith RJ, Schlievert PM, Himelright IM, Baddour LM. Dual infections with *Staphylococcus aureus* and *Streptococcus pyogenes* causing toxic shock syndrome: possible synergistic effects of toxic shock syndrome toxin 1 and streptococcal pyrogenic exotoxin C. *Diagn Microbiol Infect Dis* 1994; **19**: 245–247.

420 Schlievert PM. Enhancement of host susceptibility to lethal endotoxin shock by staphylococcal pyrogenic exotoxin type C. *Infect Immun* 1982; **36**: 123–128.

421 Crass BA, Bergdoll MS. Involvement of coagulase-negative staphylococci in toxic shock syndrome. *J Clin Microbiol* 1986; **23**: 43–45.

422 Kahler RC, Boyce JM, Bergdoll MS, Lockwood WR, Taylor MR. Case report: toxic shock syndrome associated with TSST-1-producing coagulase-negative staphylococci. *Am J Med Sci* 1986; **292**: 310–312.

423 Kreiswirth BN, Schlievert PM, Novick RP. Evaluation of coagulase-negative staphylococci for ability to produce toxic shock syndrome toxin-1. *J Clin Microbiol* 1987; **25**: 2028–2029.

424 Parsonnet J, Harrison AE, Spencer SE, Reading A, Parsonnet KC, Kass EH. Nonproduction of toxic shock syndrome toxin-1 by coagulase-negative staphylococci. *J Clin Microbiol* 1987; **25**: 1370–1372.

425 Chesney PJ. Clinical aspects and spectrum of illness of toxic shock syndrome: overview. *Rev Infect Dis* 1989; **11** (Suppl 1): S1–S7.

426 Paris AL, Herwaldt LA, Blum D, Schmid GP, Shands KN, Broome CV. Pathologic findings in twelve fatal cases of toxic shock syndrome. *Ann Intern Med* 1982; **96**: 852–857.

427 Hurwitz RM, Rivera HP, Gooch MH, Slama TG, Handt A, Weiss J. Toxic shock syndrome or toxic epidermal necrolysis? *J Am Acad Dermatol* 1982; **7**: 246–254.

428 Hurwitz RM, Ackerman AB. Cutaneous pathology of the toxic shock syndrome. *Am J Dermatopathol* 1985; **7**: 563–578.

429 Bach MC. Dermatologic signs in toxic shock syndrome—clues to diagnosis. *J Am Acad Dermatol* 1983; **8**: 343–347.

430 Deetz TR, Reves R, Septimus E. Secondary rash in toxic shock syndrome? *N Engl J Med* 1981; **304**: 174.

431 Chesney PJ, Crass BA, Polyak MB *et al*. Toxic shock syndrome: management and long-term sequellae. *Ann Intern Med* 1982; **96**: 847–851.

432 Cone LA, Woddard DR, Byrd RG, Schulz K, Kopp SM, Schlievert PM. A recalcitrant, erythematous, desquamating disorder associated with toxin-producing staphylococci in patients with AIDS. *J Infect Dis* 1992; **165**: 638–643.

433 Strausbaugh LJ. Toxic shock syndrome: are you recognizing its changing presentations? *Postgrad Med* 1993; **94**: 107–118.

434 Todd JK. Therapy of toxic shock syndrome. *Drugs* 1990; **39**: 856–861.

435 Fisher CJ Jr, Horowitz Z, Albertson TE. Cardiorespiratory failure in toxic shock syndrome: effects of dobutamine. *Crit Care Med* 1985; **13**: 160–165.

436 McIvor ME, Levin ML. Treatment of recurrent toxic shock syndrome with oral contraceptive agents. *Maryland State Med J* 1982 (Sept): 56–57.

437 Todd JK, Ressman M, Caston SA, Todd BH, Wiesenthal AM. Corticosteroid therapy for patients with toxic shock syndrome. *JAMA* 1984; **252**: 3399–3402.

438 Melish ME, Frogner K, Hirata S, Murata MS. Use of IVIG for therapy in the rabbit model of TSS (abstract). *Clin Res* 1987; **35**: 220A.

439 The Working Group on Severe Streptococcal Infections. Defining the group A streptococcal toxic shock syndrome: rationale and consensus definition. *JAMA* 1993; **269**: 390–391.

440 Stevens DL. Streptococcal toxic-shock syndrome: spectrum of disease, pathogenesis, and new concepts in treatment. *Emerg Infect Dis* 1995; **1**: 69–78.

441 Hoge CW, Schwatz B, Talkington DF, Breiman RF, MacNeill EM, Englender SJ. The changing epidemiology of invasive group A streptococcal infections and the emergence of streptococcal toxic shock-like syndrome. *JAMA* 1993; **269**: 384–389.

442 Davies HD, Matlow A, Scriver SR *et al*. Apparent lower rates of streptococcal toxic shock syndrome and lower mortality in children with invasive group A streptococcal infections compared with adults. *Pediatr Infect Dis J* 1994; **13**: 49–56.

443 Torres-Martinez C, Mehta D, Butt A, Levin M. *Streptococcus*-associated toxic shock. *Arch Dis Child* 1992; **67**: 126–130.

444 Givner LB, Abramson JS, Wasilauskas B. Apparent increase in the incidence of invasive group A beta-hemolytic streptococcal disease in children. *Pediatrics* 1991; **118**: 341–346.

445 Bradley JS, Schlievert PM, Peterson BM. Toxic shock-like syndrome, a complication of strep throat. *Pediatr Infect Dis J* 1991; **10**: 790.

446 Chapnick EK, Gradon JD, Lutwick LI *et al*. Streptococcal toxic shock syndrome due to noninvasive pharyngitis. *Clin Infect Dis* 1992; **14**: 1074–1077.

447 Herold AH. Group A beta-hemolytic streptococcal toxic shock from a mild pharyngitis. *J Family Pract* 1990; **31**: 549–551.

448 Silver RM, Heddleston LN, McGregor JA *et al*. Life-threatening puerperal infection due to group A streptococci. *Obstetr Gynecol* 1992; **79**: 894–896.

449 Dotters DJ, Katz VL. Streptococcal toxic shock associated with septic abortion. *Obstetr Gynecol* 1991; **78**: 549–551.

450 Margolis DJ, Horlick SE. Group A *Streptococcus*-induced bullous toxic shock-like syndrome. *J Am Acad Dermatol* 1991; **24**: 786–787.

451 Swingler GR, Bigrigg MA, Hewitt BG *et al*. Disseminated intravascular coagulation associated with group A streptococcal infection in pregnancy. *Lancet* 1988; **i**: 1456–1457.

452 Novotny W, Faden H, Mosovich L. Emergence of invasive group A streptococcal disease among young children. *Clin Pediatr* 1992; **31**: 596–601.

453 Begovac J, Morton E, Lisic M, Beus I, Bozinovic D, Kuzmanovic N. Group A beta-

hemolytic streptococcal toxic shock-like syndrome. *Pediatr Infect Dis J* 1990; **9**: 369–370.

454 Bradley JS, Schlievert PM, Sample TG Jr. Streptococcal toxic shock-like syndrome as a complication of varicella. *Pediatr Infect Dis J* 1991; **10**: 77–78.

455 Gonzales-Ruiz A, Ridgway GL, Cohen SL, Hunt CP, McGrouther G, Adiseshiah M. Varicella gangrenosa with toxic shock-like syndrome due to group A *Streptococcus* infection in an adult: case report. *Clin Infect Dis* 1995; **20**: 1058–1060.

456 Stevens DL. Editorial response: varicella gangrenosa with toxic shock-like syndrome. *Clin Infect Dis* 1995; **20**: 1061–1062.

457 Stevens DL. Could nonsteroidal antiinflammatory drugs (NSAIDs) enhance the progression of bacterial infection to toxic shock syndrome? *Clin Infect Dis* 1995; **21**: 977–980.

458 Holm SE, Norrby A, Bergholm AM, Norgren M. Aspects of pathogenesis of serious group A streptococcal infections in Sweden, 1988–1989. *J Infect Dis* 1992; **166**: 31–37.

459 Mahieu LM, Holm SE, Goossens HJ, Acker KJV. Congenital streptococcal toxic shock syndrome with absence of antibodies against streptococcal pyrogenic exotoxins. *J Pediatr* 1995; **127**: 987–989.

460 Johnson DR, Stevens DL, Kaplan EL. Epidemiologic analysis of group A streptococcal serotypes associated with severe systemic infections, rheumatic fever, or uncomplicated pharyngitis. *J Infect Dis* 1992; **166**: 374–382.

461 Forni AL, Kaplan EL, Schlievert PM, Roberts RB. Clinical and microbiological characteristics of severe group A *Streptococcus* infections and streptococcal toxic shock syndrome. *Clin Infect Dis* 1995; **21**: 333–340.

462 Schwartz B, Facklam RR, Breiman RF. Changing epidemiology of group A streptococcal infection in the USA. *Lancet* 1990; **336**: 1167–1171.

463 Musser JM, Kapur V, Kanjilal S *et al.* Geographic and temporal distribution and molecular characterization of two highly pathogenic clones of *Streptococcus pyogenes* expressing allelic variant of pyrogenic exotoxin A (scarlet fever toxin). *J Infect Dis* 1993; **167**: 337–346.

464 Hackett SP, Stevens DL. Superantigens associated with staphylococcal and streptococcal toxic shock syndrome are potent inducers of tumor necrosis factor-β synthesis. *J Infect Dis* 1993; **168**: 232–235.

465 Hackett SP, Stevens DL. Streptococcal toxic shock syndrome: synthesis of tumor necrosis factor and interleukin-1 by monocytes stimulated with pyrogenic exotoxin A and streptolysin O. *J Infect Dis* 1992; **165**: 879–885.

466 Fast DJ, Schlievert PM, Nelson RD. Toxic shock syndrome-associated staphylococcal and streptococcal pyrogenic toxins are potent inducers of tumor necrosis factor production. *Infect Immun* 1989; **57**: 291–294.

467 Stevens DL, Bryant AE, Hackett SP *et al.* Group A streptococcal bacteremia: the role of tumor necrosis factor in shock and organ failure. *J Infect Dis* 1996; **173**: 619–626.

468 Musser JM. Clinical relevance of streptococcal pyrogenic exotoxins in streptococcal toxic shock-like syndrome and other severe infections. *Pediatr Ann* 1992; **21**: 821–828.

469 Wolf JE, Rabinowitz LG. Streptococcal toxic shock-like syndrome. *Arch Dermatol* 1995; **131**: 73–77.

470 Yong JM. Necrotizing fasciitis. *Lancet* 1994; **343**: 1427.

Chapter 3
Skin Infections due to Other Bacteria

Anne E. Weilepp, John A.D. Leake &
Sheila Fallon-Friedlander

Cutaneous diseases caused by corynebacteria

Erythrasma (Fig. 3.1)

Definition

Erythrasma is a superficial bacterial infection of the skin which most often affects the axilla, groin or interdigital-web spaces. The lesions are generally asymptomatic, but can be pruritic. They consist of homogeneous red-brown patches. The borders are often sharply marginated and the surface possesses a diffuse fine scale.

Epidemiology

This disease is most common in warm, moist climates. It has also been found in approximately 20% of randomly selected subjects in a temperate climate [1]. Fifteen per cent of cases occur in children between 5 and 14 years of age, and the incidence increases with age [2]. Outbreaks have been documented [3], although the organism is not considered highly contagious. In a clinical and microbiological evaluation of 665 Danish recruits, the microbiological and clinical prevalence of foot erythrasma prior to induction was found to be 51%, and increased to 77% by the end of their military service [4]. Asymptomatic infection often occurs, as does coinfection with dermatophytes or *Candida*.

Aetiology

Erythrasma is caused by *Corynebacterium minutissimum*, a short Gram-positive rod possessing subterminal granules. This diphtheroid has special growth requirements and produces small white-grey shiny colonies when grown in culture.

Clinical manifestations

This disorder most commonly affects the axilla, groin and interdigital-web

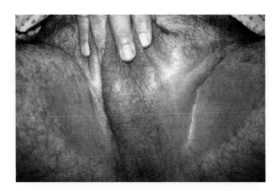

Fig. 3.1 Erythrasma.

spaces. Any moist intertriginous area may be involved, and occasionally a generalized lamellated scaling form can occur. The latter is more likely in tropical climates, or in debilitated or diabetic individuals. The scrotum and penis are usually spared but vulvar involvement occurs.

The eruption is brown-red, homogeneous and faintly scaling. A discrete symmetrical patch is frequently noted in the groin or axillae. If the inter-digital-web spaces are involved, maceration and fissuring are common. Symptoms are variable; some patients are asymptomatic, while others have significant pruritus. The disorder is often indolent and chronic, and the condition may recur despite appropriate treatment.

Diagnosis and treatment

The hallmark of infection is coral-red fluorescence, which can be seen on Wood's-lamp examination. The *Corynebacterium* elaborates a porphyrin, which results in fluorescence when the lesions are exposed to ultraviolet (UV) light. False-negative examinations may occur [5], especially following vigorous cleansing of the involved areas. Gram stain will reveal Gram-positive rods or cocci. Routine cultures are unhelpful as the organism has special growth requirements.

Differential diagnosis includes tinea, *Candida*, inverse psoriasis and streptococcal infection.

Treatment consists of oral or topical antibiotics. Oral erythromycin, 250 mg four times a day for 1–2 weeks, is often used. Topical erythromycin and clindamycin are also efficacious, but resolution may not be as rapid with these agents. Topical miconazole and antibiotic cleansers, such as chlorhexidine, have also been utilized as treatment. A Danish multipractice study evaluated the efficacy of oral erythromycin and topical fusidic acid cream, and found that both treatments used as monotherapy were signifi-cantly better than placebo [6]. Of note, there was no statistical difference in response rate between oral and topical treatment.

Trichomycosis axillaris (Fig. 3.2)

Definition/aetiology

This disorder is caused by *Corynebacterium tenuis*. Infection leads to the development of white, black, yellow or red concretions on axillary or pubic hair. Patients are usually asymptomatic and the disorder is an incidental finding.

Epidemiology

This condition is more common in tropical climates and during the summer. Adult males are more affected than females, probably reflecting the female tendency to shave axillary hair in many countries. Pubic-hair involvement is much less common than axillary disease. Individuals with hyperhidrosis are at higher risk, as are those whose work or lifestyle involves humid conditions.

Clinical manifestations/diagnosis

The condition is generally asymptomatic. Thickening of the hair shaft is noted, with either white, yellow, red or black concretions. These encrustations take the form of irregularly spaced nodules along the shaft, consisting of bacteria embedded in an amorphous matrix. Patients may complain of offensive axillary odour or red-stained perspiration. Wood's-lamp examination (in all but the red form) reveals a yellow or white-blue fluorescence. Microscopic examination reveals nodular adherent concretions of organisms. Unlike piedra, hair cuticles infected with corynebacteria do not appear weakened or easily broken.

Differential diagnosis includes white or black piedra, or deodorant or talcum-powder adherence.

Treatment

Removal of the hair, most commonly by shaving, is efficacious, as is the use

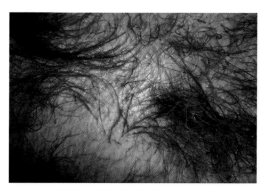

Fig. 3.2 Trichomycosis axillaris.

of topical antibiotics, such as erythromycin and clindamycin. The elimination of humidity and utilization of germicidal products and antiperspirants is often also effective in eradicating the organism.

Pitted keratolysis (Fig. 3.3)

Definition/aetiology

This bacterial infection affects the soles, lateral aspects of the toes and occasionally the palms. It is thought to result from infection with a *Corynebacterium* species, either alone or in combination with *Micrococcus sedentarius* [7, 8].

Epidemiology

As with other cutaneous corynebacterial infections, pitted keratolysis most commonly occurs in tropical climates and in the summer season. It is worldwide in distribution. Hyperhidrosis and occlusive wet environments predispose to this condition.

Clinical manifestations

Affected individuals sometimes complain of a foul-smelling odour from the feet. On examination, distinctive shallow crateriform depressions or small shallow 1–2 mm pits are noted on the soles, toes and/or palms. Erythematous or violaceous patches are occasionally noted as well. The tissue may appear boggy, macerated or eroded.

Diagnosis and treatment

The appearance of pitted keratolysis is quite distinctive and diagnosis is thus usually straightforward.

Treatment should always involve an attempt to dry the affected area. This alone will often lead to resolution of the condition. Topical drying

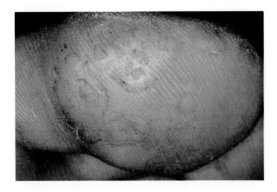

Fig. 3.3 Pitted keratolysis.

agents, such as benzoyl peroxide, and topical antibiotics, including erythromycin and clindamycin, are also useful.

Cutaneous diphtheria (Table 3.1 and Fig. 3.4)

Definition and pathophysiology

Corynebacterium diphtheriae is a non-motile, unencapsulated pleomorphic
Gram-positive bacillus. The name derives from the Greek word for leather
hide, 'diphtheria', descriptive of the grey leathery membrane which covers
both cutaneous and pharyngeal ulcers. The diphtheria bacillus was first isolated by Friedrich Loeffler in 1884. He utilized a culture medium of his own
design, which is still used for identification of the organism. The organism
grows rapidly on Loeffler's medium, composed of 75% serum and 25%
broth, producing colonies at 12–18 hours. Smears from this medium
display metachromatic granules and 'Chinese-character' palisading, which
are the microbiological hallmarks of this organism. *Corynebacterium diphtheriae* may be grouped into *gravis*, *intermedius* and *mitis* subtypes, based on differing morphology on tellurite agar, fermentation reactions and haemolytic
potential.

   Corynebacterium diphtheriae produces a potent exotoxin, its key virulence
factor. A single toxin molecule can arrest protein synthesis in a cell within

Table 3.1 Cutaneous disorders caused by corynebacteria.

Disease	Organism	Location	Cutaneous findings	Treatment
Cutaneous diphtheria	*Corynebacterium diphtheriae*	Most common: lower extremities, feet, hands	Ulcer with grey pseudomembrane	Antitoxin/systemic penicillin
Erythrasma	*C. minutissimum*	Axillae, groin, interdigital-web space	Brown-red lesions; confluent with faint scale	Topical or systemic erythromycin
Trichomycosis axillaris	*C. tenuis*	Axillary or pubic hair	Thickening and encrustation of the hair shaft ± offensive odour, red stain	Remove hair: topical erythromycin or clindamycin; germicidal products, antiperspirants
Pitted keratolysis	*Corynebacterium* species ± *Micrococcus sedentarius*	Most common: soles of feet; toes and palms occasionally	Shallow crateriform depressions, small shallow 1–2 mm pits; boggy macerated tissue	Drying the area; benzoyl peroxide, topical erythromycin or clindamycin, 40% formaldehyde in Aquaphor ointment, aluminium chloride 20%

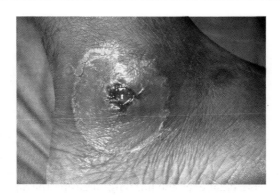

Fig. 3.4 Cutaneous diphtheria (courtesy of Dr Wolfram Hofler).

several hours, and 0.1 μg/kg is a lethal dose for susceptible animals [9]. The toxin exerts its most powerful effects on the heart (myocarditis), nerves (demyelination) and kidneys (renal tubular necrosis). Toxin production depends on the presence of a lysogenic 'β phage'. The phage carries the gene encoding the toxin. In the lysogenic phase, the phage's circular deoxyribonucleic acid (DNA) integrates as a prophage into the genome of the bacterial host. Stimuli such as UV light induce the phage to enter a lytic cycle. The toxin genome is subsequently expressed and the host cell destroyed, with release of new β phage [10].

Epidemiology

Humans are the only reservoir for *C. diphtheriae*. Although *C. diphtheriae* is a ubiquitous pathogen, disease is currently rare in developed countries, with an annual incidence of 0.1–0.2 per million [11]. Infection is spread via aerosolized respiratory droplets or by direct contact with infected skin lesions. Cutaneous diphtheria is more contagious than infection via the respiratory route, and bacterial shedding from cutaneous infections continues longer than from the respiratory tract. Skin infections are the major reservoir of *C. diphtheriae* in overcrowded endemic areas with poor hygiene. In tropical climates, cutaneous diphtheria infections prevail over respiratory infections. The organism has been isolated from 30–60% of skin ulcers of various types, including impetigo, yaws and infected abrasions, in the paediatric age-group in Tanzania, Sri Lanka and Samoa [11].

The incidence and epidemiology of diphtheria in the western hemisphere has changed dramatically in the past century. Respiratory diphtheria was the leading cause of death in Canadian children in the 1920s [12]. During the 1940s, many servicemen in the Mediterranean, South Pacific and Asian regions contracted ulcerative cutaneous diphtheria. In 1975 cutaneous diphtheria accounted for 56% of the total *C. diphtheriae* isolates reported in the USA. Since then, there has been a steady sharp decline in incidence, with less than five reported cases since 1980. Rates of infection are considerably less in immunized populations, and where infections occur within this population they are usually less severe. While immunization programmes have been in part responsible for the decreased incidence of diphtheria, toxoid administration does not fully explain the sharp decline in diphtheria incidence. Rates began to fall prior to the development of vaccination programmes and epidemics have continued to occur even in immunized populations. Factors other than toxin production may contribute to pathogenicity.

Recent outbreaks of cutaneous diphtheria have occurred in underdeveloped countries and among the homeless in North America. Despite high rates of immunization, 30–60% of adults in Western Europe have subprotective levels of antitoxin, creating the potential for resurgence [13]. Travellers to developing countries who live in close contact with the indigenous population run a particular risk of contracting cutaneous diphtheria. Of particular relevance, the Russian diphtheria epidemic of 1994, affecting 46 000 individuals, comprised mainly of immunized adults, was attributed to 'the arrival in Moscow in 1990 of infected military recruits from southern Russia where cutaneous diphtheria is endemic [14]. Such foci in overcrowded, impoverished environments may be important reservoirs of infection. Immunization with diphtheria toxoid has been reported to counteract the selective advantage for toxigenic strains. Thus it would seem prudent to administer diphtheria toxoid along with tetanus toxoid when treating skin ulcers in any patient with respiratory diphtheria.

Clinical manifestations

Cutaneous diphtheria classically presents as a chronic non-healing ulcer with undermined margins, covered by a leathery grey membrane. This is also known as ecthyma diphthericum. Sites of predilection include the lower extremities, feet and hands. The lesions are painful and covered by a dark pseudomembrane during the first several weeks. Spontaneous resolution usually occurs within 6–12 weeks, but cases lasting up to 1 year have been observed. The resulting depressed scars have a concentric pattern, due to progressive healing beginning from the margin. Only 15% of cases fit the classic description of ecthyma diphthericum, with the characteristic ulcer and grey pseudomembrane [11]. The morphology of cutaneous diphtheria can be extremely variable, due to its ability to colonize pre-existing skin lesions (e.g. surgical wounds, impetigo, dermatitis, scabies, paronychia, insect bites, psoriasis, eczema). In addition, *Staphylococcus aureus* and group A β-haemolytic *Streptococcus* are frequent copathogens, making isolation of *Corynebacterium* difficult. Cutaneous lesions are rarely associated with signs of systemic infection. Membranous pharyngitis rarely occurs, although 20–40% of the patients with cutaneous diphtheria carry *C. diphtheriae* in their upper respiratory tract. Guillain–Barré syndrome and cranial-nerve defects can occur in 3–5% of patients with skin lesions. Close supervision for changes in cardiac or neurological status is recommended [15]. Cutaneous infection produces high circulating antitoxin levels and, in addition to serving as a dangerous reservoir of infection, may also act as a natural immunizing event. In endemic conditions, 3–5% of healthy individuals may harbour the organism in their throats. In the USA, where disease incidence is very low, isolation of the organism from healthy individuals has become extremely rare [15].

Diagnosis

All suspicious lesions should be examined for *C. diphtheriae*. Characteristic beaded metachromatically staining bacilli can be found in methylene blue-stained smears of the membrane. Corynebacteria are often seen with streptococci or staphylococci as irregular, clubbed rods lying in an L, V, or Y 'Chinese-letter' configuration. Colonial morphology and microscopic appearance on selective media, such as Loeffler's or tellurite agar, remain the gold standard for diagnosis. *Corynebacterium diphtheriae* is distinguished by metachromatic granules when stained with Loeffler's medium. The laboratory must be instructed to use selective media when the disease is suspected. Rapid diagnosis with immunofluorescent staining for the organism on 4-hour cultures is available in some institutions. Toxigenicity may be demonstrated by the agar-diffusion precipitin reaction (Elek plate), which consists of development of an immunoprecipitin band on antitoxin-impregnated filter-paper laid over an agar culture of the organism. Dermonecrosis on guinea-pig inoculation is another effective gauge of toxin production [10]. Diagnosis by polymerase chain reaction (PCR) holds promise; however, this technique is not yet available for this purpose in the USA. Differential diagnosis includes pyogenic infection, which is usually more purulent and lacks the grey pseudomembrane. Fungal infection, which typically has heaped-up irregular margins, must also be considered. Early lesions of cutaneous diphtheria frequently resemble impetigo.

Treatment

Antitoxin is the treatment of choice, administered as 20 000–50 000 units intramuscularly or intravenously. As 10% of the population may be hypersensitive to horse serum, the patient must be tested with a 1 : 10 dilution of Diphtheria anti-toxin (DAT). This may be inoculated on to the conjunctiva or a 1 : 10–1 : 100 dilution injected intravenously. Adrenaline must be available for immediate administration in case of anaphylaxis.

   Diphtheria may occur in immunized individuals. Concomitant treatment with antibiotics (erythromycin 2 g per day, procaine penicillin G 600 000 units per day intramuscularly or rifampicin 600 mg per day) [16] assists in eliminating the convalescent carrier state, decreases toxin production and inhibits spread of the organism. Erythromycin is the most effective antibiotic for eliminating skin carriage. Débridement of the necrotic eschar and treatment with topical antibiotics facilitates re-epithelialization of the lesions [17].

Listeriosis

Definition

Listeriosis is an uncommon, serious bacterial infection that frequently affects neonates. Pregnancy, old age and immunosuppression are also risk factors for this disease, which often presents as sepsis or meningitis. Cutaneous findings are generally only found in neonatal disease.

Epidemiology

Listeriosis occurs in both endemic and epidemic forms. Food-borne transmission is a major cause of human disease. The organism resides in soil, vegetation and the faeces of wild animals and birds. Human faecal carriage occurs in approximately 5% of individuals, but is definitely increased in family members of afflicted individuals [18]. Contaminated food products, such as unpasteurized milk and cheese, raw fruits and vegetables and undercooked chicken, can serve as sources of infection. This was clearly demonstrated when a major epidemic occurred in the USA in 1985 associated with contaminated Mexican-style cheese [19]. Restriction-endonuclease digestion profiles can now be utilized to more accurately identify the point source in such outbreaks [20]. Hospital-acquired infections in immunosuppressed patients and neonatal units have been documented [21].

The disorder most commonly affects newborn infants. Infection may be apparent at birth or develop several weeks after delivery; the former is believed to be secondary to congenital infection while the latter is the result of acquisition at or around the time of birth.

Leukaemia, acquired immune deficiency syndrome (AIDS) or renal failure confers an approximately 1000-fold greater risk for development of disease [22]. Patients with disorders leading to iron overload and those with vascular aneurysms or grafts also appear to be at higher risk [23, 24]. An increasing number of cases have been noted presenting as spontaneous bacterial peritonitis in patients with underlying cirrhosis [25].

Aetiology

Listeria monocytogenes is a motile, aerobic, thin, Gram-positive rod that possesses a characteristic trait known as 'tumbling motility'. When grown in broth at room temperature, this distinctive motion is quite helpful in identifying the organism. It can assume a coccoid as well as rod-shaped appearance, decreasing the utility of Gram stain in arriving at the appropriate diagnosis. *Listeria* is a facultative intracellular organism, and thus competent macrophage function is crucial in eradicating the organism.

Clinical manifestations

Early-onset neonatal infection is present at birth or within the first few days of life. Infants may be acutely ill and appear growth-retarded and/or septicaemic. Granulomas on the posterior pharynx or skin are characteristic but not always present. Hepatosplenomegaly may occur, as may granulomas within multiple organs, such as the liver, spleen and lungs. Cutaneous lesions can be petechial, papular, pustular or granulomatous. Gram stain of such lesions may reveal Gram-positive rods or cocci. Late-onset disease may present as meningitis.

Adult-onset disease is generally non-specific in nature and lacks cutaneous findings. The one exception to this rule occurs in veterinarians exposed to stillborn or infected animals. In this situation, cutaneous lesions, consisting of erythematous papules or pustules, may develop, along with tender regional adenopathy. More commonly, adults present with malaise, fever, headache and signs of bacteraemia or meningitis. Joint infections and endocarditis have also been documented in adults [26, 27].

Diagnosis and treatment

Diagnosis is often difficult on clinical grounds, as the findings are non-specific. Infection in the neonatal period may be confused with congenital infections, such as herpes simplex, cytomegalovirus (CMV), rubella, toxoplasmosis and syphilis. Group B streptococcal and other bacterial infections must also be considered in such clinical situations. Culture and Gram stain of blood, cerebrospinal fluid (CSF), skin lesions and placenta must be performed. Gross examination of the placenta is also quite useful in neonatal disease. A clinicopathological study of seven cases of neonatal *Listeria* seen over a 7-year period in Minnesota revealed that placental macroabcesses were the most characteristic finding in infected placentas [28]. In addition, silver-impregnation stains were more reliable than was routine Gram stain in identifying the organism.

Penicillin or ampicillin is considered first-line therapy for this disease. Addition of gentamicin leads to synergistic killing of the organism, and this aminoglycoside is therefore often also utilized for serious disease. Bactrim is a reasonable alternative in penicillin-allergic patients, as is erythromycin in pregnancy. It is important to remember that *Listeria* is resistant to cephalosporin therapy, and thus third-generation cephalosporins, often utilized for treatment of meningitis, will be ineffective in listeriosis.

Recent investigations have centred around the role of T-cell subsets and cytokines in the elimination of *Listeria* infections. As the organism is a facultative intracellular pathogen, both macrophage and cytokine functions are crucial in eradication of the organism. Decreased interferon-γ levels have been noted in supernatants from neonatal mononuclear cells infected *in vitro* in comparison with those levels noted from adult infected cells [29]. Future therapy may therefore involve the utilization of specific cytokines to stimulate optimal macrophage function in affected infants and adults.

Cutaneous anthrax (Table 3.2)

Definition

Bacillus anthracis is a large, Gram-positive, spore-forming rod, which measures 10 μm in length. Anthrax is distributed worldwide. Infection is acquired via contact with soil-borne spores. It is primarily a disease of livestock and only incidentally infects humans who have direct contact with diseased animals or animal products, such as wool, hides or bones. Spores may remain viable for several years in the soil, as the bacillus is thermostable. Anthrax was first described in the book of Genesis as the 'fifth plague', killing the Egyptian cattle herds. An outbreak in seventeenth-century Europe was called 'the black bane'. Anthrax came to be known as 'malignant pustule' and the pulmonary form as 'wool-sorters' disease', due to the frequency of infection in industrial wool factories in the early twentieth century [30].

Microbiology

Anthrax bacilli have a complex life cycle in the soil. A vegetative phase is necessary to release the spore from dormancy and to allow anthrax spores to multiply to a sufficient population such that grazing animals can become infected. The bacteria cycle through herbivores, which release bacteria into the soil and water upon their death. *Bacillus anthracis* has three key virulence factors: a polysaccharide capsule, oedema toxin and lethal toxin. The poly-D-glutamic acid capsule inhibits phagocytosis by macrophages. Oedema toxin has two components: oedema factor (EF) and protective antigen (PA). Lethal toxin is composed of lethal factor (LF) and PA.

Table 3.2 Uncommon infectious disorders with cutaneous findings.

Organism	Cutaneous findings	Reservoir	Treatment
Bacillus anthracis	Painless eschar with peripheral oedema	Livestock	PCN/vaccine
Erysipelothrix rhusiopathiae	Acral violaceous plaques	Pigs, fish	PCN/fluoroquinolone
Pseudomonas mallei	Lymphangitic nodules ('farcy buds')	Equine	Streptomycin/TCN
Pseudomonas pseudomallei	Suppurative nodule with lymphangitis	Water, soil	Bactrim + ceftazidime

PCN, penicillin; TCN, tetracycline.

Protective antigen is required for transport of EF and LF into target cells. Lethal and oedema toxin work together to inhibit bacterial phagocytosis and the oxidative burst of polymorphonuclear neutrophils. Each of these key virulence factors increases host susceptibility to infection by depressing phagocytic function [31]. Spores are deposited in minute abrasions in the skin and multiply to produce toxin. The local chancre, with extensive gelatinous oedema, results from tissue necrosis due to elaboration of EF exotoxin.

Epidemiology

Human cutaneous anthrax is a disease rarely seen in the USA, due to vaccination of livestock and safety protocols for employees in the textile industry. Nonetheless, 80% of cases of anthrax in the USA in the past century have been due to industrial exposure [32]. The majority of the cases have resulted from contact with imported goat hair. Cases still occur in those who directly import wool for their own weaving. Since 1979 there have only been four reported cases of disease. An enzootic focus of animal anthrax exists in Texas, where animal outbreaks have occurred every year since 1974 [33]. The potential exists for additional cases of cutaneous anthrax with exposure to contaminated animals in such enzootic regions. This public-health threat underscores the need for vaccination of livestock and exposed workers in these regions.

Enzootic anthrax is still prevalent in tropical countries where veterinary control of livestock is difficult and where environmental conditions are favourable for perpetuation of the animal–soil–animal food cycle. Key affected regions include western Asia (Iran, Afghanistan, Turkey) and western Africa. The disease remains a major cause of mortality among African wildlife, which cannot be easily vaccinated. The incidence of human anthrax in the world is estimated to be 20 000–100 000 cases per annum and is confounded by underreporting. The largest agricultural outbreak occurred in Zimbabwe between 1979 and 1985. More than 10 000 cases of human infection were reported with a case–fatality ratio of 1.55% [34]. The monitoring and detection of anthrax in the environment and identification of affected grazing patterns are important public-health issues. Selective growth media are currently ineffective in inhibiting background flora. The application of PCR and monoclonal antibody techniques may greatly improve attempts to identify contaminated regions.

Anthrax bacilli have been produced as potential weapons for germ warfare. An explosion at a plant in north central Russia in 1979 produced 30 000 human cases of anthrax. Autopsy reports on 42 of the victims revealed pathological lesions diagnostic of inhalation anthrax. This underscores the potential use of *Bacillus anthracis* in biological warfare [35].

Clinical manifestations

Lesions develop after a 1–3-day incubation period as pruritic papules, which vesiculate and eventually ulcerate. Exposed sites, including the head, forearm and hands, are most commonly involved. The painless ulcer becomes covered by a thick necrotic eschar, with extensive surrounding gelatinous oedema. Lymphadenopathy, headache, fever and malaise are noted in approximately 90% of cases. At all stages, the lesion remains painless. Healing occurs within a few weeks and leaves a shallow granulating ulcer. Bacteraemia occurs rarely, accompanied by high fever and hypotension. Meningitis may occur in the setting of bacteraemia; however, more than 95% of cases in the USA are soley cutaneous. The case–fatality ratio for treated cutaneous anthrax is less than 1%. The mortality rate for untreated disease approaches 20% [36]. The differential diagnosis includes staphylococcal disease, plague and ulceroglandular tularaemia. The extensive gelatinous oedema aids in differentiation from other chancriform lesions. Staphylococcal carbuncles are characteristically tender, unlike the painless ulcer seen in anthrax.

Diagnosis

Gram stain of tissue or exudate reveals characteristic boxcar-shaped encapsulated bacilli. Methylene-blue stain visualizes the polypeptide capsule. Bacilli are usually abundant and are readily cultured on standard blood or nutrient agar. Colonies are grey-white to white and non-haemolytic. Fluorescent-antibody staining can be applied to vesicular fluid smears. An enzyme-linked immunosorbent assay (ELISA) test has been developed that measures antibodies to the lethal and oedema toxins. Diagnosis is confirmed serologically by demonstrating a fourfold change in titre between acute and convalescent sera collected 4 weeks apart. Emergency diagnostic kits were prepared for use during the Persian Gulf War (1990–1992).

Treatment

Bacillus anthracis is sensitive to penicillin, chloramphenicol, erythromycin and tetracycline. Penicillin G in a dose of 1 million units every 4–6 hours is the treatment of choice. Ciprofloxacin or doxycycline is a recommended alternative [31]. Lesions become culture-negative after several hours but therapy should be continued for 2–6 weeks. Incision and drainage are not recommended, as this may result in dissemination into the bloodstream. Person-to-person transmission has not been documented. Specific antianthrax serum should be employed in conjunction with bactericidal antibiotics in treating those with septicaemic anthrax [37]. To prevent latent infection, penicillin prophylaxis should be combined with vaccination. The highly resistant anthrax spore has been shown to persist for years in factories processing contaminated materials. Individuals at occupational risk of exposure should be immunized. Aggressive decontamination efforts include the use of paraformaldehyde vapour to kill *Bacillus anthracis* spores, autoclaving of instruments and 5% hypochlorite or carbolic acid for sterilization of laboratory surfaces.

Immunization

A killed vaccine derived from a component of the exotoxin is currently used for human prophylaxis in the USA. Vaccination of all employees of textile mills, who may have contact with contaminated materials in the environment should be routinely performed. Veterinarians and others who have potential contact with anthrax should also be immunized with human anthrax vaccine. United Nations and Allied forces were immunized against anthrax during the Persian Gulf War due to the threat of germ warfare. The recommended course consists of three parenteral injections at 2-week intervals, followed by three booster inoculations at 6-month intervals and annual booster vaccinations [38]. Recombinant DNA technology holds promise for the development of new vaccines using specific anthrax exotoxin components.

Tularaemia (Table 3.3)

Definition

First described in the early twentieth century as a 'plague-like illness

Table 3.3 Tularaemia.

Aetiology	*Francisella tularensis* (Gram-negative pleomorphic rod)
Distribution	North America, Europe, Asia
Principal vector	Ticks; less common: fleas, mites, mosquitoes, deer-flies
Reservoir	Rabbits, rodents, beavers, muskrats and insects
Modes of transmission	Contact with, inhalation of or ingestion of contaminated animal products; animal or insect bites
Incubation	Varies: average 5 days
Clinical manifestations	Ulceroglandular (>50%) Glandular (10–60%) Typhoidal (10–30%) Oculoglandular (<5%) Rare forms: pharyngeal, pneumonic
Treatment	Streptomycin Cefotaxime Fluoroquinolones Gentamicin Tetracycline Chloramphenicol

among ground squirrels' [39] in Tulare County, California, tularaemia is caused by a small, Gram-negative pleomorphic rod, *Francisella tularensis*. It has a widespread geographical distribution, numerous animal reservoirs and protean clinical manifestations. Lymphadenopathy, fever, ulcerative skin lesions and conjunctivitis are the most common findings. In atypical cases, meningitis, pharyngitis, gastroenteritis or pneumonia can also occur. Not surprisingly, other infections, such as influenza, infectious mononucleosis, typhoid fever, brucellosis, cat-scratch disease (CSD), plague or tuberculosis are often initially considered in the affected patient.

Skin involvement is a prominent finding and may be the only clue to diagnosis. Ulcerative lesions and regional lymphadenopathy are the usual skin findings. Unusually, an array of cutaneous manifestations may be present, including macular, papular, vesicular, pustular or petechial rashes, and erythema nodosum [40].

Tularaemia's severity ranges from asymptomatic infection (more often seen in endemic areas) to 30% mortality in untreated individuals with severe illness. With administration of appropriate antimicrobials, however, the clinical response is usually excellent [41, 42]. Thus, the importance of making the diagnosis of tularaemia cannot be underestimated.

Epidemiology

Tularaemia is found in North America, Europe and Asia, including Japan. It is notably absent in the UK, Africa, South America and Australia. Prior to the Second World War, it was common in the USA; thereafter, it declined rapidly, with an incidence since 1965 of approximately one case per million US inhabitants [43–45]. Over half of US cases in the late 1980s were reported in Missouri, Arkansas and Oklahoma, with sporadic outbreaks in the Great Plains and Rocky Mountain states [46].

Seasonal peaks in incidence reflect the two most important modes of tularaemia transmission: arthropods (especially ticks) and infected animals (especially rabbits). Peaks in summertime correspond with increased exposure to ticks, the most common vector in North America. A variety of *Dermacentor* and *Ixodes* species of ticks feed on infected vertebrates. The organism is transmitted to and multiplies within the tick, translocates across the gut and progresses to the salivary glands. The next blood meal exposes the new host via contact with saliva or via tick faecal material as the meal ensues. In endemic areas, such as in Alaska and Montana, ticks and their infected enzootic hosts frequently come into contact with human populations. Serological and skin-test evidence in native Americans and animal trappers in these settings indicates that asymptomatic infection is common. Less commonly, fleas, mites and mosquitoes serve as vectors. A smaller peak in late autumn relates to contact with infected animals, especially rabbits. Other temporal and climatic factors, such as unusually heavy periods of rainfall, have been reported.

Worldwide, the epidemiological pattern of tularaemia is complex, a function of multiple reservoirs of infection and modes of transmission [47]. Infection occurs in over 100 species of wild animals, including birds, Amphibia and fish, with rodents and lagomorphs most susceptible. In North America, rodents, hares, squirrels, beavers and domesticated animals, such as dogs, have most often been implicated as cofactors in disease spread. In the former USSR, voles, muskrats, mice and other rodents more frequently play a role. In Europe and Japan, hares and field mice predominate. Accordingly, tularaemia has historically been named rabbit fever, deer-fly fever, market-men's disease (USA), water-rat trappers' disease (Russia) or yato-bigo (Japan). The severity of infection with tularaemia is more variable in North America than the generally mild disease seen in Europe and Asia. Differences in *Francisella* species biogroups and their respective virulence probably contribute to the variety of disease manifestations.

Although arthropod bites or contaminated animal products account for most cases, animal bites, inhalation and ingestion are also reported modes of transmission [47, 48]. Ingestion of contaminated animal meat produces infection even when meat is frozen, although proper cooking does kill the organisms. Tissue samples from tularaemia patients pose a significant risk to non-immune laboratory personnel who are performing cultures. Despite successful isolation from the human oropharynx and sputum, person-to-person transmission has not been reported.

Aetiology

The ophthalmological surgeon Martin first reported a case of human tularaemia in 1908. Over a decade later, Dr Edward Francis demonstrated that 'deer-fly fever' was a consequence of infection with *Bacterium tularense*, an organism that had been previously isolated in squirrels [49]. Francis clearly established the deer-fly as the vector and named the human disease tularaemia to underscore the frequency of accompanying bacteraemia. His work so improved existing microbiological, serological and epidemiological knowledge of the disease that the bacterial genus was recast as *Francisella* in 1947.

Francisella tularensis is a Gram-negative rod, which sometimes appears more spherical, depending on its growth phase. Colony growth is optimal after 2–4 days on cysteine-enriched media; the organism grows poorly on routine solid culture media [50]. All strains produce catalase and β-lactamase. The cell wall has a high fatty-acid content. Wild strains also have a lipid capsule, a major determinant of the organism's virulence: capsule-negative mutants succumb to serum bactericidal factors, while wild-type capsule-possessing strains are resistant. Endotoxin activity of the lipopolysaccharide (LPS) from live vaccine strains of *F. tularensis* is one-thousandth that of *Escherichia coli*, although radiation-killed *Francisella* species have endotoxin-like properties in rabbits. Host immune activity is directed against LPS, cell-wall antigens and membrane proteins [51].

Clinical manifestations

The majority of cases of tularaemia may be classified as ulceroglandular, oculoglandular, glandular or typhoidal [52]. There are rarer pharyngeal and pneumonic forms as well. The incubation period depends upon the clinical category, averaging approximately 5 days (when a vector history is obtainable). Physical findings are determined by portal of entry, serogroup virulence and host factors. Symptoms commence abruptly, including fever, myalgia, headache and weakness. Delirium, restlessness, splenomegaly, hepatomegaly, jaundice, cough, vomiting and diarrhoea may also occur.

Ulceroglandular tularaemia is diagnosed in over half of cases. The hallmark is a papule at the inoculation site, which is swollen, painful and purulent in the centre. This lesion (0.3–2.0 cm) subsequently ulcerates, leaving a raised border. Multiple lesions may occur. The ulcer(s) may resolve over weeks in untreated patients and form a scar. Simultaneously or within a few days of the initial skin lesion, a painful regional lymphadenopathy develops. If untreated, the node may spontaneously drain. A nodular lymphangitis emanating from the inoculation site with subcutaneous nodules may falsely suggest sporotrichosis. Despite the tenderness of skin lesions and lymph nodes, most patients with ulceroglandular disease experience a benign course.

Glandular tularaemia comprises greater than 60% of cases in Japan, and 10–15% of cases in the USA. This form is almost identical to ulceroglandular disease except for the absence of skin lesions. The most commonly involved nodes are the axillary, which are red and tender. Fever is present, but other signs of systemic infection are unusual.

The gravest form is typhoidal tularemia (10–30%). These patients are toxic, with any combination of high fever, malaise, headache, meningismus, vomiting, diarrhoea, cough and sepsis. Diagnosis is routinely obscured by lack of a visible inoculation site or lymphadenopathy [41, 53]. Delays in diagnosis, the presence of pleural or pulmonary disease, and underlying medical conditions all increase the likelihood of a poor outcome. Without antibiotic therapy, up to one-third of patients succumb.

Oculoglandular tularaemia (<5%), the rarest form, consists of markedly erythematous conjunctivitis with preauricular, submandibular or cervical lymphadenopathy. Visual acuity may be decreased and photophobia, epiphora, eyelid oedema and occasional corneal ulceration may occur. As with ulceroglandular and glandular tularaemia, oculoglandular disease does not lead to advanced pathological states as a rule.

Other rare disease forms include pharyngitis and gastroenteritis. The former primarily affects children, and is characterized by a painful, exudative, pustular pharynx. Occasionally, the inflammatory exudate leads to the formation of a tonsillar membrane (similar to that of diphtheria), with the potential for airway obstruction. Gastroenteritis has most often occurred in the setting of epidemic water-borne outbreaks in the former USSR. The watery stool is sometimes bloody due to the presence of superficial ulcerations of the colon.

The outcome of tularaemia is generally good, especially with early and appropriate use of antimicrobials and supportive measures. Death occurs in less than 5% of cases, usually as a result of pneumonia or adult respiratory distress syndrome. Other rare complications include pericarditis, meningoencephalitis, disseminated intravascular coagulation and renal failure [42].

Diagnosis

In endemic areas or in the setting of an epidemic with known exposure history to risk factors, diagnosis should not be difficult. In 25–50% of patients, however, no source of infection is evident, and laboratory data may furnish additional clues. The complete blood-cell count often reveals a significant leucocytosis with a normal differential and a mild anaemia; however, these findings are not constant. The erythrocyte sedimentation rate is usually elevated. Severely ill patients with typhoidal tularaemia may have hyponatraemia, elevated creatine phosphokinase, myoglobinuria, pyuria or renal failure. Positive blood cultures are frequently seen in typhoidal and pneumonic disease forms.

A single serum agglutination titre (greater than 1:80) is strongly suggestive of infection, and diagnosis is confirmed by at least a fourfold rise in titre in acute versus convalescent serum. Peak antibody titres usually occur in the second to fourth week of illness, ranging from a usual 1:1024 to greater than 1:40000 [54].

Though not routinely performed because of potential occupational exposure to non-immune laboratory technicians, cultures of infected tissues (including blood, skin ulcer, lymph nodes or sputum) are often revealing. Fluorescent-antibody staining of infected material demonstrates intracellular organisms within neutrophils and macrophages, with extracellular organisms in necrotic areas. Finally, inoculation of infected tissue into rabbit or guinea-pigs should lead to the animal's demise within 2 weeks and, upon necropsy, hepatic and splenic necrosis is present [52]. The advent of serology and the clinical importance of prompt diagnosis has rendered such xenodiagnostic methods obsolete in most settings.

Immunity follows natural infection or administration of live attenuated vaccine strains of *F. tularensis* [55]. Killed vaccine strains confer immunity poorly. Lifelong immunity is cell-mediated. Though not widely available, an intradermal tularaemia skin test is positive in the first week of infection in over 90% of cases.

Prevention and treatment

As with other vector-mediated infections, public-health emphasis should rest on reducing exposure of high-risk populations to relevant vectors. This includes avoidance of areas with high tick burdens, such as woods and streams, and eradication of tick populations in those areas. Protective clothing should be worn, such as hats, long-sleeved shirts and full-length trousers tucked into socks. Frequent examination for adherent ticks should be performed, including hard-to-visualize areas of the scalp and back; household pets should also be searched. Vaccination should be considered for workers in laboratories or animal industries.

When infection does occur, early diagnosis and initiation of effective chemoprophylaxis is potentially life-saving. Streptomycin in adult doses of 1–2 g daily for 10–14 days is efficacious [51]. Cefotaxime, fluoroquinolones, tetracycline and chloramphenicol have also been used, with variable rates of cure. Gentamicin for 7–10 days is an acceptable alternative to streptomycin in both adult and paediatric patients [56, 57].

Response to treatment is usually rapid. With treatment delay, risk of adverse sequelae is increased and convalescence is protracted. Fever may persist for over a month and fatigue, weight loss and lymphadenopathy may ensue for many months in untreated patients with tularaemia. Presumptive treatment pending serological confirmation is clearly warranted in appropriate clinical settings.

Erysipeloid

Definition/aetiology

Erysipelothrix rhusiopathiae is the aetiological agent of erysipeloid, an acute cellulitis occurring in traumatized skin of the digits in handlers of raw fish, poultry and meat products. The organism measures 0.8–2.5 μm and is a non-spore-forming, non-motile, pleomorphic, aerobic, Gram-positive rod. *Erysipelothrix rhusiopathiae* was first isolated in mice by Robert Koch in 1878 and in pigs by Pasteur in 1882. Loeffler established *E. rhusiopathiae* as the aetiological agent of pig erysipeloid in 1886. Pigs are more frequently infected than any other animal. Rosenbach described the first case in humans in 1909 and proved the aetiological agent via self-inoculation. The localized cutaneous form is named eponymously [58].

The organism is rod-shaped and tends to form long branching filaments. *Erysipelothrix rhusiopathiae* grows both aerobically and anaerobically on standard bacteriological media, as well as in conventional blood-culture systems. Colonies grown at 37°C for 24 hours are transparent, with a shiny smooth surface. *Erysipelothrix rhusiopathiae* produces two key virulence factors — a neuraminidase and a hyaluronidase — which facilitate tissue destruction. The organism displays α-haemolysis on blood agar, a key distinguishing feature from β-haemolytic Gram-positive bacilli, such as

Corynebacterium, Listeria and *Lactobacillus,* which are frequently in the differ-ential diagnosis. Other identifying characteristics include a negative cata-lase reaction and the production of hydrogen sulphide in the butt of a triple-sugar iron-agar slant [59].

Epidemiology

Domestic pigs are the key reservoir for *E. rhusiopathiae.* The organism can persist for prolonged periods on the mucoid slime of fish; however, it is not pathogenic to fish or shellfish. The majority of cases are related to occupa-tional exposure. Those at greatest risk of infection include fishermen, butchers, slaughterhouse workers and housewives. Contact with fish poses the greatest risk of disease. Erysipeloid is widespread along the entire Atlantic sea coast among commercial fishermen who handle live fish, crabs and other shellfish. The disease is also found amongst meat packers who handle raw pork products [60].

Clinical manifestations

Cutaneous disease exists in four forms: as erysipeloid of Rosenbach, a localized cutaneous form of the disease; as a diffuse cutaneous form; as subacute bacterial endocarditis; and as a bacteraemic form without endocarditis.

Erysipeloid of Rosenbach, localized cutaneous form. The organism gains entry via a skin break, usually on the hands. After a 2–7-day incubation period, painful, violaceous, sharply marginated plaques develop, typically on the hands and proximal aspects of the digits, with sparing of the terminal pha-langes. Lesions are warm and extremely tender to palpation. Central clear-ing occurs as the lesion expands peripherally. Ulceration does not occur. As the initial lesion heals, centrifugal spread at a rate of approximately 1 cm per day may occur. Cutaneous disease is frequently accompanied by fever and malaise. Lymphadenopathy occurs in approximately 30% of cases. Arthraglia occurs in 10% of patients [60]. The violaceous colour and severe pain of these lesions serve to distinguish erysipeloid from cellulitis due to *Staphylococcus* and *Streptococcus.*

Diffuse cutaneous disease. The diffuse cutaneous form occurs secondary to proximal extension of the localized type or due to widespread, non-contiguous dissemination. Urticarial lesions with a diamond-shaped morphology are seen in the disseminated variant of human disease. This rhomboidal pattern is characteristic of infection in domestic pigs. These lesions are the result of thrombotic vasculitis of end arterioles. Fever and arthralgia are frequent accompanying symptoms. Diffuse disease com-monly recurs and runs a protracted course compared with localized erysipeloid.

Subacute bacterial endocarditis. Bacteraemia accompanied by endocarditis can occur but is rare. Septicaemia occurs most often in fishermen and in meat handlers who are occupationally exposed to the organism. Two cases have been reported to occur following ingestion of undercooked pork. Skin lesions occur in approximately 36% of cases. Endocarditis due to erysipeloid has a higher mortality rate than endocarditis due to other organisms (38% vs. 20%) [61]. Congestive heart failure due to valvular insufficiency develops in approximately 80% of patients. Other reported sequelae include myocardial abscess, meningitis and glomerulonephritis. Valve replacement is necessary in 30% of patients. The organism is readily recovered from routine blood cultures.

Bacteraemia without endocarditis. Immunosuppressed hosts may develop the bacteraemic form of the disease without endocarditis. Osteomyelitis, brain abscess and chronic arthritis are frequent sequelae. A case of fulminant bacteraemia with septic shock has been reported in a crab fisherman undergoing corticosteroid therapy for idiopathic myocarditis. Treatment consisting of 2 weeks of parenteral penicillin followed by 2 weeks of oral penicillin, combined with aggressive hydration and vasopressors, resulted in a return to haemodynamic stability [62]. *Erysipelothrix* septicaemia may be accompanied by repeated episodes of pulmonary infarction. The focus of infection in such cases lies in the venous system or in the arterial side of the cardiovascular system. Infected emboli dislodge and result in pulmonary infarction [63].

Diagnosis

The basic disease process is a cellulitis and, as such, the organism resides in the deep dermis and subcutaneous fat. Accordingly, aspirates and biopsy specimens should extend into the deep dermis in order to maximize recovery of the causative agent. Definitive diagnosis rests on isolation of *E. rhusiopathiae* from blood or tissue. Serological testing is not a reliable diagnostic tool for erysipeloid. The organism is rarely visible on Gram-stained lesional material, but may be isolated on culture of biopsy specimens taken from the advancing margin of the lesion.

Treatment

Mild forms of erysipeloid are typically self-limited and resolve spontaneously within 3–4 weeks; however, healing is hastened by antibiotic therapy. Penicillin G (12–20 million units per day for 7–10 days) is the treatment of choice for severe infections. Fluoroquinolones are effective in the penicillin allergic patient. First-generation cephalosporins provide an acceptable treatment alternative. Most strains of the organism are resistant to vancomycin, a first-line agent in the treatment of most forms of gram-positive septicaemia. Endocarditis due to *E. rhusiopathiae* should be treated with intravenous antibiotics for four to six weeks [64]. The development of a live attenuated vaccine, coupled with improved waste-disposal practices, has helped to control the porcine reservoir of *E. rhusiopathiae*.

Lyme disease (Table 3.4 and Fig. 3.5)

Definition

Lyme disease is the most common vector-borne illness in the USA [65]. The spirochete *Borrelia burgdorferi* was identified as the aetiology in 1975, when an apparent cluster of juvenile rheumatoid arthritis cases occurred in Lyme, Connecticut, prompting an exhaustive epidemiological investigation [66]. This also led to the identification of the *Ixodes scapularis* tick as the vector of the disease. Extensive clinical and laboratory investigation of the patho-physiology and treatment of Lyme disease has greatly expanded medical and public awareness of this condition.

Epidemiology

Worldwide, borreliosis syndromes similar to that first described in Con-necticut also occur in Europe, the Far East and Australia [67]. Since initia-

Table 3.4 Lyme disease.

Aetiology	*Borrelia burgdorferi*
Epidemiology	USA, Europe, Far East, Australia
Principal vector	*Ixodes* species of ticks; nymphal form principal cause of human infection
Reservoir	Deer, dogs, horses, cattle
Incubation	Up to 1 month; mean 7–10 days
Clinical manifestations	*Cutaneous* Erythema chronicum migrans (30–80% of affected patients), expanding ovoid or annular red plaque, often with central clearing. Central red papule (tick-bite site) may become indurated, vesicular, ecchymotic or necrotic. Multiple lesions occur in 50% of patients several days later and are usually smaller. Less common: malar rash, urticaria, conjunctivitis. Late: acrodermatitis chronica atrophicans: red or violaceous atrophic or sclerotic lesions; more common in Europe. *Systemic* Acute phase: fever, malaise, headache, myalgias Second stage (2 weeks to 2 years): joint involvement, meningitis, cranial neuropathy, conjunctivitis, keratitis, uveitis. Cardiac: AV dissociation, palpitations, myocarditis, pericarditis (rare)
Treatment	Uncomplicated disease: amoxycillin or doxycycline Neurological disease: parenteral penicillin or third-generation cephalosporins Penicillin-allergic patients: erythromycin, azithromycin

AV, atrioventricular.

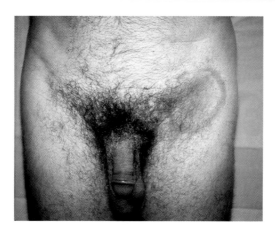

Fig. 3.5 Erythema chronicum migrans (Lyme disease).

tion of surveillance by the Centers for Disease Control and Prevention (CDC) in 1982, over 50 000 cases of Lyme disease have been reported in the USA, with almost all states represented. Three geographical foci exist: the north-east (Massachusetts to Maryland), the mid-west (Minnesota and Wisconsin) and the west (California and Oregon) [68]. Migratory birds may be involved in the spread of Lyme disease into states in which the life cycle of the vector is limited. In the north-east and the mid-west, the principle vector is *I. scapularis* (also called *Ixodes dammini*, the black-legged tick); in the west, the vector is *Ixodes pacificus* (the western black-legged tick). These ticks are closely related members of the *Ixodes ricinus* complex.

Affected individuals range from 2 to almost 90 years of age, with a median of 28 years, and age-adjusted attack rates show comparable rates of disease acquisition across all strata [69]. Subclinical infection has been shown to be the norm in serosurveys of endemic areas, such as Sweden and Switzerland, where only 2–12% of seropositive individuals reported previous symptoms [70, 71].

As with other tick-borne infections, there is a summer and autumn predominance. In the northern hemisphere, most patients experience the onset of symptoms in June or July. The disease appears to afflict adult males and females equally, although one study of childhood Lyme disease reported the relative risk to be two to four times higher in boys than in girls [72].

Geographically, subjects with Lyme disease are likely to live in suburban or rural areas. Although the organism does survive in blood, person-to-person transmission and transfusion-acquired disease have not been reported to date. Deer and numerous other fauna do not seem to become ill with *Borrelia* infestation in the wild, but domesticated dogs, horses and cattle do suffer from illnesses consistent with the classical features of human disease, and may serve as an additional reservoir of infection [73].

The natural cycle of infection in humans exclusively involves ticks, although deer-flies and mosquitoes also harbour *B. burgdorferi*. Up to half of *Ixodes* ticks carry the organism in New York State, versus one-third of ticks in Connecticut and only 2% in California [74]. The *I. scapularis* tick has a 2-year life cycle that involves progression from larva to nymph to adult. In late summer, the larvae hatch. They ingest one blood meal, usually from white-footed mice (*Peromyscus leucopus*), and the following spring they become nymphs. Nymphs in turn ingest a blood meal, and finally become larger adults the following autumn. Adults are only a few millimetres in size, making detection difficult. Nymphs are the principal cause of human infection, although all stages of tick development may feed on humans [74]. In experimental studies of tick-mediated spirochaete transmission to rodents, tick attachment for over 24 hours was crucial for successful infection to occur [75]. *Borrelia burgdorferi* live in the tick midgut and may be transmitted as the tick regurgitates while feeding.

The remarkable increase in number of cases over the last 10 years reflects increased populations of deer and perhaps mice, on which *Ixodes* ticks feed, and increasing diagnostic recognition and reporting practices.

Aetiology

Borrelia and other spirochaetes have a long cylindrical protoplasmic core surrounded successively by a cell wall, flagella and an outer membrane. *Borrelia burgdorferi* is the longest (20–30 µm) and narrowest (0.25 µm) of all spirochaetes; it appears filamentous on electron micrography. Both chromosomal and plasmid DNA encode for several membrane lipoproteins (outer-surface proteins), flagellar and protoplasmic antigens, heat-shock proteins and other antigens [76]. Several of these polypeptides determine host immune response; a succession of antibody titres develops to diverse spirochaetal antigens as the clinical course progresses [77].

The six outer-surface proteins (OspA–F) are encoded by unusual linear plasmids, whose structure is not found in other prokaryotes [78]. Sequences of DNA in these plasmids resemble African swine fever virus and other poxviruses [79]. The organism is fastidious; it is best cultured at 33°C on Barbour–Stoenner–Kelly or other solid media [74]. Although it is rarely necessary to culture the organisms, the erythema migrans skin lesions represent the optimal culture site; recovery of organisms is less likely in other tissue sites [80].

Clinical manifestations

As with other spirochaetal infections, Lyme disease evolves in stages over a period of weeks to years [74]. After injection of the spirochaete into human skin, it may spread locally and later travel haematogenously to peripheral muscle and myocardium, to joint and bone, to brain, meninges and CSF or to liver, spleen and macrophages. *In vitro*, pathogenic strains of *B. burgdorferi* may survive phagocytosis, which provides evidence of the organism's ability to escape eradication by the immune system early in infection, allowing dissemination [81].

Acute disease manifestations usually follow the bite of an infected tick by a few days to a month (mean 7–10 days) [69]. A non-specific prodrome includes intermittent fever and chills, headache, myalgia, arthralgia and fatigue).

Thirty to eighty per cent of patients develop the hallmark rash of erythema migrans. Children develop the rash more predictably than adults. Early physical findings may also include lymphadenopathy, hepatosplenomegaly and—rarely—cough, pharyngitis or orchitis.

Erythema migrans is a characteristic rash that begins as a red macula or papule at the site of the tick attachment. Typical sites include the groin, thighs and axillae, although the lesion can occur anywhere. Within 2 days, there is rapid expansion to a circular or ovoid lesion of approximately 5 cm (range 3–68 cm), whose outer margins remain bright red and are usually flat. There is an area of central clearing, which at times becomes indurated, vesicular, ecchymotic or necrotic. Usually the area is warm but not very painful. Spirochaetes can be recovered from these early skin lesions, especially from the margins.

Several days after the initial lesion, multiple annular lesions not associated with tick attachment develop in approximately 50% of patients. These secondary skin lesions are usually smaller and less indurated than the original one, with which they may coexist. Additional cutaneous features at this stage may include malar rash, urticaria or conjunctivitis [74].

Fever may accompany the rash during the acute phase and is often quite elevated. It is intermittent, as are malaise, headache and neck and muscle aches. These symptoms, along with the erythema migrans rash and its secondary annular counterparts, usually last 3 or 4 weeks and resolve even when there has been no treatment with antibiotics. Fatigue, however, may be exceptionally persistent, often lasting several months after the resolution of the rash. Respiratory or gastrointestinal symptoms are rare in the acute presentation of Lyme disease.

The second stage of Lyme disease is marked by a variable pattern of dissemination of the spirochaete to involve the joints, the nervous system, the eyes and/or the heart. These symptoms may subsequently become chronic. From 2 weeks to 2 years after acute disease symptoms, four-fifths of untreated patients experience joint symptoms and signs, which vary from migratory arthralgia to chronic erosive synovitis [74, 82]. Attacks of a few weeks to months, with periods of complete remission, are characteristic of the pattern of joint involvement. Often the knee is remarkably swollen and warm, but is rarely erythematous; pain may not be present. The incidence of chronic joint symptoms increases with age at the time of initial infection [83].

With every year after disease onset, the number of patients with joint findings decreases by 10–20% [74]. Approximately 10% of untreated patients develop chronic arthritis (defined as greater than 1 year of continuous arthritis).

Host factors probably help to determine which subset of patients will develop chronic arthritis. Patients with chronic Lyme arthritis have joint-space infiltration with mononuclear cells and *Borrelia*-specific T-cell clones, which produce cytokines consistent with a T-helper-1 (Th1) pattern (and delayed-type hypersensitivity) [84]. These patients are also more likely to possess human leucocyte antigen (HLA)-DR4 class II antigens of the major histocompatibility complex [21]. Such patients have an exaggerated humoral immune response, with persistently elevated immunoglobulin M (IgM) titres and higher IgG antibody responses to two of the outer-surface proteins of the spirochaete (OspA and OspB). Patients with the exaggerated antibody titres and HLA-DR4 are also remarkable in that they frequently fail to improve with antibiotic therapy [85].

Besides arthritis, the disseminated stage of Lyme disease includes several neurological abnormalities, which are seen in approximately 15% of all patients [86]. The most common pattern of neurological abnormality is a fluctuating meningitis with accompanying cranial neuropathy, especially of the facial nerve. The neck is typically stiff, but only upon extreme flexion. Meningeal irritation without CSF pleocytosis may occur early in the illness along with the erythema migrans rash, but patients with frank meningitis usually have a CSF white blood-cell count of approximately 100, with a lymphocytic predominance [74]. The CSF protein count is elevated, usually with a normal glucose. Conversely, in Europe, patients may have a CSF pleocytosis, with cranial neuropathy and neuritic pain in the absence of headache; this constellation has been called the Bannwarth syndrome [74, 87].

Peripheral nerves may reveal a pattern of sensory or motor radiculopathy or mononeuritis multiplex, with a perivascular lymphocytic infiltrate around the vessels that supply axons.

Chronic neurological sequelae are less common than chronic arthritis, but may last over a decade. The subacute encephalopathy caused by Lyme disease alters mood, sleep, memory or language, sometimes subtly. Conversely, borrelial encephalomyelitis (usually seen in Europe) is often severe, causing ataxia, cranial neuropathy, cognitive dysfunction, bladder abnormalities and spastic paraparesis. Intrathecal production of *B. burgdorferi*-specific IgM, IgG and IgA and oligoclonal bands has been reported in acute meningitic forms of Lyme disease, as well as in chronic encephalopathy or encephalomyelitis [87]. The pathological determinants of acute versus chronic neurological sequelae are poorly understood.

Besides late rheumatological and neurological findings, late cutaneous manifestations can also occur in untreated patients. Acrodermatitis chronica atrophicans consists of red or violaceous lesions of the extremities, which may appear atrophic or sclerotic and mimic localized scleroderma.

This skin manifestation is usually seen in patients from Europe and some-times lasts for over a decade [88].

Finally, disseminated Lyme disease may be found in the eye and heart. Conjunctivitis is the most common eye finding, but keratitis, uveitis, iritis and panophthalmitis occur as well [83]. Cardiac manifestations affect approximately 5% of patients, usually lasting less than 6 weeks [89]. Palpi-tations or mild dyspnoea may be present, and electrocardiography may reveal any degree of atrioventricular dissociation. Myocarditis and peri-carditis are rare. Valve disease and heart murmurs should prompt investiga-tion for acute rheumatic fever and other conditions.

Congenital infection is probably rare, but may be devastating. Two infants died in the first week of life whose mothers had both developed Lyme disease in the first trimester [90, 91]. As gestation continues, the risk of sequelae to the fetus diminishes, with trimester-specific risk decreas-ing from 63% to 38% to 10%. A retrospective study of Lyme disease during pregnancy showed approximately 25% adverse outcomes overall, including prematurity, blindness, syndactyly, and rash, as well as intrauter-ine fetal demise [92]. Treatment during pregnancy did not alter the incidence of adverse outcomes in this study; however, many believe that antibiotics administered to pregnant women may have a protective effect on the fetus. To add to the confusion, subsequent prospective studies have failed to document maternal–fetal transmission of the *B. burgdorferi* spirochaete [93].

Diagnosis

Criteria established by the CDC for the clinical diagnosis of Lyme disease include the rash of erythema migrans or at least one objective rheumato-logical, neurological or cardiac finding not explicable by another diagnosis that is confirmed by diagnostic laboratory findings (see below) [65]. The child or adult from an endemic region with a known tick exposure and ery-thema migrans should be treated without delay. Difficult cases to diagnose include individuals who have not been to endemic areas or who present without rash, with non-specific flu-like symptoms, with chronic fatigue or with late or atypical disease manifestations.

Laboratory data may serve as useful adjuncts and are required for diag-nosis in the absence of the erythema migrans rash. Elevated levels of IgM in serum or CSF, a significant rise in paired acute versus convalescent sera or isolation of the organism from a clinical specimen constitute diag-nostic laboratory findings. Although significant differences in serological values may result among different laboratories, most commercially avail-able ELISA, indirect immunofluorescene (IFA) and antibody-capture immunoassay (EIA) tests are both sensitive and specific [94]. As with other screening tests, the predictive value is decreased (regardless of sensitivity or specificity) in areas of low disease prevalence, underscoring the importance of knowing the epidemiology of Lyme disease when obtaining *Borrelia* serologies [95]. Titres of IgM usually peak from the third to the sixth week of illness [96]. Titres of IgG may require months, as the response to various borrelial antigens sequentially expands [77].

Although there is a correlation between late symptoms and serological findings, elevated antibody titres do not always reflect active disease. Titres remain indistinguishable in treated and untreated patients alike, and there is a high background rate of asymptomatic infection in endemic areas [83]. Furthermore, false-positive results may be due to non-borrelial spirochaetal disease (syphilis) or other infections (infectious mononucleosis, leptospirosis) or due to autoimmune disease (rheumatoid arthritis, systemic lupus erythematosus). Rapid plasma reagin (RPR) and Venereal Disease Reference Laboratory (VDRL) tests are negative in Lyme disease.

The clinical utility of PCR in blood, urine and CSF samples has still to be refined, although it appears promising. Polymerase chain reaction of synovial-fluid samples was positive in 85% of patients and 0% of controls in one study [97], although it is less sensitive and specific in blood, urine and CSF.

Routine blood values are usually non-diagnostic. Twenty per cent of patients have elevated transaminases, but these usually return to normal values within a few weeks. The peripheral white blood-cell count is occasionally elevated, with variably increased immature polymorphonuclear forms.

Overdiagnosis is common according to numerous experts, with the most common difficulty arising when attempting to distinguish Lyme disease from syndromes of chronic fatigue or fibromyalgia [74].

Treatment

Oral antibiotics are effective for most manifestations of Lyme disease; however, involvement of the nervous system usually necessitates parenteral therapy. For uncomplicated disease, amoxycillin and doxycycline in routine doses are equally efficacious [98]. Doxycycline should not be used in children, because of the risk of dental staining; amoxycillin is safer. If allergies exist, oral cefuroxime or macrolide antibiotics (erythromycin and azithromyin) can be used. *In vitro, B. burgdorferi* are routinely sensitive to penicillin and related antibiotics and to second- and third-generation cephalosporins, erythromycin and tetracycline [99]; however, resistance to aminoglycosides, fluoroquinolones and rifampicin is common.

Duration of therapy should conform to the severity of systemic manifestations. Skin infection responds to 10 days of treatment, while disseminated disease, including arthritis, mild heart block (see below) or isolated cranial nerve palsy requires 3–4 weeks of oral antibiotics. Treatment of disseminated disease may be accompanied by the Jarisch–Herxheimer reaction (fever, chills, malaise) upon initiation of therapy in approximately 15% of patients.

Except for isolated cranial neuropathy, objective neurological abnormalities warrant parenteral therapy. Intravenous third-generation cephalosporins (ceftriaxone or cefotaxime) and penicillin G for 2–3 weeks have proven effective [100, 101]. Patients with carditis or elongated P–R intervals require intravenous antibiotic therapy and close monitoring of the patient's cardiac status.

Patients with relapses of rash, fever or other symptoms may require a second course of antibiotics. Relapses are especially likely to occur when treatment is instituted before a substantial immune response has occurred (e.g. during the first 3 weeks of infection) or when there has been reinfection. In one study, 11% of children with Lyme disease appropriately treated with antibiotics developed a second episode of erythema migrans rash. When these patients received further therapy with either the original antibiotic or an alternative regimen, none of the 63 study patients had late rheumatological, neurological or cardiac recurrences after $3\frac{1}{2}$ years of follow-up [102].

Ixodes ricinus-complex ticks are also capable of transmitting the organisms that cause ehrlichiosis and babesiosis, and coinfection may explain treatment failures (e.g. persistence of fever, fatigue or arthralgia, but not erythema migrans) in a small subset of patients with Lyme disease.

Corticosteroids have a role in treating selected eye and cardiac findings. In the treatment of keratitis, topical steroids may be more beneficial than antibiotics [83]. Corticosteroids may also hasten recovery of the patients with cardiac conduction abnormalities or congestive heart failure who do not improve within 24 hours of initiating antibiotic therapy [74].

Evidence is limited regarding optimal treatment of Lyme disease in pregnancy. Standard therapy appropriate to the extent of illness is probably warranted, although its adequacy is unestablished.

Prophylactic antibiotic therapy is probably not advisable for a history of tick bite in endemic areas, unless there has been prolonged attachment of the tick (greater than 24 hours), the tick is visibly engorged upon removal or follow-up is uncertain. In this setting, 10 days of oral therapy prevents disease occurrence [103].

Natural immunity follows infection in most patients, except when they are treated early in the illness and the immune response is blunted [74]. A vaccine consisting of recombinant OspA is currently being evaluated [104]. Public-health guidelines on who should receive the vaccine (and data on its cost-effectiveness) are not yet available.

Preventive measures for Lyme disease (and other arthropod-borne illnesses) include avoiding the vector, wearing hats and long-sleeved shirts and full-length trousers tucked into socks in the woods and applying insecticide to exposed skin. Examination of the skin for ticks is important and should include the lower extremities, groin and axillae. In children, the head and neck are also frequent sites of tick attachment. If a tick is seen, it should be grasped as close to the skin as possible with fine tweezers and removed by pulling gently away from skin in a perpendicular direction. Domestic pets should also be checked for ticks. Eradication of ticks from their sylvan habitat by use of widespread chemical spraying may be partially effective but remains controversial, given lack of data on human disease reduction and potential for toxic environmental effects.

Glanders

Definition/microbiology

Glanders is a rare disease caused by *Pseudomonas mallei*, a non-motile Gram-negative aerobic bacillus. The organism is distributed widely in soil, stagnant water and marine environments. Also known as 'equinia', this organism has an equine reservoir and primarily infects humans who care for horses, mules or donkeys. *Pseudomonas mallei* is catalase- and oxidase-positive and is capable of growth over a broad range of temperatures, ranging from 4 to 43°C. Media must be supplemented with glycerol for optimal growth [105].

Epidemiology

Glanders primarily infects equine hosts. Pigs and cattle are resistant to infection. The incidence of glanders has steadily decreased worldwide, due to isolation of diseased animals. Cases continue to occur sporadically in Asia and Africa. Prominent pulmonary involvement is characteristic of equine infection; however, subcutaneous and ulcerative lesions are not uncommon. Potential mechanisms of transmission in animals include inhalation, ingestion or inoculation of skin abrasions. Humans may acquire disease via inoculation of skin breaks or contact with contaminated nasal discharge of infected horses, mules or donkeys. Due to improved sanitation measures, there have been no cases of glanders in the USA since 1938 [105]. The infectivity of aerosolized particles has been shown by the high incidence (46% in one series) of infection among personnel in cases of laboratory contamination [106].

Clinical manifestations

Primary infection of the skin occurs via inoculation of an abrasion or through the conjunctiva or nasal mucous membranes, due to contact with infected nasal secretions from infected animals. Acute localized suppurative lesions, accompanied by malaise, fever and headache, develop following an incubation period of a few days to 2 or 3 weeks. Lesions are typically erythematous papules or vesicles, which ulcerate to form a sharply defined excavations with a haemorrhagic, malodorous, purulent discharge. The regional lymphatics become swollen and tender, and dull red nodules ('farcy buds') break down to form abscesses and sinuses. The mucous membranes are particularly susceptible to infection, and a profuse nasal discharge is a clinical hallmark of glanders. Disease may present with acute epistaxis, catarrhal symptoms or a characteristic mucoid nasal discharge. Extensive necrosis of the mucous membranes, with destruction of the septum and palate, may occur. Skin lesions may progress to caseating granulomas of the periorbital or centrofacial regions. Chronic cycles of recurrent ulceration and healing may occur.

Septicaemia occurs in a small percentage of patients, accompanied by a generalized papulopustular eruption. The mortality rate is high during the first 1–2 weeks in the acute septicaemic form of glanders. Acute pulmonary infection occurs via inhalation of aerosolized particles. After a 10 to 14-day incubation period, symptoms include fever, myalgia and pleuritic chest pain. Radiography reveals well-circumscribed densities suggestive of pulmonary abscesses. Acute lobar or bronchopneumonia frequently supervenes.

Another subtype, chronic suppurative glanders, is characterized by generalized subcutaneous abscesses in 80% of cases. Fifty per cent of these patients develop lymphangitic spread and mucoid nasal discharge with ulcerations. Visceral involvement occurs in less than 25% of cases, as summarized by Robins [107]. Blood cultures are typically negative until terminal stages of the disease.

Diagnosis

Organisms are generally difficult to demonstrate, even in acute abscesses. Methylene-blue staining reveals small, irregularly staining, Gram-negative bacilli. *Pseudomonas mallei* and *Pseudomonas pseudomallei* cannot be differentiated by staining pattern. Complement fixation is the most sensitive technique for demonstrating acute infection. Positive values occur at a dilution of $>1:20$. Rising agglutination titres are sensitive but not specific, as healthy persons may have titres of $1:320$. Titres exceeding $1:640$ are considered diagnostic [87].

Treatment

Treatment consists of immediate surgical excision of inoculated lesions followed by streptomycin and tetracycline. Sulphadiazine has also been found to be effective in experimental animals and in humans at a dose of 100 mg/kg administered for a 3-week course [108]. Due to the small incidence of human infection, many of the newer antimicrobials have not been evaluated. With limited clinical experiene, sources recommend using regimens with demonstrated efficacy in treating melioidosis. Surgical débridement and drainage are essential for chronic suppurative infections. Isolation of infectious individuals and equine hosts is a key prophylactic intervention.

Table 3.5 Cutaneous disorders caused by *Bartonella*.

Disease	Organism	Location	Cutaneous findings	Systemic findings	Treatment
Cat-scratch disease	*B. henselae*; rarely *B. quintana*, *B. elizabethae*	Initial papule— extremities, Lymphadenopathy— neck, axilla. Less common: epitrochlear, inguinal, femoral, supraclavicular	*Acute*: macula, papule or vesicle at inoculation site (1–3 weeks) *Chronic*: regional lymphadenopathy, tender and erythematous (2–6 months)	Fever, malaise, headache Atypical: oculoglandular syndrome of Parinaud, encephalopathy	Unnecessary in most patients; rifampicin, trimethoprim– sulpha and ciprofloxacin for systemic symptoms
Bacillary angiomatosis	*B. henselae*	Any cutaneous surface	Erythematous to violaceous vascular papules and nodules of varying size	DIC, hypotension	Erythromycin
Bartonellosis	*B. bacilliformis*	Any cutaneous surface Less common: subcutaneous, mucous membranes Rare: viscera, bones, muscles	*Acute*: Oroya fever, jaundice, facial and pedal oedema *Chronic*: verruga peruana—red to purple vascular papules or nodules of varying size, easily bleed	Wide spectrum: fever, anorexia, headache, joint pain, anaemia, hepatosplenomegaly	Tetracycline, chloramphenicol

DIC, disseminated intravascular coagulopathy.

Cutaneous diseases caused by *Bartonella*

Bartonellosis (Table 3.5)

Definition

Bartonellosis is an infection of human erythrocytes and vascular endothelium caused by *Bartonella bacilliformis*. The Andean habitat of the major vector, the *Phlebotomus* sandfly, accounts for the limited geographical distribution of disease. Human pathogenesis of bartonellosis comprises two distinct clinical forms, Oroya fever and verruga peruana. The Incas long ago recognized the distinctive skin lesion that is the hallmark of the chronic form of bartonellosis, the haemangioma-like nodule termed a verruga peruana [109]. In 1885, Peruvian medical student Daniel Carrion underwent voluntary inoculation with blood from a patient's verruga. Tragically, he died of Oroya fever, the acute disease form. This led to the recognition of the unified aetiology of acute and chronic disease states. Bartonellosis is also referred to as Carrion's disease in his honour [110].

Epidemiology

Infection is only endemic within river valleys in Peru, Ecuador and Colombia. The sharply demarcated distribution of cases greatly facilitates the diagnosis of bartonellosis in either of its two clinical manifestations. The last great epidemic occurred in 1870, when thousands of railway workers constructing the line between Lima and Oroya died.

The sandfly *Phlebotomus verrucarum* (also called *Lutzomyia verrucarum*) plays a principal role in the transmission of bartonellosis, although the occurrence of unusual cases outside the habitat of this sandfly suggests the existence of other vectors as well [111]. The sandfly's habitat spans elevations of 700–2500 m above sea level, and this generally corresponds to the distribution of human disease. Only female sandflies seek blood meals, preferring to feed at night. The insects may live within dwellings in humid, dark niches.

Up to 10% of residents of endemic areas have blood cultures positive for the bacilli; most are asymptomatic. Humans with asymptomatic infection and chronic disease carriers are the only significant disease reservoirs; there are no known animals that carry the disease. Either or both of the human pathogenic forms may be found within given endemic areas in Peru [112].

Aetiology

Bartonella bacilliformis is a small, aerobic, Gram-negative, pleomorphic rod, which is variably bacillary or spherical. It appears red-violet upon Giemsa staining. Growth is best facilitated on solid agar enriched with rabbit serum and haemoglobin [113].

There appears to be an intriguing association between the dimorphic nature of the bacteria and the character of fever in the affected patient. The bacillary form is important in provoking the febrile response, whereas the coccoid form does not induce fever. In the first week of illness, fever correlates with the increase in bacillary forms, which parasitize nearly all circulating erythrocytes by the seventh day of illness. During the second week of illness, bacillary and coccoid forms coexist and fevers continue. Week 3 signals the resolution of fever and the predominance of the coccoid form. Both *in vivo* and *in vitro*, 'rosary-like' intermediate forms may be seen and provide evidence that bacillary multisegmentation results in the coccoid morphology [112]. The means through which the change in bacterial shape modulates host inflammatory response has not been completely elucidated.

Clinical manifestations

Bartonellosis comprises two distinct clinical disease states, Oroya fever and verruga peruana. In non-immune individuals, Oroya fever may have an indolent course, reflecting the paucibacillary nature of some infections. Indeed, most infections are asymptomatic. Conversely, the patient may be heavily parasitized and acutely toxic. The spectrum of symptoms ranges from low-grade fever, with anorexia, malaise, headache and arthralgias, to high fevers, with chills, severe headaches, bone and large-joint pains and alterations of consciousness.

Fever, anaemia and hepatosplenomegaly with lymphadenopathy are the hallmarks of the sick patient with Oroya fever. Fever typically reaches 40°C, fluctuating over several weeks. The fever lacks a predictable temporal pattern and induces considerable diaphoresis. Anaemia is acute and potentially life-threatening, the result of haemolysis and the abbreviated lifespan of parasitized red blood cells. Although the organisms are intraerythrocytic and red blood cells lack cell-surface antigen-presenting molecules, macrophages selectively engulf red cells that contain bacilli. Erythrocyte-laden macrophages are sequestered within the enlarged spleen, liver and lymph nodes. The anaemia may cause dyspnoea and angina, as well as an exaggerated proprioception of the cardiac impulse being propagated to the ears and head.

The integument assumes a characteristic hue, from combined pallor and mild jaundice. Additionally, facial and pedal oedema, resulting from hypoproteinaemia, may be seen. Mental-states changes range from insomnia to delirium, stupor and coma, these latter usually portending a fatal course.

Adverse outcomes in Oroya fever most often occur during the convalescent phase, from the third week after the onset of infection onward. Superinfection with *Salmonella* species (most commonly *Salmonella typhimurium*) and other enteric pathogens develops in approximately 40% of Oroya-fever patients. Amoebiasis, tuberculosis and malaria are also common. Signs of probable intercurrent infection include the resurgence of fever or prominent splenomegaly or leucocytosis during convalescence [114]. Anaemia, with resultant anoxia, worsens outcome from these infections, as do leucopenia, thrombocytopenic purpura and poor nutritional status. There is no chronic form of Oroya fever, and no individual with Oroya fever who is treated with appropriate antibiotics subsequently develops verruga peruana.

Verruga peruana is the cutaneous form of human bartonellosis, which can either follow Oroya fever or occur without prior symptoms. The appearance of verruga lesions following Oroya fever may coincide with the resolution of systemic symptoms, such as myalgias or arthralgias. Alternatively, joint pain may accompany the appearance of the lesions, most commonly in the knees; this is called verrucous rheumatism. Fever accompanying verruga peruana is of variable intensity, but anaemia is rare at this stage.

The verruga lesions are red to purple, appear in crops over 1–2 months and persist for months to years. They are most commonly present in the skin, but may appear in the subcutaneous tissues, the mucous membranes or, rarely, the internal viscera, bones or muscles. Verrugas vary in size from 1–2 mm in the case of the miliary form (which lasts only weeks) to slightly larger nodules (lasting up to 6 months). They may also achieve the size of giant tumours. As a rule, the larger the nodules, the fewer the lesions. The skin lesions appear pleomorphic when both miliary and nodular forms occur in the same patient.

The typical nodule is pea-sized, shiny and red, with the external surface of the nodule composed of the overlying skin as it is distended by the nodule's growth. The lesions bleed easily, which may present problems in the nasopharynx and respiratory tract. Laryngeal nodules pose a risk of airway obstruction even in the absence of bleeding. On mucous membranes, the nodules may be pedunculated. Only the miliary form exists within internal organs (spleen, intestine, meninges, gut, lungs, serosal surfaces and muscle). Larger nodules may be found in the interstices of large muscle groups. Regardless of the site of infection, *Bartonella* organisms themselves localize exclusively within the capillaries.

Given their vascular nature, it is not surprising that bleeding may be provoked by even minor trauma. Rarely, nodules may become secondarily infected, but, unless this occurs, nodules eventually fall off the skin without forming a scar.

Diagnosis

Patients with known exposure to sandflies in endemic disease areas with the clinical features of Oroya fever should be treated promptly. When the patient has not been to an endemic area, the diagnosis is more difficult. Laboratory data reflect haemolysis, reticulocytosis and hypersplenism. The anaemia is macrocytic, with Howell–Jolly bodies, nucleated forms, basophilic granulations, poikilocytosis and polychromasia seen on the peripheral smear. Serum unconjugated bilirubin is elevated, as are urobilin and stercobilin, and iron stores in the liver and spleen are increased. Erythroid precursors are increased in the bone marrow and the periphery. The white blood-cell count is variable, but the differential usually shows a shift to the left. There may be significant pancytopenia, which predisposes to complications.

For Oroya fever, the most useful diagnostic study is the eosin/thiazine stain of peripheral blood. *Bartonella* organisms may be seen within the vast majority of erythrocytes (except in paucibacillary forms of the disease, in which the recognition of the organisms may be difficult). Serology may be misleading, as elevated IgM levels have been found in acutely infected patients as well as healthy controls, and also in patients with the verrugal form of bartonellosis [115]. Polymerase chain reaction diagnostic techniques are under development [116].

The angiomatous skin lesion is the diagnostic hallmark of the verruga form of bartonellosis. Histologically, the verruga is a densely reticular lesion that is highly vascularized, rich in angioblasts and lymphatic vessels and contained within an oedematous connective-tissue matrix. Fibroblasts and phagocytic cells are present in variable numbers. The organism is rarely seen on light-microscopic examination, but electron microscopy shows cytoplasmic (Rocha–Lima) [112] inclusions within endothelial cells or neutrophils [117], and cultures of the cutaneous lesion (as well as blood and bone marrow) often grow organisms. The histopathological appearance of the verruga is suggestive of Kaposi's sarcoma or other neoplastic disorders; epidemiological, clinical or serological evidence for bartonellosis is therefore necessary to establish the diagnosis [118].

Prevention and treatment

Cases are best prevented by diminishing exposure to the sandfly. Wearing protective clothing, applying insect repellent, using bed nets and spraying insecticide around dwellings may be highly effective. With regular use of insecticides in houses, both bartonellosis and malaria were reduced considerably in Peru until spraying was discontinued [112]. There is no vaccine available against either disease form.

Tetracycline in doses as low as 250 mg every 12 hours is effective prophylaxis; as a 5-day course of treatment, it prevents both Oroya fever and verruga peruana from developing. Chloramphenicol is an excellent choice for treatment of active Oroya fever, since coinfection with *Salmonella* is common. Penicillin, tetracycline and streptomycin are acceptable alternatives [119]. When the diagnosis remains in doubt and the patient is sick, initiation of treatment pending further confirmatory data is indicated. Blood transfusion may be life-saving in acute anaemia.

The efficacy of antimicrobial therapy for verruga peruana (except for superinfected lesions) is unproved. Surgical excision or cautery of verruga may be indicated in critical anatomical sites (e.g. the eye or the larynx). Corticosteroids are of value in the treatment of verrucous rheumatism.

Cat-scratch disease (Fig. 3.6)

Definition

Cat-scratch disease (CSD) is an infection consisting of regional lymphadenopathy with variable fever and systemic symptoms. These findings occur following a bite or scratch sustained from a cat or, more commonly, a kitten. This disorder accounts for a large proportion of cases of chronic lymphadenopathy in children, who generally experience a benign clinical course. After almost a decade of controversy, there now exists substantial evidence that the cause of CSD is *Bartonella henselae*.

Epidemiology

Although CSD may occur at any age, it is generally a disease of childhood. In most case series, approximately 80% of patients acquired the infection within the first two decades of life [120]. Whether this represents increased

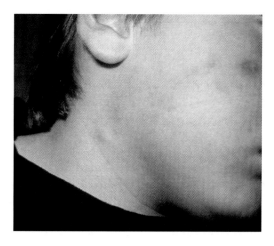

Fig. 3.6 Cat-scratch disease.

risk of exposure in younger ages or an age-specific immunological phenomenon has not been ascertained.

The disease is worldwide in distribution but occurs predominantly in temperate regions. There is a seasonal preponderance in autumn and winter months. Approximately 90% of individuals with CSD have a history of exposure to cats, with roughly three-quarters of this group reporting a known scratch, lick or bite of the skin or eye. Kittens under 1 year of age account for the majority of the cats implicated in disease transmission [121]. Depending on the region, 28–55% of cats in the USA are seropositive with antibodies against *B. henselae*; warm, humid areas had the highest prevalence [122]. Bacteraemia was detected in up to 40% of cats in another study in California, in which *B. henselae* was isolated by both DNA amplification and by culture from cat-associated fleas [123]. Cats are almost always asymptomatic; humans, too, may occasionally be exposed to the organism but remain disease-free [121]. The period of infectivity in kittens may be short-lived, as disease clusters within families most often fall within a period of a few weeks [124].

In approximately 5% of cases, dogs appear to be linked with disease transmission and, in rarer instances, thorns or wooden splinters have been implicated.

The male : female ratio reveals a slight male predominance. Person-to-person transmission does not occur; no special isolation precautions are indicated. There have been no public-health recommendations regarding the removal of infectious animals from the homes of patients.

Aetiology

Bartonella henselae (formerly known as *Rochalimaea henselae*) is a pleomorphic Gram-negative rod, which was first isolated from infected lymph nodes of CSD patients. The use of the Warthin–Starry silver stain, previously employed for spirochaetal specimens, was instrumental in the identification of the pathogens within biopsy material [125]. Non-*B. bacilliformis* species (including *B. henselae*) grow slowly in 5–30 days' time on media used for fastidious bacteria; however, the cultures must be performed specifically for isolation of *Bartonella*; this requires incubation at 35–37°C under conditions of high humidity and carbon dioxide (CO_2). Colonies have a variety of morphologies, including smooth, rough, raised and 'cauliflower-like' [126].

Other non-*B. bacilliformis* species (including *Bartonella quintana* and *Bartonella elizabethae*) are occasionally implicated in CSD transmission. Differentiating *B. henselae* from *B. quintana* is difficult, but may be performed commercially by detecting minor differences in arylamidases; *B. elizabethae* possesses a rare unsaturated fatty acid and may be thus identified. Such techniques may facilitate future detection of more CSD cases due to *B. quintana* (better known as the causal agent of trench fever) or *B. elizabethae*. To date, the vast majority of cases are due to *B. henselae* [127].

The cause of CSD was controversial at the end of the past decade. *Afipia felis*, a small pleomorphic bacillus related phylogenetically to *Bartonella*, was isolated in culture from 10 affected patients in 1988. Subsequent investigation has failed to substantiate a role for this organism. Several lines of evidence point more conclusively to the importance of *B. henselae* in the pathogenesis of this disease: (i) 84–96% of CSD study patients have elevated antibody titres of at least 1 : 64 to *B. henselae*—no titres were observed in control subjects above 1 : 16 [121, 128]; (ii) *B. henselae* has been noted in culture of lymph nodes of many patients [125]; (iii) PCR was positive for *Bartonella* DNA in 21 of 25 infected lymph-node specimens [129]; (iv) PCR exclusively amplifies *Bartonella* (and not *Afipia*) DNA within CSD skin-test preparations [130]; and (v) young cats are bacteraemic with the organism and have elevated antibody titres against it [121–123].

Clinical manifestations

In the vast majority of cases, the principal clinical manifestation of CSD consists of a chronic regional lymphadenopathy. A hallmark of the disease is a well-appearing child with tender, localized lymphadenopathy. The affected lymph node is usually located in the neck or axilla, but may instead be found in epitrochlear, inguinal, femoral or supraclavicular sites. Single-node enlargement is found in about half of all patients. In one-fifth of patients, several nodes are affected within the same region. Involved nodes may achieve a considerable size of up to 10 cm, although most measure 1–5 cm. They are frequently tender and erythematous; they suppurate in 10–15% of cases.

It is important to emphasize the chronic nature of the lymphadenopathy to patients and their concerned parents, as the duration of lymph-node swelling is generally 2–6 months or longer. Significant or rapid changes in the size of the node should prompt a search for other causes of lymphadenopathy.

Two-thirds of patients manifest a skin lesion at the inoculation site. This usually consists of a papule but may be a macula or vesicle. Diligent searching may be required in order to find it, particularly if it is obscured by hair or skin creases. The skin lesion is usually encountered distal to the affected node. The primary skin lesion arises 3–10 days after the time of the scratch and persists for 1–3 weeks.

Although CSD is often referred to as 'cat-scratch fever', less than half of patients have fever greater than 38.3°C. When it occurs, however, fever may persist for weeks. This protracted course reflects the organism's ability to survive intracellularly within phagocytic cells, a capacity common among genera that share significant 16S ribosomal ribonucleic acid (RNA) sequence homology with *Bartonella*, including *Ehrlichia*, *Rickettsia* and *Brucella* species. The means by which this survival occurs is incompletely understood.

In addition to fever, other systemic findings in large case series commonly include malaise and fatigue and, less often, headache, weight loss, emesis, sore throat or parotid swelling. Several well-described atypical manifestations of CSD occur in about 10% of cases. The most common of these is the oculoglandular syndrome of Parinaud (6%) [131, 132], which includes painless unilateral granuloma of the conjunctiva with preauricular lymphadenopathy. There is usually no discharge from the conjunctiva. The eye is probably inoculated when the patient's hands rub the eye after contacting a bacteraemic kitten. Parinaud first described this syndrome in 1889, although he was not aware of its aetiology. The eye granuloma resolves over the same time course as the lymphadenopathy, with no ocular residua.

A more serious atypical manifestation of CSD is encephalopathy. This occurs in 1–2% of patients, who present with sudden alterations in behaviour or consciousness weeks after the lymphadenopathy is first noted [126]. The CSF is often normal but may show a mild elevation of protein and/or white blood cells. Encephalopathy is sometimes complicated by seizures or coma, which may last weeks. Electroencephalographic patterns reveal non-specific diffuse slowing or, less often, focal abnormalities. Complete recovery over a period of 1–6 months is the rule. Cranial and peripheral neuropathies and neuroretinitis account for the other rare central nervous system pathology seen in less than 1% of cases.

Other extraordinary clinical manifestations of CSD have been reported in skin, liver or bone. Rashes are seen in 4% of patients, and include a diverse array of presentations: erythema nodosum, erythema marginatum, erythema multiforme, granuloma annulare, petechiae, urticaria or maculopapular exanthem [133, 134]. Hepatic granuloma (without hepatomegaly or elevated liver-function tests) and bacterial osteomyelitis (with granulomas seen in aspirate of infected bone) have been reported in very rare instances [126].

In addition to CSD *B. henselae* produces bacillary angiomatosis and bacillary peliosis in immunocompromised individuals. The former condition is characterized by vascular cutaneous lesions, which contain proliferation of blood-vessels, in the skin and sometimes the underlying bone. There may be a single lesion or hundreds; they may be papules measuring 1 mm or nodules measuring 5 cm in diameter. *Bartonella henselae* bacilli and DNA have been recovered from the lesions via culture and PCR, respectively. The clinical severity of bacillary angiomatosis ranges from spontaneous resolution to sepsis, with resultant disseminated intravascular coagulation, hypotension and death.

Bacillary peliosis appears to be a related manifestation of *B. henselae* in immunocompromised individuals that consists of numerous blood-filled cystic structures within organs of the reticuloendothelial system. Affected liver, spleen or lymph nodes contain variable numbers of these cysts. These lesions are generally quite small, only 1–2 mm in size. They are separated from the parenchyma by a collection of inflammatory cells, dilated capillaries and organisms. These lesions do not involve the skin and herald a more benign clinical course than bacillary angiomatosis [127].

Diagnosis

The development of chronic lymphadenopathy of more than 3 weeks' duration in a patient with a known exposure to a young cat strongly suggests CSD. The observation of a primary inoculation site on the skin further supports the diagnosis. Most cases of CSD in children can now usually be diagnosed solely on a clinical basis. Historically, however, three of the following four criteria were necessary to define a case: (i) contact with an infected animal, usually a cat, with a primary skin or eye lesion; (ii) lymphadenopathy and aspiration of sterile pus from the affected node and relevant laboratory data that rule out other aetiologies; (iii) positive CSD skin test; and (iv) lymph-node biopsy with histopathology consistent with CSD.

Since CSD skin tests do not contain standard amounts of antigen and are no longer routinely placed, it has been suggested that serologies and PCR should now replace the skin test in this list of criteria. Reliable serological assays include indirect fluorescent antibody [121] and enzyme immunoassay [124, 135], with IgM titres rising after a few weeks of illness. Polymerase chain reaction is also commercially available and is especially useful in the diagnosis of atypical cases (e.g. in encephalopathic patients). Warthin–Starry stains and tissue culture may be similarly employed in such patients.

Though rarely performed, biopsy of affected skin shows a central area of necrosis surrounded by lymphocytes and macrophages. On pathological sections of involved organs (e.g. lymphoid tissue), the classic finding is stellate areas of necrosis. The organisms themselves may be found within neutrophils and macrophages or extracellularly within necrotic debris.

Routine laboratory data are non-specific. Early in the illness there may be a mild elevation in the peripheral white-cell count and eosinophilia in a minority of patients. The presence of a very high white-cell count or a significant CSF pleocytosis is unlikely to be due to CSD. Imaging techniques may be of value in selected clinical settings. Ultrasound of the affected lymph node may help to differentiate between other forms of bacterial adenitis and CSD, though this is often non-diagnostic. Ultrasound examination of the liver and spleen in children with systemic findings often reveals stellate granulomas. Neuroimaging with computed tomography or magnetic resonance in encephalopathic patients shows non-specific findings, but may be useful in ruling out other causes of acute encephalopathy.

Other infectious causes of chronic lymphadenopathy include tuberculous and atypical mycobacterial infection, infections with herpes-like DNA viruses (Epstein–Barr virus, CMV and herpes simplex virus), mycotic infections (coccidioidomycosis, histoplasmosis and sporotrichosis) and —more rarely—brucellosis, syphilis, toxoplasmosis and tularaemia [131]. *Staphylococcus aureus* and streptococcal spp. are more likely to cause acute lymphadenopathy, but are common and should always be considered. For this reason, children with CSD often receive an empirical course of oral antibiotics.

Non-infectious aetiologies of chronic lymphadenopathy include abnormalities of embryogenesis (branchial arch, thyroglossal duct), malignancy (leukaemia, lymphoma) or sarcoidosis. The location of the involved node may direct suspicion toward one of these causes.

Treatment

The natural course of CSD is benign and treatment is unnecessary for most patients. No controlled clinical trials have been performed. A review of numerous antibiotic regimens found that rifampicin, trimethoprim–sulphamethoxazole and ciprofloxacin orally or gentamicin parenterally was of benefit in the treatment of systemic manifestations of CSD [132]. In immunocompromised patients with bacillary angiomatosis, erythromycin is effective if administered for an extended course [127].

Surgical procedures are rarely necessary. Needle aspiration may relieve pain due to suppurative nodes. When mycobacterial adenitis is suspected, excisional biopsy may represent a better option than fine-needle aspiration. Lifelong immunity follows infection in childhood, although there have been a few case reports of recurrences in cases acquired in adulthood. There is currently no vaccine.

Melioidosis

Definition/Etiology

Melioidosis, also known by the eponym 'Whitmore's disease', is caused by a member of the *Pseudomonas* genus, *P. pseudomallei*. The organism is a motile, Gram-negative, aerobic bacillus, which is widely distributed in water and soil. Transmission occurs by direct skin inoculation or via inhalation of aerosolized particles. Melioidosis occurs predominantly in adults with underlying disease. The disease can recur years after successful treatment or remain latent for decades prior to clinical infection. Immunosuppression, chronic disease states and stress are important factors in recurrence. Predisposing risk factors for melioidosis include alcoholism, diabetes, chronic lung disease, haematological malignancy, steroid therapy and chronic renal disease. The most common clinical presentation is a rapidly progressive pneumonia with septicaemia. This form is frequently fatal [136]. Other forms include local pulmonary infection and visceral abscesses of the liver and spleen.

Epidemiology

While clinically similar to glanders, melioidosis is epidemiologically dissimilar. Melioidosis is endemic in South-East Asia, northern Australia, Central and South America, the West Indies and Madagascar. *Pseudomonas pseudomallei* is a saprophytic inhabitant of soil, brackish water, rice paddies and market produce in South-East Asia. *Pseudomonas pseudomallei* has been isolated in up to 50% of soil samples from Thailand [136]. The correlation of melioidosis with rainfall is well recognized. A direct relationship has been shown between rainfall and increased presence of *P. pseudomallei* in surface water in Malaysia [136]. Although wild and domestic animals may become infected, it is no longer thought that animals form an important natural reservoir of infection.

Melioidosis should be suspected in military personnel or residents of endemic regions presenting with fever and subcutaneous abscesses. In one series of burn patients in South-East Asia, up to 80% had pulmonary melioidosis and all had microbiological evidence of *P. pseudomallei* on culture [137]. Subclinical infection is common, with a seroconversion rate of 24% in the paediatric age-group in Thailand. Significant haemagglutination titres have been found in 6–20% of the indigenous population in Vietnam, Malaysia and northern Australia. After 12 months in Vietnam, US army personnel returned with positive titres [138]. Melioidosis is the commonest cause of fatal bacteraemic community-acquired pneumonia in northern Australia, with only *Streptococcus pneumoniae* responsible for more bacteraemic pneumonia admissions. In a series at the Royal Darwin Hospital in northern Australia, the bacteraemic mortality rate was 26% for *S. pneumoniae* and 55% for *P. pseudomallei* [139].

Clinical manifestations

Melioidosis has a protean clinical spectrum. Four broad disease categories have been defined: acute pulmonary infection, an acute localized suppurative infection, acute septicaemia and a frequently fatal form characterized by chronic suppurative infection with multiple miliary abscesses in the viscera.

Acute pulmonary infection. Community-acquired pneumonia is the most common form of disease and may occur either in isolation or as a result of haematogenous spread. The clinical symptoms may vary from a mild bronchitis to overwhelming necrotizing pneumonia. Fever in excess of 102°F, accompanied by pleuritic chest pain, is a common presenting symptom. Pneumonia is characterized by upper-lobe consolidation. Cavitation frequently occurs. Progressive pulmonary spread with bacteraemia is not uncommon [140].

Acute localized cutaneous and soft-tissue infection. Infection occurs via inoculation of skin abrasions after a 1–2-day incubation period. A suppurative nodule surrounded by lymphangitis rapidly develops. Cutaneous infection is frequently accompanied by fever, malaise and regional lymphadenopathy. Rapid progression to the acute septicaemic form may occur. In rare cases, clinically latent infections may remain silent for many years after leaving an endemic area. Disease has been reported up to 26 years after initial exposure [141].

Acute septicaemic infection. Septicaemia may occur, with or without visceral abscess formation in the lung, spleen or liver. Whitmore's original description of melioidosis was in a narcotic addict with septicaemia. Melioidosis is still a disease predominantly of debilitated patients, with underlying immunosuppression secondary to chronic disease. Affected individuals may be immunocompromised due to renal failure, diabetes mellitus, chemotherapy and steroid-treated lupus erythematosus. The presenting symptoms depend on the site of initial organ involvement. For primary pulmonary infection, dissemination may result in dyspnoea, pharyngitis, diarrhoea and a characteristic pustular eruption of the trunk and extremities. Radiography reveals disseminated nodular densities, which may cavitate with disease progression. Confusion with tuberculosis is a frequent problem. The course is usually rapidly fatal. The overall mortality in septicaemic melioidosis remains 60–90% despite prompt administration of third-generation cephalosporins and intensive-care hospitalization [141].

Chronic suppurative infection. Residual active foci without life-threatening systemic illness develop in some patients. Clinical manifestations of this form resemble glanders, disseminated deep fungal infection and disseminated tuberculosis. Abscesses develop in skin, brain, lung, myocardium, liver, spleen, bone and lymph nodes. In a series of 126 patients with liver abscesses in Thailand, 27% were due to *P. pseudomallei*. When accompanied by splenic abscess, ultrasound is diagnostic, with multiple hypoechoic areas in the liver [142]. Such findings mandate immediate treatment.

Diagnosis

The protean clinical spectrum makes diagnosis on clinical grounds difficult. *Pseudomonas pseudomallei* has a characteristic 'safety-pin' configuration on staining with methylene blue or Wright's stain. *Pseudomonas pseudomallei* is readily grown on standard media and is easily distinguished from *P. mallei* and *Pseudomonas aeruginosa* by characteristic surface wrinkling of the colonies at 72 hours. The complement-fixation test assists in diagnosis if a fourfold or greater rise in titre is demonstrated; however, negative serological results are present in approximately one-third of culture-positive patients at the time of diagnosis [143]. Culture remains the gold standard for diagnosis. The organism may remain latent in infected individuals for many years. From this dormant state, active infection results from a variety of insults to the immune system, including diabetes, alcoholism, chronic lung disease, haematological malignancy and chronic renal disease. Tuberculosis is a key consideration in the differential diagnosis, as both diseases present with cavitating pneumonia. The index of suspicion must be high to avoid delay in bacteriological identification, which may result in inappropriate empirical antibiotic therapy. This delay in identification accounts for the high mortality noted in many published series. When an immunocompromised patient from an endemic area presents with community-acquired pneumonia and septicaemia, first-line therapy should include an agent that is effective against *P. pseudomallei*.

Treatment

Pseudomonas pseudomallei is usually sensitive *in vitro* to the tetracyclines, chloramphenicol, amoxycillin clavulanate, ticarcillin clavulanate, piperacillin, imipenem, most of the third-generation cephalosporins, sulphadiazine and trimethoprim-sulphamethoxazole. The organism is resistant to benzylpenicillin G, erythromycin, ampicillin, streptomycin and ciprofloxacin. In Thailand, resistance to trimethoprim-sulphamethoxazole is found in 12–80% of strains. Empirical therapy for severe community-acquired pneumonia consists of ceftriaxone, with gentamicin added for coverage of Gram-negative organisms. Ceftazidime is used when *P. pseudomallei* is confirmed or strongly suspected. Treatment with two antimicrobials for the initial 30 days is followed by 60–150 days of amoxycillin clavulanate or trimethoprim-sulphamethoxazole. In patients with visceral abscesses, prolonged therapy for 6–12 months is recommended. Disseminated disease with deep-seated tissue involvement and visceral abscesses is characteristically refractory to treatment. Blood cultures may remain positive despite prolonged intravenous administration of ceftazidime. Steroid therapy has not been successful. Combined therapy with three agents is recommended for septicaemic melioidosis in order to decrease resistance to ceftazidime. Parenteral therapy is given for 2 weeks, followed by oral maintenance therapy for 6 months. The current recommended daily regimen consists of trimethoprim 8 mg/kg, sulphamethoxazole 40 mg/kg, plus ceftazidime 120 mg/kg. Imipenem 4 g/day or piperacillin–tazobactam is an effective alternative for strains that are resistant to ceftazidime or trimethoprim-sulphamethoxazole [144]. The respective roles of toxin production and host immune activation in the pathogenesis and progression to disseminated pyogenic infection remain controversial. Prophylaxis against melioidosis must centre upon the following: prevention and control of the two major risk factors, diabetes and alcoholism; decreasing exposure to wet-season soils by use of protective footwear and gloves, which prevent direct inoculation; prevention of delay in therapy for suspected melioidosis; and maximizing compliance with maintenance therapy to minimize relapse.

References

1 Swartz MN, Weinberg AN. Infections due to Gram-positive bacteria. In: Fitzpatrick TB, Elsen AZ, Wolff K *et al.* (eds) *Dermatology in General Medicine.* McGraw-Hill, New York, 1993, pp. 2331–2332.

2 Hurwitz S. *Clinical Pediatric Dermatology.* Saunders, Philadelphia, 1993, p. 293.

3 Munro-Ashman D, Wells RS, Clayton YM. Erythrasma in adolescence. *Br J Dermatol* 1963; **75**: 401–404.

4 Svejgaard E, Christophersen J, Jelsdorf HM. Tinea pedis and erythrasma in Danish recruits: clinical signs, prevalence, incidence, and correlation to atopy. *J Am Acad Dermatol* 1986; **14** (6): 99–103.

5 Mattox TF, Rutgers J, Yoshimori RN *et al.* Nonfluorescent erythrasma of the vulva. *Obstetr Gynecol* 1993; **81** (5, part 2): 862–864.

6 Hamann K, Thorn P. Systemic or local treatment of erythrasma? A comparison between erythromycin tablets and Fucidin cream in general practice. *Scand J Primary Health Care* 1991; **91** (1): 35–39.

7 Zaias N. Pitted and ringed keratolysis. *J Am Acad Dermatol* 1982; **7**: 787–791.

8 Nordstrom KM, McGiuley KH, Cappiello L *et al.* Pitted keratolyses: the role of *Micrococcus sedentarius. Arch Dermatol* 1987; **123**: 1320–1325.

9 Englich PC. Diphtheria and theories of identification: centennial appreciation of the role of diphtheria in the history of medicine. *Pediatrics* 1985; **76**: 1–9.

10 Pappenheimer AM, Murphy JR. Studies on the molecular epidemiology of diphtheria. *Lancet* 1983; **ii**: 923–926.

11 Hofler W. Cutaneous diphtheria. *Int J Dermatol* 1991; **30**: 845–847.

12 Halsey NA, Smith MH. Diphtheria. In: Warren KS, Mahmoud AAK (eds) *Tropical and Geographic Medicine.* McGraw-Hill, New York, 1984, pp. 810–815.

13 Kwantes W. Diphtheria. *Eur J Hyg* 1989; **493**: 433–437.

14 Maurice J. Belated attempts to contain Russia's diphtheria. *Lancet* 1995; **345**: 715.

15 Kalapothaki V, Sapounas T, Xirouchake H *et al.* Prevalence of diphtheria carriers in a population with disappearing clinical diphtheria. *Infection* 1984; **12**: 387–389.

16 Sanford JP, Gilbert DN, Sande M. *Sanford Guide to Antimicrobial Therapy.* Antimicrobial Therapy, Inc. Dallas, Texas, 1995. 1995, p. 38.

17 Karzon DT, Edwards LM. Diphtheria outbreaks in immunized populations. *N Engl J Med* 1988; **4**: 1–43.

18 Fitzpatrick T, Eisen A, Wolff K. Bacterial diseases with cutaneous involvement. Diptheria: Dermatology in General Medicine, 3rd edn. McGraw-Hill, New York, 1993. p. 2365.

19 Ewert DP, Lieb L, Hayes PS *et al. Listeria monocytogenes* infection and serotype distribution among HIV-infected persons in Los Angeles County, 1985–1992. *J AIDS*

& Hum Retrovirol 1995; **8** (5): 461–465.

20 Proctor ME, Brosch R, Mellen JW *et al.* Use of pulsed-field gel electrophoresis to link sporadic cases of invasive listeriosis with recalled chocolate milk. *Appl Env Microbiol* 1995; **61** (8): 3177–3179.

21 Paul ML, Dwyer DE, Chow C *et al.* Listeriosis—a review of eighty-four cases (review). *Med J Aust* 1994; **160** (8): 489–493.

22 Jensen A, Fredericksen W, Gerner-Smidt P. Risk factors for listeriosis in Denmark, 1989–1990. *Scand J Infect Dis* 1994; **262** (2): 171–178.

23 Lee AC, Ha SY, Yuen KY *et al. Listeria* septicemia complicating bone marrow transplantation for Diamond–Blackfan syndrome. *Pediatr Hematol Oncol* 1995; **12** (3): 295–299.

24 Gauto AR, Cone LA, Woodard DR *et al.* Arterial infections due to *Listeria monocytogenes*: report of four cases and review of world literature [see comments] (review). *Clin Infect Dis* 1992; **14** (1): 23–28.

25 Kent SJ, Van Scoy MS, Skerrett S. *Listeria monocytogenes* peritonitis with review of literature (review). *Aust NZ J Med* 1994; **24** (4): 405.

26 Ellis LC, Segreti J, Gitelis S *et al.* Joint infections due to *Listeria monocytogenes*: case report and review (review). *Clin Infect Dis* 1995; **20** (6): 1548–1550.

27 Speeleveld E, Muyldermans L, Van den Bruel A *et al.* Prosthetic valve endocarditis due to *Listeria monocytogenes*: a case report with review of the literature (review). *Acta Clin Belg* 1994; **49** (2): 95–98.

28 Topalovski M, Yang SS, Boonpasat Y. Listeriosis of the placenta: clinicopathologic study of seven cases. *Am J Obstetr Gynecol* 1993; **169** (3): 616–620.

29 Serushago B, Macdonald C, Lee SH *et al.* Interferon-gamma detection in cultures of newborn cells exposed to *Listeria monocytogenes*. *J Interferon Cytokine Res* 1995; **15** (7): 633–635.

30 Tiggert WD. Anthrax. William Smith Greenfield, MD, FRCP, Professor Superintendent, The Brown Animal Sanatory Institution (1878): concerning the priority due to him for the production of the first vaccine against anthrax. *J Hyg* 1980; **85**: 415–420.

31 O'Brien J, Friedlander A, Prier T *et al.* Effects of anthrax toxin components on human neutrophils. *Infect Immun* 1985; **47**: 306–330.

32 Brachman PS. Anthrax. *Ann NY Acad Sci* 1970; **174**: 577–582.

33 Taylor J, Dimmit DC, Ezzell F *et al.* Indigenous human cutaneous anthrax in Texas. *South Med J* 1993; **86**: 1–4.

34 Lamarque D, Haessler C, Champion R *et al.* Le charbon au Tchad: une zoonose encore d'actualité. *Med Trop* 1989; **49**: 245–251.

35 Nettleman MD. Biological warfare and infection control. *Infect Cont Hosp Epidem* 1991; **12**: 368–372.

36 Christie AB. Anthrax. In: *Infectious Diseases: Epidemiology and Clinical Practice.* Livingstone, Edinburgh, 1969, pp. 751–779.

37 Burnett JW. Anthrax. *Cutis* 1991; **18**: 112–114.

38 Turnbull PC. Anthrax vaccines: past, present and future. *Vaccine* 1991; **9**: 19533–19539.

39 McCoy GW. A plaguelike disease of rodents. *Publ Health Bull* 1911; **43**: 53–71.

40 Cerny Z. Skin manifestations of tularemia. *Int J Dermatol* 1994; **33**: 468–470.

41 Evans ME, Gregory DW, Schaffner *et al.* Tularemia: a 30 year experience with 88 cases. *Medicine* 1985; **64**: 251–269.

42 Penn RL, Kinasewitz GT. Factors associated with a poor clinical outcome in tularemia. *Arch Intern Med* 1985; **147**: 265–268.

43 Centers for Disease Control and Prevention. Summary of notifiable diseases, United States, 1991. *MMWR* 1991; **40**: 51.

44 Centers for Disease Control and Prevention. Summary of notifiable diseases, United States. *MMWR* 1987–1991.

45 Boyce JM. Recent trends in the epidemiology of tularemia in the United States.

J Infect Dis 1975; **131**: 197–199.

46 Taylor JP, Istre GR, McChesney TC *et al.* Epidemiologic characteristics of tularemia in the southwest-central states, 1981–1987. *Am J Epidemiol* 1991; **133**: 1032–1038.

47 Morner T. The ecology of tularemia. *Rev Sci Tech* 1992; **11**: 1123–1130.

48 Syrjälä H, Kujala P, Myllylä V *et al.* Airborne transmission of tularemia in farmers. *Scand J Infect Dis* 1985; **17**: 371–375.

49 Francis E. The occurrence of tularemia in nature as a disease of man. *Publ Health Rep* 1921; **36**: 1731–1738.

50 Payne MP, Morton RJ. Effect of culture media and incubation temperature on growth of selected strains of *Francisella tularensis*. *J Vet Diagn Invest* 1990; **4**: 264–269.

51 Penn RL. *Francisella tularensis* (tularemia). In: Mandell GL, Douglas RG, Bennett JE (eds) *Principles and Practice of Infectious Diseases*, 4th edn. Churchill Livingstone, New York, 1995, pp. 2060–2068.

52 Bates JH. Tularemia. In: Braude AI, Davis CE, Fierer J (eds) *Infect Dis Med Microbiol*, 2nd edn. WB Saunders, Philadelphia, 1986, pp. 1503–1506.

53 Ohara Y, Sato T, Fujita H *et al.* Clinical manifestations of tularemia in Japan—analysis of 1355 cases observed between 1924 and 1987. *Infection* 1991; **19**: 14–17.

54 Snyder MJ. Immune response to *Francisella tularensis*. In: Rose NR, Friedman H, Fahey JL (eds) *Manual of Clinical Laboratory Immunology*. American Society for Microbiology, Washington, DC, 1986, pp. 377–378.

55 Tärnvik A. Nature of protective immunity to *Francisella tularensis*. *Rev Infect Dis* 1989; **11**: 440–450.

56 Enderlin G, Morales L, Jacobs RF *et al.* Streptomycin and alternative agents for the treatment of tularemia: review of the literature. *Clin Infect Dis* 1994; **19**: 42–47.

57 Cross JT Jr, Schutze GE, Jacobs RF. Treatment of tularemia with gentamicin in pediatric patients. *Pediatr Infect Dis J* 1995; **14**: 151–152.

58 Griecom A, Sheldon C. *Erysipelothrix rhusiopathiae*. *Ann NY Acad Sci* 1970; **174**: 523–532.

59 Sneath PHA, Abbott JD, Cunliffe AC. The bacteriology of erysipeloid. *Br Med J* 1951; **2**: 1063–1066.

60 Erlich JC. *Erysipelothrix rhusiopathiae* infection in man. *Arch Intern Med* 1946; **78**: 565–577.

61 Gorby GL, Peacock JE. *Erysipelothrix rhusiopathiae* endocarditis: microbial, epidemiologic, and clinical features of an occupational disease. *Rev Infect Dis* 1988; **10**: 317–325.

62 Ognibene FP, Cunnion RE, Gill V *et al.* Erysipelothrix rhusiopathial bacteremia presenting as septic shock. *Am J Med* 1985; **78**: 861–864.

63 Townshend RH, Jephcott AE, Yekta MH. *Erysipelothrix* septicemia without endocarditis. *Br Med J* 1973; **1**: 464.

64 Venditti M, Gelfusa V. Antimicrobial susceptibilities of *Erysipelothrix rhusiopathiae*. *Antimicrob Agents Chemother* 1984; **25**: 385–386.

65 Centers for Disease Control and Prevention. Lyme Disease—United States, 1991–1992. *MMWR* 1993; **42**: 345–348.

66 Steere AC, Malawista SE, Snydman DR *et al.* Lyme arthritis: an epidemic of oligoarticular arthritis in children and adults in three Connecticut communities. *Arthritis Rheum* 1977; **20**: 7–17.

67 Schmid GP. The global distribution of Lyme disease. *Rev Infect Dis* 1985; **7**: 41–50.

68 Steere AC, Malawista SE. Cases of Lyme disease in the United States: locations correlated with distribution of *Ixodes dammini*. *Ann Intern Med* 1979; **91**: 730–733.

69 Steere AC, Bartenhagen NH, Craft JE *et al.* The early clinical manifestations of Lyme disease. *Ann Intern Med* 1983; **99**: 76–82.

70 Gustafson R, Svenungsson B, Forsgren M, Gardulf A, Granstrom M. Two-year survey of the incidence of Lyme borreliosis and tick-borne encephalitis in a high-risk population in Sweden. *Eur J Clin Microbiol Infect Dis* 1992; **11**: 894–900.

71 Fahrer H, van der Linden S, Sauvain M-J *et al*. The prevalence and incidence of clinical and asymptomatic Lyme borreliosis in a population at risk. *J Infect Dis* 1991; **163**: 305–310.

72 Williams CL, Strobino B, Lee A *et al*. Lyme disease in childhood: clinical and epidemiologic features of ninety cases. *Pediatr Infect Dis J* 1990; **9**: 10–14.

73 Anderson JF, Magnarelli LA, Burgdorfer W *et al*. Spirochetes in *Ixodes dammini* and mammals from Connecticut. *Am J Trop Med Hyg* 1983; **32**: 818–824.

74 Steere AC. *Borrelia burgdorferi* (Lyme disease, Lyme borreliosis). In: Mandell GL, Douglas RG, Bennett JE (eds) *Principles and Practice of Infectious Diseases*, 4th edn. New York, Churchill Livingstone, 1995, pp. 2143–2155.

75 Piesman J, Mather TN, Sinsky RJ. Duration of tick attachment and *Borrelia burgdorferi* transmission. *J Clin Microbiol* 1987; **25**: 557–558.

76 Barbour AG, Hayes SF. Biology of *Borrelia* species. *Microbiol Rev* 1986; **50**: 381–400.

77 Craft JE, Fischer DK, Shimamoto GT *et al*. Antigens of *Borrelia burgdorferi* recognized during Lyme disease: appearance of a new IgM response and expansion of the IgG response late in the illness. *J Clin Invest* 1986; **78**: 934–939.

78 Barbour AG, Garon CF. Linear plasmids of the bacterium *Borrelia burgdorferi* have covalently closed ends. *Science* 1987; **237**: 409–411.

79 Hinnebusch J, Barbour AG. Linear plasmids of *Borrelia burgdorferi* have a telomeric structure and sequence similar to those of a eukaryotic virus. *J Bacteriol* 1991; **173**: 7233–7239.

80 Berger BW, Johnson RC, Kodner C *et al*. Cultivation of *Borrelia burgdorferi* from erythema migrans lesions and perilesional skin. *J Clin Microbiol* 1992; **30**: 359–361.

81 Georgilis K, Steere AC, Klempner MS. Infectivity of *Borrelia burgdorferi* correlates with resistance to elimination by phagocytic cells. *J Infect Dis* 1991; **163**: 150–155.

82 Steere AC, Schoen RT, Taylor E. The clinical evolution of Lyme arthritis. *Ann Intern Med* 1987; **107**: 725–731.

83 Szer IS, Taylor E, Steere AC. The long-term course of Lyme arthritis in children. *N Engl J Med* 1991; **325**: 159–163.

84 Shanafelt MC, Anzola J, Soderberg C *et al*. Epitopes on the outer surface protein A of *Borrelia burgdorferi* recognized by antibodies and T cells of patients with Lyme disease. *J Immunol* 1992; **148**: 218–224.

85 Kalish RA, Leong JM, Steere AC. Association of treatment-resistant chronic Lyme arthritis with HLA-DR4 and antibody reactivity to OspA and OspB of *Borrelia burgdorferi*. *Infect Immun* 1993; **61**: 2774–2779.

86 Reik L, Steere AC, Bartenhagen NH *et al*. Neurologic abnormalities of Lyme disease. *Medicine* 1979; **58**: 281–294.

87 Wilske B, Schierz G, Preac-Mursic V *et al*. Intrathecal production of specific antibodies against *Borrelia burgdorferi* in patients with lymphocytic meningoradiculitis (Bannwarth's syndrome). *J Infect Dis* 1986; **153**: 304–314.

88 Asbrink E, Hovmark A. Early and late cutaneous manifestations of *Ixodes*-borne borreliosis (erythema migrans borreliosis, Lyme borreliosis). *Ann NY Acad Sci* 1988; **539**: 4–15.

89 Steere AC, Batsford WP, Weinberg M *et al*. Lyme carditis: cardiac abnormalities of Lyme disease. *Ann Intern Med* 1980; **93**: 8–16.

90 Schlesinger PA, Duray PH, Burke BA *et al*. Maternal–fetal transmission of the Lyme disease spirochete, *Borrelia burgdorferi*. *Ann Intern Med* 1985; **103**: 67–68.

91 Weber K, Bratzke HJ, Neubert U *et al*. *Borrelia burgdorferi* in a newborn despite oral penicillin for Lyme borreliosis during pregnancy. *Pediatr Infect Dis J* 1988; **7**: 286–289.

92 Markowitz LE, Steere AC, Benach JL *et al.* Lyme disease in pregnancy. *JAMA* 1986; **256**: 3394–3396.

93 Strobino BA, Williams CL, Abid S, Chalson R, Spierling P. Lyme disease and pregnancy outcome: prospective study of two thousand pre-natal patients. *Am J Obstet Gynecol* 1993; **169**: 367–375.

94 Magnarelli LA. Current status of laboratory diagnosis for Lyme disease. *Am J Med* 1995; **98** (4A): 10S–14S.

95 Dennis DT. Lyme disease. *Dermatol Clin* 1995; **13**: 537–551.

96 Steere AC, Hardin JA, Ruddy S *et al.* Lyme arthritis: correlation of serum and cryoglobulin IgM with activity and serum IgG with remission. *Arthritis Rheum* 1979; **22**: 471–483.

97 Nocton JJ, Dressler F, Rutledge BJ *et al.* Detection of *Borrelia burgdorferi* DNA by polymerase chain reaction in synovial fluid from patients with Lyme arthritis. *N Engl J Med* 1994; **330**: 229–234.

98 Massarotti EM, Luger SW, Rahn DW *et al.* Treatment of early Lyme disease. *Am J Med* 1992; **92**: 396–403.

99 Johnson RC, Kodner C, Russell M. *In vitro* and *in vivo* susceptibility of the Lyme disease spirochete, *Borrelia burgdorferi*, to four antimicrobial agents. *Antimicrob Agents Chemother* 1987; **31**: 164–167.

100 Pfister HW, Preac-Mursic V, Wilske B *et al.* Randomized comparison of ceftriaxone and cefotaxime in Lyme neuroborreliosis. *J Infect Dis* 1991; **163**: 311–318.

101 Steere AC, Pachner AR, Malawista SE. Neurologic abnormalities of Lyme disease: successful treatment with high-dose intravenous penicillin. *Ann Intern Med* 1983; **99**: 767–772.

102 Salayar JC, Gerber MA, Goff CW. Long-term outcome of Lyme disease in children given early treatment. *J Pediatr* 1993; **122**: 591–593.

103 Shapiro ED, Gerber MA, Holobird NB *et al.* A controlled trial of anitmicrobial prophylaxis for Lyme disease after tick bites. *N Engl J Med* 1992; **327**: 1769–1773.

104 Fikrig E, Barthold SW, Kantor FS *et al.* Protection of mice against the Lyme disease agent by immunizing with recombinant OspA. *Science* 1990; **250**: 553–556.

105 Mandell SG, Bennett J, Dolin R. *Principles and Practice of Infectious Diseases*, 4th edn. Churchill Livingstone, New York, 1995; **2**: 2003–2007.

106 Howe C, Miller WR. Human glanders: report of six cases. *Ann Intern Med* 1947; **26**: 93–96.

107 Robins GD. A study of chronic glanders in man with report of a case. In: *Studies from the Royal Victoria Hospital, Montreal*, 1906, 29–38 Vol. 2.

108 Miller WR, Pannell L, Ingalls MS. Experimental chemotherapy in glanders and melioidosis. *Am J Hyg* 1948; **47**: 205–208.

109 Alexander B. A review of bartonellosis in Ecuador and Colombia. *Am J Trop Med Hyg* 1995; **52**: 354–359.

110 Garcia-Caceres U, Garcia FU. Bartonellosis: an immunosuppressive disease and the life of Daniel Alcides Carrion. *Am J Clin Pathol* 1991; **95**: S58–S66.

111 Caceres AG. Distribution geographica de *Lutzomyia verrucarum* (Townsend, 1913) (Diptera, Psychodidae, Phlebotominae), vector de la bartonellosis humana en el Peru. *Rev Inst Med Trop Sao Paulo* 1993; **35**: 485–490.

112 Cuadra M. Bartonellosis. In: Braude AI, Davis CE, Fierer J (eds) *Infectious Diseases and Medical Microbiology*, 2nd edn. WB Saunders, Philadelphia, 1986, pp. 1219–1225.

113 Kreier JP, Ristic M. The biology of hemotropic bacteria. *Ann Rev Microbiol* 1981; **35**: 325–338.

114 Ricketts WE. Clinical manifestations of Carrion's disease. *Arch Intern Med* 1949; **84**: 751–781.

115 Knobloch J, Solano L, Alvarez O *et al.* Antibodies to *Bartonella bacilliformis* as determined by fluorescence antibody test, indirect haemagglutination and ELISA. *Trop Med Parasitol* 1985; **36**: 183–185.

116 Maass M, Schreiber M, Knobloch J. Detection of *Bartonella bacilliformis* in cultures,

blood, and formalin preserved skin biopsies by use of the polymerase chain reaction. *Trop Med Parasitol* 1992; **43**: 191–194.

117 Bhutto AM, Nonaka S, Hashiguchi Y *et al.* Histopathological and electron microscopical features of skin lesions in a patient with bartonellosis (verruga peruana). *J Dermatol* 1994; **21**: 178–184.

118 Matteelli A, Castelli F, Spinetti A *et al.* Short report: verruga peruana in an Italian traveler from Peru. *Am J Trop Med Hyg* 1994; **50**: 143–144.

119 Roberts NJ Jr. *Bartonella bacilliformis* (bartonellosis). In: Mandell GL, Douglas RG, Bennett JE (eds) *Principles and Practice of Infectious Diseases*, 4th edn. Churchill Livingstone, New York, 1995, pp. 2209–2210.

120 Jackson LA, Perkins BA, Wenger JD. Cat scratch disease in the United States: an analysis of three national databases. *Am J Publ Health* 1993; **83**: 1707–1711.

121 Zangwill KM, Hamilton DH, Perkins BA *et al.* Cat-scratch disease in Connecticut: epidemiology, risk factors and evaluation of a new diagnostic test. *N Engl J Med* 1993; **329**: 8–12.

122 Jameson P, Greene C, Regnery R *et al.* Prevalence of *Bartonella henselae* antibodies in pet cats throughout regions of North America. *J Infect Dis* 1995; **172**: 1145–1149.

123 Koehler JE, Glaser CE, Tappero JW. *Rochalimaea henselae* infection: new zoonosis with the domestic cat as reservoir. *JAMA* 1994; **271**: 531–535.

124 Regnery RL, Olson JG, Perkins BA *et al.* Serological response to *Rochalimaea henselae* antigen in suspected cat-scratch disease. *Lancet* 1992; **339**: 1443–1445.

125 Wear DJ, Margileth AM, English CK *et al.* Cat-scratch disease. Isolation and culture of the bacterial agent. *JAMA* 1988; **259**: 1347–1352.

126 Fischer GW. Cat scratch disease. In: Mandell GL, Douglas RG, Bennett JE (eds) *Principles and Practice of Infectious Diseases*, 4th edn. Churchill Livingstone, New York, 1995, pp. 1310–1312.

127 Slater LN, Welch DF. *Rochalimaea* species (recently renamed *Bartonella*). In: Mandell GL, Douglas RG, Bennett JE (eds) *Principles and Practice of Infectious Diseases*, 4th edn. Churchill Livingstone, New York, 1995, pp. 1741–1747.

128 Demers DM, Vincent JM, Bass JW *et al.* Serologic evidence of *Rochalimaea henselae* (Rh) infection and cat scratch disease (CSD) in humans scratched by Rh bacteremic kittens. *Pediatr Res* 1994; **35**: 177A (abstract 1050).

129 Anderson B, Sims K, Regnery T *et al.* Detection of *Rochalimaea henselae* DNA in specimens from patients with cat-scratch disease by PCR. *J Clin Microbiol* 1994; **32**: 942–948.

130 Anderson B, Kelly C, Threlkel R. Detection of *Rochalimaea henselae* in cat scratch disease skin test antigens. *J Infect Dis* 1993; **168**: 1034–1036.

131 Margileth AM. Sorting out the causes of lymphadenopathy. *Contemp Pediatr* 1995; **12**: 23–40 (first of two parts).

132 Margileth AM. Cat scratch disease as a cause of the oculoglandular syndrome of Parinaud. *J Pediatr* 1957; **20**: 1000–1005.

133 Margileth AM. Cat scratch disease. In: Wyngarden JB, Smith JH Jr (eds) *Cecil Textbook of Medicine*, 17th edn. Saunders, Philadelphia, 1985, p. 1618.

134 Miller P, Bell W. Cat scratch disease with encephalopathy. *Clin Pediatr* (*Philadelphia*) 1980; **19**: 233–234.

135 Barka NE, Hadfield T, Patnaik M *et al.* EIA for detection of *Rochalimaea henselae*-reactive IgG, IgM, and IgA antibodies in patients with suspected cat-scratch. *J Infect Dis* 1993; **167**: 1503–1504.

136 Chaowagul W, White NJ. Melioidosis: a cause of community-acquired septicemia in northern Thailand. *J Infect Dis* 1989; **159**: 890–899.

137 Lumbiganon P, Viengondha S. Clinical manifestations of melioidosis in children. *Pediatr Infect Dis* 1995; **14**: 136–140.

138 Strauss JM, Alexander AD, Rapmund G *et al.* Antibodies to *Pseudomonas pseudomallei* in the human population. *Trop Med Hyg* 1969; **18**: 703–704.

139 Mays EE, Rickets EA. Melioidosis: recrudescence associated with bronchogenic carcinoma twenty-six years following initial geographic exposure. *Chest* 1975; **68**: 261–264.

140 Everett ED, Nelson R. Pulmonary melioidosis: observations in fifty-five cases. *Am Rev Respir Dis* 1975; **112**: 331–340.

141 Tanphaichitra D. Tropical disease in the immunocompromised patient. *Rev Infect Dis* 1989; **11** (Suppl. 7): 535–545.

142 Vatcharapreechasakul T, Supputomongkol Y. *Pseudomonas pseudomallei* liver abscesses: a clinical, laboratory and ultrasonagraphic study. *Clin Infect Dis* 1992; **14**: 412–417.

143 Guard RW, Khafagi FA, Brigden MC *et al.* Melioidosis in the district of Queensland. *Am J Trop Med Hyg* 1984; **33**: 467–473.

144 Kanaphun P, Thirawattanusak N, Supputtamongkol Y *et al.* Epidemiology of *Pseudomonas pseudomallei*: prospective study in the children of northeast Thailand. *J Infect Dis* 1993; **167**: 230–233.

Chapter 4
Mycobacterial Skin Infections

Marwali Harahap & M. Reza P. Marwali

Tuberculosis of the skin

Definition and classification

Tuberculosis of the skin is caused by *Mycobacterium tuberculosis* of the human, the bovine and, very rarely, the avian type [1]. The skin manifestations comprise a considerable number of skin changes.

The classification used in this chapter is simple and does not attempt to introduce immunological considerations [2, 3]. This classification distinguishes between exogenous infections and endogenous infections (Table 4.1). Exogenous infections arise from direct inoculation with *M. tuberculosis* through a break in the skin. Endogenous infections arise from infection elsewhere in the body. A group of eruptions, the tuberculids, which are pathogenically less well understood, will be briefly mentioned.

Epidemiology

The prevalence of tuberculosis was declining the world over, because of affluence, advanced public health measures and effective antituberculosis drugs. In spite of the dramatic decline of tuberculosis in the well-developed countries from 1970, the infection has increased markedly since 1985 because of a number of problems: firstly, the influx of infected immigrants from developing countries; secondly, the increased numbers of problem groups in the indigenous population: middle-aged and elderly men, immunocompromised patients, drug addicts, diabetics and patients with acquired immune deficiency syndrome (AIDS) [4, 5], and thirdly, in some areas tuberculosis has become so uncommon that it may be overlooked [6]. In developing countries of Africa and South-East Asia, the increase of tuberculosis cases has paralleled the epidemic caused by the human immunodeficiency virus (HIV) [7].

In the tropics cutaneous tuberculosis is still seen from to time. The predominant forms of cutaneous tuberculosis in the tropics are scrofuloderma, tuberculosis verrucosa cutis and lupus vulgaris [8–13].

Table 4.1 Classification of cutaneous tuberculosis.

True tuberculosis
Exogenous infection
    Primary inoculation tuberculosis
    Tuberculosis verrucosa cutis
Endogenous infection
    Lupus vulgaris
    Scrofuloderma
    Tuberculosis orificialis
    Miliary tuberculosis of the skin
    Tuberculous gumma

Tuberculids
    Papulonecrotic tuberculid
    Lichen scrofulosorum
    Erythema induratum

Aetiology

Mycobacterium tuberculosis, Mycobacterium bovis and, very rarely, the avian type [1] cause all forms of skin tuberculosis. The incidence of skin tuberculosis elicited by these organisms varies and is determined by the probability of exposure to either human, bovine or avian tuberculosis. In humans, *M. tuberculosis* and *M. bovis* caused identical skin manifestations. The skin changes elicited by *M. tuberculosis/bovis* infection are polymorphous, depending upon the interplay of host immunity and bacterial virulence.

In many forms of skin tuberculosis, the number of bacteria in the lesions is so small that it may be difficult to find them in histological sections, whereas, in the primary inoculation tuberculosis (tuberculous chancre) or in acute miliary tuberculosis, large numbers of bacteria can be demonstrated in the affected tissue.

Diagnosis

The diagnosis of cutaneous tuberculosis is based on the following [3, 14].
1   Lesions which are clinically typical of one of the validated types of cutaneous tuberculosis.
2   Microscopic examination of the tissue section may exhibit a tuberculoid/tuberculous granuloma.
3   A positive Mantoux test.
4   Demonstration of acid-fast bacilli on Ziehl–Nielsen staining of the smear from lesions and recovery of *M. tuberculosis* in culture.

Primary inoculation tuberculosis (tuberculous chancre)

Definition

Primary inoculation tuberculosis or tuberculous chancre develops as a result of inoculation into the skin of a host not previously infected with tuberculosis.

Incidence

This is now a very uncommon primary presentation of tuberculosis [2]. In some regions, particularly in Asia, where the incidence of tuberculosis is still high and the socio-economic condition is low, primary inoculation tuberculosis is not unusual.

Clinical manifestations

All parts of the body may be affected, but the face and the extremities exhibit the most frequent sites of inoculation.

The earliest lesion is a nondescript, brownish papule, which develops into an indurated nodule or plaque that may ulcerate. This is the tuberculous chancre. The ulcer is painless with an undermined edge and granular haemorrhagic base (Fig. 4.1). In time, the edge becomes firmer, with thick adherent crusts. There is prominent regional lymphadenopathy, which occurs about 3–4 weeks or longer after the development of the ulcer. The ulcer and the affected regional lymph nodes constitute the primary tuberculous complex of the skin. This primary complex has great diagnostic value.

The primary tuberculosis complex occurs on the mucous membranes of the conjunctiva and oral cavity in about one-third of patients [15]. Lesions on the conjunctiva cause oedema and irritation [16] or develop into shallow ulcers or fungating granulations [15]. In the mouth, painless ulcers, often misdiagnosed, may occur on the gingiva or the palate. Inoculation around the nail may present as painless paronychia [17].

The chancre will heal slowly, taking many months; the regional lymph-node enlargement subsides slowly, often calcifying. Less often, after weeks or months the lymph nodes form abscesses, which perforate the surface of the skin, forming sinuses.

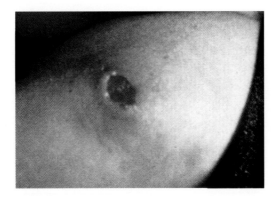

Fig. 4.1 The tuberculous chancre. The ulcer is painless with an undermined edge and granular base. (Reprinted with permission of the Upjohn Company, Kalamazoo, Michigan, USA.)

Diagnosis

Any painless, unilateral ulcer with regional lymphadenopathy in a child should always arouse suspicion. Acid-fast bacilli can be seen in histological section or in smears in the initial stages of the disease. The diagnosis can be confirmed by bacterial culture.

Primary inoculation tuberculosis may be confused with the primary complex of syphilis, tularaemia, sporotrichosis or actinomycosis [18]. Cat-scratch fever and ulcerative lesions of other mycobacterioses as well as other forms of skin tuberculosis may resemble primary tuberculosis, but are distinguished both clinically and by laboratory procedures.

Tuberculosis verrucosa cutis (warty tuberculosis)

Definition

Tuberculosis verrucosa cutis is a warty granulomatous form of tuberculosis occurring as a result of the inoculation of organisms into the skin of a previously infected individual who has a moderate or high degree of immunity.

Incidence

In Western countries, tuberculosis verrucosa cutis is a rare form of skin tuberculosis, but it is not uncommon in the East [8, 13, 19].

Clinical manifestations

Tuberculosis verrucosa cutis usually occurs on the dorsa of the fingers (Fig. 4.2) and hands, the knees (Fig. 4.3), the ankles and the buttocks [8, 9, 13]. The lesion starts as a symptomless, small papule, indurated with a purple inflammatory halo. Slow growth and gradual extension lead to the formation of a verrucous plaque with irregular outline and a papillomatous horny surface (Fig. 4.4). The centre may involute, leaving a thin white scar,

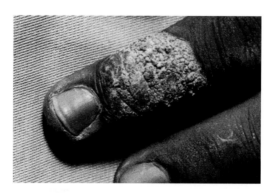

Fig. 4.2 Tuberculosis verrucosa cutis on the dorsum of a finger. (From Department of Dermatology, University of Indonesia.)

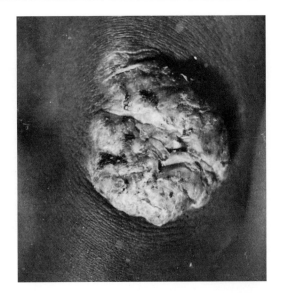

Fig. 4.3 Tuberculosis verrucosa cutis on the knee. (From Department of Dermatology, University of Indonesia. Reprinted by permission of Kluwer Academic Publishers.)

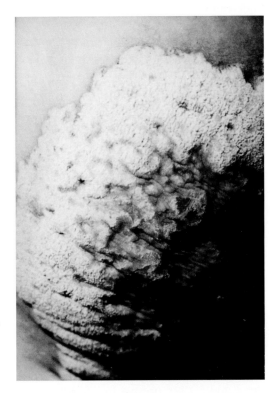

Fig. 4.4 Tuberculosis verrucosa cutis. Slow growth and gradual extension lead to formation of a verrucous plaque with papillomatous horny surface. (From Department of Dermatology, University of Indonesia. Reprinted by permission of Kluwer Academic Publishers.)

or the whole lesion may become very papillomatous. The plaques tend to be single, but multiple lesions may occur. The consistency is usually firm, but there may be areas of softening. Pus and keratinous material may sometimes be expressed from these soft areas or from fissures. Because of the usual presence of good immunity, the regional lymph nodes are rarely affected. Enlargement of regional lymph nodes may be due to pyococcal infection.

Diagnosis

Early subungual and digital lesions resemble warts or keratoses. Lupus vulgaris is not usually hyperkeratotic and it exhibits 'apple-jelly' nodules at the periphery. Tuberculosis verrucosa cutis must also be distinguished from blastomycosis, chromoblastomycosis and actinomycosis. Negative fungal cultures and small tuberculoid foci are diagnostic aids. The lesions caused by atypical mycobacteria may be difficult to exclude except by culture. Tertiary syphilis and yaws can be distinguished by serological changes.

Prognosis

Tuberculosis verrucosa cutis responds to antituberculosis therapy. Without treatment, the evolution of the lesions is usually slow and lesions may remain inactive for many years. Spontaneous involution sometimes occurs.

Lupus vulgaris

Definition

Lupus vulgaris is a progressive form of cutaneous tuberculosis occurring in individuals with a moderate to high degree of immunity.

Incidence

The incidence of lupus vulgaris has shared the steady decline of cutaneous tuberculosis and is now rare in the USA and Europe [20]. There is a greater prevalence of the disease in regions with a cool, moist, dull climate. Lupus vulgaris occurs two to three times more often in females than in males [21]. It affects all ages equally.

Clinical manifestations

The characteristic lesion is a plaque composed of reddish-brown nodules. If these nodules are pressed by a glass slide (diascopic examination), they show a diagnostic brownish yellow or 'apple-jelly' colour. They tend to heal slowly in one area with simultaneous irregular expansion in another (Fig. 4.5). The lesions are usually solitary, but two or more sites may be involved simultaneously. Multiple lesions are uncommon. The head and neck are involved most frequently (Fig. 4.6). Next in frequency are the arms and legs

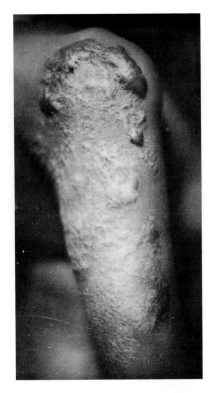

Fig. 4.5 Lupus vulgaris tends to heal slowly in one area with simultaneous irregular expansion in another. (From Department of Dermatology, University of Indonesia.)

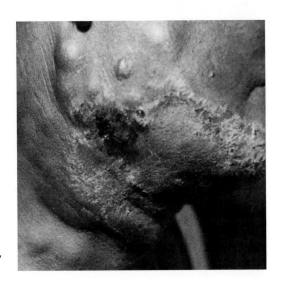

Fig. 4.6 Lupus vulgaris involves the head and neck most frequently. (From Department of Dermatology, University of Indonesia.)

but involvement of the trunk is rare. The course of this disease is destructive, frequently causes ulceration and on involution leaves deforming scars (Fig. 4.7), as it slowly spreads peripherally over many years. The sequelae of this destructive and mutilative disease are disfigurement due to scars,

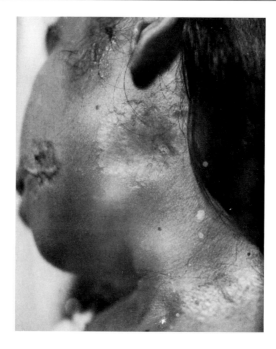

Fig. 4.7 Lupus vulgaris leaves ugly scars. (From Department of Dermatology, University of Indonesia.)

ectropion, microstomia and keloid and functional impairment due to contracture of the scars.

The nasal, buccal and conjunctival mucosa may be involved, with rapid formation of papillary and vegetative lesions, which ulcerate owing to moisture and contamination with other microorganisms.

The association of lupus vulgaris with other forms of tuberculosis cutis is not unusual. Lupus vulgaris occurred with tuberculosis verrucosa cutis in the same patient and was also found in 12 patients with papulonecrotic tuberculid [22, 23].

Diagnosis

Sometimes lesions of sarcoidosis, leprosy, syphilis, lymphocytoma, discoid lupus erythematosus, blastomycosis or other deep mycotic infections may simulate lupus vulgaris. Criteria helpful in the diagnosis of lupus vulgaris are the softness of the lesions, the brownish-red colour and the slow progress. The typical 'apple-jelly' nodules revealed by diascopy are distinctive. Finding them, especially in ulcerated, crusted or hyperkeratotic lesions, is decisive.

The nodules of sarcoidosis resemble grains of sand rather than 'apple jelly' and the nodules of leprosy are firmer and other signs are present. Papular syphilids are monomorphic and bilateral, and spirochaetes may be demonstrated in the serum from the lesions. The histological features and culture results will separate the deep mycoses and lupus erythematosus. In some cases, sparse acid-fast bacilli can be demonstrated in histological sections of lupus vulgaris, and a positive culture for *M. tuberculosis/bovis* confirms the diagnosis.

Treatment

Standard antituberculosis therapy is effective. Plastic surgery may be helpful to correct the disfigurement and mutilating effects of the disease.

Scrofuloderma

Definition

Scrofuloderma results from the tuberculous involvement and breakdown of the skin secondary to an underlying tuberculous focus, usually a lymph gland but sometimes a bone or joint.

Incidence

Scrofuloderma appears to be the most common form of cutaneous tuberculosis in tropical countries [6, 9, 12].

Clinical manifestations

The process usually begins with a deep purplish induration of the skin on the lateral aspects of the neck overlying an enlarged node or group of discrete or matted palpable nodes. The lymph nodes that are fixed to the skin suppurate and burrow to the skin surface, with fistula and ulcer formation (Fig. 4.8). Scrofuloderma occurs most frequently over the cervi-

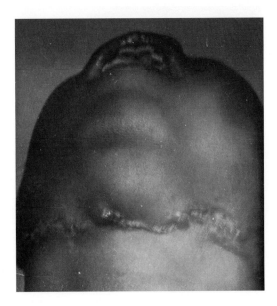

Fig. 4.8 Scrofuloderma on the neck with nodules and fistula. (From Department of Dermatology, University of Indonesia.)

cal lymph node, but it may occur over an infected bone or joint. Ulcers and sinuses discharge watery and purulent or caseous material. Soft undermined ulcers tend to be linear or serpiginous, with granulating floors (Fig. 4.9). As a result of progression and scarring, irregular cord-like scars develop and soft gummatous nodules, bulky crust and irregular pale granulations form.

Diagnosis

An underlying tuberculous lymphadenitis or bone or joint disease provides the best mean of diagnosis. The clinical diagnosis is confirmed by bacterial culture. Syphilitic gumma, sporotrichosis, blastomycosis and lymphogranuloma venereum (LGV) may resemble scrofuloderma. When ulcerated, syphilitic gummas create deep craters, and sporotrichosis and blastomycosis yield the typical fungus when cultured. Lymphogranuloma venereum is excluded by a negative LGV complement-fixation test and occurs usually in the inguinal and perineal areas. Dental sinus, hydradenitis suppurativa and severe forms of acne conglobata must be ruled out. Actinomycosis and tularaemia should be differentiated by culture.

Orificial tuberculosis

Definition

Orificial tuberculosis is tuberculous infection of the mucous membranes and the adjoining skin of the orifices in a patient with advanced underlying pulmonary, intestinal or urogenital tuberculosis.

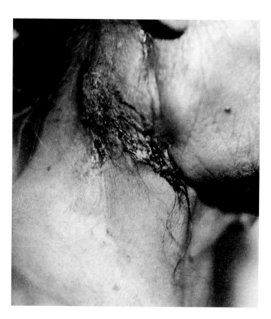

Fig. 4.9 Scrofuloderma on the lateral aspect of the neck with linear ulcer and granulating floor. (From Department of Dermatology, University of Indonesia.)

Incidence

The condition is now very rare. Most of those affected are middle-aged or older men [24].

Clinical manifestations

The initial lesion is a small oedematous red nodule, which rapidly breaks down to form a painful shallow ulcer with undermined bluish edges. Lesions occur most frequently in the mouth, especially the tip and lateral margins of the tongue [25]. Oral and pharyngeal involvement can result in dysphagia and inability to eat. In patients with active genitourinary disease, lesions develop on the penis or vulva and, in those with intestinal tuberculosis, on and around the anus.

Diagnosis

Painful ulcers in and around the orifices in patients with advanced internal tuberculosis should arouse strong suspicion. The diagnosis is confirmed by smears and bacterial culture. Syphilitic lesions, aphthosis and carcinoma must be ruled out.

Miliary tuberculosis of the skin

Definition

Miliary tuberculosis of the skin is a rare form of tuberculosis, which appears as an acute generalized eruption and which most often occurs in infants and children, due to haematogenous dissemination of mycobacteria.

Clinical manifestations

The skin lesions are often brownish-red acuminate papules, vesicles and pustules, which may become necrotic to form numerous small ulcers [26]. Tubercle bacilli have been demonstrated in these lesions.

Exanthematous miliary tuberculosis usually occurs in infants following intercurrent illness or some type of severe infection that reduces immunological responsiveness. Miliary tuberculosis is occasionally seen in adults who have diseases such as AIDS that have an immunosuppressant effect or who are taking immunosuppressant chemotherapeutic agents.

Diagnosis

The appearance of an unusual skin eruption in a gravely ill patient with known tuberculosis or tuberculous contacts suggests the diagnosis. Biopsy of a skin lesion showing acid-fast bacilli confirms the diagnosis. Many other skin diseases with a multitude of maculopapular and vesicular rashes must be ruled out, but the diagnosis is usually substantiated by the evidence of acute miliary disease of the internal organs.

Tuberculous gumma (metastatic tuberculous abscess)

Definition

Tuberculous gumma is due to haematogenous dissemination of mycobacteria from a primary focus during a period of lowered resistance, resulting in firm, non-tender erythematous nodules, which soften, ulcerate and form sinuses. These are seen particularly in undernourished children of low socioeconomic status or in immunodeficient or severely immunosuppressed patients, as in AIDS or due to therapy.

Clinical manifestations

Tuberculous gumma presents as a firm, single or multiple non-tender subcutaneous nodule, which slowly softens and breaks down, forming undermined ulcers and sinuses [27] (Fig. 4.10). The lesions affect the extremities

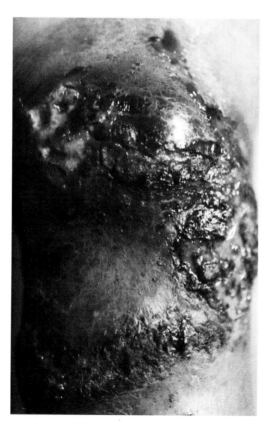

Fig. 4.10 Tuberculous gumma with undermined ulcers. (From Department of Dermatology, University of Indonesia. Reprinted by permission of Kluwer Academic Publishers.)

more frequently than the trunk. Similar lesions may occur, rarely, along the course of lymphatics.

Diagnosis

This condition must be differentiated from syphilitic gumma, deep fungal infections, hydradenitis suppurativa and panniculitides. The diagnosis is confirmed by histopathology, acid-fast stain of the tissue and smears and bacterial culture.

Bacillus Calmette–Guérin vaccination

Bacillus Calmette–Guérin (BCG) vaccine is an *in vitro* attenuation of a strain of *M. bovis*, used to enhance immunity to tuberculosis.

Untoward reactions to BCG vaccination are rare in relation to the number of vaccinations carried out. Non-specific reactions to BCG include keloid formation, urticaria, erythema multiforme [28], general maculopapular or purpuric rashes associated with myalgia or arthralgia and abdominal pain [29, 30]. Extensive ulceration may occur. Specific lesions originating from BCG vaccination include lichen scrofulosorum, papular tuberculids, lichen nitidus [29], lupus vulgaris [31] and scrofuloderma [29].

BCG can cause progressive mycobacteriosis in AIDS patients [32].

The tuberculids

Definition

Tuberculids represent recurrent disseminated or systemic skin eruptions, which arise in response to haematogenous dissemination of antigen from an internal focus of tuberculosis.

Incidence

Tuberculids have become rare because of the sharp decline in tuberculosis and its effective multidrug therapy in the developed countries; however, they are being reported more frequently because of the recent resurgence of tuberculosis in some Western countries.

Diagnosis

In general, the diagnosis of tuberculids rests on the following.
1   Lesions which have the clinical characteristics of the tuberculids.
2   The tuberculid exhibits tuberculoid structure on histological examination.
3   A positive tuberculin test.
4   Previous and concomitant tuberculous focus is desirable.

Lichen scrofulosorum

Definition

Lichen scrofulosorum is an eruption of grouped, closely set, minute lichenoid papules, occurring in children most frequently but also in adults with tuberculosis.

Clinical manifestations

The eruption tends to be follicullar and consists of symptomless yellow, pink or reddish-brown papules or they may be of normal skin colour, 1–2 mm in diameter (rarely exceeding 5 mm) (Fig. 4.11). They are sometimes slightly scaly and occasionally surmounted by a minute pustule. The lesions may be sparse or develop in groups, forming discoid plaques. The eruption persists for weeks, and then involutes slowly over a period of months, without scarring.

It usually occurs in children who have tuberculosis of bones [33] or lymph nodes [34] or with specific pleurisy.

Diagnosis

Lichen nitidus, lichen planus, keratosis spinulosa, lichenoid sarcoidosis, secondary syphilis and drug eruption should be ruled out.

The lesions of lichen nitidus are more shiny and tend to be peripheral. The lesions of keratosis spinulosa are more skin-coloured and more truly follicular. The tuberculin reaction in patients with lichen scrofulosorum is usually positive.

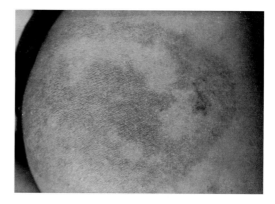

Fig. 4.11 Lichen scrofulosorum tends to be follicular and consists of symptomless, yellow, pink, reddish-brown papules. (From Department of Dermatology, University of Indonesia. Reprinted by permission of Kluwer Academic Publishers.)

Papulonecrotic tuberculid

Definition

Papulonecrotic tuberculid is a symmetric eruption of necrotizing papules, which appear in crops and heal spontaneously with scarring.

Incidence

Young adults are frequently affected but it also occurs in children and infants.

Clinical manifestations

The eruption recurs in successive crops, usually on the extensor aspects of the extremities, particularly on the elbows, knees, buttocks and lower trunk (Fig. 4.12), and also on the face. Localized papulonecrotic tuberculids appear also on the penis [35, 36]. The papules, which may initially be colourless, are dusky red and symptomless and vary in size from a pinhead to a pea. They undergo central necrosis and heal spontaneously, with depressed pigmented scarring. New crops may continue over the course of a few weeks to a few months, to be followed by fresh outbreaks. Healing is by the formation of pitted scars. The lesions do not itch and usually there are no systemic symptoms. Papulonecrotic tuberculid should be considered in the differential diagnosis of all symmetric, chronic, papulopustular lesions that occur in an acral distribution [37].

Diagnosis

Papulonecrotic tuberculid is distinguished from acne varioliformis and papular syphilis by the absence of pustules and the stigmata of syphilis, respectively. Insect bites are itchy and usually less symmetrical. The distinction from prurigo and excoriated papules is easily established because of the itch and because they are not as peripherally distrib-

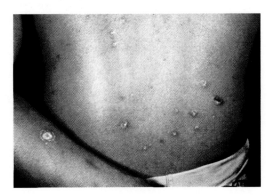

Fig. 4.12 Papulonecrotic tuberculid papules on the lower trunk and arms. (Reprinted with permission of the Upjohn Company, Kalamazoo, Michigan, USA.)

uted. The diagnosis of papulonecrotic tuberculid should be confirmed by histology.

Erythema induratum

Definition

Erythema induratum (Bazin's disease, tuberculosis cutis indurativa) is a chronic vasculitis, which causes persistent or recurrent nodules secondary to active or inactive foci of tuberculosis.

Incidence

The disease is found predominantly in women. Only 5–10% of cases reported have been in males [38]. Erythema induratum is most often seen in the winter and early spring.

Clinical manifestations

The lesions are usually symmetric and indolent, affecting the lower calf of middle-aged or younger females with an erythrocyanotic circulation. The disease rarely occurs on the front of the leg, on the arms or elsewhere. In the period of evolution, the lesions are slightly tender erythematous indurations, which gradually become deep nodules. The nodules slowly progress into ulceration. The ulcers are irregular and shallow, with under-mined edges.

Diagnosis

Erythema nodosum, gumma, nodose lesions caused by iodides and bromides and nodular vasculitis should be excluded.

Erythema nodosum chiefly affects the shins instead of the calves and is of short duration and the lesions do not usually ulcerate. Gummatous syphilis is usually unilateral and single. A confirmation of the clinical diagnosis is obtained by serological, microscopic and therapeutic tests. The lesions due to iodides or bromides and nodular vasculitis can be ruled out by histology, a history of halide ingestion and the presence of elevated serum bromide.

Therapy of skin tuberculosis

General measures

Chemotherapy is usually the treatment of choice, but attention to the patient as a whole may be required to provide the patient with optimal care. A careful search for an underlying focus of disease and the improvement of general health and nutrition are important factors to be considered. Skin tuberculosis associated with mycobacterial disease of other organs requires a combined approach with other specialists.

Chemotherapy

The aims of chemotherapy are to cure the disease as rapidly as possible, to prevent relapses and to avoid the emergence of resistant strains. The basic principles of tuberculosis treatment are as follow [39].

1   Never treat with a single drug. A combination of drugs must be used.
2   Never treat less than 6 months.
3   Ensure that the patient takes the drug for an adequate length of time.
4   Review other drugs that the patient is taking and anticipate drug interactions.

Treatment regimens do not differ for pulmonary and extrapulmonary tuberculosis [40]. Short-course chemotherapy (6 or 9 months) has become the standard treatment [41, 42]. The daily long-term regimen (18–24 months) is a long time for any patient to take medication. Problems with expense and patient compliance account for the high failure rate.

The first-line drugs used for previously untreated disease are isoniazid, rifampicin, streptomycin, pyrazinamide, ethambutol, thiacetazone and *p*-aminosalicyclic acid (PAS). They represent the first choice because of their effectiveness, relatively low toxicity and relatively low cost. The second-line drugs, used mainly in the treatment of patients whose first-line treatment has failed, are ethionamide or prothionamide, cycloserine, kanamycin, capreomycin and viomycin. In general, the second-line drugs are less effective, more toxic and more expensive than the first-line drugs [43, 44].

Isoniazid. Isoniazid remains the mainstay of antituberculous therapy, given in all regimens because of its efficacy, cheapness and low toxicity. The daily dosages are 300 mg for adults and 10 mg/kg for children. Pyridoxine 10 mg per dose should be given concomitantly to prevent neurotoxicity.

Rifampicin. Rifampicin is bactericidal for *M. tuberculosis* and for many other pathogens. Rifampicin rarely causes serious toxicity and seldom necessitates an interruption of treatment. It is used in an antituberculosis regimen to prevent the emergence of strains resistant to drugs. The drug may accumulate in patients with severe liver disease or biliary obstruction and should be used with care in treating patients with chronic liver disease. Patients should be warned that it may impart a red stain to their urine and other body secretions, including saliva.

The daily dosages are 600 mg/day for adults and 10–20 mg/kg for children.

Streptomycin. Streptomycin is bactericidal for *M. tuberculosis*. It is used as a companion drug for isoniazid and other bactericidal drugs. The toxicity of streptomycin prohibits continuous long-term therapy, because patients develop vestibular disturbances, including impairment of hearing. It should be avoided in the treatment of pregnant women because it may occasionally damage the eighth nerve of the fetus.

The daily dosages are 750 mg–1 g for adults and 20 mg/kg for children.

Ethambutol. Ethambutol is bacteriostatic for *M. tuberculosis*, and is used in combination with other drugs, usually rifampicin and isoniazid. It should not be used alone, as mycobacteria rapidly develop resistance. Ethambutol can cause a dose-related retrobulbar neuritis, with diminished visual acuity and other visual disturbances. Because ocular toxicity from ethambutol in children is difficult to monitor, it should not be given to children under age 13. Streptomycin or pyrazinamide is substituted. The dosages are 15–25 mg/kg.

Pyrazinamide. Pyrazinamide (pyrazinoic acid amide) is bactericidal for *M. tuberculosis*. It may cause arthralgia and, rarely, hepatitis. Care should be taken in treating patients with chronic liver disease or alcoholism.

The daily dosages are 40 mg/kg for adults and children.

The following guidelines for the treatment of tuberculosis have been established [41, 42].

1 Extrapulmonary tuberculosis (including tuberculosis of the skin) should be treated with the same standard course as pulmonary tuberculosis.

2 A 9-month regimen of isoniazid and rifampicin, usually supplemented with a third drug (ethambutol, streptomycin or pyrazinamide) during the initial phase (first 2–3 months).

3 Infants, children and adolescents with tuberculosis should receive a 9-month course of isoniazid and rifampicin, supplemented with ethambutol, streptomycin or pyrazinamide in the initial phase. This initial-phase treatment is only necessary when drug resistance is suspected.

4 A 6-month course of treatment is acceptable if four drugs (isoniazid, rifampicin, pyrazinamide and streptomycin or ethambutol) are given for 2 months and followed by 4 months of isoniazid and rifampicin, with all drugs given under close supervision.

5 Tuberculosis during pregnancy should be treated with a 9-month course of isoniazid and rifampicin, supplemented by ethambutol (streptomycin and pyrazinamide should not be used) in the initial phase.

6 Immunosuppressed patients with tuberculosis should be treated with 9–12 months of isoniazid and rifampicin, supplemented by ethambutol, streptomycin or pyrazinamide in the initial phase.

Small lesions of lupus vulgaris or tuberculosis verrucosa cutis are best excised, but chemotherapy should also be given. Plastic surgery may help to repair the disfigurement left by long-standing lupus vulgaris.

In developing countries, the incidence of tuberculosis is high, medical services are limited and drug costs are a limiting factor. Compromises must be made with drug regimens and treatment measures in general. It is to be hoped that in the near future research into short-course chemotherapy will make it possible to provide a regimen which would be applicable and economical for developing countries [45]. Regimens recommended by the World Health Organization (WHO) [46] are given in Table 4.2.

The incidence of drug-resistant tuberculosis isolates is also increasing [47, 48]. This has greatly affected the choice of therapy. Both the Infectious Disease Society of America and the Centers for Disease Control (CDC) have strongly recommended the use of 'second-line' drugs, such as amikacin and fluoroquinolones (ciprofloxacin and ofloxacin), together with ethamb-

Table 4.2 Recommended treatment regimens for tuberculosis* (reproduced by permission of WHO).

	6-month regimens	
Drug	Phase 1: 2 months	Phase 2: 4 months
Isoniazid	5 mg/kg daily	5 mg/kg daily
Rifampicin	10 mg/kg daily	10 mg/kg daily
Pyrazinamide	30 mg/kg daily	
Supplemented, in areas where resistance to one of these drugs is demonstrated, by		
Streptomycin	15 mg/kg daily	
or		
Ethambutol	25 mg/kg daily†	
OR		
Isoniazid	15 mg/kg 3 times weekly	15 mg/kg 3 times weekly
Rifampicin	10 mg/kg 3 times weekly	10 mg/kg 3 times weekly
Pyrazinamide	50 mg/kg 3 times weekly	50 mg/kg 3 times weekly
Together with		
Streptomycin	15 mg/kg 3 times weekly	15 mg/kg 3 times weekly
or		
Ethambutol	40 mg/kg 3 times weekly‡	40 mg/kg 3 times weekly‡
	8-month regimens	
	Phase 1: 2 months	Phase 2: 6 months
Isoniazid	5 mg/kg daily	5 mg/kg daily
Rifampicin	10 mg/kg daily	
Pyrazinamide	30 mg/kg daily	
Thioacetazone		2.5 mg/kg daily
Together with		
Streptomycin	15 mg/kg daily	
or		
Ethambutol	25 mg/kg daily†	

* Unless otherwise indicated, doses are suitable for both adults and children.
† 15 mg/kg for children.
‡ Not suitable for children.

utol and pyrazinamide in persons in whom drug-resistant isolates are suspected or found [49]. The daily dose of amikacin is 15 mg/kg intramuscularly (i.m.) and it is 500–1000 mg four times a day (qid) by mouth (p.o.) for ciprofloxacin and 400–800 mg qid p.o. for ofloxacin.

Skin infections with atypical mycobacteria

Mycobacterium marinum

Mycobacterium marinum is acquired after trauma while in contact with fresh or salt water, e.g. in a swimming pool and working with aquariums (fish tanks). It was identified for the first time in 1951 as the causative organism of a granulomatous skin eruption of swimmers using a contaminated swimming pool [50].

Its distribution appears to be worldwide and, depending on the source of infection, the disease occurs sporadically or in small community outbreaks.

Clinical manifestations

About 2 to 3 weeks after inoculation, the initial lesion is usually a violaceous plaque or nodules at the site of a trauma: hands, elbows, knees or feet (Fig. 4.13). As a rule, lesions are solitary, but occasionally sporotrichoid forms, with one or more nodules along the line of lymphatic drainage, are found (Fig. 4.14). The regional lymph nodes infrequently become slightly enlarged but never break down. Multiple lesions occur rarely.

Diagnosis

The history should raise suspicion. A history of handling fish or the use of swimming pools and the presence of a tuberculoid granuloma in histological section are suggestive. The diagnosis can only be confirmed by the demonstration of *M. marinum* in culture. Other conditions considered in

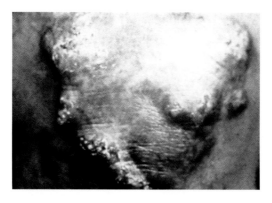

Fig. 4.13 *Mycobacterium marinum* infection. Plaques or nodules at the site of trauma. (Reprinted with permission of the Upjohn Company, Kalamazoo, Michigan, USA.)

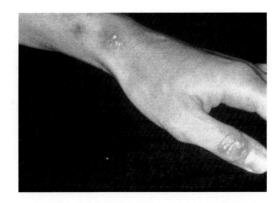

Fig. 4.14 Nodules along the line of lymphatic drainage. (Reprinted with permission of the Upjohn Company, Kalamazoo, Michigan, USA.)

the differential diagnosis are: cutaneous leishmaniasis, sporotrichosis, tertiary syphilis and other mycobacterial infections.

Treatment

No controlled trials of therapy have studied treatment regimens for atypical mycobacteria. Tetracycline 500 mg four times a day may be effective. Minocycline 100 mg twice daily for 1–2 months is effective in many cases. If there is no response, rifampicin 600 mg, usually with ethambutol, 15 mg/kg body weight, daily for 18 months is useful.

Mycobacterium ulcerans

The chronic necrotizing, painless skin ulceration due to *Mycobacterium ulcerans* occurs frequently on the extremities. This is also known as Buruli ulcer, as most patients in the first report from Uganda were from Buruli County [51]. Human infections with *M. ulcerans* have been recorded from many parts of the world: Bolivia, Mexico, Australia, Nigeria, Zaïre, Uganda, Sumatra and Malaysia.

Aetiology

Mycobacterium ulcerans is regarded as an environmental saprophyte. It is cultured in Löwenstein–Jensen medium at 33°C, and has a marked tendency to clump, especially to fibrous bundles [52].

Clinical manifestations

Most cases occur in children and young adults; the incidence is greater in women than in men. Microtrauma by pricks or cuts has been advanced as the possible means of inoculation into the skin. After an incubation period of about 3 months, the lesions begin as solitary, painless subcutaneous nodules, which subsequently enlarge and eventually ulcerate. The ulcer is deeply undermined. The floor of the ulcer is formed of necrotic fat, with sometimes clear mucoid discharge. Both the nodule and ulcer are painless and there is little or no constitutional disturbance if the disease is not complicated by bacterial superinfection. The lesions may occur anywhere on the body, but in adults the extremities are the sites of predilection. The course is variable. Spontaneous healing, when it occurs, begins at the proximal end of the ulcer while active necrosis is still present at the distal end (Fig. 4.15). The ulcers take months to years to heal spontaneously, with sometimes a disabling degree of scarring, complicating contraction and lymphoedema.

Diagnosis

Diagnosis is confirmed on the basis of histopathology and bacteriological examination of smears and culture from a subcutaneous node or an ulcer in a patient with an appropriate history. The differential diagnosis of the subcutaneous nodule includes foreign-body granuloma, phycomycosis, nodular fasciitis, panniculitis, nodular vasculitis, sebaceous cyst, injection abscess, myiasis and appendageal tumours. The differential diagnosis of the ulcer includes necrotizing cellulitis, blastomycosis and other deep fungus infections, pyoderma gangrenosum, gumma (syphilis, yaws) and suppurative panniculitis.

Treatment

Excision of the early lesion is curative. With ulceration, wide excision and skin grafting is probably the best form of therapy.

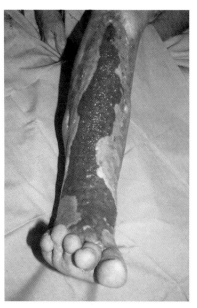

Fig. 4.15 Buruli ulcer caused by *Mycobacterium ulcerans* on the leg. Spontaneous healing at the proximal end of the ulcer and active necrosis at the distal end. (Reprinted with permission of Elsevier Science.)

Despite initial reports that *M. ulcerans* is sensitive to rifampicin *in vitro* and that some infections may respond to it, chemotherapy appears to be of limited value. Local therapy [53], hyperbaric oxygenation [54] and a combination of trimethoprim and sulphamethoxazole are probably of some value.

Mycobacterium kansasii

Skin lesions due to *Mycobacterium kansasii* usually occur in adults. The organism is possibly introduced into the skin by minor trauma, such as a puncture wound.

Clinical manifestations

Skin disease due to *M. kansasii* may present in several forms: verrucous, nodular or sporotrichoid [55, 56]. Localized granulomatous lesions or cellulitis-like lesions of the leg are also found.

Diagnosis

Diagnosis is confirmed on microbial culture. Histopathologically it is indistinguishable from tuberculosis.

Treatment

Successful chemotherapy can often be accomplished with antituberculous drugs: streptomycin, rifampicin and ethambutol. Minocycline 200 mg daily may be effective.

Mycobacterium scrofulaceum

Mycobacterium scrofulaceum is widely distributed and has been found in water, soil and dairy products. The cervical lymphadenitis caused by this organism occurs in children [57] but it may occasionally cause pulmonary infection or skin abscesses [58]. The involved lymph nodes are frequently unilateral, with mild pain. The nodes enlarge slowly over several weeks and eventually soften and drain. They are located high up in the neck and just below the mandible and maxilla. They heal with fibrosis and calcification. There are no constitutional symptoms and the disease is benign and self-limited.

Diagnosis

Unilateral cervical lymphadenitis in a child should evoke suspicion. The histopathology is similar to that of tuberculosis. The diagnosis can only be confirmed by the demonstration of *M. scrofulaceum* in culture from a biopsy specimen. The condition has to be distinguished from sporotrichosis, tuberculosis, *M. marinum*, *Mycobacterium cheilonei* and other granulomatous infections of the skin.

Treatment

In localized lesions or in cervical lymphadenitis, surgical excision should be performed. For more extensive disease, combined therapy with isoniazid, ethambutol and rifampicin has to be tried, because *M. scrofulaceum* is not very sensitive to antituberculous drugs.

Mycobacterium avium–intracellulare

Mycobacterium avium–intracellulare (MAI) comprises strains of two species, *Mycobacterium avium* and *Mycobacterium intracellulare*. They are usually grouped together with *M. scrofulaceum* and have been described as the *M. avium–intracellulare scrofulaceum* (MAIS) complex. They usually cause lung or lymph-node diseases, but *M. scrofulaceum* produces only a benign, self-limited lymphadenopathy without involvement of organs.

Clinical manifestations

Skin involvement is less common. Skin lesions may be multiple purulent ulcer [59] or ulcers and papules histologically resembling lepromatous leprosy [60]. Sometimes, involvement of the skin occurs secondary to disseminated infection with *M. avium–intracellulare*. These skin lesions may be ulcerations, multiple skin granulomas, infiltrated erythematous lesions, pustular lesions or soft-tissue swelling. Such disseminated infection with *M. avium–intracellulare* is one of the commonest opportunistic infections in AIDS patients [61].

Diagnosis

The diagnosis can only be confirmed by the demonstration of *M. avium–intracellulare* in bacterial culture.

Treatment

Localized lesions may be best excised, as the organism seems to be poorly susceptible to chemotherapeutic drugs. More extensive infections need combination therapy with multiple antituberculous drugs [60]. A randomized study comparing clarithromycin with a four-drug treatment regimen clearly showed that clarithromycin 1500–2000 mg/day was superior [62]. Rifamycin (ansamycin) and clofazimine may be effective in AIDS patients [63, 64].

Mycobacterium szulgai

Mycobacterium szulgai can cause diffuse cellulitis, draining nodules and cervical lymphadenitis [65]. It has also been isolated from patients with bursitis and pneumonia.

It is more susceptible to several antituberculous drugs than are most of the other atypical mycobacteria.

Mycobacterium fortuitum and Mycobacterium chelonae

Mycobacterium fortuitum and *Mycobacterium chelonae* seem to be widely distributed and are commonly found in water or soil.

Clinical manifestations

Infection usually occurs after a puncture wound or surgical procedure [66]. Postinjection abscesses are the most frequent lesions caused by either organism [20]. Cold abscesses after injection, especially in the tropics, may also be due to these organisms. *Mycobacterium fortuitum* and *M. chelonae* have infected median sternotomy [67], augmentation mammoplasty [68] and other surgical procedures.

Diagnosis

These infections should be remembered in all cases of resistant or unusual cold abscesses in the tropics. *Mycobacterium fortuitum* and *M. chelonae* may be identified by culture of biopsy material.

Treatment

These infections are commonly resistant to most standard antituberculosis drugs [69]. Excision for localized lesions and surgical débridement for widespread disease are best combined with an appropriate antibiotic, such as amikacin or doxycycline [70].

Erythromycin, cefoxitin and tobramycin may be useful for *M. chelonae* infections [69, 71, 72], and amikacin, doxycycline and sulphonamide for those due to *M. fortuitum* [69]. The wide variability in antibiotic susceptibility means that a rational treatment has to await results of identification of the organism and *in vitro* sensitivity testing.

Mycobacterium infection in HIV-infected patients

In the USA, new cases of tuberculosis declined steadily to a low until 1985. Subsequently, the incidence of infection caused by *M. tuberculosis* rose in some areas where AIDS patients were concentrated [73]. Most cases of tuberculosis seem to be the reactivation of latent infection, and the incidence of extrapulmonary tuberculosis is usually high.

The WHO estimated in 1990 that 1.7 billion people were or had been infected by the tuberculosis bacillus [74]. In addition, 4 million people had coinfection with HIV and the tuberculosis bacillus [75]. Tuberculosis in HIV-infected patients has also been found in Africa [74, 76]. It is estimated that 3 million of these patients lived in sub-Saharan Africa [75].

The clinical presentation of cutaneous tuberculosis is highly variable in patients with chronic tuberculosis. Most patients with coinfection with HIV and tuberculosis have no specific mucocutaneous lesions. Acute miliary tuberculosis, presenting as erythematous papules on the trunk and extremities, in patients with AIDS has been reported. Miliary tuberculosis of the skin is an extremely rare manifestation of infection with *M. tuberculosis* [77, 78].

Mycobacterium avium–intracellulare infection in HIV-infected patients

Disseminated MAI infection occurs frequently in HIV-infected patients with advanced immunodeficiency, but symptomatic cutaneous MAI involvement is rare. Resolution occurred after a short course of routine antituberculosis treatment [79, 80].

The use of clarithromycin or azithromycin has been recommended, in association with ethambutol and one of the following drugs: clofazimine, rifampicin, rifabutin, ciprofloxazin or amikacin [81, 83]. Rifabutin at a daily dose of 300 mg could be proposed as prophylaxis for disseminated *M. avium* complex (MAC) disease for patients with fewer than 100 CD4 lymphocytes/mm^3 [81, 83].

Mycobacterium haemophilum

Mycobacterium haemophilum infection of the skin is rare and has been reported to cause erythema, swelling, painful nodules and abscess formation in immunosuppressed patients. No standardized susceptibility tests and no recommended therapy are yet available. Response to antituberculous therapy has been poor [82, 84].

Mycobacterium fortuitum

Mycobacterium fortuitum infection has been reported in patients with HIV disease. Cutaneous lesions include multiple subcutaneous nodules, ulceration and abscess formation. The therapeutic response to antituberculous drugs was poor [85].

References

1 Christiansen JV. Lupus vulgaris gigantea caused by *Mycobacterium avium*. In: Jadassohn W, Schirren CG (eds) *Proceedings of the 13th International Congress of Dermatology*, Vol. II. Springer Verlag, Berlin, 1968, pp. 1319–1320.

2 Beyt BE, Ortbals DW, Santa Cruz DJ *et al*. Cutaneous mycobacteriosis: analysis of 34 cases with a new classification of the disease. *Medicine* 1981; **60**: 95–109.

3 Harahap M. Tuberculosis of the skin: clinical aspects. In: Harahap M (ed.) *Mycobacterial Skin Diseases*. New Clinical Applications: Dermatology, Kluwer Academic Publishers, Dordrecht, 1989, pp. 79–104.

4 James DG, Mishra BB. The changing pattern of tuberculosis. *Postgrad Med J* 1984; **60**: 92–97.

5 Genewein A, Telenti A, Bernasconi C *et al*. Molecular approach to identifying route of transmission of tuberculosis in the community. *Lancet* 1993; **342**: 841–844.

6 McNicol M. Trends in the epidemiology of tuberculosis—a physician's view. *J Clin Pathol* 1983; **36**: 1087–1090.

7 Narain JP, Raviglione MC, Kochi A. *HIV-associated Tuberculosis in Developing Countries: Epidemiology and Strategies for Prevention*. WHO document, WHO/TB/92. 166, WHO, Geneva. 1992.

8 Harahap M. Tuberculosis of the skin. *Int J Dermatol* 1983; **22**: 542–545.

9 Kim YP, Sohn HS. Cutaneous tuberculosis in Korea. In: *Proceedings of the Third Regional Conference of Dermatology, Denpasar Bali, Indonesia*. Indonesian Society of Dermatology and Venereology, Jakarta 1978, pp. 499–513.

10 Goh YS, Ong BH, Rajan VS. Tuberculosis cutis in Singapore: a two year experience. *Singapore Med J* 1974; **15**: 223–226.

11 Sehgal VN, Srivastava G, Khurana VK, Sharma VK, Bhalla P, Beohar PC. An appraisal of epidemiologic, clinical, bacteriologic, histopathologic, and immunologic parameters in cutaneous tuberculosis. *Int J Dermatol* 1987; **26**: 521–526.

12 Wirjohatmodjo NT, Djuanda A, Wiryadi BE, Wirawan R. Multiple tuberculosis cutis (lupus vulgaris or tuberculosis verrucosa cutis). In: *Proceedings of the Third Regional Conference of Dermatology, Denpasar Bali, Indonesia*. Indonesian Society of Dermatology and Venereology, Jakarta 1978, pp. 518–522.

13 Wong KO, Lee KP, Chin SF. Tuberculosis of the skin in Hong Kong (a review of 160 cases). *Br J Dermatol* 1968; **80**: 287–292.

14 Sehgal VN, Bhattacharya SN, Jain S *et al*. Cutaneous tuberculosis: the evolving scenario. *Int J Dermatol* 1994; **33**: 97–104.

15 Miller FJW. Recognition of primary tuberculous infection of skin and mucosae. *Lancet* 1953; **i**: 5.

16 Miller FJW, Cashman JM. Peripheral tuberculous lymphadenitis associated with a visible primary focus. *Lancet* 1955; **i**: 1286–1289.

17 Goette DK. Primary inoculation of tuberculosis of the skin: Prosector's paronychia. *Arch Dermatol* 1978; **114**: 567.

18 Pereira CA, Webber B, Orson JM. Primary tuberculosis complex of the skin. *JAMA* 1976; **235**: 942.

19 Ramesh V, Misra RS, Jain RK. Secondary tuberculosis of the skin: clinical features and problems in laboratory diagnosis. *Int J Dermatol* 1987; **26**: 578–581.

20 Grange JM, Noble WC, Yates MD *et al*. Inoculation mycobacterioses. *Clin Exp Dermatol* 1988; **13**: 211–220.

21 Horwitz O, Christensen S. Numerical estimates of the extent of the lesion of lupus vulgaris cutis and their significance for epidemiologic and clinical research. *Am Rev Respir Dis* 1960; **82**: 862–872.

22 Pramatarov K, Balabanova N, Miteva L *et al*. Tuberculosis verrucosa cutis associated with lupus vulgaris. *Int J Dermatol* 1993; **32**: 815–817.

23 Wilson-Jones E, Winkelmann R. Papulonecrotic tuberculid: a neglected disease in Western countries. *J Am Acad Dermatol* 1986; **14**: 815–826.

24 Sheingold MA, Sheingold H. Oral tuberculosis. *Oral Surg* 1951; **4**: 239.

25 Weaver RA. Tuberculosis of the tongue. *JAMA* 1976; **235**: 2418.

26 Sahn SA, Neff TA. Miliary tuberculosis. *Am J Med* 1974; **56**: 459–505.

27 Bolgert M. La tuberculose cutanée: historique, clinique, et évolution thérapeutique. Semin Hosp Paris 1967; **43**: 868–888.

28 Tschen EH, Jessen T, Robertson G *et al*. Erythema multiforme as a complication of BCG scarification technique. *Arch Dermatol* 1979; **115**: 614–615.

29 Dostrovsky A, Sagher F. Dermatological complications of BCG vaccination. *Br J Dermatol* 1963; **75**: 181–192.

30 Machtey I, Bandmann M, Palant A. Unusual reaction to BCG. *Lancet* 1968; **i**: 114–116.

31 Izumi AK, Matsunaga J. BCG vaccine-induced lupus vulgaris. *Arch Dermatol* 1982; **118**: 171–172.

32 Centers for Disease Control. Disseminated *Mycobacterium bovis* infection from BCG vaccination of a patient with AIDS. *Morb Mort Weekly Rep* 1985; **34**: 227–229.

33 Graham-Brown RA, Sarkany I. Lichen scrofulosorum with tuberculous dactylitis. *Br J Dermatol* 1980; **103**: 561.

34 Wandall JH, Nissen BK, Krabbe S *et al*. Et tilfaede of lichen scrofulosum. *Ugeskr-Laeger* 1975; **137**: 1538–1540.

35 Nishigori C, Taniguchi S, Hyakawa M. Penis tuberculides: papulonecrotic tuberculides on the glans penis. *Dermatologica* 1986; **172**: 93–97.

36 Morrison JGL, Fourie ED. The papulonecrotic tuberculid—from Arthus reaction to lupus vulgaris. *Br J Dermatol* 1974; **91**: 263–270.

37 Sloan JB, Medenica M. Papulonecrotic tuberculid in a 9-year-old American girl: case report and review of the literature. *Pediatr Dermatol* 1990; **7**: 191–195.

38 Montgomery H. Nodular vascular diseases of the legs. *JAMA* 1945; **128**: 335–341.

39 American Thoracic Society. Treatment of tuberculosis and tuberculosis infection in adults and children. *Am Rev Respir Dis* 1986; **134**: 355–363.

40 Corsella BF. New approach to treatment of pulmonary and extrapulmonary tuberculosis: possible ramifications of cutaneous mycobacterial infections. *Int J Dermatol* 1987; **26**: 185–189.

41 Iseman MD, Sbarbaro JA. National ACCP Consensus Conference on Tuberculosis. *Chest* 1985; **87**: 115S–149S.

42 American Thoracic Society. Treatment of tuberculosis and other mycobacterial diseases. *Am Rev Respir Dis* 1983; **127**: 790–796.

43 Harahap M. Tuberculosis of the skin: clinical aspects. In: Harahap M (ed.) *Mycobacterial Skin Diseases*. New Clinical Applications: Dermatology, Kluwer Academic Publishers, Dordrecht, 1989, pp. 100–101.

44 Citron KM, Girling DJ. Tuberculosis. In: Weatherall DJ, Ledingham JGG, Warrell DA (eds) *Oxford Textbook of Medicine*, Vol. 1, Part 5. Oxford University Press, Oxford, 1987, pp. 291–292.

45 Ramesh V, Misra RS, Saxena U *et al*. Comparative efficacy of drug regimens in skin tuberculosis. *Clin Exp Dermatol* 1991; **16**: 106–109.

46 Anonymous. *WHO Model Prescribing Information: Drugs Used in Mycobacterial Disease*. World Health Organization, Geneva, 1991, pp. 12–13.

47 Dooley SW, Jarvis WR, Marton WJ *et al*. Multidrug resistant tuberculosis. *Ann Intern Med* 1993; **117**: 257–259.

48 Small PM, Shafer RW, Hopewell PC *et al*. Exogenous reinfection with multidrug-resistant *Mycobacterium tuberculosis* in patients with advanced HIV infection. *N Engl J Med* 1993; **328**: 1137–1144.

49 Iseman MD. Treatment of multidrug resistant tuberculosis. *N Engl J Med* 1993; **329**: 748–749.

50 Norden A, Linell FA. A new type of pathogenic mycobacterium. *Nature* 1951; **168**: 826.

51 Clancey JK, Doge OG, Lunn HF *et al*. Mycobacterial skin ulcers in Uganda. *Lancet* 1961; **ii**: 951.

52 Tyrell DAS, McLauchlan SL, Goodwin CS. The growth of some mycobacteria on cultured human tissues. *Br J Exp Pathol* 1975; **56**: 99–102.

53 Meyers WM, Shelly WM, Connor DH. Heat treatment of *M. ulcerans* infections without surgical excision. *Am J Trop Med Hyg* 1974; **23**: 924–929.

54 Krieg RE, Walcott JH, Confer A. Treatment of *M. ulcerans* infection by hyperbaric oxygenation. *Aviation Space Environ Med* 1975; **46**: 1241–1245.

55 Dore N, Collins JP, Mankiewicz E. A sporotrichoid-like *M. kansasii* infection of the skin treated with minocycline hydrochloride. *Br J Dermatol* 1979; **101**: 75–79.

56 Owens DW, McBride ME. Sporotrichoid cutaneous infection with *M. kansasii*. *Arch Dermatol* 1969; **100**: 54–58.

57 Lai KK, Sottmeier KD, Sherman IH *et al*. Mycobacterial cervical lymphadenopathy: relation of etiologic agents to age. *JAMA* 1984; **251**: 1286–1288.

58 Murray-Leisure KA, Egan N, Weitekamp MR. Skin lesions caused by *M. scrofulaceum*. *Arch Dermatol* 1987; **123**: 369–370.

59 Noel SB, Ray MC, Greer DL. Cutaneous infection with *M. avium intracellulare scrofulaceum* intermediate: a new pathogenic entity. *J Am Acad Dermatol* 1988; **19**: 492–495.

60 Cole GW, Gerhard J. *M. avium* infection of the skin resembling lepromatous leprosy. *Br J Dermatol* 1979; **101**: 71–74.

61 Lerner CW, Tapper MC. Opportunistic infection complicating acquired immune deficiency syndrome. *Medicine* 1984; **63**: 155–164.

62 Dautzenberg B, Saint Marc T, Meyohas M *et al*. Clarithromycin and other anti-microbial agents in the treatment of disseminated *Mycobacterium avium* infections in patients with acquired immunodeficiency syndrome. *Arch Intern Med* 1993; **153**: 368–372.

63 Masur H, Tuazon C, Gill V *et al*. Effect of combined clofazimine and ansamycin therapy on *Mycobacterium avium–Mycobacterium intracellulare* bacteremia in patients with AIDS. *J Infect Dis* 1987; **155**: 127–129.

64 Agins BD, Berman DS, Spicehandler D *et al*. Effect of combined therapy with ansamycin, clofazimine, ethambutol and isoniazid for *Mycobacterium avium* infections in patients with AIDS. *J Infect Dis* 1989; **159**: 784–787.

65 Sybert A, Tsou E, Garagusi VF. Cutaneous infection due to *M. szulgai*. *Am Rev Respir Dis* 1977; **115**: 695–698.

66 Johnson S, Weir TW. Multiple cutaneous ulcers of the legs. *Arch Dermatol* 1993; **129**: 1190–1191, 1193.

67 Hoffman PC, Fraser DW, Robiesek F *et al*. Two outbreaks of sternal wound infections due to organisms of *M. fortuitum* complex. *J Infect Dis* 1981; **143**: 533–542.

68 Centers for Disease Control. Mycobacterial infections associated with augmentation mammoplasty—Florida, North Carolina, Texas. *Morb Mort Weekly Rep* 1978; **27**: 513.

69 Wallace RJ. The clinical presentation, diagnosis and therapy of cutaneous and pulmonary infections due to rapidly growing mycobacteria, *M. fortuitum* and *M. chelonae*. *Clin Chest Med* 1989; **10**: 419–429.

70 Dalovisio JR, Wallace RJ. Clinical usefulness of amikacin and doxycycline in the treatment of infection due to *M. fortuitum* and *M. chelonei*. *Rev Infect Dis* 1981; **3**: 1068–1074.

71 Fenske NA, Millns JL. Resistant cutaneous infection caused by *M. chelonei*. *Arch Dermatol* 1981; **117**: 151–153.

72 Swetter SM, Kindel SE, Smoller BR. Cutaneous nodules of *Mycobacterium chelonae* in an immunosuppressed patient with preexisting pulmonary colonization. *J Am Acad Dermatol* 1993; **28** (2): 352–355.

73 Rieder HL, Cauthen GM, Kelly GD *et al.* Tuberculosis in the United States. *JAMA* 1989; **262**: 385–389.

74 Kochi A. The global tuberculosis situation and the new control strategy of the World Health Organization. *Tubercle* 1991; **72**: 1–6.

75 De Cock K, Soro B, Coulibaly I *et al.* Tuberculosis and HIV infection in sub-Saharan Africa. *JAMA* 1992; **268**: 1581–1587.

76 Meeran K. Prevalence of HIV infection among patients with leprosy and tuberculosis in rural Zambia. *Br Med J* 1989; **298**: 364–365.

77 Stack RJ, Bickley LK, Coppel IG. Miliary tuberculosis presenting as skin lesions in a patient with acquired immunodeficiency syndrome. *J Am Acad Dermatol* 1990; **23** (2): 1031–1035.

78 Rohatgi PK, Palazzolo JV, Saini NB. Acute miliary tuberculosis of the skin in acquired immunodeficiency syndrome. *J Am Acad Dermatol* 1992; **26**: 356–359.

79 Friedman BF, Edwards D, Kirkpatrick CH. *Mycobacterium avium–intracellulare*: cutaneous presentations of disseminated disease. *Am J Med* 1988; **85**: 257–263.

80 Inwald D, Nelson M, Cramp M *et al.* Cutaneous manifestations of mycobacterial infection in patients with AIDS. *Br J Dermatol* 1994; **130**: 111–114.

81 Bassiri A, Chan NB, Mc Leod A *et al.* Disseminated cutaneous infection due to *Mycobacterium tuberculosis* in a person with AIDS. *Can Med Assoc J* 1993; **148**: 577–578.

82 Dever LL, Martin JW, Seaworth B *et al.* Varied presentations and responses of treatment of infections caused by *Mycobacterium haemophilum* in patients with AIDS. *Clin Infect Dis* 1992; **14**: 1195–1200.

83 Masur H, Public Health Service Task Force on Prophylaxis and Therapy for *Mycobacterium avium* Complex. Recommendations on prophylaxis and therapy for disseminated *Mycobacterium avium* complex disease in patients infected with the human immunodeficiency virus. *N Engl J Med* 1993; **329**: 898–904.

84 Kristjansson M, Bieluch VM, Byeff PD. *Mycobacterium haemophilum* infection in immunocompromised patients: case report and review of the literature. *Rev Infect Dis* 1991; **13**: 906–910.

85 Shafer RW, Sierra MF. *Mycobacterium xenopi, Mycobacterium fortuitum, Mycobacterium kansasii,* and other nontuberculous mycobacteria in an area of endemicity for AIDS. *Clin Infect Dis* 1992; **15**: 161–162.

Chapter 5
Viral Infections

Monica L. McCrary, Martha S. Paterson &
Stephen K. Tyring

Many viral diseases have a skin component at some time during their course. While some are readily diagnosable by virtue of their characteristic appearance, others require the presence of other clues from the history, physical examination or laboratory data. In years past, it was not uncommon to simply diagnose 'viral exanthem', since little could be done other than supportive treatment. With the emergence of new antiviral therapies, however, arriving at the correct diagnosis is of increased importance, and to simply say 'viral exanthem' is not nearly enough.

Herpes simplex viruses 1 and 2

The herpes simplex viruses type 1 (HSV-1) and type 2 (HSV-2), although most known for causing cold sores and genital herpes, respectively, cause several other mucocutaneous infections seen in humans. These infections include: gingivostomatis, herpes gladiatorum, eczema herpeticum, herpes whitlow, lumbrosacral herpes, herpetic keratoconjuntivitis and herpes encephalitis. Typically, these viruses cause a primary mucocutaneous infection, followed by a latent infection, when the virus remains dormant in the neuronal ganglia. Later, recurrent disease can occur, with viral reactivation and movement down the nerve to produce active mucocutaneous infections. While herpes encephalitis is potentially fatal, most herpetic infections are simply painful, socially embarrassing or psychologically devastating. Therefore, finding a way to prevent or treat herpes simplex infections is of paramount importance to the health-care profession.

Aetiology

Herpes simplex viruses 1 and 2 have a double-stranded deoxyribonucleic acid (DNA) genome, with a surrounding protein coat and lipid envelope. Approximately half of HSV-1 and HSV-2 nucleotide sequences are identical, but the rest are unique to the particular virus. Of the 50 viral-specific proteins encoded by the genome, five to six are glycoproteins located on viral surfaces and infected cell surfaces. These glycoproteins are important in inducing an antibody response in the infected individual.

197

Other proteins encoded by the genome are used in viral DNA replication. These viral enzymes, such as viral DNA polymerase, thymidine kinase and ribonucleotide reductase, can be recognized by antiviral drugs. Therefore, antiviral chemotherapy is often effective in treating herpes viral infections.

Primary infection

Herpes simplex viruses usually cause primary infections in mucocutaneous locations, can cause asymptomatic infections while shedding viral particles from the neuronal ganglia and can later re-emerge as recurrent infections. Primary infection most often results from exposure via mucocutaneous contact with an infected individual. Transmission can occur when the infected person has active disease or is asymptomatic but shedding viral particles. In one study, subclinical (asymptomatic) HSV shedding accounted for nearly one-third of the total days of reactivation of HSV infection [1]. Respiratory transmission has not been documented, and there have been no documented cases of herpes viral infection acquired through water or from damp surfaces, even though the virus is able to survive for some time outside the infected host. Also, it is well known that halogenated compounds can immediately inactivate the virus.

Initial infections with either HSV-1 or HSV-2 can be the most disabling, and could involve widespread blistering, severe pain and an extended healing time of 3–4 weeks if no treatment occurs. However, it should be noted that an individual's first symptomatic episode may not be the actual 'primary infection', since the virus may have been unnoticed but within the infected person's body for some time before the clinically obvious outbreak occurs. Not everyone who develops a primary infection will have recurrent episodes; the virus can remain asymptomatic without therapy. Also, antibodies to HSV-1 and 2 are found in millions of adults who deny ever having an outbreak of either cold sores or genital herpes. Even so, most individuals do have recurrent infections after the primary outbreak, and some require antiviral treatment to encourage the healing process or to prevent these episodes entirely.

Recurrent infections

As previously mentioned, the HSV-1 and 2 have the ability to remain dormant in neuronal ganglia after the primary infection, but can later cause recurrent disease through viral reactivation. Recurrent infections arise after the latent virus is awakened by particular triggering events, such as emotional or physical stress, nerve manipulation or even sunlight. However, the triggering effect can be unknown or unclear. Next, the resulting new viral particles travel down the ganglia and start the replication process, inducing an outbreak. This event is common in most recurrent herpes viral infections. Recurrent infections are usually less severe than the initial episode, with lesions often healing in less than 2 weeks without therapy, but can still be quite bothersome. In immunocompromised individuals, such as those with acquired immune deficiency syndrome (AIDS), cancer or organ transplants, the HSV recurrences can be chronic, in that one episode does not completely heal before another begins.

Facial–oral herpes simplex

Recurrent facial–oral herpes infection, also termed herpes labialis, cold sores or fever blisters, is a common worldwide problem that affects 20–40% of the population [2]. It is estimated that at least 80% of adults have evidence of HSV-1 infection detected via serology. Although at least 90% of recurrent facial–oral herpes are caused by HSV-1, some are actually caused by HSV-2. Recurrent outbreaks are variable among individuals, with some experiencing multiple episodes each year.

The clinical course of herpes labialis usually progresses from a prodromal stage of burning, tingling and itching to erythema and papule formation. Next, the papule forms a vesicle, which later ulcerates and finally crusts before completely healing (Fig. 5.1). These lesions usually occur somewhere on the lip, especially on the vermilion border, but they can occur in the nose and on other areas near the lip. Occasionally, the regional lymph nodes are painful and enlarged. The entire episode, from prodromal stage to complete healing, can last days to weeks, but usually lasts 8–9 days [3]. It is important to note that lesions continue to be infectious until all crusts are gone. Virus can be isolated from cold sores for about 3.5 days [3]. Some individuals experience a triggering event before developing an outbreak. These events include stress (both physical and emotional), trauma to the area, sunlight and even fatigue. However, many patients do not know what caused their outbreak and deny experiencing the typical triggering events.

Since most recurrent episodes of herpes labialis are mild and self-limited, many individuals do not seek treatment and require only topical antiseptics to prevent possible secondary infections [2]. Also, treatment of mild infections or those late in the course of disease with antiviral chemotherapy does not seem to benefit the patient [4]. However, antiviral

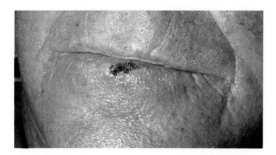

Fig. 5.1 Herpes labialis due to herpes simplex type 1.

chemotherapy does have a role in preventing outbreaks in those patients who experience frequent recurrences and in patients with an early infection. The antibodies produced by HSV-1 infection do not render the individual immune to recurrences, but infected individuals are known to have an increased amount of circulating antibody during an active outbreak.

The complications of recurrent facial–oral herpes include secondary infection, herpes gladiatorum, herpes whitlow, keratoconjuctivitis and life-threatening encephalitis.

Primary gingivostomatitis

The primary infection of HSV in children and young adults can often present as acute gingivostomatitis. The peak years of incidence usually occur between ages 1 and 5 [3]. Primary gingivostomatitis, usually caused by HSV-1, presents with sore throat, painful ulcers, fever and denuded ulcers on the tongue, palate, gingival, buccal mucosa and lips [5]. The time from exposure to onset of symptoms is 5–10 days [3]. Most often the infection starts as a single cluster of lesions on the buccal mucosa, which later spreads to involve much of the buccal mucosa and other areas. Although herpetic gingivostomatitis is generally self-limited and rarely requires treatment, the infection can resemble other infections, such as streptococcal pharyngitis, ulcerative stomatitis, diphtheria or Coxsackie virus, and differentiation may be necessary for treatment purposes.

Genital herpes

The most common cause of genital ulcerations worldwide is HSV infection. Currently, recurrent genital herpes affects approximately 25 million adults in the USA [6]. Genital herpes is transmitted via mucocutaneous contact with an infected individual, usually during sexual contact. However, asymptomatic individuals, with no evidence of active disease, can shed HSV and can transmit the virus. The infection, most often HSV-2, generally appears within 3–14 days after exposure. Roughly 85% of these infections are caused by HSV-2, and these tend to be more severe and recur more often than those caused by HSV-1. Men with HSV-2 infection have 20% more recurrences than do women, a factor that may contribute to the higher rate of HSV-2 transmission from men to women than from women to men [7].

The primary infection presents as a small group of vesicles, which ulcerate after several days and eventually crust after 18–21 days. New lesions can continue to develop throughout the first week. Typical viral shedding lasts about 10 days in men and 8–14 days in women. Symptoms can include itching, pain, dysuria, tender inguinal lymph nodes and discharge. As previously mentioned, the primary episode is the most disabling and can involve widespread blistering and severe pain. Complications of primary genital herpes infection include aseptic meningitis and severe dysuria, requiring catherization. About 30% of women and 13% of men develop aseptic meningitis, with fever, stiff neck, photophobia, headache and pleocytosis in the spinal fluid [8].

Recurrent genital infection occurs when the virus is reactivated after a latent stage in the sacral ganglia. Typically these recurrent episodes occur three to four times per year, but have shorter and lessened severity when compared with the original outbreak. More than 35% of patients that have recurrences have frequent recurrences. These rates are especially high in individuals who had extended primary episodes [7]. Many patients experience a prodrome of pain and tingling in the thigh and buttock area before vesicle formation (Fig. 5.2). The time from vesicle formation to crusting is about 5 days, with complete healing within 10 days. Although the virus can only rarely be isolated from crusted lesions, patients should be instructed to avoid sexual contact until lesions have completely healed.

Most individuals have recurrent episodes that last only a few days and only require supportive care, such as comforting soaks or compresses and mild analgesics. However, as in other herpetic infections, oral antiviral chemotherapy is beneficial when given during the prodromal stage or at the onset of vesicle formation. Unfortunately, topical antiviral treatment has not been found to have much effect. Suppression of infection with oral antiviral drugs is appropriate when recurrences are frequent (> six per year) or debilitating. Patients with aseptic meningitis should receive parenteral antiviral chemotherapy and most often should be seen by a neurologist as well.

Some complications of genital herpes include aseptic meningitis, impotence, constipation, perianal numbness, neurogenic bladder, pharyngitis and viral cervicitis; genital herpes is also a risk factor for acquisition of human immunodeficiency virus (HIV). Pregnant women with genital herpes can have an increased risk of birth defects or even fetal death, and should receive appropriate prenatal care and counselling if needed.

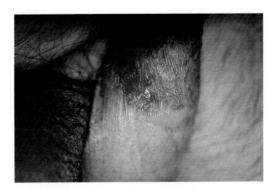

Fig. 5.2 Genital herpes due to herpes simplex type 2.

Diagnosis

Most of the time the diagnosis of a herpes infection is made from the individual's history and clinical findings. However, there are tools to aid in diagnosing HSV infection when the history and findings are not typical. The Tzanck smear is a useful test to rapidly screen for HSV. This procedure involves taking a sample of a suspected lesion and smearing it on to a slide. The slide is stained with Giemsa's or Wright's stain, and then is examined for large multinucleated epithelial giant cells. This finding, termed a positive Tzanck smear, represents probable HSV infection. However, false-positive Tzanck smears do occur. The viral culture is a more precise method for identifying HSV, although not as rapid. In a particular clinical trial, lesions that appeared to be herpes produced positive virus culture about 85–90% of the time. Monoclonal antibodies against HSV and immunofluorescence techniques are also being employed to make rapid and precise diagnoses, and may soon replace the above methods.

Other herpetic infections

The herpes virus can cause other infections than just facial–oral herpes and genital herpes. Herpetic whitlow is a herpes infection of the hand or fingers. This infection occurs most often in health-care professionals that work in or around the mouths of patients that shed facial–oral herpes. However, it can also be a result of contact with genital herpes. Acquisition occurs when the virus comes in contact with broken skin around the hands and fingers. The primary infection resembles typical herpetic infection, with the appearance of painful vesicles, erythema that can involve the forearm and sometimes even tender axillary lymph nodes. The lesions do eventually heal within 6 weeks, but recurrences are common. This infection can be avoided by the proper use of gloves when contact with human body fluids is anticipated.

Herpes gladiatorum is a herpetic infection found most often in wrestlers. This infection, usually caused by HSV-1, is transmitted by direct skin-to-skin contact. Abrasions and breaks in the skin at the site of inoculation are common but are not found in all cases. The usual location of these lesions is the head, trunk and extremities. Identification of affected individuals is crucial to avoid the rapid spread to other team players.

Herpes keratoconjunctivitis is currently one of the leading causes of blindness due to an infectious agent. This infection can cause repeated ulcerations and erosions of the cornea and the conjuctiva. Recurrences can ultimately cause stromal scarring, leading to blindness. Diagnosis requires a slit-lamp examination. Early therapy with topical antiviral drugs is used to heal and to prevent stromal scarring.

The most common cause of encephalitis today is HSV. This disease, which can be fatal, can affect all ages at any time of the year. The affected individual does not always have a prior diagnosis of herpes infection, and may be otherwise healthy. Fever, headache, confusion and other neurological findings can occur. Diagnosis is suggested by pleocytosis and elevated protein in the cerebrospinal fluid (CSF) or enhancement of the brain on computed tomography or magnetic resonance imaging. Unfortunately, viral culture of the CSF is usually negative. However, brain biopsy and culture can ensure a diagnosis. Recently, the polymerase chain reaction (PCR) has been used to isolate HSV DNA in the CSF and may offer a more rapid diagnosis [8]. Untreated herpes encephalitis has a significant mortality; therefore patients should receive antiviral chemotherapy even before a definitive diagnosis is made.

Some individuals with other underlying skin disorders can develop a cutaneous herpetic infection in this same area. This widespread cutaneous infection, known as eczema herpeticum, is associated with fever and lymphadenopathy (Fig. 5.3). Often the lesions coalesce and become secondarily infected with a bacterial agent. This infection can be recurrent, but these infections will be milder and will not have systemic involvement.

In a small group of individuals, recurrent herpes infections are followed by erythema multiforme. Erythema multiforme usually develops within 10 days of a recurrent herpes infection. The rash starts as erythematous papules, which develop into targetoid lesions on the skin and ulcerations on the mucosa (Fig. 5.4). Recurrences are variable and studies suggest that antiviral therapy may be successful when given early [9].

Treatment

Antiviral therapy can shorten the healing time of herpetic lesions. Some

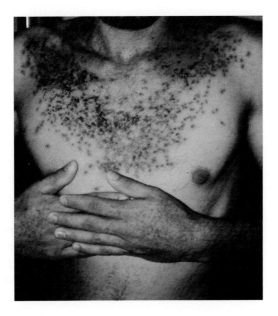

Fig. 5.3 Eczema herpeticum associated with herpes simplex type 1 in a patient with Darier's disease.

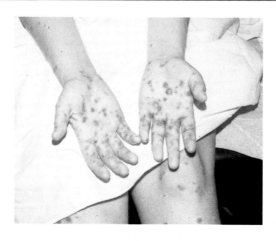

Fig. 5.4 Erythema multiforme following an outbreak of herpes labialis.

episodes can be prevented if therapy is initiated early during the prodromal stage or if suppressive therapy is given to individuals who have frequent recurrences. Currently there are several antiviral agents approved for use against herpes viral infections, such as iododeoxyuridine, vidarabine, trifluorothymidine, foscarnet, acyclovir, famciclovir and valaciclovir. Of these antivirals, acyclovir, famciclovir and valaciclovir use viral thymidine kinase to terminate viral DNA strands, and therefore are the safest and most effective antiherpetic drugs. Since these drugs are activated by viral-specific enzymes, they only act where they are needed and have few side-effects. Oral and intravenous acyclovir is effective, but topical acyclovir has little to no effect. The primary drawbacks are the low bioavailability and frequent dosing needed with acyclovir. However, acyclovir does reduce healing time and viral shedding. The recently approved antiviral drugs famciclovir and valaciclovir may soon replace acyclovir as the first-line treatments.

The usual treatment of initial episodes of herpes virus infection requires 200 mg by mouth five times per day for 10 days. Recurrent episodes require 200 mg by mouth five times per day for 5 days. An alternative to the inconvenient five-times-daily dosing is acyclovir 400 mg three times daily. Even more convenient, and in some cases more effective, are the recently approved alternatives to acyclovir: valaciclovir 500 mg twice daily or famciclovir 125 mg twice daily (both taken orally). Individuals that need suppressive therapy take acyclovir 400 mg by mouth twice a day. Patients with herpes encephalitis, severe herpetic infection or aseptic meningitis may require acyclovir 5 mg/kg intravenously every 8 hours for at least 5 days. Unfortunately, acyclovir-resistant HSV infection has become an increasing problem, especially in the AIDS population. Intravenous forcarnet is currently the treatment of choice for acyclovir-resistant strains. Recombinant HSV vaccinations, both therapeutic and preventive, are currently under investigation.

Varicella zoster

Both primary varicella (chickenpox) and herpes zoster (shingles) derive from a single aetiological agent, varicella-zoster virus (VZV). While herpes zoster occurs in persons who have previously been infected with varicella, it is not believed that it can be acquired from contact with persons with varicella or herpes zoster [10–12]. Instead, herpes zoster is thought to occur as the result of a reactivation of a latent VZV infection, most often in those dermatomes which had the highest density of chickenpox lesions [10, 13].

Varicella (chickenpox)

Aetiology

Varicella-zoster virus is a member of the viral herpes family Herpesviridae. It has an icosahedral capsid and linear molecule of double-stranded DNA. It is surrounded by a lipoprotein envelope to form a roughly spherical virion, approximately 150–200 nm in diameter [14].

Diagnosis

Varicella is usually diagnosed clinically and the diagnosis is particularly easy when there is a history of exposure within the preceding 2–3 weeks [15–17].

Pathogenesis

The initial site of VZV infection is the conjunctiva or the upper respiratory-tract mucosa, followed sequentially by viral replication in regional lymph nodes. Next, a primary viraemia develops within 4–6 days, followed by viral replication in the liver, spleen, lungs and possibly other organs. In most individuals (who are not immunocompromised), a secondary viraemia occurs about 2 weeks after infection [18–22]. This causes fever and malaise and results in VZV infection of the epidermis.

Immunity

In immunocompetent individuals, one attack of varicella generally imparts lifelong immunity to the disease. However, this does not protect against herpes zoster, which is probably the source of the rarely reported 'second attacks'. However, persons who develop a more limited infection, due to the presence of maternal antibody, or persons who received a live attenuated varicella vaccine may respond to future exposure by developing a second outbreak of chickenpox [23–25]. Administration of zoster immune globulin (ZIG) to susceptible normal children can prevent varicella when administered within 3 days of exposure. However, ZIG only modifies the disease in immunosuppressed children. Varicella-zoster immune globulin (VZIG) shows better results in immunocompromised patients. Recently, a live attenuated vaccine (Oka varicella vaccine) for VZV received Food and Drug Administration (FDA) approval. This vaccine was shown to be 100% efficacious in preventing varicella in the vaccine-immunized group in one clinical trial [26].

Epidemiology

Varicella-zoster virus is highly contagious, with 87% of susceptible siblings in households being affected [27]. It is seen worldwide, but with greater numbers of seropositive individuals in the USA (>95% of parturient women in New York City) than in Latin America (approximately 84% [28]). Even greater numbers of seronegative individuals exist in Asia, Africa and the Middle East [29, 30]. Most people in urban USA are exposed early, as 90% of cases occur in children less than 10 years of age and less than 5% of cases occur in individuals greater than age 15 [27, 29]. Patients are usually infectious for 1–2 days before the onset of the rash and thereafter for approximately 4–5 days or until it has completely crusted. The incubation period is generally 14–15 days, with a range of 10–23 days [27, 31]. Occasionally, the rash is so scarce and transient as to go unnoticed by the patient.

Clinical manifestations

The hallmark of varicella is simultaneous presence of lesions in all stages (i.e. vesicles, pustules and crusts) (Fig. 5.5). The early vesicle on an erythematous macula has been likened to a 'dewdrop on a rose petal'. In young children, a prodrome is not commonly reported and primary varicella infection is usually not associated with extracutaneous involvement. After an initial rash, maculae and papules develop on the face and trunk, leading to vesicles, which eventually crust. Vesicles usually show relative sparing of the extremities, but may involve the mucous membranes. In adults and older children, the rash may be preceded by fever, chills, malaise, headache, anorexia, backache, sore throat and dry cough. However, the symptom causing the most distress is generally pruritus. In adults, primary varicella is generally more severe, occasionally involving internal organs, such as the lungs.

Complications

The most common complication is secondary bacterial infection of the rash, most commonly by staphylococci or streptococci. Rarely, this may lead to septicaemia, with infection of other organs [16, 32–34], such as the lungs. However, this secondary bacterial pneumonia usually occurs in children

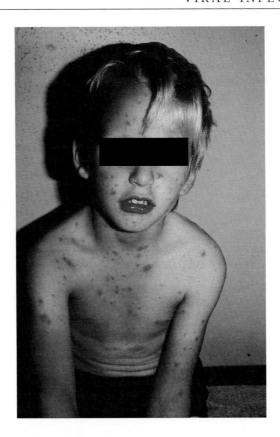

Fig. 5.5 Primary varicella (chickenpox) in a child.

less than 7 years of age and is usually readily responsive to appropriate antibiotic therapy. In adults, the major complication is primary varicella pneumonia, with radiographic evidence of pneumonia being present in 3–16% [35, 36]. This is associated with significant mortality, with estimates ranging from 10 to 30%. However, if immunocompromised patients are excluded, the number is probably less than 10% [16, 37–40]. Of particular concern is congenital infection. A rare syndrome of hypoplasia of an extremity, cicatricial skin scarring, cortical atrophy, ocular abnormalities and low birth weight has been described in infants exposed between the seventh and twentieth weeks of gestation [41–44]. Some infants, however, show no evidence of infection, only to later develop shingles at an early age [41–43, 45]. Even more worrisome are infants whose mother develops varicella less than 5 days before or within 2 days after delivery. Their immature immune systems are sometimes unable to control VZV infection and, without sufficient quantities of maternal antibody, the result can be devastating, with mortalities as high as 30% reported. In addition, central nervous system (CNS) complications can occur (less than 1 in 1000), including Reye's syndrome, acute cerebellar ataxia, encephalitis or meningoencephalitis, acute ascending or transverse myelitis and Guillain–Barré syndrome. Other rare complications include hepatitis (usually subclinical), orchitis, glomerulonephritis, gastritis, pancreatitis, myocarditis, arthritis, Henoch–Schönlein vasculitis and such ocular complications as iritis, keratitis and optic neuritis [35, 46–50]. Of course, immunocompromised patients are more likely to experience severe complications and suffer from a high morbidity and mortality [51–64].

Treatment

Historically, normal children have received only symptomatic treatment for varicella, such as calamine lotion, cool compresses, tepid bath and antipyretics (avoiding aspirin due to the association with Reye's syndrome) [65, 66]. Recently, acyclovir (20 mg/kg four times per day for 5 days) has been shown to reduce the duration and severity of chickenpox when it is started within 24 hours of rash onset [67–69]. However, due to the usually benign nature of the disease and the low rate of complications in this population, as well as the cost of treatment, difficulty in rapid institution of therapy and concern of development of acyclovir-resistant strains of VZV, acyclovir use in normal children has not received widespread acceptance.

However, acyclovir is frequently used in the treatment of immuno-compromised patients with varicella infection [70, 71]. In addition, vidarabine and parenteral human interferon-α have been shown to be efficacious in the population [63, 72–76]. However, due to the neurotoxicity associated with vidarabine use and uncomfortable side-effects (fever, myalgias) associated with interferons (contrasted with few side-effects associated with acyclovir), acyclovir continues to be the drug of choice for treatment of varicella in immunocompromised patients (intravenous (i.v.) dosing of 500 mg/m² every 8 hours for 7–10 days) [72]. Of course, the prevention of varicella is of paramount importance in this patient population. Historically, VZIG has been used in immunocompromised patients who have had significant exposure to varicella-zoster (the recommended dose is 125 units/10 kg). However, one-third to one-half of these patients will still develop clinical infection [77]. Therefore, there has been much interest in the live attenuated VZV vaccine (Oka strain), which has recently received FDA approval. It produced seroconversion in 96% of healthy children in one study [78], although a few vaccinated patients have developed a mild breakthrough varicella after known exposure to VZV [79]. Of concern was the development of shingles in vaccinated patients. However, while several mild self-limiting cases of zoster in healthy vaccinated children have been reported [80–82], the incidence of zoster following vaccination appears to be decreased relative to that following natural infection [83]. Side-effects of vaccine include mild varicelliform rash, fever or injection-site reactions [84, 85]. These seem to be outweighed by the large savings in time off from work to care for sick children and the cost of caring for varicella-related complications.

Herpes zoster (shingles)

Aetiology

Von Bokay was the first to notice the relationship of herpes zoster to chickenpox, noting that susceptible children acquired varicella after exposure to patients with zoster [27, 29, 86]. Next Kundratiz produced varicella-like lesions and generalized varicella in children by inoculation with vesicle fluid from patients with zoster [86]. The relationship between the two diseases was finally cemented by Weller *et al.* [87, 88], who showed that the viruses recovered from the two diseases had identical biological, physical and immunological characteristics.

Pathogenesis

While not completely understood, it is thought that, during the primary infection with varicella, VZV travels from the skin and mucosal lesions to the endings of the sensory nerves and from there up to the sensory ganglion, where a latent infection begins [10]. There, the virus remains until it reverts to infectivity. This can be brought on by any number of conditions, including immunosuppression by chemotherapeutic agents, corticosteroids, HIV infection, tumour involvement, surgical manipulation, irradiation of the spinal cord or even local trauma [10, 51, 89–97]. On reactivation, VZV will replicate in the ganglion, causing necrosis and inflammation, which manifest as neuralgia. Varicella-zoster virus then travels down a sensory nerve and infects the area of skin within the respective dermatome.

Immunity

Immunosuppressed and immunocompromised persons have an increased incidence and severity of herpes zoster infection, accompanied by greater complications, especially dissemination, often involving internal organs. It is estimated that 20–50% of patients with Hodgkin's disease develop herpes zoster [95, 98–104]. In fact, the greatest risk among cancer patients of acquiring zoster appears to be among patients with leukaemia or lymphoma. Usually, zoster occurs shortly after initiation of chemotherapy (1 month) or radiotherapy (7 months) [105]. In addition, 20–40% of bone-marrow transplant patients develop zoster in the first year after receiving their transplants [106–109]. Finally, herpes zoster is greatly increased in HIV patients, often occurring as the first sign of infection [89, 110]. In contrast to patients without HIV infection, it can often recur and the lesions associated with it can have an unusual appearance [53, 90, 111–115]. The increased incidence and severity of herpes zoster observed in older patients can be explained by a selective decline in cellular immune response to VZV [106, 116–120].

Epidemiology

Herpes zoster shows no seasonal, racial or gender preference. While patients with zoster are infectious (virus can be isolated from vesicles for up to 7 days in non-immunocompromised patients), they are much less so than patients with varicella [10, 11, 27, 86] and there is no evidence that herpes zoster can be acquired through contact with patients with either varicella or zoster [10–12]. While previously thought by some to be a heralding sign of a subclinical malignancy, a study of 590 patients with zoster showed the incidence of cancer to be no different from that in the general population in the first 5 years after diagnosis [121]. These results have been confirmed by Fueyo and Lookingbill [122] and by Wurzel *et al.* [123], who showed similar findings in healthy children with zoster. As mentioned previously, however, it can be a sign of occult HIV infection [88, 108].

Diagnosis

Laboratory findings are usually not helpful in the diagnosis of either varicella or herpes zoster, as the latter is also a clinical diagnosis. However, viral cultures or Tzanck smears may be performed, with the presence of multinucleated giant cells or epithelial cells with acidophilic intranuclear inclusions suggestive of VZV or HSV infection.

Clinical manifestations

Usually, a prodrome of pain and paraesthesia in the involved dermatome precedes the onset of the rash by several days. Occasionally, patients will experience this neuralgia without ever breaking out in vesicles, a condition known as zoster sine herpete [17, 98, 124–126]. The pain of zoster may be intense and misdiagnoses of myocardial infarction, glaucoma, cholecystitis, nephrolithiasis, appendicitis, prolapsed disc or pleurisy are often made. However, once the rash appears, it is pathognomonic, consisting of a cluster of vesicles on an erythematous base confined to one dermatome (Fig. 5.6). This rash is usually unilateral and does not cross the midline. The most fre-

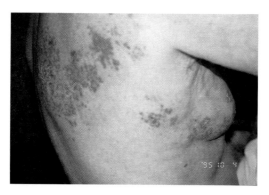

Fig. 5.6 Herpes zoster (shingles) in a thoracic dermatome.

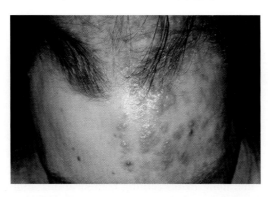

Fig. 5.7 Herpes zoster (shingles) of the ophthalmic branch of the trigeminal nerve.

quently affected areas are the trunk from T3 to L2 and the trigeminal region, particularly the ophthalmic division (Fig. 5.7) [10, 12, 91, 98, 127, 128]. It is of particular concern when the nasociliary branch of the ophthalmic division is affected, manifested by vesicles on the tip and the side of the nose. The vesicles associated with zoster usually evolve into pustules by the third day, form crusts within 7–10 days and finally lose their crusts within 2–3 weeks.

Complications

Acute neuritis and postherpetic neuralgia (PHN) are the most debilitating complications of zoster infection. When defined as pain that remains after lesions have healed, PHN occurs in 10–15% of zoster patients [129]. However, this incidence increases with age, occurring in greater than one-third of patients greater than 60 years old [22, 98, 127, 129, 130]. This pain can be reduced by appropriate antiviral therapy, although no agent is 100% effective in preventing PHN. Luckily, however, it generally remits spontaneously within 1–6 months; although some patients continue to suffer severe pain for years.

Ophthalmic zoster has a relatively high complication rate, with 20–70% of cases with eye involvement. These complications consist of conjunctivitis, scleritis, iridocyclitis, extraocular muscle palsies, ptosis, mydriasis, cicatricial lid retraction, keratitis, uveitis, secondary glaucoma, chorioretinitis, optic neuritis and secondary bacterial infection, which occasionally result in panophthalmitis.

Other less frequent complications include motor paralysis, Ramsay Hunt syndrome, meningoencephalitis or myelitis and granulomatous angiitis of the cerebral arteries. Motor paralysis has been reported in 1–5% of patients with zoster [17, 98, 131, 132]. Ramsay Hunt syndrome resulting from involvement of the facial or auditory nerves consists of facial palsy, in combination with zoster of the external ear or tympanic membrane, and can result in tinnitus, vertigo or deafness [133]. The incidence of acute clinically apparent meningoencephalitis and myelitis is low, occurring in 0.2–0.5% [134–139]. Granulomatous angiitis of the cerebral arteries is probably underdiagnosed, as the onset of symptoms may occur weeks to months after the attack of ophthalmic zoster. It may present as transient ischaemic attacks, stroke in evolution, an isolated cerebral infarction or even multiple cerebral infarctions. The mortality has been reported to be approximately 15%.

Treatment

Acute herpes zoster. Acyclovir, famciclovir, vidarabine, foscarnet, valaciclovir and interferon-α have all shown efficacy in treating VZV infections. Foscarnet is used in cases of acyclovir-resistant zoster. Acyclovir has been shown to decrease the time of neuralgia [140] and has been found to be superior to vidarabine in preventing complications and decreasing the time of viral shedding [141]. In addition, both vidarabine and interferon are associated with some toxicity [142–145]. Recently, both famciclovir and valaciclovir have received FDA approval for use in the treatment of herpes zoster and both have shown greater efficacy than acyclovir in decreasing the incidence of postherpetic neuralgia [146, 147], although clinical trials comparing these drugs with one another are still ongoing.

Postherpetic neuralgia. No antiviral drug has demonstrated any efficacy in the treatment of PHN. However, analgesics, narcotics, cutaneous stimulation [148], amitriptyline, capsaicin (only on healed skin, never on acute zoster) [149], biofeedback or nerve blocks may be tried, often with good relief.

Prevention

Immunization with Oka vaccine of healthy adults greater than 50 years of age, with a history of primary varicella, has been attempted, with an increase of VZV-specific T lymphocytes and VZV immunity [150, 151]. Whether this would correspond to a reduction in the incidence and severity of zoster infections is unknown. While suppressive use of acyclovir in the peritransplant periods in patients with bone-marrow transplant may be useful [152], in HIV patients long-term use of acyclovir has been associated with the development of acyclovir-resistant strains of VZV [52, 53, 111, 114, 153].

Epstein–Barr virus

Aetiology

Several conditions are associated with the presence of Epstein–Barr virus (EBV): infectious mononucleosis (IM) African Burkitt lymphoma, nasopharyngeal carcinoma, lymphoma and lymphoproliferative diseases in immunocompromised patients and chronic fatigue syndrome. Epstein–Barr virus is a DNA virus of the herpesvirus family, which is trophic for B lymphocytes. We shall limit our discussion to IM.

Pathogenesis

B lymphocytes seem to become infected in the oropharynx through salivary exchange. These infected B cells then circulate in the blood until they become incorporated in the bone marrow and lymph glands.

Epidemiology

Age at acquisition of EBV infection is determined by environmental, hygienic and socioeconomic factors. While in higher socioeconomic settings only about 50–60% of older children and young adults have antibodies to EBV, in tropical regions and developing countries almost all children under 3 years of age are antibody-positive [154–156].

Clinical manifestations

After an incubation period of 30–50 days, a prodrome of headache, malaise and fever develops and lasts for 3–5 days. Next, acute disease develops, with symptoms of fever, sore throat and lymphadenopathy (most commonly cervical). Splenomegaly occurs in approximately 50% and hepatomegaly in 10–15%. Although serum transaminase and lactic acid dehydrogenase (LDH) are usually abnormally elevated, clinical hepatitis is relatively rare, with only 5–10% of patients exhibiting jaundice. An extensive greyish-white exudative tonsillitis is characteristic. In addition, periorbital and eyelid oedema occur in 30–50% of patients and may be the presenting sign of the infection [157–159]. Another highly characteristic manifestation of EBV infection is discrete red petechiae, which appear at the border of the hard and soft palates in 25–30% of patients and fade to brown in approximately 2 days. An exanthem occurs in 3–16% of patients and may appear macular or maculopapular, morbilliform, urticarial, vesicular, petechial or even erythema multiforme-like [160–164]. It most commonly involves the trunk and upper arms and lasts for 1–7 days. The percentage with cutaneous eruptions increases almost fivefold in patients treated with certain penicillin derivatives, such as ampicillin. These hypersensitivity rashes persist for approximately 1 week and may be followed by desquamation. However, they do not recur when penicillin derivatives are used again after IM has subsided [165–168]. Finally, oral hairy leucoplakia (OHL) is associated with an EBV infection in HIV-positive persons, and it is a prognostic marker for progression to AIDS.

Complications

Central nervous system complications are rare, including aseptic meningitis, meningoencephalitis, cerebellar ataxia, tranverse myelitis, Bell's palsy and acute psychosis, but recovery is usually complete. Haematological complications are also rare, but marked neutropenia, thrombocytopenia and haemolytic anaemia have been described [169–172]. Splenic rupture is also very rare, but warrants emergency splenectomy and may be fatal. Finally, the proposed relationship between EBV infection and the development of chronic fatigue syndrome has been questioned lately [173, 174].

Diagnosis

While based on both clinical and laboratory findings, elevated titres (>1:112) of heterophil antibodies or a positive monospot test have long been used to confirm a diagnosis of IM. However, approximately 10% of adults are heterophil antibody-negative and children younger than age 4 have a high incidence of false negatives as well [175]. Another common laboratory finding is lymphocytosis, with atypical lymphocytes. For the 10% of patients with IM who test negative for heterophils, EBV-specific antibodies can confirm the diagnosis.

Treatment

Acyclovir is not usually used in the treatment of EBV infection, although it does decrease the level of viral replication during the period of drug administration [176]. However, it has not been found to be effective in reducing the symptoms of IM, possibly because the half-life is not long enough and acyclovir exerts most of its effects at the lytic phase of EBV replication. Therefore, treatment is largely symptomatic. However, a subunit vaccine, consisting of EBV gp350 envelope glycoprotein, has been effective in animal studies and is awaiting clinical trials [177].

Cytomegalovirus

The majority of people are infected with cytomegalovirus (CMV) and carry the virus in a latent stage. While immunocompetent hosts rarely have symptoms of clinical disease, neonates and immunocompromised patients are at risk for symptomatic CMV disease and account for the majority of persons with cutaneous manifestations.

Aetiology

Cytomegalovirus is a member of the herpesvirus family and can be isolated from urine, tears, breast milk, faeces, semen, cervical secretions, blood and saliva in healthy persons [178].

Pathogenesis

It is believed that the initial reactivation of CMV leads to viraemia in an immunosuppressed host [179]. The virus then infects the vascular endothelium, which results in an exanthem. Then, as the vessels become more involved, a vasculitis and then ulceration result, as vessels become destroyed [178].

Epidemiology

Cytomegalovirus infection shows no seasonal preference, and humans are its only known host. Rates of CMV seropositivity vary in different populations around the world. There appear to be two periods of increased risk of acquiring CMV infection: the perinatal and the reproductive years [180]. Infants with CMV-positive mothers may acquire the virus during birth or through breast-feeding, and seroconversion while at day-care centres has been well documented [181]. Sexual intercourse accounts for the majority of adult transmissions of CMV, with 80% of women in one study showing cervical shedding of CMV [182].

Diagnosis

While often asymptomatic, cutaneous infection with CMV will show preferential involvement of endothelial and ductal cells, with relative sparing of the epithelium. While a false-negative rate of 12% has been reported [183], the basophilic intranuclear inclusions, known as 'owl's eyes', are pathognomonic [184]. However, if these inclusions are not seen, the infection can be confirmed by viral cultures, most commonly urine, blood and throat.

Clinical manifestations

Dermatological manifestations of CMV are rare and diverse, with perianal ulcerations being the most specific and present in 30% of cases of cutaneous CMV [183]. Other cutaneous manifestations include the 'blueberry-muffin' baby, seen with congenital CMV infection (Fig. 5.8), urticarial and/or morbilliform rashes in the CMV mononucleosis-like syndrome (after ampicillin therapy) and everything from vesicles [185–188] to verrucous lesions [189–192] seen particularly in immunocompromised patients. Also in this population, pneumonitis, gastroenteritis, hepatitis, encephalitis, chorioretinitis or mononucleosis may occur as a result of CMV infection [193]. In congenital CMV infection, infants may have microcephaly, hepatomegaly, splenomegaly, chorioretinitis, deafness, thrombocytopenia, jaundice or purpura as a part of the toxoplasmosis, other (syphilis), rubella, cytomegalovirus, herpes simplex (TORCH) syndrome [178]. Cytomegalovirus is believed to be the most common congenital viral infection, with 1% of babies born in the USA infected *in utero* [179]. Luckily, however, less than 10% of those infected will show clinical signs of disease

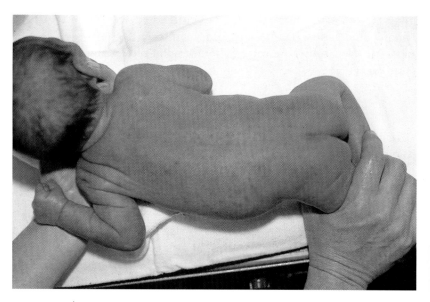

Fig. 5.8 Congenital cytomegalovirus infection ('blueberry-muffin' baby).

[178]. Sadly, 65% of these who do show clinical evidence of disease will develop mental retardation, learning disabilities, sensorineural hearing loss and seizures [194]. In CMV mononucleosis, pharyngitis, lymphadenopathy and splenomegaly may occur (though usually less severe than EBV mononucleosis) [178, 195]. In addition, fever, abnormal liver-function tests and blood smears with atypical lymphocytes may be seen, although the heterophil-antibody test is negative [196].

Immunity

Primary infection or reactivation of latent CMV infection in immunocompromised patients with HIV or solid-organ or bone-marrow transplants remain a major public-health concern. In patients with AIDS, 77–90% have CMV at the time of their death. Death from CMV occurs from viraemia, with resultant pneumonia and necrotizing adrenalitis [192, 197]. In addition, CMV retinitis occurs in 30% of patients with AIDS and may result in blindness [198]. In renal-transplant patients, 50% experience CMV disease, with CMV being responsible for 25% of deaths, 20% of graft failure, 30% of febrile episodes and 35% of leucopenic episodes [199].

In bone-marrow transplant patients, CMV pneumonia is the most common adverse effect of CMV infection, with a mortality rate of nearly 85% [200]. In contrast, CMV hepatitis is more commonly seen after liver transplants [180] and gastrointestinal disease is the most common manifestation of CMV in heart and lung transplants [201, 202].

Treatment

Both ganciclovir and foscarnet (trisodium phosphonoformate) are indicated for the treatment of CMV retinitis. However, ganciclovir is virostatic,
not virocidal, and patients with CMV retinitis usually relapse within a
month of discontinuing therapy [201]. Foscarnet has been reported to be
associated with longer patient survival than ganciclovir, but both drugs are
associated with significant toxicity. For prophylaxis, high-dose acyclovir is
somewhat effective, although it is useless for treatment of active disease
[201]. In addition, interferon-α [182] or CMV hyperimmune globulin
confers partial prophylactic [203, 204, 205] effects in transplant patients.

Human herpesvirus type 6: Exanthem subitum/ roseola infantum/sixth disease

Although this disease has been described for some time as roseola infantum
('the pink rash of infants') or exanthem subitum (ES) ('sudden rash'), the
aetiological agent responsible — human herpesvirus type 6 (HHV-6) — was
not isolated until 1986 [206] and was proved to be causal in 1988 [207].
Recently, evidence has been obtained indicating that HHV-7 may also be a
causative agent of ES.

Aetiology

Human herpesvirus type 6 is a member of the herpesvirus family, which,
after a primary infection in childhood, persists or stays dormant in asymptomatic adults [208].

Epidemiology

Since ES is a mild and self-limited disease, it is probably frequently unre-
ported or misdiagnosed. However, it is thought by some to be the most
common exanthem of children less than 2 years of age. Moreover, it
appears that only a small percentage of those infected with the virus
develop clinical signs and symptoms. There appears to be no seasonal or
gender preference, but the majority of patients affected are between 6
months and 2 years of age.

Clinical manifestations

After an incubation period of 5–15 days [209–212], a high fever develops,
which lasts from 3 to 5 days. Usually on the fourth day, the fever will
suddenly break and the rash will suddenly appear. The rash consists of
discrete rose-pink maculae to maculopapules, usually 2–3 mm in diameter,
which may be tender, will blanch with pressure, rarely coalesce and
may resemble rubella or measles. It normally appears on the trunk first,

and may then spread to the neck and extremities, before resolving in 1–2 days. Another clinical sign is periorbital oedema, although pharyngitis, tonsillitis, otitis or lymphadenopathy may also be present. Particularly characteristic is the alert and playful appearance of the child in spite of the high fever.

Diagnosis

While the clinical course is highly characteristic, serological tests are available for diagnostic purposes [213, 214] and PCR may become the test of choice, due to its sensitivity, specificity and efficiency [215].

Complications

The disease is usually mild and self-limited and with no permanent sequelae. However, meningoencephalitis [216, 217], hepatitis [218] and intussusception [219] have been reported in association with HHV-6 infection. Most commonly, seizures are reported, probably as a result of the associated high fever.

Treatment

Due to the benign self-limited nature of the disease, treatment has been largely symptomatic. However, both ganciclovir and foscarnet have shown efficacy against HHV-6 [220].

Human herpesvirus type 8 (Kaposi's sarcoma-associated herpesvirus)

Recently, DNA sequences from an agent believed to represent a new member of the herpesvirus family have been found in HIV-positive and negative patients with Kaposi's sarcoma (Fig. 5.9) [221, 222]. In addition, HHV-8 DNA has been found in body-cavity-based B-cell lymphomas in AIDS [223] patients and in squamous-cell carcinomas in transplant patients [224]. Whether immunosuppression (endogenous or exogenous) combined with viral reactivation leads to malignant transformation is unknown. (For more information on Kaposi's sarcoma, see 'Human immunodeficiency virus' below).

Human papillomavirus warts

Warts are benign tumours caused by infection with human papillomavirus (HPV). There are several clinical varieties of warts, including verruca vulgaris, verruca plantaris, verruca plana, laryngeal papillomas and condyloma acuminata (genital warts). In addition, epidermodysplasia verruciformis is a rare autosomal recessive disease associated with HPV infection

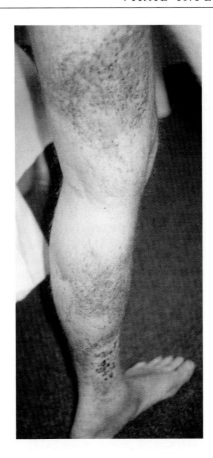

Fig. 5.9 Kaposi's sarcoma associated with human herpesvirus 8 in an HIV-seropositive man.

and the presence of multiple, flat, wart-like lesions, some with malignant potential.

Aetiology

Human papillomavirus is a DNA virus of the papovavirus family, of which more than 70 different genotypes are recognized. Commonly three categories encompass the different genotypes of HPV trophic for non-genital regions (e.g. HPV-1, 2, 3, 4, 10, 28, 29 and 57); trophic for the genital–mucosal regions (e.g. HPV-6, 11, 16, 18, 31, 33 and 35); and those types associated with epidermodysplasia verruciformis (e.g. HPV-5 and 8). Of these, HPV types 16, 18, 31, 33 and 35 (for cervical and genital-tract cancers) and types 5 and 8 (in epidermodysplasia verruciformis-associated squamous-cell carcinomas) are thought to have the highest malignant potential.

Pathogenesis

While the interactions between HPV infection and the immune system are not well understood, patients with defective cell-mediated immunity (CMI) are at particular risk of HPV infection, and the power of suggestion (or 'charming'), as well as cimetidine therapy, for warts has long been felt to have immunostimulatory effects as their mode of action. Human papillomavirus infection is felt to occur after inoculation of the virus through epithelial defects. A fairly long incubation period (1–9 months or longer) follows before clinically apparent disease develops.

Epidemiology

While found in 7–10% of the population, warts are most commonly found in patients between 10 and 19 years of age [225]. Patients with both clinical and subclinical infections may serve as reservoirs for HPV, with transmission of virus probably dependent upon a variety of factors, including the location of lesions, quantity of infectious virus present, degree and nature of contact and the general and HPV-specific immunological status of the exposed individual [226].

Diagnosis

While usually made on the basis of clinical appearance, an epidermis with acanthosis, papillomatosis, hyperkeratosis and parakeratosis seen on histopathology aids in diagnosis. In addition, the large keratinocytes with pyknotic nuclei and perinuclear haloes known as koilocytes are characteristic of HPV infection. Application of 3–5% acetic acid may aid detection of genital warts [227]. Finally, DNA hybridization may become widely used.

Clinical manifestations

The clinical appearance of warts varies with their location. Verruca vulgaris (Fig. 5.10), which commonly appears on the dorsal surface of the hands (particularly in the periungual region), occurs as single or grouped papules, which may enlarge and become increasingly keratotic or verrucous. Often, punctate black dots are seen (commonly called 'seeds'), which represent thrombosed capillaries. Verrucae planae are 2–5-mm flat papules, which are usually flesh-coloured to brown. Several hundred of these warts may be found on a given individual, as they can be spread by shaving. The presence of warts in a line at the site of a scratch (the Koebner phenomenon) is characteristic of these lesions as well. These warts occur primarily on the face, neck, arms and legs. Verrucae plantaris (plantar warts) occur on the plantar surfaces of the feet (Fig. 5.11) and can be quite painful with pressure. They are thick hyperkeratotic lesions, which are pressed inward by walking. They also frequently exhibit thrombosed capillaries. Laryngeal papillomas are HPV-associated tumours, which usually involve the larynx

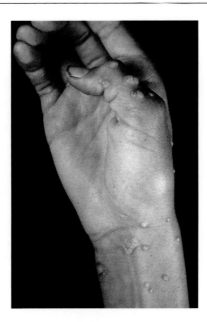

Fig. 5.10 Verruca vulgaris due to human papillomavirus type 2.

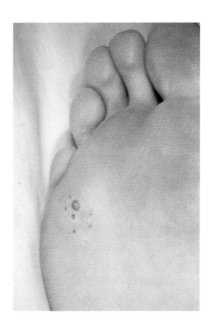

Fig. 5.11 Plantar warts associated with human papillomavirus type 1.

but may also involve the oropharynx, trachea, bronchi or even pulmonary epithelium. The presenting signs are often hoarseness or stridor, and diagnosis is made by direct laryngoscopy. It is thought that infection is acquired during delivery from exposed maternal condyloma acuminata or cervical papillomas [228]. Condylomata acuminata (genital warts) usually present

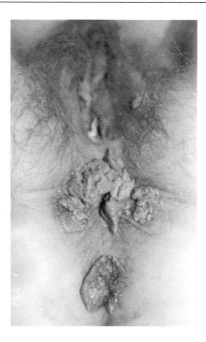

Fig. 5.12 Condyloma acuminatum due to human papillomavirus type 6.

as soft, flesh-coloured papules or nodules, which are found on the genitalia or the perineum in the crural folds or around the anus (Fig. 5.12). They can multiply and coalesce until large cauliflower-like masses result. They are usually spread by sexual contact.

Treatment

Treatment of warts is dependent on the location, number, size and type of warts. Common warts (verruca vulgaris) can be treated with liquid nitrogen, cantharidin, salicylic acid, lactic acid or trichloroacetic acid. Plantar warts are frequently treated with liquid nitrogen or salicylic or lactic acid in flexible collodion. Flat warts may be treated with topical retinoids, salicylic acid in propylene glycol or cautery. While interferon is not approved for use in non-genital warts, some have reported efficacy with its use [229]. In addition, some success has been reported with cimetidine [230, 231].

Therapy available for genital warts is also extensive, and includes cytodestructive techniques (e.g. laser, cryotherapy, caustic chemicals, surgery), chemotherapeutic regimens (e.g. 5-fluorouracil cream, podofilox, bichloroacetic acid and trichloroacetic acid) and interferon-α. In fact, intralesional interferon-α has been found to be safe and effective in the treatment of condylomata acuminata resistant to conventional therapy [232]. Some of the best results have been obtained by the use of interferon-α in combination with cytodestructive or chemotherapeutic agents [233]. The recent availability of imiquimod, a topical inducer of endogenous interferon-α and a variety of other cytokines, has the potential to markedly reduce the use of exogenous interferon-α in the therapy of condyloma acuminatum.

Measles (rubeola)

Measles is a universal and highly contagious disease, whose epidemiology was altered by the licensing of measles vaccine in the USA in 1963 (prior to this, measles was the most common viral exanthem of childhood). Having been previously associated with a high incidence and fatality rate (500 000 cases per year with 400–500 deaths), this was reduced to a low of 1497 cases in 1983. However, due to a variety of causes (particularly low vaccination rates among the urban poor), the number of measles cases again began rising, with 25 672 cases and 89 suspected measles-associated deaths in 1990 [234, 235].

Aetiology and pathogenesis

The measles virus is a paramyxovirus (ribonucleic acid (RNA) virus), which is spread by direct contact with infected droplets. While the mechanism of the formation of the rash is not completely clear, it is thought that it may be either a direct effect of viral invasion into epithelial and endothelial cells or, alternatively, a result of damage from a virus–antibody complex [236].

Epidemiology

Measles is a worldwide illness affecting children, without preference as to race or sex. However, the age at infection depends on the environmental setting, with children in urban areas primarily infected in infancy and early childhood and children in rural areas primarily infected between ages 5 and 10 [236]. Measles shows a peak incidence in winter and spring for temperate areas, and the attack rate approaches 100% in susceptible individuals [236]. However, infants under 4 months are usually protected by transplacentally acquired maternal antibody [236]. Due to declining immunization rates among the urban poor, black and Hispanic children have comprised the majority of patients in recent epidemics [236].

Diagnosis

The clinical course (see 'Clinical manifestations') is highly characteristic. Multinucleated giant cells may be found in skin lesions, as well as in respiratory and lymphoid tissues and nasal secretions.

Clinical manifestations

After an asymptomatic incubation period of 10–14 days, a prodromal phase of 3–4 days is entered. The measles prodrome is characterized by fever (up to 40–40.5°C) and chills, barking cough refractory to antitussives, conjunctivitis (primarily palpebral, giving the eyes a red-rimmed appearance), coryza, malaise and headache. Photophobia may accompany the conjunctivitis, and generalized adenopathy is often seen. Approximately 1–2 days before the onset of the rash, Koplik's spots appear, which are the pathognomonic lesions of measles. These are 1–3 mm bluish-white specks on an erythematous background ('grains of sand on a red background'), which occur in greatest numbers on the buccal mucosa opposite the second molars, but can be found on the conjunctiva, on the gums and lips and all over the inside of the cheeks and have even been found in the large intestine [237]. They usually begin to fade as the rash appears. The rash of measles is an erythematous maculopapular exanthem, which usually appears 3–4 days after the onset of the illness (Fig. 5.13). It appears first on the scalp, forehead and behind the ears, and spreads downward to involve the face, neck and trunk and then the superior portion of the lower extremities. Confluence of lesions on the face and neck is often seen. Then, the rash begins fading in the order in which it appeared, occasionally with some degree of bran-like desquamation.

Complications

Perhaps the most feared complications of measles are encephalitis and sub-

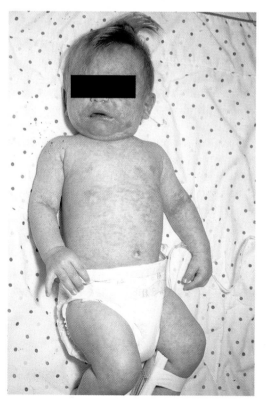

Fig. 5.13 Measles in an infant.

acute sclerosing panencephalitis (SSPE). Encephalitis occurs in about 1 in 1000 cases. Of these, a significant minority (about 15%) die as a result of their illness and about 45% of the survivors are left with permanent CNS damage (e.g. hearing loss, mental retardation or seizure disorder) [223]. Subacute sclerosing panencephalitis occurs in patients who seem to recover completely from their illness, only to present months or years later with motor and mental deterioration and myoclonic seizures, with a characteristic spike-and-wave pattern on the electroencephalogram (EEG). Fortunately, this condition is rare (approximately 5–10 cases per million cases of measles), since it is progressive and usually fatal. More common are bacterial secondary infections, such as otitis media or pneumonia caused by *Pneumococcus*, group A haemolytic *Streptococcus*, *Haemophilus influenzae* or *Staphylococcus aureus*. A secondary fever spike or prolongation of a fever should alert the practitioner to look for such a secondary cause.

Treatment

Treatment of measles is limited to supportive care. Rest, diet, hydration, antipyretics and the use of a vaporizer may be helpful.

Prevention

The live attenuated measles vaccine produces detectable levels of antibody in 95% of the population after a single dose. However, the remaining 5% who fail to respond undoubtedly provide a reservoir for continued out-breaks. Therefore, public-health authorities in the USA have adopted a two-dose measles immunization schedule, with the first dose given at 15 months and the second dose given just prior to school entry. Of concern is the poor (less than 50%) rate of vaccination among 2-year-old children in the USA. Human immunodeficiency virus infection is not a contraindica-tion for measles vaccination.

Among children who received the killed virus vaccine and were then exposed to natural measles, an atypical infection has been reported. Some became quite sick, with high fever, extreme prostration, pneumonia, swollen hands and feet and urticarial, vesicular or petechial rashes. Another variety of measles, known as modified measles, has been reported in children who have been immunized with γ-globulin after exposure and in infants who have lost some protection from transplacentally acquired maternal antibody. This is characterized by a longer incubation period, absent or diminished prodrome, low-grade to normal temperature, minimal to absent cough, coryza, conjunctivitis, Koplik's spots and mild rash [225].

Immune serum globulin (ISG) may modify or prevent measles if given within 6 days of exposure, with doses of 0.25 ml/kg intramuscularly (i.m.) given to normal patients and 0.5 ml/kg for immunosuppressed patients, to a maximum dose of 15 ml.

Rubella (German measles)

Rubella is a common viral infection of children and young adults, which would have little significance were it not for the congenital rubella syndrome. Like measles, the number of cases decreased to an all-time low of 225 cases in 1988 after the licensing of the vaccine in 1969. However, it too has staged a comeback, with 1093 provisional cases reported in 1990 [238].

Aetiology and pathogenesis

Rubella is caused by an RNA virus and is spread via respiratory secretions. Generally, a single attack results in lifelong immunity, but a few subclinical reinfections can occur. Fortunately, congenital rubella syndrome is unlikely in children whose mothers acquire a reinfection during pregnancy [239].

Epidemiology

Rubella is a worldwide disease, with epidemics frequently occurring in 6–9-year cycles. It most commonly affects school-age children, adolescents and young adults and usually occurs in the spring months in North America.

Clinical manifestations

After an incubation period ranging from 14 to 21 days, a prodrome of lymphadenopathy, headache, low-grade fever, sore throat, rhinitis, conjunctivitis and cough may occur in older children, adolescents and adults (in young children, prodromal signs are rare). At the end of the prodrome, an exanthem, consisting of pink-red maculae and papules, begins on the face and rapidly spreads to involve the neck, trunk and extremities. The lesions on the trunk may coalesce and the rash is usually gone within 2–3 days. The face generally clears first and clearing may be followed by fine desquamation. In addition, an enanthema called Forchheimer's sign may be seen in up to 20% of the patients, consisting of petechiae or reddish pinpoint spots on the soft palate and occurring during the prodrome or on the first day of the rash [225]. Another notable characteristic of rubella infection is the lymphadenopathy which can occur, most commonly suboccipital, postauricular and anterior and posterior cervical. In addition, splenomegaly, arthritis (more frequently in adults) and thrombocytopenic purpura can occasionally occur.

Diagnosis

Diagnosis is usually made clinically but, if indeterminate, pharyngeal viral cultures can be performed from 7 days before rash onset to 14 days after. Alternatively, serological studies demonstrating a fourfold or greater rise of rubella titre between the first (soon after rash is noted) and second (2 to 4 weeks later) blood tests is diagnostic.

Complications

Encephalitis has been found in approximately 1 in 6000 cases. However, this is usually followed by complete recovery.

Treatment and prevention

Treatment is supportive due to the benign and self-limited nature of the disease. In the USA, rubella vaccine is given as measles/mumps/rubella (MMR) at 15 months and a second dose before entering school (age 5–6 years). Pregnant women should not be vaccinated, as rubella vaccine virus has been found in fetal membranes and amniotic fluid (although no cases of congenital rubella syndrome have been found). However, care should be taken in the immunization of adolescent and young women, and pregnancies are not recommended for 3 months postimmunization. There is no problem in vaccinating children in a family in which their mother is pregnant, as they do not shed sufficient virus to be infective.

Congenital rubella

Due to the devastating effects of congenital rubella syndrome, the vaccine to prevent rubella was developed, as rubella itself is usually a benign illness. Almost 50% of infants who acquire rubella during the first trimester will show evidence of congenital rubella syndrome, with the most severe malformations seen in infants infected in the first few weeks of intrauterine life [239]. These infants are themselves infectious, with 85% shedding virus at 1 month of age and 1–3% still shedding virus up to 2 years of age [239]. This syndrome consists of low birth weight, microcephaly with mental retardation, deafness, cataracts, congenital heart disease (most often patent ductus arteriosus or ventricular septal defect), a 'blueberry muffin' appearance (due to petechiae and ecchymoses) and retinopathy. If infected later *in utero*, pneumonitis, myocarditis, encephalitis, hepatitis, osteomyelitis or splenomegaly may occur.

Parvovirus B19 (fifth disease, erythema infectiosum)

Parvovirus B19 is the aetiological agent of erythema infectiosum (fifth disease), as well as aplastic crisis in patients with chronic haemolytic anaemias, chronic anaemia in immunocompromised patients, fetal hydrops and a type of arthritis in adults similar to rheumatoid arthritis.

Aetiology

While previously thought to only infect animals, a parvovirus was discovered in the serum of blood donors in England in 1975 [240] and discovered to be the cause of erythema infectiosum in 1983 [241]. Parvovirus B19 is a single-stranded DNA virus of the family parvoviridae and genus parvovirus [242]. Unlike other parvoviruses, it does not require coinfection with a helper virus in order to replicate [243].

Pathogenesis

Parvovirus B19 is believed to be spread by the aerosolization of respiratory droplets [244]. Since B19 is not found in the respiratory secretions after the appearance of the rash [245], it is thought that patients with fifth disease are infectious only before the onset of the rash [244]. While the pathogenesis of erythema infectiosum is not completely understood, it is thought that the mechanism may involve the formation and deposition of immune complexes [246]. The ability of parvovirus to infect and lyse erythroid precursor cells [247] may lead to the aplastic crises, chronic anaemias and fetal hydrops [248].

Epidemiology

Fifth disease is found worldwide, with 15–60% of children ages 5–19 years and 30–60% of adults demonstrating serological evidence of past infection [240, 244, 249]. While it can occur at any time of the year, epidemics among schoolchildren in the late winter and early spring are common [246].

Diagnosis

While the diagnosis is generally made on the basis of the clinical features, special arrangements (in the USA) can be made through the state health departments for assays for immunoglobulin M (IgM) antibody by radioimmunassay (RIA) or enzyme-linked immunosorbent assay (ELISA) techniques. Even better are the techniques of dot–blot hybridization [250] or PCR [251] for identifying viral DNA in various tissues and secretions.

Clinical manifestations—erythema infectiosium

After an incubation period of 4–14 days [241, 244, 252, 253], headache, low-grade fever and coryza may begin [254]. After approximately 2 days of the non-specific symptoms, the characteristic rash appears and, with it, symptoms of headache, malaise, myalgias, arthralgias, pharyngitis, low-grade fever, coryza, cough, conjunctivitis, nausea, diarrhoea and (in children) rarely arthritis [254]. The rash usually begins as an erythematous malar blush and gives the child a 'slapped-cheek' appearance. The facial rash generally fades over 1–4 days as an erythematous eruption appears on the trunk, neck and particularly the extensor surfaces of the extremities (Fig. 5.14) [244]. This rash usually lasts 5–9 days and the lesions often have an area of central clearing, giving them a lacy or reticulated appearance [254]. The rash can reappear, after it subsides, in response to exercise, temperature change, stress, friction, bathing or sun exposure [254]. It is often quite pruritic [252, 253]. An enanthema has been reported, consisting of red maculae on the buccal mucosa and palate in association with erythema of the tongue and pharynx [255].

Complications

In chronic haemolytic anaemia. In patients with hereditary spherocytosis [256], sickle-cell anaemia [257, 258], autoimmune haemolytic anaemia [259], pyruvate kinase deficiency [260] and heterozygous β-thalassaemia [261], a transient aplastic crisis can develop, which can be fatal if untreated [246]. Patients usually present with fever, followed by fatigue, pallor and worsening anaemia, although rarely the crisis may be the presenting sign of haematological disease [259, 261].

In immunocompromised patients. In HIV-infected patients [262], acute leukaemias [263], congenital immunodeficiencies [264], lupus erythematosus [263] and normal infants during the first year of life [265], B19 infection can cause a prolonged anaemia from chronic lysis of red-cell precursors [266].

In fetuses. B19 infection can result in fetal hydrops and death due to extensive haemolysis of red-cell precursors, leading to severe anaemia, high-output cardiac failure and hydrops (oedema) [267]. However, the risk of this in a woman of unknown serological status is estimated to be

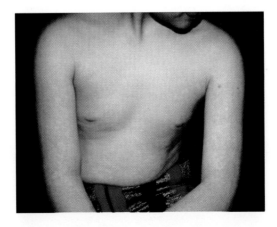

Fig. 5.14 Erythema infectiosum secondary to parvovirus B19.

less than 2.5% after a household exposure and less than 1.5% after work exposure [267]. After maternal infection, the risk is thought to still be less than 10% in the first half of pregnancy and even less in the second half [267, 268].

In adults. In adults (primarily women), acute symmetric polyarthritis, involving mainly the small joints of the hands, wrists, knees, ankles and feet [269], occurs as the main symptom of B19 infection. It is usually self-limited but may persist for months [269, 270]. Adults rarely have the 'slapped-cheek' appearance of erythema infectiosum seen in children [270] but may have a lacy rash of the extremities or severe pruritis without any evidence of a rash [271]. Adults often have more constitutional symptoms, with fever, adenopathy, fatigue, malaise and even depression [272]. Men frequently report only flu-like symptoms, without joint involvement [270].

Treatment and prevention

Erythema infectiosum is a benign condition without a specific treatment. Chronic anaemias can be successfully treated with γ-globulin [262, 263, 273], aplastic crisis with blood transfusions and oxygen therapy [274] and fetal hydrops with intrauterine blood transfusions [268, 275]. At the present time, there is no vaccine to prevent parvovirus B19 infection, and whether i.v. immunoglobulin given after exposure would prevent infection is unknown.

Poxviruses (molluscum contagiosum, orf and milker's nodules)

With the elimination of smallpox (Fig. 5.15) (the last reported case occurred in Somalia in 1977), none of the remaining poxviruses infecting humans seem as awe-inspiring or deadly (up to 40% mortality rate with

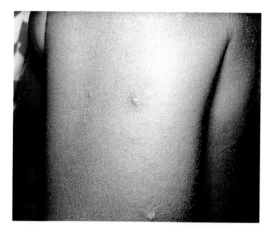

Fig. 5.15 Vesiculopustule from vaccinia virus, the vaccine responsible for the worldwide eradication of smallpox.

smallpox). However, molluscum contagiosum (MC), orf and milker's nodules (MN) continue to infect a significant portion of the population at various times in their lives.

Molluscum contagiosum

Aetiology

Molluscum contagiosum is the most common poxvirus infection. The cause of MC is MC virus (MCV), which is a large DNA virus of the poxvirus group, of which two strains have been identified (MCV I and MCV II) [276, 277]. Of these, MCV I has been seen more often [278, 279], but no differences have been demonstrated between the two strains as to clinical presentation. Studies of MCV have been limited by its failure to be propagated in tissue culture.

Pathogenesis

There is indirect evidence that MCV synthesizes an epidermal growth factor (EGF)-like growth factor [277]. In addition, there is an apparent increase in the number of receptors for EGF in infected cells [280], causing the rate of cell division in infected cells to be doubled [281]. The disease is believed to be spread both by direct person-to-person contact and also by fomites (e.g. swimming pools). In adults, lesions are probably spread by sexual contact [282, 283].

Epidemiology

Molluscum contagiosum has a worldwide distribution and may be seen at any age, although children are primarily infected (greatest incidence occurs between the ages of 3 and 16). Boys are more commonly affected than girls.

Diagnosis

Although the diagnosis is usually easily made by the distinctive clinical appearance of the lesions, stained smears may be made of the curd-like material extracted from the umbilicated papules. This material consists primarily of enlarged epidermal cells containing molluscum bodies, which are large intracytoplasmic inclusion bodies. The histological appearance of lobular proliferation of epidermal cells into the dermis is also highly characteristic.

Clinical manifestations

Molluscum contagosium presents on mucocutaneous surfaces as dome-shaped papules with a central umbilication (Fig. 5.16). While initially firm,

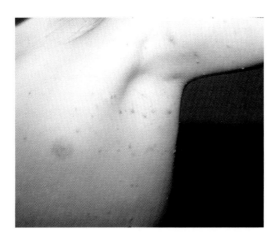

Fig. 5.16 Molluscum contagiosum in a child.

solid and flesh-coloured, they may become softer and waxy to pearly grey in colour. The curd-like core may be expressed with a sterile needle or comedo extracto [225]. While lesions generally range from 2 to 5 mm in diameter, they have been reported to reach 2–3 cm in diameter [284]. The lesions are usually asymptomatic.

Complications

Occasionally a chronic conjunctivitis may complicate lesions located on the conjunctive or at the eyelid margin [225]. Up to 10% of affected patients develop an area of dermatitis surrounding the molluscum lesions, which may represent a delayed hypersensitivity to molluscum virus antigen [285].

Immunity

The presentation of MC is generally more aggressive in immunocompromised patients. Patients with AIDS are at very high risk, with prevalence rates of 9–18% reported [286, 287].

Treatment

While treatment is often not necessary, due to the self-limited nature of the infection and the tendency for lesions to heal with little to no scarring, various techniques have demonstrated effectiveness in promoting healing of the molluscum lesions. Some of the techniques that have been used include removal by liquid nitrogen, curettage, electrodesiccation, silver nitrate, salicylic acid, canthardin, iodine (7–9%), phenol (1%) and trichloroacetic acid (30–50%) [225]. The intralesional injection of interferon-α is effective in eliminating MC in immunocompetent patients, but has been found to be less effective in patients with AIDS.

Orf (contagious ecthyma)

This zoonotic infection is endemic among sheep and goats and can be transmitted from them to humans. In affected animals, the lesions appear as nodules on the mouth and nose.

Aetiology and epidemiology

The infection is caused by a parapox virus, the orf virus, which is very hardy and can survive long periods of time on fomites. For obvious reasons, sheepherders are often affected, as well as farmers and veterinarians, with patients varying from 10 to 72 years of age [288]. Strangely, the disease has been reported only in Caucasians, although this may be due to reporting anomalies rather than a race predilection. The disease occurs predominantly in the spring, when the majority of susceptible lambs are born.

Clinical manifestations

After an incubation period of 3–6 days, single to multiple papules or nodules (Fig. 5.17) appear [225], most commonly on the dorsal aspect of the right index finger. Lesions vary from 1.5 to 5.0 cm in diameter, with an average of 1.6 cm [288]. Regional lymphadenopathy, fever and lymphangitis may also occur. Lesions heal slowly over 35 days, going through a papular, target, acute, regenerative, papillomatous and finally regressive stage [288].

Diagnosis

The diagnosis is made by the clinical appearance of the lesions combined

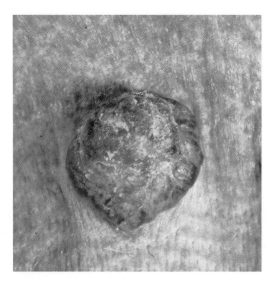

Fig. 5.17 Nodular stage of orf in a shepherd.

with a history of contact with affected animals. However, the virus can be grown in sheep cultures or alternatively fluorescent antibody tests or electron microscopy (EM) can be performed. On EM, encapsulated viroplasm and nucleoids are seen.

Complications

Rarely, erythema multiforme, ocular involvement, widespread papulovesicular rashes or secondary bacterial infections may occur.

Treatment

Treatment of orf is largely symptomatic, with excision and cautery helping to promote healing [289]. Corticosteriods should be avoided, but compresses and culture-specific antibodies may be helpful in the treatment of superficial bacterial infections [288].

Milker's nodule

Milker's nodule (MN) is a zoonotic viral infection, seen in areas where there is human contact with cattle. Like orf, person-to-person spread has not been observed in the wild, although human-to-human and human-to-cow spread has occurred experimentally [290].

Aetiology

Milker's nodule is caused by the paravaccinia virus. Infection with paravaccinia is endemic among cows, in which the condition is called pseudocowpox. Like other poxviruses, paravaccinia virus is a large brick-shaped DNA virus, which induces hyperplasia of infected cells.

Epidemiology

Milker's nodules occur wherever humans are in contact with cows. Therefore milkers have been primarily infected, but stock-handlers and slaughterhouse workers have also been infected.

Clinical manifestations

After an incubation period of 4–7 days, single to multiple maculae (usually no more than four) may appear on the finger, hand or forearm. These maculae progress slowly to papules, vesicles and finally nodules and are usually asymptomatic, although they may be slightly painful [291, 292]. After approximately 4–6 weeks, they heal, usually without scarring.

Diagnosis

While the diagnosis is generally made on the basis of the history, combined with the clinical appearance, biopsy may be performed if it is questionable. The biopsy will often show vacuolization of cells with eosinophilic bodies and multilocular vesicles in the upper third of the stratum malpighii, if taken during the maculopapular stage.

Complications

Lymphadenopathy, lymphangitis, erythema multiforme or secondary infections may occasionally complicate MN [289].

Treatment

Due to the self-limited nature of the disease, treatment is not required. However, surgical removal by razor-blade transection may reduce the healing time and minimize complications [289].

Enteroviruses (hand-foot-and-mouth disease and herpangina)

Hand-foot-and-mouth disease

Hand-foot-and-mouth disease (HFMD) is characterized by vesicular lesions on the mouth and extremities and is caused by enteroviruses.

Aetiology and epidemiology

Epidemic cases of HFMD are associated with Coxsackie virus A16 or enterovirus 71 [293], while sporadic cases are associated with other Coxsackie virus types. During epidemics (more common in late summer and autumn), the virus is spread both horizontally (from child to child) and vertically (from child to adults) by either the oral–oral or the faecal–oral route. These epidemics tend to occur approximately every 3 years and cases are most commonly seen in patients younger than 15 years of age.

Pathogenesis

Following viral implantation in the buccal mucosa and ileum, the regional lymph nodes are affected, usually within 24 hours. After 72 hours, a viraemia follows, with viral seeding of other areas, most commonly the hands, feet and oral mucosa [294].

Clinical manifestations

After an incubation period of 3–6 days, a prodrome of 12–24 hours begins, consisting of malaise, low-grade fever, anorexia, sore mouth, abdominal pain or respiratory symptoms. The oral lesions are very characteristic and occurred in 100% of patients in one series [295]. In fact, sore mouth and refusal to eat were the presenting symptoms in 80% of the patients [295]. The lesions start as small red maculae and then progress to vesicles 1–3 mm to 2 cm in diameter on an erythematous base. The vesicles are typically short-lived and are followed by shallow, yellow-grey ulcerations surrounded by a red halo. These usually heal within 1–6 days. Most commonly, the lesions are found on the hard palate, tongue and buccal mucosa, but they may also be seen on the soft palate, gingivae, uvula or anterior tonsillar pillars. The exanthem usually begins either along with or shortly after the enanthema. These lesions begin as erythematous maculae or papules, which develop into grey vesicles on an erythematous base. They occur more commonly on the hands than on the feet, and usually on the dorsal surfaces of either. Often, they involve the lateral aspects of fingers, toes, hands or feet. These lateral lesions on the feet frequently have a characteristic football shape. The vesicles may be either pruritic, painful, tender or asymptomatic, and usually heal in approximately 1 week. Rarely, high fever, marked malaise, diarrhoea or joint pains may occur with HFMD and marked cervical or submandibular adenopathy may also be present.

Diagnosis

Usually the diagnosis is made on the basis of the clinical appearance. However, the virus may be grown in suckling mice or in tissue culture after swabbing the throat, vesicles or stools.

Complications

Rarely, myocarditis [296, 297], meningoencephalitis [296], pneumonia [296, 298, 299], aseptic meningitis [296, 300], paralytic disease [301] and an illness resembling rubeola [302] have occurred after HFMD.

Treatment

While there is no specific treatment for HFMD, patient comfort may be improved with the use of topical lidocaine or dyclonine hydrochloride (HCl) solution.

Herpangina

Herpangina is a disease characterized by oropharyngeal lesions, which can be caused by any of six or seven types of group A Coxsackie virus.

Aetiology, pathogenesis and epidemiology

Coxsackie virus types A2, A4, A5, A6, A8, A10 and, in one cluster of cases, A3 have been associated with herpangina. The most common method of spread is believed to be through oropharyngeal secretions, with epidemics usually occurring in the summer months. Herpangina is believed to be worldwide in distribution, with no sex or race predilection.

Clinical manifestations

After an incubation of approximately 4 days, the child experiences a sudden onset of fever, often accompanied by headache, myalgias, fatigue, anorexia, vomiting, abdominal pain, sore throat and dysphagia. Grey-white papulovesicular lesions appear most commonly on the tonsils and the anterior pillars of the tonsillar fauces, the soft palate and the uvula. These lesions subsequently ulcerate and are surrounded by a zone of erythema. These heal in approximately 4–6 days and may be accompanied by conjunctivitis and or an exanthem.

Complications

Approximately 5% of patients experience convulsions with the onset of fever.

Diagnosis

While primarily made on the basis of the characteristic oral lesions, the diagnosis may be confirmed by viral culture (in suckling mice) from swabs of the oropharyngeal lesions or the anus. Alternatively, serological studies may be performed comparing antibody titres taken early in the illness with those drawn during convalescence.

Treatment

There is no specific treatment for herpangina.

Human retroviruses—human T-cell leukaemia virus and human immunodeficiency virus

Retroviruses are RNA viruses that contain an RNA-dependent DNA polymerase, which gives rise to the DNA provirus species. The important retroviruses that lead to disease are human T-cell leukaemia virus (HTLV) types 1 and 2 and HIV types 1 and 2. Human T-cell leukaemia virus type 2 has yet to be linked to a certain disease, but has been isolated from cells derived from two patients with a rare hairy-cell leukaemia [303]. It is important to remember that the dermatological manifestations of HIV and HTLV can be unusual and difficult to treat and may even be the presenting sign of infection.

Human T-cell leukaemia virus type 1

Human T-cell leukaemia virus type 1 is strongly associated with the development of adult T-cell leukaemia/lymphoma (ATL). Although the exact mechanism is not known, HTLV-1 is able to transform normal T lymphocytes into ones unable to control their own growth. The result is a fatal, adult-onset T-cell malignancy.

Endemic patterns of HTLV-1 were found in southern Japan [304], the Caribbean [304] and equatorial Africa [305, 306]. The virus is transmitted in a manner similar to HIV, but is not nearly as infectious as HIV.

Infection with either HTLV type can be determined by seroepidemiological methods. However, to distinguish between HTLV-1 and HTLV-2, the PCR is required [307].

Typically, ATL develops 20 years or more after the acquisition of HTLV-1 [308]. However, infection with HTLV-1 does not always lead to the development of ATL, and many individuals remain lifelong asymptomatic carriers. Adult T-cell leukaemia/lymphoma is characterized by multilobate lymphocytes in the peripheral blood and multiorgan involvement. Organs that can be involved include spleen, liver, CNS and lungs. Skin involvement is common and is present in all forms of ATL. The skin manifestations of ATL vary in each patient and may precede the onset of acute ATL for up to two decades [309]. Infective dermatitis, recently linked to infection with HTLV-1 [310], can be found in children who may later develop ATL as adults.

Common dermatological findings in patients with ATL are papular infiltrates, nodular tumours and erythroderma, some of which may be mistaken for mycosis fungoides. Sometimes patients present with specific skin infiltrates without any evidence of malignant T cells; it is proposed that this condition be termed cutaneous-type ATL [311]. Patients with acute ATL have a variety of clinical findings, according to specific organ involvement and the condition of the immune system. Refractory hypercalcaemia is a common finding in these patients and may be noticed on presentation. However, patients may present with many different complaints, due to particular organ involvement, which can make the diagnosis difficult unless a leukaemia is suspected.

Adult T-cell leukaemia/lymphoma has a poor prognosis, and findings of hypercalcaemia, high LDH level and high white blood-cell count predicts a 50% survival time of less than 6 months [312]. Combination cytotoxic chemotherapy is a common treatment, but remission has not been documented. Other therapeutic approaches are currently under investigation.

Human immunodeficiency virus

Human immunodeficiency virus is a retrovirus that infects human CD4+ T cells and monocyte/macrophages, and is the aetiological agent of AIDS. Cutaneous manifestations of HIV occur in up to 92% of those individuals infected with the virus [313]. The dermatological findings are most often due to an underlying immune deficiency and can be categorized as neoplastic, infectious and non-neoplastic/non-infectious lesions. Some of the cutaneous findings associated with HIV will be described.

Neoplastic lesions

Kaposi's sarcoma (KS) is the most common malignant manifestation of HIV infection. Ninety-five per cent of AIDS-related KS appears in homosexual or bisexual men [314]. Clinically, KS presents as erythematous maculae or papules, which progress to violaceous nodules or plaques. Peripheral oedema, most often in the lower legs, and disseminated cutaneous KS can also occur. Recently, KS has been found to be associated with a new member of the herpesvirus family known as herpesvirus type 8 [221]. Treatment can include local radiotherapy, cytodestructive procedures or intralesional administration of vincristine sulphate, bleomycin or interferon-α. Currently, interferon-α is the most efficacious systemic approach to treatment [314].

B-cell and T-cell lymphomas are common in AIDS patients, the majority of which are of the B-cell lineage. Both forms can present with cutaneous manifestations.

Other cutaneous malignancies found in AIDS patients include squamous-cell carcinomas (which often contain HPV if the carcinoma presents in the anogenital area) and basal-cell carcinomas. Melanomas have a much poorer prognosis in AIDS patients compared with immunocompetent patients [313].

Infectious lesions

The majority of the cutaneous disorders found in HIV-infected individuals are in the form of infections. Herpesviruses, HPV and MC are the most common secondary infecting viruses found in these patients. *Staphylococcus aureus* is the most common infecting bacterium and can cause a variety of dermatological disorders. In general, candidiasis is the most common mucocutaneous fungal infection in HIV disease. Although the immunodeficient state predisposes to infection, most conditions will resemble those found in the normal population, but they will be more severe or recurrent. However, there can be differences in the presentation or type of infection that ensues. In this section, some infections unique to the HIV-infected population, either due to an unusual agent or an unusual presentation, will be discussed.

Bacterial infections. Human immunodeficiency virus disease has many effects on the immune system which yield the infected individuals more susceptible to bacterial infections [315]. Most patients have a functional neutropenia late in the course of HIV disease for a number of reasons, and then are susceptible to most bacteria.

A variety of *S. aureus* infections are seen in HIV-infected individuals, with an increasing incidence with the degree of immunocompromise. Primary infections include impetigo, folliculitis, furuncles, carbuncles and cellulitis. Catheter and other line sites commonly become infected, and bacteraemia can be a serious, fatal complication. Treatment requires anti-staphylococcal antibiotics for eradication and suppression of recurrent infections. Rifampicin can be used to eradicate *S. aureus* from the nares, thereby preventing continuous autoinoculation. In addition, patients with AIDS suffer from an increased incidence of bacillary angiomatosis, which has been associated with *Bartonella henselae* and *Bartonella quintana* [316].

Fungal infections. Mucosal candidiasis occurs in almost every HIV-infected individual. The oropharynx is the usual site of infection; however, spread to the trachea or oesophagus is not uncommon. Mucosal candidiasis most often develops in patients with a reduction in the CD4 cell count; and oesophageal candidiasis, which is associated with retrosternal burning and odynophagia, only occurs in those with a CD4 cell count of $<100/mm^3$. Oropharyngeal candidiasis may be asymptomatic or can cause burning and soreness of the mouth, often during a spicy meal. This condition has four different forms: erythematous candidiasis, hyperplastic candidiasis, pseudomembranous candidiasis and angular chelitis. Erythematous candidiasis can be easily overlooked, since it occurs as erythematous patches, on the hard and soft palate, within normal-appearing mucosa. It can also affect the tongue, giving it a smooth red appearance. Hyperplastic lesions most often appear as a white coating of the dorsum of the tongue. Thrush can be quite impressive, and may produce cheesy white plaques or dusting flecks in any area of the oropharynx. Erythema or plaque formation in the corners of the mouth is termed angular chelitis. Candidiasis should be differentiated from OHL, which can also be seen in HIV-positive individuals. This is accomplished by demonstrating multiple pseudohyphae on a potassium hydroxide-stained slide of the affected area or by a lesional biopsy. Treatment of candidiasis is directed against acute attacks and possible recurrences. Topical agents are the first-line therapies, but are not always the treatment of choice, due to the necessity of frequent dosing (four to five times per day). Systemic therapies currently available include ketoconazole, fluconazole, imidazoles and itraconazole. Fluconazole is more effective than ketoconazole for the treatment of both oropharyngeal [317] and oesophageal [318] candidiasis. However, fluconazole is more expensive than the other agents, and this may cause problems when chronic, suppressive treatment is required.

Onychomycosis is an infection of the nail plates, caused by superficial dermatophytes, yeasts or moulds. Although this condition is quite common in the immunocompetent population, it can affect HIV-infected individuals differently, both in location of infection and in severity. The proximal subungual nail is the typical location of onychomycosis in HIV disease. This infection, usually caused by *Trichophyton rubrum* [319] in HIV patients, causes a white, chalky appearance of the outer nail plates, starting at the proximal portion of the toenail, which may extend to involve the entire nail. This proximal pattern is the least common variant in the immunocompetent population. Another finding unique to HIV-infected individuals is involvement of both hands. Usually onychomycosis is limited to one hand and most often only one nail. Treatment is not always required, since most patients are already taking systemic antifungal agents to prevent other more serious fungal infections.

Viral infections. Viruses can cause many infections in HIV-infected individuals, many of which are recurrent, are difficult to treat and cause more serious illnesses and sequelae.

Herpes simplex viruses are not only risk factors for acquiring HIV, but recurrences are one of the most common viral illnesses in those infected with HIV. At some point the recurrent HSV infections may become chronic and unremitting. Multiple large ulcerations with angulated borders may form, which can be confused with neurotic excoriations [320]. Some herpetic lesions may not respond to antiviral chemotherapy and may contain acyclovir-resistant strains of HSV, which are sometimes found in HIV-infected individuals [321]. If a resistant strain is suspected, i.v. foscarnet is currently effective [322].

Varicella-zoster virus causes a primary infection in children (chickenpox) and a reactivated infection in adults (zoster). Children with HIV have an increased risk of severe primary infection, VZV dissemination and even death [51]. Adults with HIV may suffer a reactivation of the primary infection (zoster) due to the immunocompromised state. Zoster usually occurs early in the course of HIV disease, and most patients have an uneventful recovery. However, the disease may be multidermatomal, disseminated, and recurrent, which does not usually occur in the normal population. As in HSV infection, VZV may be resistant to acyclovir, which requires treatment with i.v. foscarnet [53].

Oral hairy leucoplakia, caused by EBV, is a lesion unique to individuals with HIV. This condition, most often asymptomatic, presents as hyperplastic, white or grey plaques on the tongue. One typical finding in OHL is a white lesion on the lateral portion of the tongue, which cannot be removed. These lesions are often mistaken for candidiasis, but will not respond to antifungal agents. Biopsy can ensure a proper diagnosis. The lesions vary in number and location, but usually affect the lateral tongue.

Treatment with topical podophyllin is effective, but recurrence is common [323].

Human papillomavirus affects a large portion of the population, but HIV-infected individuals have an increased risk of developing warts, neoplasia and possibly invasive squamous-cell carcinoma [324]. In advanced HIV disease, the warts may become more numerous and more difficult to treat. Condyloma acuminata—warts in anal areas—are common in HIV-infected homosexual males and can be refractory to treatment. Of considerable importance is the fact that some strains of HPV may have oncogenic potential. Treatment, most often cytodestructive, is not curative and may cause more harm than good, unless the patient has early HIV disease with little immunodeficiency. In this case, the usual treatments can be used, but recurrences should be expected.

Molluscum contagiosum is a poxvirus transmitted by skin-to-skin contact, and is usually found in children and adolescents who play contact sports. This condition, which resolves spontaneously in the immunocompetent host, has a different course in HIV-infected individuals. Clinically, the patient has multiple, umbilicated papules covering the face and neck, especially in shaved areas. Most of the papules have a 'cobblestone' appearance on side-view. Recurrence is the rule, and treatment is directed at minimizing the number of lesions, since a cure is not likely. Treatment with liquid nitrogen or lasers may be effective. Also, patients should be encouraged to quit shaving not only to prevent autoinoculation, but also to disguise existing lesions.

Disseminated fungal infections. Some cutaneous findings in HIV-infected patients are the result of disseminated fungal infections. Dissemination causes a multiorgan illness, which can include fever, weight loss, meningitis, hepatomegaly and pulmonary symptoms. Although fungal dissemination does not always demonstrate cutaneous manifestations, these findings may be of importance for proper diagnosis.

Cryptococcus neoformans usually causes a pulmonary infection, which eventually resolves. However, *C. neoformans* is able to remain within the body only to re-emerge when the immune system is depressed, and is currently the second most common fungal infection in HIV-infected patients. When the infection is reactivated, haematogenous spread can occur, which may involve the skin. The skin lesions often resemble MC, since there can be multiple papules or nodules on the face. The lesions are numerous and flesh-coloured, but are not umbilicated. Since this infection is not just a cosmetic problem and can be fatal, it should be differentiated from MC. A biopsy of the lesion that demonstrates yeast forms yields the diagnosis [325]. Other methods of diagnosis include Giemsa stain and Indian-ink stains to show yeast forms. Treatment of disseminated *Cryptococcus* is i.v. amphotericin B. The lesions usually resolve during treatment but typically recur.

Coccidioides immitis, only seen in the western hemisphere, usually causes a subclinical pulmonary infection in the normal host. However, similar to *Cryptococcus*, the infection can re-emerge in the HIV-infected individual as a result of the immunodeficient state. Dissemination can involve the skin, bones, meninges and lungs. The skin lesions, which can also mimic MC, are multiple papules, which develop into nodules or plaques on an erythematous base. The lesions may become secondarily infected, with abscess formation. Diagnosis is made by biopsy or fungal culture. It should be noted that the mucosal surfaces are spared in this infection, and can aid in distinguishing this entity from cryptococcosis and histoplasmosis, which both have mucocutaneous involvement. Treatment is i.v. amphotericin B.

Histoplasma capsulatum, primarily in the Ohio and Mississippi River valleys, can cause disseminated histoplasmosis in HIV-infected patients. The cutaneous findings are varied and can include erythematous, keratin-plugged papules and nodules, folliculitis, psoriasis-type eruptions, ulcers and plaques. The lesions occur most often on the face, extremities and trunk. Tissue biopsy is used to identify the organism. Treatment is i.v. amphoterecin B or oral fluconazole. However, recurrences are common.

Sporotrix schenkii, a fungus found in organic matter that causes sporotrichosis, has a different presentation in HIV-infected individuals. The cutaneous findings are due to dissemination and include papulosquamous eruptions [326] or papulonodular lesions, which are crusted, ulcerated or eroded [327]. The lesions are usually generalized and spare the mucosal surfaces. The organism can be identified by either Gram stain or culture of the lesion. Treatment is i.v. amphotericin B, but relapse is common.

Non-infectious lesions

Seborrhoeic dermatitis is a common skin disease in HIV-infected individuals. The condition is similar to that found in immunocompetent individuals, but can behave differently in the HIV population. The condition may be more severe and often involves hair-bearing areas of the body, such as the scalp, eyebrows, beard, chest and pubic areas. Treatment is topical steroids or topical antifungals, but relapse occurs. *Pityrosporum ovale* may have a significant role in this condition, but this is still unclear at this time [328].

Eosinophilic folliculitis is a chronic, pruritic condition that is unique to those infected with HIV. It is characterized by numerous follicular and non-follicular papules on the face, trunk and extremities. Extreme pruritus is the main complaint of those affected. The lesions are culture-negative and do not respond to antibiotics. Eosinophilia, increased IgE levels and a peripheral leucocytosis are common findings; however, the diagnosis is most often made histologically. Treatment with antihistamines (such as cetirizine) [329], topical steroids or phototherapy may help eliminate the pruritus and lesions, but complete eradication of the disease is unlikely.

Psoriasis vulgaris is not known to be more common in HIV disease; however, many individuals have their first episode after HIV seroconversion. Also, those with pre-existing psoriasis can have an increased severity of the lesions. The lesions can resemble those found in the normal population, but the histology differs. The HIV-infected patient's skin has a dermal infiltrate of mostly plasma cells rather than T cells [330]. Treatments are varied and some respond to the antiretroviral agent, zidovudine [331]. Other treatments include topical steroids, tar and phototherapy. Treatment of psoriasis with immunosuppressive agents is usually contraindicated in HIV disease and should be used with caution.

Treatment of HIV

Currently, there are three classes of antiretroviral agents approved for use in the treatment of HIV. The first class of drugs approved for the treatment of HIV was the nucleoside analogues, which selectively inhibit HIV reverse transcriptase. These include zidovudine (AZT), didanosine (ddI), zalcitabine (ddC), stavudine (d4T) and lamivudine (3TC). The second class of drugs for the fight against HIV was the protease inhibitors. These agents, which block the HIV protease used late in replication, include indinavir, nelfinavir, ritonavir and saquinavir. The third class of drugs approved for therapy of HIV infection was the non-nucleoside reverse transcriptase inhibitors; only one member of this class, nevirapine, has been approved thus far.

As patients become refractory to AZT, ddI can be effective. Combination therapy with both AZT and ddC is useful in deteriorating patients who have not responded to other therapy. Lamivudine is also recommended for use in combination with AZT. The treatment of choice for therapy of HIV infection is one protease inhibitor in combination with two nucleoside inhibitors. This combination may prevent the resistance that is commonly seen when nucleoside inhibitors are used as long-term monotherapy. Other treatments, such as therapeutic vaccinations, are under investigation but have remained unsuccessful, due to the marked capacity of HIV to mutate.

References

1 Wald A *et al.* Virologic characteristic of subclinical and symptomatic genital herpes infections. *N Engl J Med* 1995; **333**: 770.
2 Higgins CR *et al.* Natural history, management and complications of herpes labialis. *J Med Virol* 1993; Suppl 1: 22.
3 Beutner KR. Rational use of acyclovir in the treatment of mucocutaneous herpes simplex virus infections. *Semin Dermatol* 1992; **11**: 256.
4 John RE *et al.* A seroepidemiologic study of the prevalence of herpes simplex virus type 2 infection in the United States. *N Engl J Med* 1989; **321**: 7.

5 Benedetti J *et al*. Recurrence rates in genital herpes after symptomatic first-episode infection. *Ann Intern Med* 1994; **12**: 847.
6 Corey L *et al*. Genital herpes simplex virus infections: clinical manifestations, course, and complications. *Ann Intern Med* 1993; **98**: 958.
7 Bader C *et al*. The natural history of recurrent facial–oral infection with herpes simplex virus. *J Infect Dis* 1978; **138**: 897.
8 Aurelius E *et al*. Rapid diagnosis of herpes simplex encephalitis by nested polymerase chain reaction assay of cerebrospinal fluid. *Lancet* 1991; **337**: 189.
9 Molin L. Oral acyclovir prevents herpes simplex associated erythema multiforme. *Br J Dermatol* 1987; **116**: 109.
10 Hope-Simpson RE. The nature of herpes zoster: a long term study and a new hypothesis. *Proc Roy Soc Med* 1965; **58**: 9.
11 Seiler HE. A study of herpes zoster particularly in its relationship to chickenpox. *J Hyg (Cambridge)* 1949; **47**: 253.
12 Burgoon CF *et al*. The natural history of herpes zoster. *JAMA* 1957; **164**: 265.
13 Stern ES. The mechanism of herpes zoster and its relation to chickenpox. *Br J Dermatol Syphilol* 1937; **49**: 263.
14 Almeida JD *et al*. Morphology of varicella (chickenpox) virus. *Virology* 1962; **16**: 353.
15 Wesselhoeft C. The differential diagnosis of chickenpox and smallpox. *N Engl J Med* 1944; **230**: 15.
16 Krugman S *et al*. Varicella-zoster infections. In: *Infectious Diseases in Children*, 8th edn. Mosby, St Louis, 1985, p. 433.
17 Christie AB. Chickenpox (varicella), herpes zoster. In: *Infectious Diseases: Epidemiology and Clinical Practice*, 3rd edn. Churchill Livingstone, Edinburgh, 1980, pp. 262–278.
18 Asano Y *et al*. Viremia is present in incubation period in nonimmunocompromised children with varicella. *J Pediatr* 1985; **106**: 69.
19 Asano Y *et al*. Severity of viremia and clinical findings in children with varicella. *J Infect Dis* 1990; **161**: 1095.
20 Ozaki T *et al*. Viremic phase in nonimmunocompromised children with varicella. *J Pediatr* 1984; **104**: 85.
21 Feldman S, Epp E. Detection of viremia during inoculation of varicella. *J Pediatr* 1979; **94**: 746.
22 Asano Y *et al*. Viral replication and immunologic responses in children naturally infected with varicella-zoster virus and in varicella vaccine recipients. *J Infect Dis* 1985; **152**: 863.
23 Baba K *et al*. Immunologic and epidemiologic aspects of varicella infection acquired during infancy and early childhood. *J Pediatr* 1982; **100**: 881.
24 Gershon AA *et al*. Clinical reinfection with varicella-zoster virus. *J Infect Dis* 1984; **149**: 137.
25 Gershon AA. Liver attenuated varicella vaccine: protection in healthy adults compared with leukemic children. *J Infect Dis* 1990; **161**: 661.
26 Takahachi M. Current status and prospects of live varicella vaccine. *Vaccine* 1992; **10**: 1007–1014.
27 Gordon JE. Chickenpox: an epidemiological review. *Am J Med Sci* 1962; **244**: 362.
28 Gershon AA *et al*. Antibody to varicella-zoster virus in parturient women and their offspring during the first year of life. *Pediatrics* 1976; **58**: 692.
29 Weller TH. Varicella-herpes zoster virus. In: Evans AS (ed.) *Viral Infections of Humans: Epidemiology and Control*, 3rd edn. Plenum, New York, 1989, p. 659.
30 Weller TH. Varicella and herpes zoster: changing concepts of the natural history, control, and importance of a not-so-benign virus. *N Engl J Med* 1983; **309**: 1362–1434.
31 Ross AH. Modification of chickenpox in family contacts by administration of gamma globulin. *N Engl J Med* 1962; **267**: 369.

32 Bullowa JGM *et al.* Complications of varicella I. Their occurrences among 2534 patients. *Am J Dis Child* 1935; **49**: 923.

33 Smith EW *et al.* Varicella gangrenosa due to group A-hemolytic *Streptococcus.* *Pediatrics* 1976; **57**: 306.

34 Fleischer G *et al.* Life-threatening complications of varicella. *Am J Dis Child* 1981; **135**: 896.

35 Wallace MR *et al.* Treatment of adult varicella with oral acyclovir: a randomized, placebo-controlled study. *Ann Intern Med* 1992; **117**: 358.

36 Haake DA *et al.* Early treatment with acyclovir for varicella pneumonia in otherwise healthy adults: retrospective controlled study and review. *Rev Infect Dis* 1990; **12**: 788.

37 Triebwasser JH *et al.* Varicella pneumonia in adults. *Medicine (Baltimore)* 1967; **46**: 409.

38 Guess H *et al.* Population-based studies of varicella complications. *Pediatrics* 1986; **78**: 723.

39 Schlossberg D, Littman MI. Varicella pneumonia. *Arch Intern Med* 1988; **148**: 1630.

40 Sargent EN *et al.* Varicella pneumonia: a report of 20 cases, with postmortem examination in six. *Calif Med* 1967; **107**: 141.

41 Brunell PA. Varicella in pregnancy, the fetus, and the newborn: problems in management. *J Infect Dis* 1992; **166** (Suppl): S42.

42 Oxman MN *et al.* Management at delivery of mother and infant when herpes simplex, varicella-zoster, hepatitis or tuberculosis have occurred during pregnancy. In: Remington JS, Swartz MN (eds) *Current Topics in Infectious Diseases*, Vol. 4. McGraw-Hill, New York, 1983, p. 224.

43 Gershon AA. Chickenpox, measles, and mumps. In: Remington JS, Klein JO (eds) *Infectious Diseases of the Fetus and Newborn Infant*, 3rd edn. Saunders, Philadelphia, 1990.

44 Williamson AP. The varicella-zoster virus in the etiology of severe congenital defects. *Clin Pediatr* 1975; **14**: 553.

45 Brunell PA, Kotchman GS. Zoster in infancy: failure to maintain virus latency following intrauterine infection. *J Pediatr* 1981; **98**: 71.

46 Pitel BA *et al.* Subclinical hepatic changes in varicella infection. *Pediatrics* 1980; **65**: 631.

47 Myers MG. Hepatic cellular injury during varicella. *Arch Dis Child* 1982; **57**: 317.

48 Ey JL *et al.* Varicella hepatitis without neurologic symptoms or findings. *Pediatrics* 1981; **67**: 285.

49 Sherman RA *et al.* Fatal varicella in an adult: case report and review of the gastrointestinal complications of chickenpox. *Rev Infect Dis* 1991; **13**: 424.

50 Baird RE *et al.* Varicella arthritis diagnosed by polymerase chain reaction. *Pediatr Infect Dis J* 1990; **10**: 950.

51 Jura E *et al.* Varicella-zoster virus infections in children infected with human immunodeficiency virus. *Pediatr Infect Dis J* 1989; **8**: 586.

52 Pahwa S *et al.* Continuous varicella-zoster infection associated with acyclovir resistance in a child with AIDS. *JAMA* 1988; **260**: 2879.

53 Jacobson MA *et al.* Acyclovir-resistant varicella zoster infection after chronic oral acyclovir therapy in patients with the acquired immunodeficiency syndrome (AIDS). *Ann Intern Med* 1990; **112**: 187.

54 Cheatham WJ *et al.* Varicella: report of two fatal cases with necropsy, virus isolation, and serologic studies. *Am J Pathol* 1956; **32**: 1015.

55 Feldman S *et al.* Varicella in children with cancer: seventy-seven cases. *Pediatrics* 1975; **56**: 388.

56 Haggerty RJ, Eley RC. Varicella and cortisone. *Pediatrics* 1956; **18**: 160.

57 Gershon A *et al.* Steroid therapy and varicella. *J Pediatr* 1972; **81**: 1034.

58 Finkel KC. Mortality from varicella in children receiving adrenocorticosteroids and adrenocorticotropin. *Pediatrics* 1971; **28**: 436.

59 Scheinman JI, Stamler FW. Cyclophosphamide and fatal varicella. *J Pediatr* 1969; **74**: 117.

60 Lux SE *et al.* Chronic neutropenia and abnormal cellular immunity in cartilage–hair hypoplasia. *N Engl J Med* 1970; **282**: 231.

61 Hattori A *et al.* Use of live varicella vaccine in children with acute leukemia or other malignancies. *Lancet* 1976; **ii**: 210.

62 Feldhoff CM *et al.* Varicella in children with renal transplants. *J Pediatr* 1981; **98**: 25.

63 Whitley RJ *et al.* Vidarabine therapy of varicella in immunosuppressed patients. *J Pediatr* 1982; **101**: 125.

64 Whitley RJ *et al.* Early vidarabine therapy to control the complications of herpes zoster in immunosuppressed patients. *N Engl J Med* 1982; **307**: 971.

65 Lichtenstein PK *et al.* Grade I Reye's syndrome: a frequent cause of vomiting and liver dysfunction after varicella and upper-respiratory-tract infection. *N Engl J Med* 1983; **309**: 133.

66 Fulginiti VA *et al.* Aspirin and Reye syndrome. *Pediatrics* 1982; **69**: 810.

67 Dunkle LM *et al.* A controlled trial of acyclovir for chickenpox in normal children. *N Engl J Med* 1991; **325**: 1539.

68 Rothe MJ *et al.* Oral acyclovir therapy for varicella and zoster infections in pediatric and pregnant patients: a brief review. *Pediatr Dermatol* 1991; **8**: 236.

69 Balfour HH *et al.* Acyclovir treatment of varicella in otherwise healthy children. *J Pediatr* 1990; **116**: 633.

70 Prober CG *et al.* Acyclovir therapy of chickenpox in immunosuppressed children: a collaborative study. *J Pediatr* 1982; **101**: 622.

71 Nyerges G *et al.* Acyclovir prevents dissemination of varicella in immunocompromised children. *J Infect Dis* 1988; **157**: 309.

72 Whitley RJ. Therapeutic approaches to varicella-zoster virus infections. *J Infect Dis* 1992; **166** (Suppl 1): S51–S57.

73 Arvin AM *et al.* Human leukocyte interferon in the treatment of varicella in children with cancer. *N Engl J Med* 1982; **306**: 761.

74 Whitley RJ, Gnann JW. Acyclovir —a decade later. *N Engl J Med* 1992; **327**: 782.

75 Nyerges G, Meszner Z. Treatment of chickenpox in immunosuppressed children. *Am J Med* 1988; **85** (Suppl 2A): 94.

76 McGregor RS *et al.* Varicella in pediatric orthotopic liver transplant recipients. *Pediatrics* 1989; **83**: 256.

77 Anon. Varicella-zoster immune globulin for the prevention of chickenpox. *Morb Mort Weekly Rep* 1984; **33**: 84–90, 95–99.

78 White CJ *et al.* Varicella vaccine (VARIVAX) in healthy children and adolescents: results from clinical trials, 1987 to 1989. *Pediatrics* 1991; **87**: 604.

79 Gershon AA *et al.* Immunization of healthy adults with live attenuated varicella vaccine. *J Infect Dis* 1988; **158**: 132.

80 Andre FE. Summary of clinical studies with the Oka live varicella vaccine produced by Smith Kline-RIT. *Biken J* 1984; **27** (2–3): 89.

81 Plokin SA *et al.* Zoster in normal children after varicella vaccine (letter). *J Infect Dis* 1989; **159**: 1000.

82 White CJ. Varicella vaccine reflux (letter). *Pediatrics* 1992; **89**: 354.

83 Guess HA *et al.* Epidemiology of herpes zoster in children and adolescents: a population based study. *Pediatrics* 1985; **76**: 512.

84 Gershon AA. Viral vaccines of the future. *Pediatr Clin North Am* 1990; **37**: 689.

85 Gershon AA. Live attenuated varicella vaccine. *Ann Rev Med* 1987; **38**: 41.

86 Bruusgaard E. The mutual relation between zoster and varicella. *Br J Dermatol Syphilol* 1932; **44**: 1.

87 Weller TH, Witton HM. The etiologic agents of varicella and herpes zoster: serologic studies with the viruses as propagated *in vitro. J Exp Med* 1958; **108**: 869.

88 Weller TH *et al.* The etiologic agents of varicella and herpes zoster: isolation, propagation, and cultural characteristics *in vitro. J Exp Med* 1958; **108**: 843.

89 Colebunders R *et al.* Herpes zoster in African patients: a clinical predictor of human immunodeficiency virus infection. *J Infect Dis* 1988; **157**: 314.

90 Cohen PR *et al.* Disseminated herpes zoster in patients with human immunodeficiency virus infection. *Am J Med* 1988; **84**: 1076.

91 Head H, Campbell AW. The pathology of herpes zoster and its bearing on sensory localization. *Brain* 1900; **23**: 353.

92 Armstrong RW *et al.* Cutaneous interferon production in patients with Hodgkin's disease and other cancers infected with varicella or vaccinia. *N Engl J Med* 1970; **283**: 1182.

93 Ruckdeschel JC *et al.* Herpes zoster and impaired cell-associated immunity to the varicella-zoster virus in patients with Hodgkin's disease. *Am J Med* 1977; **62**: 77.

94 Patel PA *et al.* Cell-mediated immunity to varicella-zoster virus infection in subjects with lymphoma or leukemia. *J Pediatr* 1979; **94**: 223.

95 Shanbrom E *et al.* Herpes zoster in hematologic neoplasias: some unusual manifestations. *Ann Intern Med* 1960; **53**: 523.

96 Wilson A *et al.* Subclinical varicella-zoster virus viremia, herpes zoster, and T lymphocyte immunity to varicella-zoster viral antigens after bone marrow transplantation. *J Infect Dis* 1992; **165**: 119.

97 Dolin R *et al.* Herpes zoster-varicella infections in immunosuppressed patients. *Ann Intern Med* 1978; **89**: 375.

98 Juel-Hensen BE, MacCallum FO. *Herpes Simplex, Varicella and Zoster.* Lippincott, Philadelphia, 1972.

99 Sokal JE, Firat D. Varicella-zoster infection in Hodgkin's disease. *Am J Med* 1965; **39**: 452.

100 Schimpff S *et al.* Varicella-zoster infection in patients with cancer. *Ann Intern Med* 1972; **76**: 241.

101 Feldman S *et al.* Herpes zoster in children with cancer. *Am J Dis Child* 1973; **126**: 178.

102 Goffinet DR *et al.* Herpes zoster-varicella and lymphoma. *Ann Intern Med* 1972; **76**: 235.

103 Goodman R *et al.* Herpes zoster in children with stage I–III Hodgkin's disease. *Radiology* 1976; **118**: 429.

104 Reboul F *et al.* Herpes zoster and varicella infections in children with Hodgkin's disease. *Cancer* 1978; **41**: 95.

105 Rusthoven JJ *et al.* Varicella-zoster infection in adult cancer patients—a population study. *Arch Intern Med* 1988; **148**: 1561.

106 Arvin AM. Cell-mediated immunity to varicella zoster virus. *J Infect Dis* 1992; **166**: S35.

107 Ljungman P *et al.* Clinical and subclinical reactivations of varicella-zoster in immunocompromised patients. *J Infect Dis* 1986; **153**: 840.

108 Meyers JD *et al.* Cell-mediated immunity to varicella-zoster virus after allogenic marrow transplant. *J Infect Dis* 1980; **141**: 479.

109 Locksley RM *et al.* Infection with varicella-zoster virus after bone marrow transplantation. *J Infect Dis* 1985; **152**: 1172.

110 Friedman-Kien AE *et al.* Herpes zoster: a possible early clinical sign for development of acquired immunodeficiency syndrome in high-risk individuals. *J Am Acad Dermatol* 1986; **14**: 1023.

111 Linnemann CC *et al.* Emergence of acyclovir-resistant varicella zoster virus in an AIDS patient on prolonged acyclovir therapy. *AIDS* 1990; **4**: 577.

112 LeBoit PE *et al.* Chronic verrucous varicella-zoster virus infection in patients with the acquired immunodeficiency syndrome (AIDS)—histologic and molecular biologic findings. *Am J Dermatopathol* 1992; **14**: 1.

113 Gilson IH *et al.* Disseminated ecthymatous herpes varicella-zoster infection in patients with acquired immunodeficiency syndrome. *Arch Dermatol* 1990; **126**: 1048.

114 Hoppenjans WB *et al.* Prolonged cutaneous herpes zoster in acquired immunodeficiency syndrome. *Arch Dermatol* 1990; **126**: 1048.

115 Alessi E *et al.* Unusual varicella zoster virus infection in patients with the acquired immunodeficiency syndrome (letter). *Arch Dermatol* 1988; **124**: 1011.

116 Levin MJ *et al.* Immune responses of elderly individuals to live attenuated varicella vaccine. *J Infect Dis* 1992; **166**: 253.

117 Takahashi M *et al.* Immunization of the elderly and patients with collagen vascular diseases with live varicella vaccine and use of varicella skin antigen. *J Infect Dis* 1992; **166**: S58.

118 Miller AE. Selective decline in cellular immune response to varicella-zoster in the elderly. *Neurology* 1980; **30**: 582.

119 Berger R *et al.* Decrease of the lymphoproliferative response to varicella zoster virus antigen in the aged. *Infect Immun* 1981; **32**: 24.

120 Burke BL *et al.* Immune response to varicella-zoster in the aged. *Arch Intern Med* 1982; **142**: 291.

121 Ragozzino MW *et al.* Risk of cancer after herpes zoster: a population-based study. *N Engl J Med* 1982; **307**: 393.

122 Fueyo MA, Lookingbill DP. Herpes zoster and occult malignancy. *J Am Acad Dermatol* 1984; **11**: 480.

123 Wurzel CL *et al.* Prognosis of herpes zoster in healthy children. *Am J Dis Child* 1986; **140**: 477.

124 Lubey JP *et al.* A longitudinal study of varicella-zoster virus infection in renal transplant recipients. *J Infect Dis* 1977; **135**: 659.

125 Easton HG. Zoster sine herpete causing trigeminal neuralgia. *Lancet* 1970; **ii**: 1065.

126 Lewis GW. Zoster sine herpete. *Br Med J* 1958; **2**: 418.

127 Ragozzino MW *et al.* Population-based study of herpes zoster and its sequelae. *Medicine (Baltimore)* 1982; **61**: 310.

128 Brown GR. Herpes zoster: correlation of age, sex, distribution, neuralgia, and associated disorders. *South Med J* 1976; **59**: 576.

129 Hope-Simpson RE. Postherpetic neuralgia. *J Roy Coll Gen Pract* 1975; **25**: 571.

130 de Moragas JM, Kierland RR. The outcome of patients with herpes zoster. *Arch Dermatol* 1957; **75**: 193.

131 Grant BD, Rowe CR. Motor paralysis of the extremities in herpes zoster. *J Bone Joint Surg* 1961; **43A**: 885.

132 Thomas JE, Howard FM. Segmented zoster paresis—a disease profile. *Neurology* 1972; **22**: 459.

133 Denny-Brown D *et al.* Pathologic features of herpes zoster: a note on 'geniculate herpes.' *Arch Neurol Psychiatr* 1944; **51**: 216.

134 McKendall RR, Klawans HL. Nervous system complications of varicella-zoster virus. In: Vinken PJ, Bruyn GW (eds) *Handbook of Clinical Neurology*, Vol. 34. North-Holland, Amsterdam, 1978, pp. 161.

135 McCormick WF *et al.* Varicella zoster encephalomyelitis. *Arch Neurol* 1969; **21**: 559.

136 Gold E, Robbins FC. Isolation of herpes zoster virus from spinal fluid of a patient. *Virology* 1958; **6**: 293.

137 Applebaum E *et al.* Herpes zoster encephalitis. *Am J Med* 1962; **32**: 25.

138 Norris FH *et al.* Herpes zoster meningoencephalitis. *J Infect Dis* 1970; **122**: 335.

139 Jemsek J *et al.* Herpes zoster-associated encephalitis: clincopathologic report

of 12 cases and review of the literature. *J Neurol Neurosurg Psychiatry* 1985; **48**: 122.

140 Huff JC *et al*. Effect of oral acyclovir on pain resolution in herpes zoster: a reanalysis. *J Med Virol* 1993; Suppl 1: 93.

141 Shepp DH *et al*. Current therapy of varicella zoster infection in immunocompromised patients. *Am J Med* 1988; **85** (Suppl 2A): 96.

142 Dolin R. Antiviral chemotherapy and chemoprophylaxis. *Science* 1985; **227**: 1296.

143 Savoia M, Oxman MN. Guidelines for antiviral therapy. In: Kass EH, Platt R (eds) *Current Therapy in Infectious Disease: 1985–1986*. BC Dekker, Toronto/Philadelphia, 1986, p. 1.

144 Nicholson KG. Antiviral therapy: varicella-zoster virus infections, herpes labialis and mucocutaneous herpes, and cytomegalovirus infection. *Lancet* 1984; **ii**: 677.

145 Winston DJ *et al*. Recombinant interferon alpha-2a for treatment of herpes zoster in immunosuppressed patients with cancer. *Am J Med* 1988; **85**: 147.

146 Tyring SK *et al*. Famciclovir for the treatment of acute herpes zoster: effects on acute disease and post-herpetic neuralgia. *Ann Intern Med* 1995; **123**: 89.

147 Beutner KR *et al*. Valaciclovir compared with acyclovir for improved therapy for herpes zoster in immunocompetent adults. *Antimicrob Agents Chemother* 1995; **39**: 1546.

148 Price RW. Herpes zoster: an approach to systemic therapy. *Med Clin North Am* 1982; **66**: 1105.

149 Bernstein JE *et al*. Treatment of chronic postherpetic neuralgia with topical capsaicin. *J Am Acad Dermatol* 1987; **17**: 93.

150 Hayward A *et al*. Varicella-zoster virus-specific immunity after herpes zoster. *J Infect Dis* 1991; **163**: 873.

151 Hayward A *et al*. Varicella-zoster virus (VZV) specific cytotoxicity after immunization of nonimmune adults with Oka strain attenuated VZV vaccine. *J Infect Dis* 1992; **166**: 260.

152 Perren TJ *et al*. Prevention of herpes zoster in patients by long-term oral acyclovir after allogeneic bone marrow transplantation. *Am J Med* 1988; **85** (Suppl 2A): 99.

153 Safrin S *et al*. Foscarnet therapy in five patients with AIDS and acyclovir-resistant varicella zoster virus infection. *Ann Intern Med* 1991; **115**: 19.

154 Evans AS *et al*. Seroepidemiologic studies of infectious mononucleosis with EB virus. *N Engl J Med* 1968; **279**: 1123.

155 Niederman JC *et al*. Prevalence, incidence, and persistence of EB virus antibody. *N Engl J Med* 1970; **282**: 361.

156 University Health Physicians *et al*. Infectious mononucleosis and its relationship to EB virus antibody. *Br Med J* 1971; **4**: 643.

157 Bernstein A. Infectious mononucleosis. *Medicine* 1940; **19**: 85.

158 McCarthy JT, Hoaglund RJ. Cutaneous manifestations of infectious mononucleosis. *JAMA* 1964; **187**: 153.

159 Decker GR, Berberian BJ, Sulica VI. Periorbital and eyelid edema: the initial manifestation of acute infectious mononucleosis. *Cutis* 1991; **47**: 323–324.

160 Sadusk JF. The skin eruption and false-positive Wasserman in infectious mononucleosis. *N Intern Clin* 1941; **1**: 239.

161 Paul JR. Infectious mononucleosis. *Bull NY Acad Med* 1939; **15**: 43.

162 Contratto AN. Infectious mononucleosis: a study of one-hundred and ninety-six cases. *Arch Intern Med* 1944; **73**: 449.

163 Milne J. Infectious mononucleosis. *N Engl J Med* 1945; **233**: 727.

164 Petrozzi JW. Infectious mononucleosis manifesting as a palmar dermatitis. *Arch Dermatol* 1971; **104**: 207.

165 Bjorg M *et al*. Temporary skin reactions to penicillins during the acute stage of infectious mononucleosis. *Scand J Infect Dis* 1975; **7**: 21.

166 Mulroy R. Amoxicillin rash in infectious mononucleosis. *Br Med J* 1973; **1**: 554.

167 Morris J. Infectious-mononucleosis rash after talampicillin (letter). *Lancet* 1976; **i**: 423.

168 Fields DA. Methicillin rash in infectious mononucleosis (letter). *West J Med* 1980; **133**: 521.

169 Carter RL. Granulocyte changes in infectious mononucleosis. *J Clin Pathol* 1966; **19**: 279.

170 Clarke BF, Davies SH. Severe thrombocytopenia in infectious mononucleosis. *Am J Med Sci* 1964; **248**: 703.

171 Cantow EK, Kostinas JE. Studies on infectious mononucleosis IV. Changes in the granulocyte series. *Am J Clin Pathol* 1966; **46**: 43.

172 Penman G. Extreme neutropenia in glandular fever. *J Clin Pathol* 1968; **21**: 48.

173 Straus SE. The chronic mononucleosis syndrome. *J Infect Dis* 1988; **157**: 405.

174 Holmes GP *et al.* Chronic fatigue syndrome: a working case definition. *Ann Intern Med* 1988; **108**: 387.

175 Sumaya CV, Ench Y. Epstein–Barr virus infectious mononucleosis in children. II. Heterophile antibody in viral specific responses. New perspectives on infectious mononucleosis. *Pediatrics* 1985; **75**: 1011.

176 Ernberg I, Anderson J. Acyclovir efficiently inhibits oropharyngeal excretion of Epstein–Barr virus in patients with acute infectious mononucleosis. *J Gen Virol* 1986; **67**: 2267.

177 Pearson GR, Levine PH. Epstein–Barr virus vaccine: the time to proceed is now. In: Roizman B, Whitley RJ, Lopez C (eds) *The Human Herpesviruses.* Raven Press, New York, 1993, pp. 349–356.

178 Lesher JL. Cytomegalovirus and the skin. *J Am Acad Dermatol* 1988; **18**: 1333.

179 Pariser RJ. Histologically specific skin lesions in disseminated cytomegalovirus infection. *J Am Acad Dermatol* 1983; **9**: 937.

180 Ho M. Cytomegalovirus. In: *Principles and Practices of Infectious Diseases,* 3rd edn. Churchill Livingstone, New York, p. 1159.

181 Ho M. Epidemiology of cytomegalovirus infections. *Rev Infect Dis* 1990; **12**: 5701.

182 Smiley L, Huang ES. Cytomegalovirus as a sexually transmitted infection. In: *Sexually Transmitted Diseases,* 2nd edn. McGraw-Hill, New York, 1990, p. 415.

183 Toome BT *et al.* Diagnosis of cytomegalovirus infection: a review and report of a case. *J Am Acad Dermatol* 1991; **24**: 857.

184 Drew WL. Diagnosis of cytomegalovirus infection. *Rev Infect Dis* 1988; **10**: S468.

185 Blatt J *et al.* Cutaneous vesicles in congenital cytomegalovirus infection. *J Pediatr* 1978; **92**: 509.

186 Bhawan J *et al.* Vesiculobullous lesions caused by cytomegalovirus infection in an immunocompromised adult. *J Am Acad Dermatol* 1984; **11**: 743.

187 Feldman PS *et al.* Cutaneous lesions heralding cytomegalovirus infection. *J Am Acad Dermatol* 1982; **7**: 545.

188 Lee JY. Cytomegalovirus infection involving the skin in immunocompromised hosts. *Am J Clin Pathol* 1989; **92**: 96.

189 Fenoglio CM *et al.* Kaposi's sarcoma following chemotherapy for testicular cancer in a homosexual man: demonstration of cytomegalovirus RNA in sarcoma cells. *Hum Pathol* 1982; **15**: 53.

190 Sugiura H. Successful treatment of disseminated cutaneous cytomegalic inclusion disease with Hodgkin's disease. *J Am Acad Dermatol* 1991; **24**: 346.

191 Bournerias I *et al.* Unusual cutaneous cytomegalovirus involvement in patients with acquired immunodeficiency syndrome. *Arch Dermatol* 1989; **24**: 346.

192 Smith KJ *et al.* Concurrent epidermal involvement of cytomegalavirus and herpes simplex virus in two HIV-infected patients. *J Am Acad Dermatol* 1991; **25**: 500.

193 Jacobson MA, Mills J. Serious cytomegalovirus disease in the acquired

immunodeficiency syndrome. *Ann Intern Med* 1988; **108**: 585.

194 Alford CA, Britt WJ. *Cytomegalovirus in Virology*, 2nd edn. Raven, New York, 1990, p. 1981.

195 Wergand DA *et al*. Vasculitis in cytomegalovirus infection. *Arch Dermatol* 1980; **116**: 1174.

196 Horwitz CA *et al*. Clinical and laboratory evaluation of cytomegalovirus induced mononucleosis in previously healthy individuals. *Medicine (Baltimore)* 1986; **65**: 124.

197 Lerner CW, Tapper ML. Opportunistic infection complicating acquired immune deficiency syndrome. *Medicine (Baltimore)* 1984; **63**: 155.

198 Buhles WC *et al*. Ganciclovir treatment of life or sight threatening cytomegalovirus infection: experience in 314 immunocompromised patients. *Rev Infect Dis* 1988; **10**: S495.

199 Marker SC *et al*. Cytomegalovirus infection: a quantitative prospective study of three hundred twenty consecutive renal transplants. *Surgery* 1981; **89**: 660.

200 Schmidt GM *et al*. A randomized controlled trial of prophylactic ganciclovir for cytomegalovirus pulmonary infection in recipients of allogeneic bone marrow transplants. *N Engl J Med* 1991; **324**: 1005.

201 Rubin RH. Impact of cytomegalovirus infection on organ transplant recipients. *Rev Infect Dis* 1990; **12**: S754.

202 Kaplan CS *et al*. Gastrointestinal cytomegalovirus infection in heart and heart–lung transplant recipients. *JAMA* 1989; **149**: 2095.

203 Bloom JN, Palestine AG. The diagnosis of cytomegalovirus retinitis. *Ann Intern Med* 1988; **109**: 963.

204 Bowden RA, Meyers JD. Prophylaxis of cytomegalovirus infection. *Semin Hematol* 1990; **27**: 17.

205 Bowden RA *et al*. Cytomegalovirus (CMV)-specific intravenous immunoglobulin for the prevention of primary CMV infection and disease after marrow transplant. *J Infect Dis* 1991; **164**: 483.

206 Salahuddin SZ *et al*. Isolation of a new virus, HBVL, in patients with lymphoproliferative disorders. *Science* 1986; **234**: 596.

207 Yamanashi K *et al*. Identification of human herpesvirus-6 as a causal agent for exanthem subitum. *Lancet* 1988; **i**: 1065.

208 Takahashi K *et al*. Human herpesvirus-6 and exanthem subitum. *Lancet* 1988; **i**: 1463.

209 Zahorsky J. Roseola infantum. *JAMA* 1913; **61**: 1446.

210 Zahorsky J. Roseola infantilis. *Pediatrics* 1910; **22**: 60.

211 Clemens HH. Exanthem subitum (roseola infantum): report of 80 cases. *J Pediatr* 1945; **26**: 66.

212 James U, Freier A. Roseola infantum: an outbreak in a maternity hospital. *Arch Dis Child* 1948–1949; **23–24**: 54.

213 Suga S *et al*. Neutralizing antibody assay for human herpesvirus-6. *J Med Virol* 1990; **30**: 14.

214 Irving WL, Cunningham AL. Serologic diagnosis of infection with human herpesvirus type 6. *Br Med J* 1990; **300**: 156.

215 Kondo K *et al*. Detection of polymerase chain reaction amplification of human herpes virus-6 DNA in peripheral blood of patients with exanthem subitum. *J Clin Microbiol* 1990; **28**: 970.

216 Burnstine RC, Paine RS. Residual encephalopathy following roseola infantum. *Am J Dis Child* 1959; **98**: 144.

217 Ishiguro N *et al*. Meningo-encephalitis associated with HHV-6 related exanthem subitum. *Acta Paediatr Scand* 1990; **79**: 987.

218 Sobue R *et al*. Fulminant hepatitis in primary herpes-6 infection. *N Engl J Med* 1991; **324**: 1290.

219 Asano Y *et al*. Simultaneous occurrence of human herpesvirus 6 infection and intussusception in three infants. *Pediatr Infect Dis J* 1991; **10**: 335.

220 Burns WH, Sandford GR. Susceptibility of human herpes 6 to antivirals *in vitro*. *J Infect Dis* 1990; **162**: 634.

221 Chang Y *et al*. Identification of herpesvirus-like DNA sequences in AIDS-associated Kaposi's sarcoma. *Science* 1994; **266**: 1865.

222 Moore PS, Chang Y. Detection of herpesvirus-like DNA sequences in Kaposi's sarcoma in patients with and those without HIV infection. *N Engl J Med* 1995; **332**: 1181.

223 Cesarman E *et al*. Kaposi's sarcoma-associated herpesvirus-like DNA sequences in AIDS-related body-cavity-based lymphomas. *N Engl J Med* 1995; **332**: 1186.

224 Rady PL *et al*. Herpesvirus-like DNA sequences in non-Kaposi's sarcoma skin lesions of transplant patients. *Lancet* 1995; **345**: 1339.

225 Hurwitz S. *Clinical Pediatric Dermatology*, 2nd edn. Saunders, Philadelphia, 1993, p. 328.

226 Lowry DR, Androphy EJ. Warts. In: Fitzpatrick TB *et al*. (eds) *Dermatology in General Medicine*, 4th edn. McGraw-Hill, New York, 1993; pp. 2611–2620.

227 Barrasso R *et al*. High prevalence of papillomavirus-associated penile intraepithelial neoplasia in sexual partners of women with cervical intraepithelial neoplasia. *N Engl J Med* 1987; **317**: 916.

228 Mounts P, Shah KV. Respiratory papillomatosis: etiologic relation to genital tract papillomaviruses. *Prog Med Virol* 1984; **29**: 90.

229 Schoenfield A *et al*. Treatment of flat facial warts with interferon-beta cream. *J Dermatol Surg Oncol* 1987; **13**: 299–301.

230 Orlow SJ, Paller A. Cimetidine therapy for multiple viral warts in children. *J Am Acad Dermatol* 1993; **28**: 794.

231 Choi YS *et al*. The effect of cimetidine on verruca plana juvenilis: clinical trials in six patients. *J Dermatol* 1993; **20** (8): 497.

232 Reichman RC *et al*. Treatment of condyloma acuminatum with three different interferon-α preparations administered parenterally: a double-blind, placebo-controlled trial. *J Infect Dis* 1990; **162**: 1270.

233 Reid R *et al*. Superficial laser vulvectomy: V. Surgical debulking is enhanced by adjuvant systemic interferon. *Am J Obstet Gynecol* 1992; **166**: 815.

234 Hutchins SS *et al*. Measles outbreak among unvaccinated preschool-aged children: opportunities missed by health care providers to administer measles vaccine. *Pediatrics* 1989; **83**: 369–374.

235 Morbidity and Mortality Weekly Report. Measles—United States, 1990. *JAMA* 1991; **265**: 3227.

236 Cooper LZ. Measles. In: Fitzpatrick TB *et al*. *Dermatology in General Medicine*, 4th edn. McGraw-Hill, New York, 1993; pp. 2516–2520.

237 Corbett EU. The visceral lesions in measles. *Am J Pathol* 1945; **21**: 905.

238 Morbidity and Mortality Weekly Report. Increase in rubella and congenital rubella syndrome—United States, 1988–1990. *Arch Dermatol* **127**: 465.

239 Gellis SE. Rubella (German measles). In: Fitzpatrick TB *et al*. (eds) *Dermatology in General Medicine*, 4th edn. McGraw-Hill, New York, 1993; pp. 2513–2515.

240 Cossart YE *et al*. Parvovirus-like particles in human sera. *Lancet* 1975; **i**: 72.

241 Anderson MJ *et al*. An outbreak of erythema infectiosum associated with human parvovirus infection. *J Hyg (Lond)* 1984; **93**: 85.

242 Siegl G *et al*. Characteristics and taxonomy of parvoviridae. *Intervirology* 1985; **23**: 61.

243 Anderson MJ, Pattison JR. The human parvovirus. *Arch Virol* 1984; **82**: 137.

244 Anderson LJ. Role of parvovirus B19 in human disease. *Pediatr Infect Dis J* 1987; **6**: 711.

245 Anderson MJ *et al*. Experimental parvoviral infection in humans. *J Infect Dis* 1985;

152: 257.

246 Anon. Risks associated with human parvovirus B19 infection. *Morb Mort Weekly Rep* 1989; **38**: 81.

247 Young N *et al*. Direct demonstration of the human parvovirus in erythroid progenitor cells infected *in vitro*. *J Clin Invest* 1984; **74**: 2024.

248 Anand A *et al*. Humans parvovirus infection in pregnancy and hydrops fetalis. *N Engl J Med* 1987; **316**: 183.

249 Cohen BJ, Buckley MM. The prevalence of antibody to human parvovirus B19 in England and Wales. *J Med Microbiol* 1988; **25**: 151.

250 Anderson MJ *et al*. Diagnosis of human parvovirus infection by dot–blot hybridization using cloned viral DNA. *J Med Virol* 1985; **15**: 163.

251 Salimans MMM *et al*. Rapid detection of human parvovirus B19 DNA by dot–blot hybridization and the polymerase chain reaction. *J Virol Methods* 1989; **23**: 19.

252 Plummer FA *et al*. An erythema infectiosum-like illness caused by human parvovirus infection. *N Engl J Med* 1985; **313**: 74.

253 Ager EA *et al*. Epidemic erythema infectiosum. *N Engl J Med* 1966; **275**: 1326.

254 Feder HM, Anderson J. Fifth disease: a brief review of infections in childhood, in adulthood, and in pregnancy. *Arch Intern Med* 1989; **149**: 2176.

255 Condon FJ. Erythema infectiosum-report of an area-wide outbreak. *Am J Publ Health* 1959; **49**: 528.

256 Tsukada T *et al*. Epidemic of aplastic crisis in patients with hereditary spherocytosis in Japan. *Lancet* 1985; **i**: 1401.

257 Pattison JR *et al*. Parvovirus infections and hypoplastic crisis in sickle-cell anemia (letter). *Lancet* 1981; **i**: 664.

258 Serjeant GR *et al*. Outbreak of aplastic crises in sickle cell anemia associated with parvovirus-like agent. *Lancet* 1981; **ii**: 595.

259 Bertrand Y *et al*. Autoimmune haemolytic anaemia revealed by human parvovirus-linked erythroblastopenia. *Lancet* 1985; **ii**: 382.

260 Duncan JR *et al*. Aplastic crisis due to parvovirus infection in pyruvate kinase deficiency. *Lancet* 1983; **ii**: 14.

261 Lefrere JJ *et al*. Familial human parvovirus infection associated with anemia in siblings with heterozygous β-thalassemia. *J Infect Dis* 1986; **153**: 977.

262 Frickhofen N *et al*. Persistent B19 parvovirus infection in patients infected with human immunodeficiency virus type 1 (HIV-1): a treatable cause of anemia in AIDS. *Ann Intern Med* 1990; **113**: 926.

263 Koch WC *et al*. Manifestations and treatment of human parvovirus B19 infection in immunocompromised patients. *J Pediatr* 1990; **116**: 355.

264 Kurtzman GJ *et al*. Chronic bone marrow failure due to persistent B19 parvovirus infection. *N Engl J Med* 1987; **317**: 287.

265 Belloy M *et al*. Erythroid hypoplasia due to chronic infection with parvovirus B19 (letter). *N Engl J Med* 1990; **322**: 633.

266 Anderson LJ. Human parvovirus. *J Infect Dis* 1990; **161**: 603.

267 Torok TJ. Human parvovirus B19 infections in pregnancy. *Pediatr Infect Dis J* 1990; **9**: 772.

268 Public Health Laboratory Service Working Party on Fifth Disease. Prospective study of human parvovirus (B19) infection in pregnancy. *Br Med J* 1990; **300**: 1166.

269 White DG *et al*. Human parvovirus arthropathy. *Lancet* 1985; **i**: 419.

270 Woolf AD *et al*. Clinical manifestations of human parvovirus B19 in adults. *Arch Intern Med* 1989; **149**: 1153.

271 Jacks TA. Pruritus in parvovirus infection. *J Roy Coll Gen Pract* 1987; **37**: 210.

272 Thurn J. Human parvovirus B19: historical and clinical review. *Rev Infect Dis* 1988; **10**: 1005.

273 Kurtzman G *et al*. Pure red cell aplasia of 10 years duration due to persistent

parvovirus B19 infection and its cure with immunoglobulin therapy. *N Engl J Med* 1990; **322**: 633.

274 Ware R. Human parvovirus infection. *J Pediatr* 1989; **114**: 343.

275 Schwarz TF *et al*. Human parvovirus B19 infection in pregnancy (letter). *Lancet* 1988; **ii**: 566.

276 Darai G *et al*. Analysis of the genome of molluscum contagiosum virus by restriction endonuclease analysis and molecular cloning. *J Med Virol* 1986; **18**: 29.

277 Porter CD, Archard LC. Characterization and physical mapping of molluscum contagiosum virus DNA and location of a sequence capable of encoding a conserved domain of epidermal growth factor. *J Gen Virol* 1987; **68**: 673.

278 Porter CD *et al*. Molluscum contagiosum virus types in genital and non-genital lesions. *Br J Dermatol* 1989; **120**: 37.

279 Scholz J *et al*. Epidemiology of molluscum contagiosum using genetic analysis of the viral DNA. *J Med Virol* 1989; **27**: 87.

280 Viac J, Chardonnet Y. Immunocompetent cells and epithelial cell modifications in molluscum contagiosium. *J Cutan Pathol* 1990; **17**: 202.

281 Epstein WL, Fukuyama K. Maturation of molluscum contagiosum virus (MCV) *in vivo*: quantitative electron microscopic autoradiography. *J Invest Dermatol* 1973; **60**: 73.

282 Brown ST *et al*. Molluscum contagiosum: sexually transmitted disease in 17 cases. *J Am Vener Dis Assoc* 1974; **1**: 35.

283 Wilkin JK. Molluscum contagiosum venereum in a women's outpatient clinic: a venereally transmitted disease. *Am J Obstetr Gynecol* 1977; **128**: 531.

284 Lynch PJ, Minkin W. Molluscum contagiosum of the adult: probably venereal transmission. *Arch Dermatol* 1969; **98**: 141–143.

285 DeOrea GA *et al*. An eczematous reaction associated with molluscum contagosium. *Arch Dermatol* 1956; **74**: 344.

286 Goodman DS *et al*. Prevalence of cutaneous disease in patients with acquired immunodeficiency syndrome (AIDS) or AIDS-related complex. *J Am Acad Dermatol* 1987; **17**: 210.

287 Matis WL *et al*. Dermatologic findings associated with human immunodeficiency virus infection. *J Am Acad Dermatol* 1987; **17**: 746.

288 Leavell UW Jr, Jacob RJ. Orf. In: Fitzpatrick TB *et al*. (eds) *Dermatology in General Medicine*, 4th edn. McGraw-Hill, New York, 1993; pp. 2603–2605.

289 Shelley WB, Shelley EP. Surgical treatment of farmyard pox: orf, milker's nodules, bovine papular stomatitis pox. *Cutis* 1983; **31**: 191–192.

290 Sonck CE, Penttinen K. Milker's nodules: transmission from man to man. *Acta Dermatol Venereol (Stockh)* 1954; **34**: 420.

291 Wheeler CE, Cawley EP. The etiology of milker's nodules. Arch Dermatol 1967: **75**: 249.

292 Leavell UW Jr, Phillip IA. Milker's nodules: pathogenesis, tissue culture, electron microscopy, and calf inoculation. *Arch Dermatol* 1975; **111**: 1307.

293 Ishimaru Y *et al*. Outbreaks of hand, foot, and mouth disease by enterovirus 71. *Arch Dis Child* 1980; **55**: 583.

294 Hood AF, Mihm MC Jr. Hand–foot and mouth disease. In: Fitzpatrick *et al*. (eds) *Dermatology in General Medicine*, 4th edn. McGraw-Hill, New York, 1993; pp. 2521–2523.

295 Evans AD, Waddington E. Hand, foot, and mouth disease in South Wales, 1964. *Br J Dermatol* 1967; **79**: 309.

296 Wright HT Jr *et al*. Fatal infection in an infant associated with Coxsackie virus group A, type 16. *N Engl J Med* 1963; **268**: 1041.

297 Baker DA, Phillips CA. Fatal hand-foot-and-mouth disease in an infant caused by Coxsackie virus A$_7$. *JAMA* 1979; **242**: 1065.

298 Tindall JP, Miller GD. Hand, foot and mouth disease. *Cutis* 1972; **9**: 457.

299 Goldbery MF, McAdams AJ. Myocarditis possibly due to Coxsackie group A, type 16, virus. *J Pediatr* 1963; **62**: 762.

300 Froeschie JE *et al*. Hand, foot and mouth disease (Coxsackie A$_{16}$) in Atlanta. *Am J Dis Child* 1967; **114**: 278.

301 Magoffin RL, Lenette EH. Nonpoliovirus and paralytic disease. *Calif Med* 1962; **97**: 1.

302 Gohd RS, Faigel HC. Hand-foot-and-mouth disease resembling measles. A life-threatening disease: case report. *Pediatrics* 1966; **37**: 644.

303 Kalyanaraman VS *et al*. A new subtype of human T-cell leukemia virus (HTLV-2) associated with a T-cell variant of hairy cell leukemia. *Science* 1982; **218**: 571.

304 Blattner WA. Retroviruses. In: Evans AS (ed.) *Viral Infections of Humans: Epidemiology and Control*. Plenum, New York, 1989, p. 545.

305 Saxinger WC *et al*. Human T-cell leukemia virus (HTLV-1) antibodies in Africa. *Science* 1984; **225**: 1473.

306 de The G *et al*. Human retroviruses HTLV-1, HIV-1, and HIV-2 and neurological diseases in some equatorial areas of Africa. *AIDS* 1989; **2**: 550.

307 Kwok S *et al*. Enzymatic amplification of HTLV-1 viral sequences from peripheral blood mononuclear cell and infected tissues. *Blood* 1988; **72**: 1117.

308 Greaves MF *et al*. Human T-cell leukemia virus (HTLV) in the United Kingdom. *Int J Cancer* 1984; **33**: 795.

309 Bunder CB *et al*. Indolent cutaneous prodrome of fatal HTLV-1 infection. *Lancet* 1990; **335**: 426.

310 La Grenade L *et al*. Infective dermatitis of Jamaican children: a marker for HTLV-1 infection. *Lancet* 1990; **336**: 1345.

311 Jono M *et al*. ATL and skin eruptions. *Hihubyou-shinryou (Japan)* 1987; **9**: 206.

312 Shimoyama M *et al*. Major prognostic factors of adult patients with advanced T-cell lymphoma/leukemia. *J Clin Oncol* 1988; **68**: 169.

313 Zalla MJ *et al*. Dermatologic manifestations of human immunodeficiency virus infection. *Mayo Clin Proc* 1992; **67**: 1089.

314 Stickler MC *et al*. Kaposi's sarcoma. *Clin Dermatol* 1991; **9**: 39.

315 Zugar JM *et al*. Bacterial infections in AIDS: Part 1. *AIDS Clin Care* 1992; **4**: 69.

316 Cockerell CJ *et al*. Clinical, histologic, microbiologic, and biochemical characterization of the causative agent of bacillary (epithelioid) angiomatosis: a rickettsial illness with features of bartonellosis. *J Invest Dermatol* 1991; **97** (5): 812.

317 De Wit S *et al*. Comparison of fluconazole and ketoconazole for oropharyngeal candidiasis in AIDS. *Lancet* 1989; **i**: 746.

318 Laine L *et al*. Fluconazole compared with ketoconazole for the treatment of *Candida* esophagitis in AIDS: a randomized trial. *Ann Intern Med* 1992; **117**: 655.

319 Lee MM *et al*. Onychomycosis (letter). *Arch Dermatol* 1990; **126**: 402.

320 Don PC *et al*. Herpetic infection mimicking chronic neurotic excoriation. *Int J Dermatol* 1991; **30**: 136.

321 Erlich KS *et al*. Acyclovir-resistant herpes simplex virus infections in patients with the acquired immunodeficiency syndrome. *N Engl J Med* 1989; **320**: 293.

322 Sall RK *et al*. Successful treatment of progressive acyclovir-resistant herpes simplex virus using intravenous foscarnet in a patient with the acquired immunodeficiency syndrome. *Arch Dermatol* 1989; **125**: 1548.

323 Sanchez M *et al*. Treatment of oral hairy leukoplakia with podophyllin. *Arch Dermatol* 1992; **28**: 1659.

324 Palefsky J *et al*. Anal intraepithelial neoplasia and papillomavirus infection among homosexual males with group IV HIV disease. *JAMA* 1990; **263**: 2911.

325 Porges DY *et al*. A novel use of the cryptococcal latex agglutination test for rapid presumptive diagnosis of cutaneous cryptococcosis. *Arch Dermatol* 1992; **128**: 461.

326 Oscherwitz SL *et al*. Disseminated sporotrichosis in a patient infected with human immunodeficiency virus. *Clin Infect Dis* 1992; **15**: 568.

327 Bibler MR *et al*. Disseminated sporotrichosis in a patient with HIV infection after treatment of acquired VII inhibitor. *JAMA* 1986; **256**: 125.

328 Wikler JR *et al*. Quantitative skin cultures of *Pityrosporum* yeasts in patients seropositive for the human immunodeficiency virus with and without seborrheic dermatitis. *J Am Acad Dermatol* 1992; **27**: 37.

329 Harris DWS *et al*. Eosinophilic pustular follucilitis in an HIV-positive man: response to cetirizine. *Br J Dermatol* 1992; **126**: 392.

330 Horn TD *et al*. Characterization of the dermal infiltrate in human immunodeficiency virus-infected patients with psoriasis. *Arch Dermatol* 1990; **126**: 1462.

331 Duvic M *et al*. Remission of AIDS-associated psoriasis. *Lancet* 1987; **ii**: 627.

Chapter 6
Parasitic Infections

Ectoparasites
Mervyn L. Elgart

We share our environment with many species of invertebrates: insects, mites, ticks, crabs, clams, worms and lobsters. For the most part, we live parallel lives and do not intrude on each other. But there are some invertebrates that have the ability to cause disease in humans, and this chapter addresses this group of creatures.

Arthropods

Arthropods harm humans for two reasons: as a necessary blood meal for a moult or procreation and for food, especially when their usual source of supply is unavailable. Occasional insects bite or sting in anger, but usually this is a defensive mechanism and, despite our unreasonable fears, not purposely aggressive behaviour. Arthropods are divided into two groups: the insects, six-legged creatures, and arachnids, eight-legged creatures.

Insects

Insects are six-legged creatures that can produce pathology in a number of ways. In this chapter, we shall discuss the direct attack of the insects, rather than concern ourselves with the transmission of bacterial, viral or rickettsial disease. However, a table of arthropod transmission of these diseases is given (Table 6.1).

Papular urticaria

Papular urticaria is an allergic reaction to a bite, usually seen as an erythematous papule. Alexander [1] (quoting Mellanby) states that, when a person is bitten by a 'new' insect, there is initially no reaction. After a variable period of time, the patient develops delayed hypersensitivity, and a papular response with a surrounding halo appears after a 24-hour delay (Fig. 6.1). When this occurs, papular urticaria is seen clinically. Again, after

Table 6.1 Insect and mite vectors of disease.

Common name	Scientific name	Disease
Sandfly	*Phlebotomus* spp.	Leishmaniasis (Europe, Africa, Asia); sandfly fever
Sandfly	*Lutzomyia* and sometimes *Psychodopygus*	Leishmaniasis (North and South America); bartonellosis
Tsetse fly	*Glossina* spp.	Trypanosomiasis
Reduviid bug	Reduviidae	Chagas' disease
Assassin bug		(American trypanosomiasis)
Black flies	*Simulium* flies *Chrysops* fly	Onchocerciasis Loiasis (Calabar swellings)
Flies	*Tabanus* spp.	Tularaemia, anthrax
Fleas	*Xenopsylla cheopis*, *Xenopsylla braziliensis*	*Rickettsia mooseri* typhus
Body lice	*Pediculosis hominis* var. *corporis*	Typhus, tick fever, trench fever Brill–Zinser disease
Rat flea	*Xenopsylla cheopis*	Bubonic plague
Mosquitoes	*Aëdes aegypti*	Yellow fever
Mosquitoes	*Anopheles* spp.	Malaria
Mosquitoes	*Psorophora* spp.	*Dermatobia hominis* eggs
Mosquitoes	Various species of *Culex*, *Aëdes*, *Anopheles*, *Culicoides*, and *Mansonia*	Bancroftian and Malayan filariasis; viral encephalitis: Eastern equine, western equine, Venezuela, Japanese B, St Louis, West Nile, Rift Valley fever
Mosquitoes		Malaria
Mosquitoes		Dengue fever
Various small mammal mites	Trombiculid mites	Scrub typhus
Mouse mite	*Liponyssoides sanguineus*	Rickettsialpox
Hard ticks: deer-tick	*Ixodes scapularis, Ixodes pacificus* and other *Ixodes* spp.	Lyme disease
Hard ticks: dog tick and others	*Dermacentor andersoni* and other *Dermacentor* species	Rocky Mountain, eastern, western and South American spotted fever; Siberian tick typhus
Soft ticks	*Ornithodorus* spp.	Endemic relapsing fever

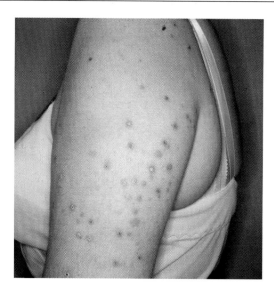

Fig. 6.1 Papular urticaria from flea bites.

another variable period of time, the patient develops immediate hypersensitivity. At that time, there is an immediate weal after the bite, followed in 24 hours by the delayed response. Slowly, the delayed hypersensitivity disappears and there is only an immediate weal. Finally, even the immediate response disappears after several months, and there is no longer any response to the insects. In this way, children seem to be the most common victims, and adults who have been in the endemic area for years are being bitten but are no longer sensitive.

Each lesion of papular urticaria represents a bite and a sensitivity response to the bite. Mellanby's original work was done with mosquitoes, but fleas and bedbugs (various species of *Cimex*) are frequent causes. Bedbugs usually prefer exposed skin and often produce several bites in a linear arrangement. Other haematophagous insects include the triatomes, particularly the Reduviidae. These usually feed once, instead of producing linear papules.

Phlebotomus and *Lutzomyia* flies can carry leishmaniasis, but, even in the absence of this, can produce a papular urticaria-like response in exposed areas to newcomers to a region. In Israel, this has been called harara [1]. These flies, biting midges and *Simulium* flies (buffalo flies or black flies) attack in large numbers, and produce many erythematous papules.

Bites are treated with topical corticosteroids or oral antihistamines. The use of insect repellents, such as DEET (N,N-diethyl-m-toluamide), or toxins, such as permethrin (Elimite), on the skin before exposure can prevent the insects from biting.

Pustules

Pustules are characteristic of stings from the fire ant (*Solenopsis*). These creatures are abundant in Central and South America and have been spreading over the south-eastern portion of the USA. They live in mounds in fields, but cannot live where a hard frost will take place. Both red (*Solonopsis invicta*) and black (*Solonopsis richardi*) (Fig. 6.2) fire ants are present in the involved area.

When a fire ant is disturbed, the worker ant bites the offending skin with its teeth. It then bends the body around and stings the adjacent areas, depositing a venom. It may move around, producing several stings around a central petechial mark from teeth. A small papule develops after each sting. In 4 hours, it is a vesicle and, in 8–10 hours, a pustule. The pustules crust and heal over 3–10 days [2]. When an individual falls asleep near a fire anthill and it overrun with fire ants, many pustules are noted.

Pustules may also be noted as a secondary phenomenon — secondary infection after the skin has been broken by the bites of the insect or by the scratching of the victim. In these instances, bacteria can be seen on Gram stain and cultured, whereas, with primary pustules, the lesions are sterile.

Bullae

Bullous reactions occur in several insect-bite situations. Most are caused by oedema and severe immunological reaction to the insect. They can be seen from a variety of insects and sometimes in scabies infestations (see below).

The blister beetle is a South American insect in the Meloidae family that contains cantharidin. This substance produces acantholysis, causing bullae if the insect is crushed against the skin. If the beetle is not crushed or damaged, no reaction takes place. The beetle, *Lytta vesicatoria*, is also known as the Spanish fly. Other beetles cause blisters, including those in the *Paederus* genus. The mechanism is the same as for the blister beetle [1].

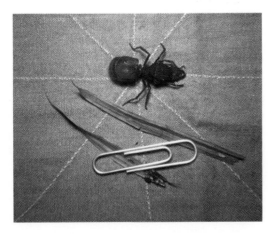

Fig. 6.2 The black fire ant, *Solonopsis richardi.*

Vicious biters

These are insects that tear at the skin, producing a painful bite. *Chrysops* (deer-flies), *Tabanus* (horse flies) and Hematopota (clegs) cause these kinds of bites, tearing tissue, which often becomes secondarily infected [1]. The reduviid bug bites and then defecates into the open wound. The contamination is responsible for the transmission of American trypanosomiasis.

Stings

Insect stings are the property of the Hymenoptera—bees, ants, wasps and hornets. Although not often a dermatological problem, the extreme sensitivity of some individuals to these insects causes respiratory failure and is probably the cause of death for as many as 40 persons a year in the USA. Treatment is adrenaline if the patient has an immediate reaction and desensitization to prevent future problems.

Wasps and hornets sting and remove the stinger from the skin. Bees, however, sting and the stinging mechanism is torn from their bodies. The stinger and attached poison sacs may be seen in the patient. It is important in trying to remove the stinger not to further empty the poison sacs. This is done by taking a scalpel blade and working the stinger free with this, rather than trying to grasp the top and risk squeezing material from the poison sacs into the patient [3].

Pruritus

Pruritus can be caused by many things, including medical diseases, such as renal failure and jaundice, and psychogenic causes. Insects or mites can cause pruritus, but often there are other signs, such as papules or burrows of scabies. Lice, especially head lice or pubic lice in individuals who bathe frequently, may only cause pruritus, with no obvious lesions. Animal mites may produce similar symptoms. The causative organisms may be found only by careful inspection.

Lice

There are three forms of lice (Anoplura). Head lice and body lice are indistinguishable, except that the body lice are larger. Pubic lice are shorter and resemble crabs (crab lice, *Phthirus pubis*).

Head lice and pubic lice produce mostly pruritus, but bites may be observed. Lice are easily found in the pubic area, at the base of the hair, where they lay their eggs (nits) on the hair. Head lice are much harder to locate, but the nits may be obvious, especially in warm areas, such as the occiput. Pubic lice prefer short hair, and may be seen on other short body hair, such as the eyebrows, eyelashes, axillary hair and the short hair at the nape of the neck. In each instance, nits require 5 days to develop and for a young nymph to hatch. The length of the infestation may be determined by measurement of the length of hair on the nit which is the most distant from the surface of the skin. Since hair grows approximately 1 cm per month, the length of time of the infestation can be determined. Treatment with permethrin (Nix shampoo) or gamma benzyl hexachloride (Kwell) is usually effective. Treatment of disease on the eyelashes is difficult, but physostigmine ointment may be used [4].

Body lice are an increasing presence in our emergency rooms, as there is an increasing number of homeless patients. The lesions are excoriated, usually secondarily infected, papules, pustules or ulcers in covered areas (Fig. 6.3). The organisms are found not on the patient but in seams of clothing (Fig. 6.4). A shower, a change of clothing and a course of antibiotics are needed. In time of war or movement of large numbers of persons, body lice can transmit typhus, or trench fever.

Caterpillar dermatitis

This is manifested by urticarial lesions and sometimes dermatitis (Fig. 6.5). The caterpillars have hollow hairs on the dorsum, which may contain histamine and other compounds to be deposited into the skin. Initially, there may be a burning or pain, followed by itch and the appearance of erythematous papules or, sometimes, weals. These lesions may be limited to the

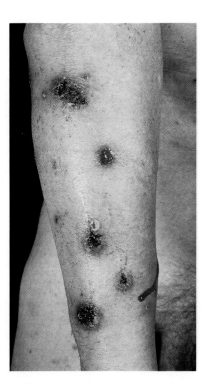

Fig. 6.3 Infected bites in covered areas in a patient with body lice.

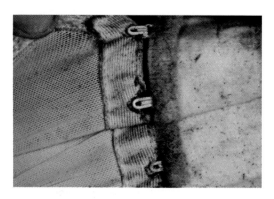

Fig. 6.4 Body lice on a brassière that has not been changed for several weeks.

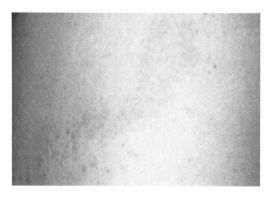

Fig. 6.5 Caterpillar dermatitis caused by the woolly bear caterpillar.

area of contact or may be widespread. Exposed areas are most commonly involved. Although the dermatitis fades in several days, lichenification and persistance may rarely develop [5].

The only caterpillar dermatitis that is different from the above is that caused by the asp, or *Megalopyge* larva. The sting of this caterpillar produces pain that radiates, erythema, lymphangitis and systemic symptoms. Weakness, shock and death have been reported rarely [6].

The *Hylesia* moth has also caused contact dermatitis from touching individuals. The moths are attracted to light, and swarm several times a year. Large numbers may therefore appear, and even the dust released from these may cause a dermatitis in selected areas near the coast of Venezuela.

Temporary parasitism

Tunga penetrans. The burrowing flea, *Tunga penetrans*, is found in Africa and South America. Rapid modern transportation has led to reports of the disease in more temperate climates [7].

The female *Tunga* flea mates and then must find a source of food to feed its developing brood. It begins to jump, and does so until it locates the soft keratin on the palm or sole or around nails. Here, it works its body into the

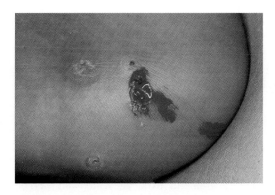

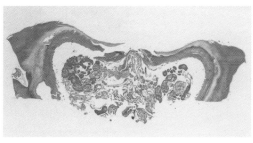

Fig. 6.7 Biopsy of *Tunga penetrans* infestation (courtesy George Elgart, MD, Department of Dermatology, University of Miami School of Medicine).

Fig. 6.6 *Tunga penetrans* infestation in a young adult who had been hiking in Panama for the summer.

flesh, in such a way that its head is in the viable dermis and its cloacal opening is still exposed to the air (Figs 6.6 & 6.7). This it must do to continue to breathe and, eventually, to lay its fully developed eggs. As the eggs develop, it becomes large and almost completely changed to a sac containing a huge ovary. As the eggs mature, they are extruded through the anal opening. Finally, the *Tunga* flea body collapses and it dies [8].

Tungiasis, also known as the 'jigger', has given rise to the expression, 'I'll be jiggered.' Other common names include nigua, chica, pico, pique and chigoe. In many countries, there is confusion with the chigger (species of *Eutrombicula*) and patients are concerned that the chigger has burrowed into the flesh. Chigger mites, however, simply bite and drop off.

Tunga can be removed by curettage. At one clinic in Brazzaville, such treatment left an opening through which 25% of cases developed tetanus [9]!

Cutaneous myiasis. Myiasis is caused when developing fly larvae burrow into flesh to undergo several developmental changes. This is known as furuncular myiasis, as opposed to wound myiasis (see below).

Dermatobia hominis is the organism often seen as a cause of furuncular myiasis in the western hemisphere, although *Cuterebra* spp. and *Hypoderma* spp. can also cause difficulty. In Africa, the tumbu fly, *Cordylobia anthropophaga*, produces similar lesions. Animals are the primary hosts, but humans are occasionally accidentally involved.

The female *Dermatobia hominis* lays its eggs on the underside of a mosquito. When the mosquito lands on a prospective host, the warmth of the host causes the eggs to hatch and the *Dermatobia* larvae burrow into the skin of that host. Usually, the recipient is cattle, but humans are an accidental host, usually on the scalp or shoulders. The larva burrows down, but always maintains a breathing tube that is in contact with the surface (Fig. 6.8). Initially, there is a small reddened papule in 24 hours, which enlarges over 3 weeks to a dome-shaped papule with a central opening, which may have a discharge. The larva goes through four instars, or moults, and portions of the cast larval skin may be present in the discharge. Marked erythema, oedema and even lymphadenopathy may result. If left alone, it takes about 49 days before the mature larva extrudes itself from the skin and drops to the ground to pupate.

Treatment of this condition takes advantage of the necessity of the larva to be in contact with the air. A slab of fat or bacon can be placed over the papule, and the larva must then raise itself so that the air tube is in contact with the air. The fat is then removed—with the larva. Alternatively, xylocaine can be used to anaesthetize the area and the larva, which can then be removed easily (Fig. 6.9). Attempts to remove the larva without anaesthesia are fruitless.

Dermatobia and *Cuterebra* are obligate screw-worms—that is, they must burrow into a vertebrate to complete their life cycle. The animal host often produces an immune response, so that animals that have survived the first season may be immune to further attacks. This fact has been taken advantage of in producing a vaccine for cattle to prevent further attacks of myiasis. The vaccination has been moderately successful.

Cordylobia anthropophaga lays its eggs on the ground in shady areas. The newly hatched larva seeks an animal in which to develop—usually the

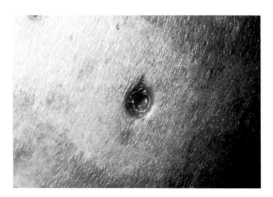

Fig. 6.8 Myiasis caused by *Cuterebra* larva. Note tiny breathing tube. (Photo courtesy Dr Nancy McCallum.)

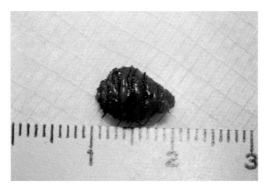

Fig. 6.9 Extruded larva of *Cuterebra* species. (Photo courtesy Dr Nancy McCallum.)

brown rat. In areas of human habitation, the human sleeps on the area and multiple lesions develop. Alternatively, clothing may be dried on the ground, and the larva then invades the next wearer. It is important to remove the larvae in ways similar to that used for *Dermatobia*. Wounds from removed larvae heal relatively quickly, while those from which the larvae emerge themselves often take a long time to heal and leave permanent depressed scars.

The Congo floor maggot, or *Auchmeromyia luteola* fly, is somewhat similar, producing maggots that live in the ground. These burrow up at night and suck blood from sleeping victims, but never burrow into the skin and drop off in 20 minutes or so.

Hypoderma spp. attack cattle around the ankles. They are seen in Europe, North America, South Africa and Australia. These flies are different, because they migrate from the original area of penetration to some body cavity and later to the skin, where a 'warble' is formed. In humans, the affected individual is usually one in contact with cattle or sheep. The recurrent swellings may be incised under anaesthesia to make the diagnosis.

In addition to the above, some flies will lay their eggs in dead matter and produce an 'accidental' myiasis. The common housefly can do this and, indeed, sterile maggots, United States Pharmacopeia (USP), were sold to physicians in the early part of the twentieth century to débride wounds. They would eat the dead matter and leave the live tissue alone [10].

Another form of wound myiasis is produced by species of *Callitroga* or *Chrysomyia*. These parasites live in wounds of animals and, rarely, humans. They can cause the death of animals by parasitizing nasal passages. The treatment involves cleansing wounds with chloroform, so as to destroy the larva, and then irrigating the wound.

Arachnids

Spiders

Spiders have two distinct regions, a cephalothorax, which contains mouthparts, and an abdomen. There are four sets of legs. Although there are many spiders that can occasionally bite humans, only two produce significant disease in the USA. They may produce three types of venom: neurotoxic, cytotoxic and haemolytic.

The black widow spider, *Latrodectus mactans*, is characterized by a red mark on the ventral abdomen. This mark has been called a 'shoe button' or 'hourglass' pattern. The female spends its time in hidden areas, most characteristically in lavatories. The spider can sometimes bite, if disturbed. The skin lesion is usually noted to be barely visible. However, there are serious systemic symptoms present. They begin with severe pain, which may be cramping and is not relieved by morphine. Shock or hypotension may follow. The reaction rarely lasts more than 24 hours, and may be treated with an antivenin. Calcium gluconate may provide immediate, if brief, respite.

There are several species of brown recluse spider. The most common in the USA is *Loxosceles reclusa*, otherwise known as the 'fiddle spider', because of the violin-like mark on the top of the thorax/abdomen. She bites only when disturbed, and produces a reaction in which there is a necrotic centre, surrounded by an area of vasoconstriction, surrounded by an area of erythema. This is the 'red, white and blue' sign, which takes 8–12 hours to develop. Dapsone has been used to treat the intense inflammatory reaction, but must be used early in the course, of the disease [11, 12]. High-voltage direct current [13] and surgical curettage [14] have also been recommended.

Necrotic arachnidism is the title given to this form of necrotic reaction thought to be due to a variety of spiders worldwide. In Australia, several species have been implicated, although *Loxosceles* species, as above, are the organisms most commonly responsible. In Africa, sac spiders (*Chiracanthium* spp.) are more frequent [15]. In the north-western part of the USA, *Tegenaria agrestis*, a spider introduced from Europe, is often the cause [16]. In some instances, there may have been secondary infection with *Mycobacterium ulcerans* [17].

Viscerocutaneous arachnidism may develop after some bites. These patients develop chills, restlessness, headache and fever and later ecchymoses, jaundice and pulmonary congestion.

Red-back spiders in Western Australia have caused several deaths. The venom contains a neurotoxin, and the treatment is a tourniquet and antivenom. One report reviews a 6-year experience and estimates 830–1950 cases per year in Australia [18].

The golden orb weaver, a large spider, may cause pain on biting. The jumping spiders have caused local pain and swelling. The huntsman spiders (Sparassidae) are found in Australia, and may cause pain and, occasionally, malaise, headache, nausea and vomiting [19].

Mites

Scabies. Of the many mites in our environment, *Sarcoptes scabiei* var. *hominis* causes the most concern. There is a worldwide epidemic, in which the scabies mite has caused a great amount of infestation.

The adult female scabies mite measures 0.4mm in diameter. It has four pairs of legs (Fig. 6.10). The male is about two-thirds the size, and its most posterior pair of legs is modified so as to allow it to grasp the female better. After mating, the male dies, while the female burrows into the keratin, usually on the hands, near the nipples, in the axilla or close to the genitalia. As it burrows, it lays eggs. Burrows can be several millimetres to 1–2cm in diameter. New larvae have only three pairs of legs, and moult twice through two nymph stages in 10 days before becoming adults. The entire process takes 10–15 days [20].

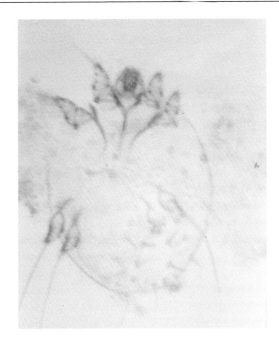

Fig. 6.10 An adult female *Sarcoptes scabiei* var. *hominis*. She has been partially damaged by the process of scraping the burrow.

When a human scabies mite lands on the skin of a person who has not previously been infested, there is no response by the patient. A response of itching requires an intact immune system, and takes approximately 30 days. When the sensitivity is established, the mite has already established itself in many areas, and severe itching intervenes. The patient works furiously to excoriate the mites and, eventually, in 90–120 days, will do so. Thereupon, the patient is clear, but, if he/she is ever exposed again to the mite, it is scratched off before the mite has a chance to develop [21].

If an animal scabies mite lands on a human, there is immediate itching and the mite cannot establish burrows. If a human does not have an intact immune system, the scabies mites can multiply without restriction, producing 'Norwegian scabies' (see below).

The disease is usually transmitted by close body contact. Since the mite is present on the hands, as well as the genitalia, simple touching may be enough to transmit the disease. Many cases are transmitted by sexual contact, but scabies is not an obligatory venereal disease.

The disease presents with severe itching and excoriations. Burrows are found especially on the wrists and between the fingers and around the breasts, axillae and genitalia. Sometimes, bullae are prevalent [22]. In children, the feet and sometimes the face may be involved. In some patients, a severe inflammatory reaction produces deep nodules, which may remain for several months after the scabies are removed. In Third-World nations, secondary impetigo is common, and this may lead to glomerulonephritis [23]. In the USA, the disease is more annoying than terrible, and simple treatment is effective.

When the immune response is lacking, mites continue to multiply, leading to a crusted scabies with millions of mites evident. This was first described in Norway, and has been called Norwegian scabies (Fig. 6.11) [24]. In a case that demonstrates the importance of the immune response, a child who was to receive a bone-marrow transplant presumably developed scabies while undergoing radiation and chemotherapy. There were no symptoms until day 23 following bone-marrow transplant, when engraftment had definitely taken place [25]. Patients with acquired immune deficiency syndrome (AIDS) have shown a predilection for this type of scabies [26].

Treatment of the disease consists of treating all exposed individuals, whether or not they have symptoms. To my mind, the best available treatment in the USA is permethrin (Elimite). This is a modified pyrethrin, an insect toxin from chrysanthemums. The lotion is applied once, from the neck down, including all folds of skin. In prepubertal children, the face, ears and neck must also be treated. The material is substantive to the skin and remains in place through several washings. It is therefore present if new organisms hatch out or if there is inadvertent contact with an untreated person. The product kills mites on contact and is therefore quite useful [27, 28].

Other treatments include the use of crotamiton (Eurax), or lindane (Kwell), which some have found to produce neurotoxic symptoms [29]. The use of lindane has been both decried and defended [30]. It seems a reasonable drug if used properly. It should not be used on extremely open skin wounds or moist skin. It should not be left on over 8 hours. Ten per cent

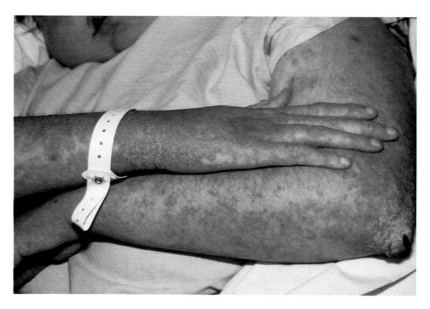

Fig. 6.11 Crusted (Norwegian) scabies in a patient with renal transplantation and on immunosuppressive drugs.

precipitated sulphur in petrolatum is a cheap alternative treatment; it smells bad but works well. It must be reapplied daily for 3 days.

Ivermectin orally has been proved to be very useful, but is not available for such use in the USA. It is used in the USA for animals. Ivermectin has been given to hundreds of thousands for the treatment of onchocerciasis, with very little toxicity [31–33]. Clothes should be washed or dry-cleaned. Since the mite cannot exist for long without human contact, leaving clothing for 5 days is safe. The mite probably survives longer when the temperature and humidity are elevated [34].

Much has been written about resistant scabies. In my personal experience, I have never seen a case. When I have suspected resistance, it has always turned out that an additional person was exposed who was not treated and who reinfected the patient.

Other human mites. The only other mites seen normally in humans are the *Demodex* mites, *Demodex brevis* and *Demodex follicularis*. These mites exist in follicles. the *D. follicularis* in hair follicles and *D. brevis* in sebaceous follicles. They spend their lives in groups of two to four with their heads down toward the deeper portions of the follicle [35].

These mites do not seem to cause disease, although some blame them for acne rosacea and others have found proliferation of these mites in the face of a lack of immunity, as in AIDS patients. This is similar to demodectic mange seen in dogs as a manifestation of reduced natural immunity. Treatment with metronidazole has helped rosacea, and some have attributed this response to a lowering in the number of *Demodex* organisms.

Non-human mites. There are many other mites in nature. Almost every other species of vertebrate has scabies mites of one type or another, which causes grief to that particular organism, but which, under suitable circumstances, can also affect humans. Although there are plant mites, humans do not seem to be a frequent recipient of trauma from these organisms (see below).

Animal scabies mites cause disease in humans as a secondary phenomenon. Dog scabies (*S. scabiei* var. *canis*) attacks dogs and produces mange (Fig. 6.12). When there is a severe infestation, the mite can attack the dogs' caretakers as well. These infestations are noteworthy for a series of interesting symptoms.

Because all animal mites produce pruritus as soon as they are in contact with the skin, patients scratch at the mites before the mites have an opportunity to burrow. Therefore, one sees symptoms of pruritic papules in areas in contact with the dog. The itching generally improves when the dog is removed from immediate contact. While mites are rarely found on the human, the diagnosis is usually made by finding the offending dog and doing a scraping on the mange which it possesses. Treatment of the dog is generally sufficient to take care of the human patient. Some, however,

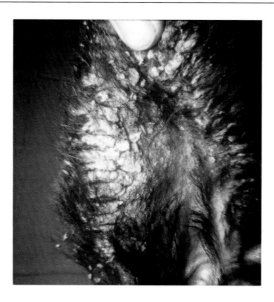

Fig. 6.12 *Sarcoptes scabiei* var. *canis* in the ear of a black spaniel.

would treat the human with permethrin (Elimite), which would protect the skin against the biting of dog mites for several days. Topical steroids and other antipruritic measures would be of value.

Other animals have scabies—cats, horses, lions, wolves, etc. Vets and animal trainers often note that they get itching after exposure to animals, and careful examination allows them to discover mange in the animals. Treatment of the animals, usually with ivermectin, is curative.

Cheyletiella is a mite which is similar to scabies, but has a slightly 'cinched in' waist (Fig. 6.13). It lives on rabbits and sometimes cats or dogs, particularly young rabbits, puppies and kittens. In these species, there is no mange, but, rather, a form of scaling, which has been called 'walking dandruff'. The human disease consists of bites in exposed areas (Fig. 6.14). Diagnosis is difficult without seeing the pet, but may be made on examination of groomings from the pet. The treatment of the animal may require ivermectin, while the patient may use permethrin (Elimite) and topical steroids.

Bird mites come in two varieties: *Ornithonyssus* mites, which remain on the bird's body at all times, and *Dermanyssus* mites, which remain in the nest during the day and bite the bird at night. The mites that remain in the nest are caught in a bind in May or June, when certain birds do not return to their nests. The mites, now quite hungry, seek other food. If the nests have been on trees near windows or in chimneys, the nearby humans may be bitten. Often, they will bring mites in with them, since there are many mites to be found. To treat this infestation, the nest needs to be removed and the house needs to be sprayed [36].

Ornithonyssus mites occur in birds and mammals. When the *Ornithonyssus* mites are involved in human disease, the host bird or animal has

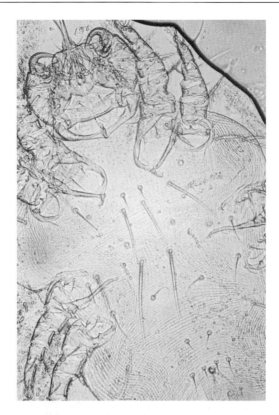

Fig. 6.13 Demonstration of a *Cheyletiella* organism from the cat pictured in Fig. 6.14.

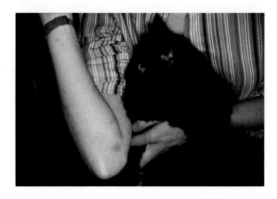

Fig. 6.14 Cat and owner. Although the cat has no evidence of mange, the owner had many bites on exposed areas. The cat's 'dandruff' was examined to reveal the organism pictured in Fig. 6.13.

usually died. As the temperature drops, the mites wander off in search of warm hosts. Birds, rats and mice have been reported. They may inadvertently find humans and bite [37]. Treatment is the same as for other mites.

In addition to the infestations produced by these mites, occasional mites may carry disease, such as *Liponyssoides sanguineus*, the mouse mite, which can carry rickettsialpox.

Plant mites. While plant mites generally do not affect humans, there are plant mites that have caused disease. When flour and other foods were sold in bulk, *Tyroglyphus* and *Pyemotes* mites were common and caused itching in individuals who handled the flour—grocer's itch, grain itch, etc. These have generally affected only the hands.

The other mite generally found on plants that bothers humans is the eutrombiculid mites. There are many species in different parts of the world, including harvest mite in the USA and UK, orange tawney in Ireland, tlalzutal in Mexico, alamushi in Japan, etc. All produce similar disease. These are six-legged larval forms of the eight-legged mature mites. They stand on vegetation and grab on to whatever animal — human or four-legged — that goes by. When an appropriate animal passes, the mite attaches itself, climbs as high as it can and generally bites and falls off. The mite bites are often in folds of skin—axillae, near the belt line, etc. They do not transmit disease and, although they are sometimes confused with the jigger, do not burrow. Only symptomatic treatment for the bites is needed [1].

Dust mites. The house-dust mite, including various species of *Dermatophagoides*, have sometimes been blamed for pruritus in the absence of obvious cause [38]. Some have been thought to be a cause for atopic dermatitis.

Ticks

Ticks are eight-legged creatures that are divided into ixodid (hard) or argasid (soft) ticks. The body is not segmented. The mouth-parts of hard ticks extend anteriorly and they can be seen from the dorsal view. Soft ticks have a leathery body. The mouth-parts are hidden from view from the dorsal aspect. The dog tick, *Dermacentor variabilis*, and the deer tick, *Ixoides scapularis*, are representative of hard ticks.

There are four stages in development of a tick: egg, larva, nymph and adult. A blood meal is necessary for a change from one stage to another. There may be more than one nymph stage, depending on the species.

The tick has the unique ability to attach itself to its prey without producing symptoms. There, it can have a blood meal, and perhaps infect its host with a rickettsial or spirochaetal disease. It does this by biting and then secreting a cement that holds the head in place while blood and other products are extracted from the host.

While most of these ticks produce only local irritation, there are diseases particularly attributed to ticks. Tick-bite fever and tick-bite paralysis are two of these. Unless the tick is found and removed, the symptoms will continue. In Australia, it is estimated that tick-bite paralysis has killed more persons than either latrodectism or funnel-web spider bites. *Ixodes* ticks are most often responsible. Tick-bite paralysis has been reported in South Africa, Algeria, Somalia, Europe, Mexico and Russia, as well as in the USA.

Dermacentor andersoni and *D. variabilis*, as well as *Ixodes* ticks, have been implicated [17].

In addition, there are viral and rickettsial diseases transmitted by ticks (see Table 6.1). Permethrin and DEET are helpful as repellents and have few adverse effects [39].

Scorpions

There are large arthropods that can measure as long as 18 cm. The tail contains a stinger, which can be bent around to sting anteriorly. They have a worldwide, although mainly tropical, distribution.

Initially, there may be pain and numbness. There may be erythema and oedema and, in some patients, restlessness, agitation, tightness of chest, dilated pupils, tachycardia and vomiting. Death may result. The venom contains a neurotoxin with adrenergic and cholinergic properties. Treatment includes antivenom serum and local anaesthetic injections. Morphine is contraindicated.

Aquatic creatures

Coelenterates: jellyfish and Portugese man-of-war

These coelenterates produce disease by nematocysts in their extraordinary tentacles. The nematocysts discharge on contact and produce an instant stinging sensation and erythema and inflammation after contact. In some situations, fragments of nematocysts may remain on the skin of the victim. Although they function similarly, nematocysts from different species are different so that the species can be identified. In cases in Australia, where the largest collection of venomous marine animals exist, one can obtain 'box-jellyfish antivenom', made in sheep, which has been credited with being partly effective against the cardiotoxicity of *Chronex fleckeri* venom.

Box jellyfish, or class Cubozoa, can be divided into an order with four tentacles, order Carybdeidea, and one with multiple tentacles, order Chirodropidea. *Chronex fleckeri* is the most deadly, producing massive stings and cardiotoxicity. Two others of medical significance include *Chiropsalmus quadrigatus* and *Chiropsalmus quadrumanus*. They favour the Indo-Pacific, Okinawa and the Gulf of Mexico.

The Portuguese man-of-war is an Atlantic Ocean animal, frequenting the coasts of Florida but sometimes extending across to Europe. It is actually not a single organism, but a colony of symbiotic animals. The tentacles may extend as far as 100 feet. The nematocysts contain phospholipases and proteolytic enzymes. There may be sharp pain, coryza, muscular pains and chest tightness. Despite the symptoms, collapse and death are unusual [40].

Other coelenterates, such as hard and soft coral and the sea anemone, also sting with nematocysts, but the sting is usually not as severe [17].

Echinoderms

These spiny creatures include starfish, sea cucumbers and sea urchins (Fig. 6.15). They produce disease by scraping the skin with their sharp points. There may be an acute or chronic reaction, but the most reported dermatitis is a granulomatous process that occurs after spines from these creatures are embedded in the skin.

Swimmer's itch and sea-bather's eruption

Swimmer's itch is the disease produced by exposure to the avian form of schistosomiasis. The infected bird drops eggs in its stool. The eggs hatch and miracidia find freshwater snails as hosts. They mature and cercariae are formed. The cercariae penetrate the skin of birds — and unfortunate humans — who swim in the freshwater lakes which they inhabit. The disease affects exposed areas and is immediate. It occurs as the water evaporates, rather than while the victim is in the water. The head (schistosomule) penetrates the papillary dermis, but cannot travel further, and inflammation is produced as the avian schistosomule dies. There are immediate weals, followed later by inflammatory papules and pustules.

Sea-bather's eruption is traditionally produced in salt water. Clinically, it is just the opposite of what is seen in swimmer's itch: it affects covered areas and the reaction is delayed. At least three different classes of organisms have been reported to cause this syndrome. These include contact dermatitis from algae off the coast of Hawaii (*Lyngbya* species),

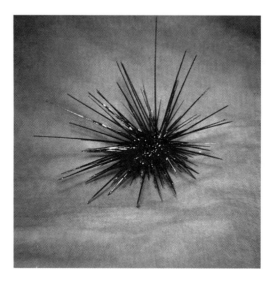

Fig. 6.15 A sea urchin. Note the spines, which are easily broken off into the flesh of a nearby swimmer.

Linuche unguiculata, a coelenterate organism that can sting, off the coast of Florida and a larva of the sea anemone, *Edwardsiella lineata*, off the coast of Long Island, New York [41–44]. Some of these have been directly due to stings from nematocysts, while others have been clear-cut contact dermatitis.

Octopuses and squids

These organisms may have suckers that cause some skin damage. Only one, the blue-ringed octopus, *Hapalochaena maculosa*, produces a neurotoxin, which it introduces by biting with its parrot-like beak. Most of the cases have been attributed to biting after the octopus was removed from the water and placed on the skin. All the reported cases recovered [17].

References

1 Alexander JOD. *Arthropods and Human Skin*, 1st edn. Springer-Verlag, Berlin, 1984.
2 deShazo M. Fire ants. *N Engl J Med* 1990; **323**: 462–466.
3 Elgart GW. Ant, bee, and wasp stings. *Dermatol Clin* 1990; **8** (2): 229–236.
4 Burns D. The treatment of *Phthirus pubis* infestation of the eyelashes. *Br J Dermatol* 1987; **117**: 741–743.
5 Rosen T. Caperpillar dermatitis. *Dermatol Clin* 1990; **8** (2): 245–252.
6 El-Mallakh RS, Baumgartner DG, Fares N. 'Sting' of the puss caterpillar, *Megalopyge opercularis*. *J Florida Med Assoc* 1986; **73**: 521.
7 D'Antuono A, Gatti M, Negosanti M, Passarini B, Pauluzzi P, Reggiani M. [Tungiasis: a clinical case]. *G Ital Dermatol Venereol* 1990; **125** (6): 259–261.
8 Sanusi ID, Brown EB, Shepard TG, Grafton WD. Tungiasis: report of one case and review of the 14 reported cases in the United States. *J Am Acad Dermatol* 1989; **20** (5, Part 2): 941–944.
9 Obengui. [Tungiasis and tetanus at the University Hospital Centre in Brazzaville]. *Dakar Med* 1989; **34** (1–4): 44–48.
10 Seaver J. Maggots took charge of this homeless patient's hygiene (letter; comment). RN 1992; **55** (5): 9.
11 DeLozier JB, Reaves L, King LE Jr, Rees RS. Brown recluse spider bites of the upper extremity. *South Med J* 1988; **81** (2): 181–184.
12 King LE Jr. Spider bites. *Arch Dermatol* 1987; **123** (1): 41–43.
13 Osborn CD. Treatment of spider bites by high voltage direct current. *J Oklahoma State Med Assoc* 1991; **84** (6); 257–260.
14 Hollabaugh RS, Fernandes ET. Management of the brown recluse spider bite. *J Pediatr Surg* 1989; **24** (1): 126–127.
15 Newlands G, Atkinson P. Behavioural and epidemiological considerations pertaining to necrotic araneism in southern Africa. *S Afr Med J* 1990; **77** (2): 92–95.
16 Vest DK. Necrotic arachnidism in the northwest United States and its probable relationship to *Tegenaria agrestis* (Walckenaer) spiders. *Toxicon* 1987; **25** (2): 175–184.
17 Meier J, White J. *Clinical Toxicology of Animal Venoms and Poisons*, 1st edn. CRC Press, Boca Raton, New York, London, Tokyo, 1995.
18 Jelinek GA, Banham ND, Dunjey SJ. Red-back spider-bites at Fremantle Hospital, 1982–1987. *Med J Aust* 1989; **150** (12): 693–695.
19 Wong RC, Hughes SE, Voorhees JJ. Spider bites. *Arch Dermatol* 1987; **123** (1): 98–104.

20 Mellanby K. Biology of the parasite. In: Orkin M, Maibach HI, Schwartzman RM (eds) *Scabies and Pediculosis*. JB Lippincott, Philadelphia, 1977; 8–16.

21 Cabrera R, Agar A, Dahl MV. The immunology of scabies. *Semin Dermatol* 1993; **12** (1): 15–21.

22 Bhawan J, Milstone E, Malhotra R, Rosenfeld T, Appel M. Scabies presenting as bullous pemphigoid-like eruption. *J Am Acad Dermatol* 1991; **24** (2, Part 1): 179–181.

23 Takiguchi Y, Kusama K, Nagao S, Iijima S. A case of scabies complicated by acute glomerulonephritis. *J. Dermatol* 1987; **14** (2): 163–166.

24 Magee KL, Hebert AA, Rapini RP. Crusted scabies in a patient with chronic graft-versus-host disease. *J Am Acad Dermatol* 1991; **25** (5, Part 2): 889–891.

25 Barnes L, McCallister RE, Lucky AW. Crusted (Norwegian) scabies: occurrence in a child undergoing a bone marrow transplant. *Arch Dermatol* 1987; **123** (1): 95–97.

26 Orkin M. Scabies in AIDS. *Semin Dermatol* 1993; **12** (1): 9–14.

27 Taplin D, Meinking TL, Porcelain SL, Castillero PM, Chen JA. Permethrin 5% dermal cream: a new treatment for scabies. *J Am Acad Dermatol* 1986; **15** (5, Part 1): 995–1001.

28 Taplin D, Porcelain SL, Meinking TL *et al.* Community control of scabies: a model based on use of permethrin cream. *Lancet* 1991; **337** (8748): 1016–1018.

29 Haustein UF, Hlawa B. Treatment of scabies with permethrin versus lindane and benzyl benzoate. *Acta Dermatol Venereol (Stockh)* 1989; **69** (4): 348–351.

30 Rasmussen J. Lindane, a prudent approach. *Arch Dermatol* 1987; **123**: 1008–1010.

31 Meinking T, Taplin J, Hermida R, Kerdel F. The treatment of scabies with ivermectin. *N Engl J Med* 1995; **333** (1): 26–31.

32 Dunne C, Malone C, Whitworth J. A field study of the effects of ivermectin on ectoparasites of man. *Trans Roy Soc Trop Med Hyg* 1991; **85** (4): 550–551.

33 Marty P, Gari-Toussaint M, Le-Fichoux Y, Gaxotte P. Efficacy of ivermectin in the treatment of an epidemic of sarcoptic scabies. *Ann Trop Med Parasitol* 1994; **88** (4): 453.

34 Arlian LG, Estes SA, Vyszenski-Moher DL. Prevalence of *Sarcoptes scabiei* in the homes and nursing homes of scabietic patients. *J Am Acad Dermatol* 1988; **19** (5, Part 1): 806–811.

35 Desch D, Nutting W. *Demodex folliculorum* (Simon) and *D. brevis* Akbulatova of man: redescription and reevaluation. *J Parasitol* 1972; **58** (1): 169–177.

36 Blankenship M. Mite dermatitis other than scabies. *Dermatol Clin* 1990; **8** (2): 265–275.

37 Hetherington G, Holder W, Smith E. Rat mite dermatitis. *JAMA* 1971; **215** (9): 1499–1500.

38 Woodford P. The house dust mite: *Dermatophagoides farinae*, as a causative agent of delusive dermatitis. *Ann Allergy* 1980; **45**: 248–250.

39 Couch P, Johnson CE. Prevention of Lyme disease. *Am J Hosp Pharm* 1992; **49** (5): 1164–1173.

40 Fisher AA. *Atlas of Aquatic Dermatology*. Grune and Stratton, New York, San Francisco, London, 1978.

41 Grauer F, Arnold H. Seaweed dermatitis. *Arch Dermatol* 1961; **84**: 720–732.

42 Burnett JW, Burnett MG, Kauffman CL. Another sea pest. *Arch Dermatol* 1995; **131** (8): 965.

43 Wong D, Meinking T, Rosen L. Seabathers' eruption. *J Am Acad Dermatol* 1994; **30**: 399–406.

44 Freudenthal A. Seabather's eruption: range extended northward and a causative organism identified. *Rev Int Oceanogr Med* 1991; **101**: 137–147.

Protozoan and helminth infections
Paul D. Wortman

Protozoan infections

Amoebiasis

Definition

Amoebiasis refers to disease caused by *Entamoeba histolytica* [1].

Epidemiology

Entamoeba histolytica and the recently discovered *Entamoeba dispar* infect approximately 500 million people worldwide. Most infections (over 90%) are caused by the non-pathogenic *E. dispar* and result in an asymptomatic carrier state. The majority of infections due to *E. histolytica* are also asymptomatic; however, about 10% of cases have symptomatic invasive disease. Risk factors for *E. histolytica* infection include poverty, institutionalization and emigration from an endemic area [1, 2].

Aetiology

Amoebiasis is acquired when infective cysts (passed in the faeces) are ingested in contaminated water or food or transmitted directly by faecal–oral contact. Disease is caused by the trophozoite stage of *E. histolytica* [3]. *Entamoeba dispar* and *E. histolytica* are morphologically identical but genetically distinct [1].

Clinical manifestations

Invasive amoebic colitis manifests as diarrhoea containing blood and mucus. Intestinal perforation, toxic megacolon, strictures and granulomatous masses may occur [4, 5]. The most common extraintestinal complication is a liver abscess [3].

Cutaneous amoebiasis is uncommon. Necrotic, foul-smelling ulcers with bloody, purulent discharge may occur in the anogenital area, at sites of fistulous tracts from the colon or liver or around abdominal surgical wounds or stomata [4, 6–8].

Diagnosis

The diagnosis of cutaneous amoebiasis is made by finding trophozoites in a wet mount of lesional fluid [2] or in a skin-biopsy specimen [6]. Active colitis due to *E. histolytica* is indicated by the presence of faecal trophozoites containing ingested erythrocytes [1].

Treatment

Amoebic colitis and extraintestinal disease (including cutaneous infection) are treated with metronidazole (750 mg by mouth (p.o.) three times a day (tid) for 10 days), tinidazole (600 mg p.o. twice a day (bid) or 800 mg p.o. tid for 5 days) or dehydroemetine (1–1.5 mg/kg/day intramuscularly (i.m.) for up to 5 days) [9].

African trypanosomiasis

Definition

African trypanosomiasis, or sleeping sickness, is a life-threatening illness caused by *Trypanasoma brucei gambiense* and *T. b. rhodesiense* [10].

Epidemiology

Numerous endemic areas of sleeping sickness are scattered in sub-Saharan Africa between the latitudes 14°N and 29°S. Approximately 25 000 cases occur annually [10, 11].

Aetiology

Tryopanosoma brucei gambiense and *T. b. rhodesiense* are transmitted from their principal reservoir hosts (humans and wild game, respectively) to humans by the bite of the tsetse fly (*Glossina* spp.) [10].

Clinical manifestations

The first stage of sleeping sickness is an indurated, erythematous nodule (chancre), which appears at the site of the tsetse-fly bite (Fig. 6.16). It lasts for 2–3 weeks [10, 12].

The second stage occurs when trypanosomes enter the blood and lymphatic systems. Patients typically have irregular cycles of fever (corresponding to waves of parasitaemia) and generalized lymphadenopathy. Prominent posterior cervical lymph nodes (Winterbottom's sign) are common in patients with *T. b. gambiense* infections. Transient morbilliform eruptions (trypanids), hepatosplenomegaly, oedema, arthralgias, pancarditis, haemolytic anaemia and disseminated intravascular coagulopathy (DIC) may occur [10, 13–16].

The third and final stage of sleeping sickness occurs with trypanosome invasion of the central nervous system (CNS). Neuropsychiatric manifestations (headaches, seizures, abnormal reflexes, psychosis, sleep disturbances and coma) [10, 13, 15] and endocrine abnormalities (amenorrhoea and impotence) are common [17].

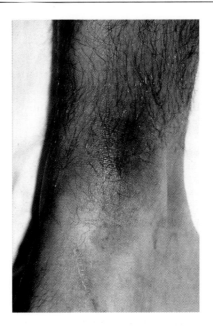

Fig. 6.16 Trypanosomal chancre caused by *Trypanosoma rhodesiense* (from: Bryceson ADM, Hay RJ. Parasitic worms and protozoa. In: Champion RH, Burton JL, Ebling FJG (eds) *Textbook of Dermatology*, 5th edn. Blackwell Scientific Publications, Oxford, 1992.)

Diagnosis

The diagnosis of African trypanosomiasis requires the demonstration of trypanosomes in chancre fluid, blood, lymph-node aspirate, bone marrow or cerebrospinal fluid. Immunological tests are helpful in confirming the diagnosis [15].

Treatment

Patients in the second stage of African trypanosomiasis are treated with suramin (test dose of 100–200 mg intravenously (i.v.) then 1 g i.v. on days 1, 3, 7, 14 and 21); pentamidine isethionate (4 mg/kg/day i.m. for 10 days); or eflornithine (400 mg/kg/day i.v. in four divided doses for 14 days, then 300 mg/kg/day p.o. for 3–4 weeks) [9]. Patients with CNS involvement have traditionally been treated with the arsenical compound melarsoprol (2–3.6 mg/kg/day i.v. for 3 days, wait a week, then 3.6 mg/kg/day i.v. for 3 days, and repeat in 10–21 days) [9, 10]. Melarsoprol causes a life-threatening arsenical encephalopathy in 5–10% of patients [10, 18]. Eflornithine may be used as an alternative in patients with CNS-stage disease due to *T. b. gambiense* [9, 18].

American trypanosomiasis

Definition

American trypanosomiasis, or Chagas' disease, is a potentially debilitating and life-threatening disease caused by *Trypanosoma cruzi* [19, 20].

Epidemiology

Approximately 15–20 million people are infected with *T. cruzi* in Latin America. The infection is particularly common in rural areas. Acute Chagas' disease affects mainly children, while chronic disease is seen in adults [20].

Aetiology

Trypanosoma cruzi is taken up by reduviid-bug vectors (genera *Triatoma*, *Panstrongylus* and *Rhodnius*) during blood meals on wild and domestic mammalian reservoir hosts, including humans [19, 20]. The parasite is transmitted to humans in the reduviid-bug faeces during a blood meal [19]. *Trypanosoma cruzi* can also be transmitted by blood transfusions [21].

Clinical manifestations

Acute Chagas' disease is often mildly symptomatic, allowing the disease to go undiagnosed. When symptomatic, patients are febrile and have generalized lymphadenopathy and hepatosplenomegaly. An inflammatory papule (chagoma) or unilateral periorbital oedema (Romaña's sign) may occur at bite sites on the skin and conjunctival mucosae, respectively. Complications of acute Chagas' disease include myocarditis and meningoencephalitis [19, 20].

   In most cases, the symptoms of acute Chagas' disease subside over weeks to months. Patients then enter an asymptomatic indeterminate phase characterized by lifelong parasitaemia. Approximately 10–30% of these patients will progress over years or decades to the chronic stage of disease, in which the heart, oesophagus and colon can be affected. Patients with cardiac disease may develop congestive heart failure, ventricular aneurysms, conduction defects, rhythm disturbances and thromboembolic events. Involvement of the oesophagus and colon ('megadisease') leads to dilatation and dysfunction, with resultant dysphagia, regurgitation, constipation, volvulus and possible perforation [19, 22].

   Some patients with chagasic cardiomyopathy who have undergone heart transplantation have developed a 'reactivation' of Chagas' disease, characterized by fever, deteriorating cardiac status and cellulitis-like lesions of the skin that have contained trypanosomes [23, 24].

Diagnosis

Acute Chagas' disease is diagnosed by demonstrating trypanosomes in concentrated wet-blood mounts of anticoagulated blood or the buffy coat. Serological tests and xenodiagnosis are used to diagnose indeterminate and chronic infections [15, 22].

Treatment

Acute Chagas' disease is treated with nifurtimox (8–10 mg/kg/day p.o in four doses for 120 days) or benznidazole (5–7 mg/kg/day for 30–120 days) [9]. These medications decrease the severity and duration of symptoms and reduce the mortality rate of acute disease but effect parasitological cure in only 50% of cases. Nifurtimox and benznidazole are of limited, if any, benefit in the treatment of chronic disease [19, 22].

Leishmaniasis

Definition

Leishmaniasis refers to a spectrum of cutaneous, mucosal and systemic (visceral) illnesses caused by different species of *Leishmania* protozoa. The manifestations of disease depend on the species of infecting parasite and on host immunity [25].

Epidemiology

Leishmaniasis affects approximately 12 million people throughout Latin America, Africa, southern Europe, the Middle East, southern Russia and the Indian subcontinent [11].

Aetiology

The leishmaniases are generally zoonoses, which affect such mammalian reservoir hosts as rodents, dogs, sloths, foxes, hyraxes and jackals. The parasites are transmitted to humans by the bite of female sandflies (genus *Phlebotomus* in the Old World and *Lutzomyia* in the New World) [26].

Clinical manifestations

Visceral leishmaniasis is caused by *Leishmania (Leishmania) donovani*, *L. (L.) infantum* and *L. (L.) chagasi*. Most patients are asymptomatic or mildly symptomatic and the disease is self-limited. Progressive disease (kala-azar), seen most often in children, has a gradual or sudden onset of fever, malaise, hepatosplenomegaly and weight loss. Hyperpigmentation of the face, abdomen and acral areas may occur. Anaemia, leucopenia and hyperglobu-linaemia are common. Pneumonia, dysentery and haemorrhage are the main causes of death [25, 26].

Post-kala-azar dermal leishmaniasis (PKDL) occurs in a small percent-age of patients months to years after treatment of visceral leishmaniasis caused by *L. (L.) donovani*. It is seen most often in India. Patients develop hypopigmented or erythematous macules and erythematous to yellowish papules, nodules or plaques. Lesions, which may be solitary or multiple, occur on the face, trunk, genitalia and extremities [27, 28].

Old World acute cutaneous leishmaniasis caused by *L. (L.) tropica* and *L. (L.) aethiopica* starts weeks to months after the sandfly bite as an erythematous papule or nodule, which enlarges into a plaque in about 6 months and then ulcerates. A shallow, 'dry', crusted ulcer forms in the centre, giving the lesion the appearance of a volcano. The ulcer usually heals with scarring within a year. Old World cutaneous leishmaniais caused by *L (L.) major* tends to develop more rapidly after the sandfly bite, to ulcerate sooner and to produce a necrotic crust which separates easily, leaving a 'wet' eroded base. Healing with a scar occurs in about 6 months. Satellite lesions and lymphatic involvement can occur [29, 30].

Leishmaniasis recidivans refers to the ocurrence of yellowish or red-brown translucent papules within or around a resolving or healed scar of cutaneous leishmaniasis. This form of infection is chronic, often occurs on the face and closely resembles lupus vulgaris. It is difficult to treat successfully [29–31].

New World acute cutaneous leishmaniasis is caused by *L. (L.) mexicana, L. (L.) amazonensis, L. (L.) venezuelensis, L. (L.) pifanoi, L. Viannia braziliensis, L. (V.) panamensis, L. (V.) guyanensis* and *L. (V.) peruviana*. It usually has an incubation period of several weeks and begins as an erythematous papule or nodule, which may progress to form an ulcer similar to that seen in Old World cutaneous leishmaniasis (Fig. 6.17). However, granulomatous, verrucous (Fig. 6.18) and lymphatic (sporotrichoid) lesions also occur. Satellite lesions and involvement of regional lymphatics are more common in New World than Old World leishmaniasis. Lesions are slow to heal and leave a scar [25, 32, 33].

Patients infected with *L. (V.) braziliensis* and *L. (V.) panamensis* are at risk of developing infection in the nasal or oropharyngeal mucosae years or decades later. This mutilating form of infection (espundia) begins in the nasal cartilage and may destroy the gums, tongue, floor of the mouth, palate, tonsils, pharynx and larynx (Fig. 6.19). Patients may die of pneumonia or malnutrition [26, 34, 35].

Diffuse cutaneous leishmaniasis (DCL) is a rare, chronic disease that occurs in patients who are anergic to the infecting *Leishmania* parasites. Widespread non-ulcerative nodules appear on the face, trunk and extremities but there is no systemic involvement. Diffuse cutaneous leishmaniasis is caused by *L. (L.) aethiopica* in Ethiopia and Kenya, *L. (L.) mexicana* in the Dominican Republic, Mexico and Central America and *L. (L.) amazonensis* and *L. (L.) pifanoi* in areas of northern South America. This form of infection is usually refractory to therapy [26, 30, 33, 36].

Diagnosis

The definitive diagnosis of leishmaniasis requires the visualization of parasites in tissue samples or the isolation of organisms in culture or after inoculation into laboratory animals. The diagnosis of cutaneous and mucosal

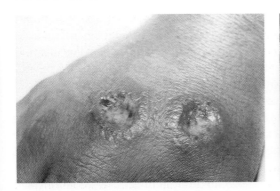

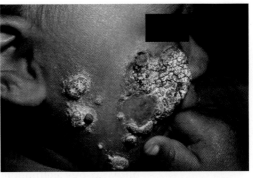

Fig. 6.17 Ulcers of New World cutaneous leishmaniasis (from: Schaller KF (ed.) *Colour Atlas of Tropical Dermatology and Venerology*. Springer-Verlag, Berlin, 1994. Published with the permission of Dr Med. Herbert Lieske, Hamburg, Germany).

Fig. 6.18 Verrucous, hyperkeratotic lesions of New World cutaneous leishmaniasis (courtesy of Marcia Ramos-e-Silva, MD, PhD, Rio de Janeiro, Brazil).

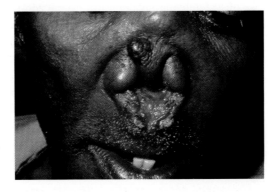

Fig. 6.19 Destructive lesion of New World mucosal leishmaniasis (espundia) (courtesy of Marcia Ramos-e-Silva, MD, PhD, Rio de Janeiro, Brazil).

infection may be difficult, depending on the species of *Leishmania*, the duration of the lesion, the form of cutaneous infection and the diagnostic tests used [37, 38].

Specimens for direct visualization or culture are obtained by scraping the base of an ulcer; by making a slit in the active border of a lesion and scraping the dermis; or by performing fine-needle aspiration or a biopsy from an active part of a lesion. Scraped or aspirated material should be smeared on a glass slide, allowed to air-dry, fixed with methanol and stained with Giemsa stain. Touch imprints from a biopsy specimen are prepared in the same way. Processed biopsy specimens should be stained with haematoxylin and eosin and Giemsa stains. Smears, touch imprints and histological sections are examined for aflagellate *Leishmania* amastigotes (2–4 μm) located within macrophages or extracellularly. The cytoplasmic kinetoplast stains red with Giemsa stain [37, 38].

To culture *Leishmania*, modified Evan's medium or Nicolle–Novy–McNeal (NNN) medium is used, often with a liquid overlay of Schneider's *Drosophila* medium. The fusiform, flagellated promastigote forms may be identified within a week but might take longer [38].

The leishmanin (Montenegro) skin test is not helpful in diagnosing acute cutaneous leishmaniais, since it is positive in a large percentage of the population in endemic areas, is negative in early cases of cutaneous leishmaniasis (less than 1 month's duration) and does not discriminate between past and current infection. It is negative in acute visceral leishmaniasis, PKDL and DCL, but strongly positive in leishmaniasis recidivans [37–39].

Serological tests are helpful mainly in epidemiological studies. New techniques, such as hybridization with deoxyribonucleic acid (DNA) probes directed against *Leishmania* kinetoplast DNA (kDNA) and polymerase chain reaction amplification of kDNA are more sensitive and specific than conventional diagnostic methods. Identification of *Leishmania* species is done primarily by electrophoretic isoenzyme analysis of cultured promastigotes [38, 38].

Treatment

The most effective treatment for all forms of leishmaniasis consists of the use of systemic pentavalent antimonial compounds. Antimonials (sodium stibogluconate or meglumine antimoniate) are recommended for visceral leishmaniasis (20 mg/kg/day i.v. or i.m. for 28 days), mucosal and cutaneous leishmaniasis known or suspected to be caused by *L. (V.) braziliensis* (20 mg/kg/day i.v. or i.m. for 28 days), PKDL (20 mg/kg/day i.v. or i.m. for at least 4 months) and extensive or severe cases of Old or New World cutaneous leishmaniasis (20 mg/kg/day i.v. or i.m. for 20 days).

The antimonial compounds may cause myalgias, arthralgias, elevations of hepatic transminases and numerous electrocardiographic (ECG) abnormalities. The response to systemic antimonials is variable and may be incomplete. Retreatment may be necessary. Patients who are not able to tolerate or do not respond to antimonials may be treated with amphotericin B or pentamidine.

Other variably effective treatments for Old and New World cutaneous leishmaniasis (not caused by *L. (V.) braziliensis*) include localized heat, cryotherapy, topical 15% paromomycin sulphate and 12% methylbenzethonium chloride in soft white paraffin, ketoconazole (especially for *L. (L.) major* and *L. (L.) mexicana*), dapsone and rifampicin plus isoniazid. Allopurinol has been reported to be more effective than systemic antimony in the treatment of *L. (V.) panamensis* infection, although this has been questioned [35, 40, 41].

Helminth infections: nematodes (roundworms)

Onchocerciasis

Definition

Onchocerciasis (river blindness) is a chronic disease of the skin and eyes caused by *Onchocerca volvulus* [20, 42].

Epidemiology

Onchocerciasis affects approximately 20 million people in equatorial Africa, Yemen and areas of southern Mexico, Guatemala, Venezuela, Brazil, Colombia and Ecuador. It is the fourth leading cause of blindness worldwide [42, 43].

Aetiology

Onchocerca volvulus is transmitted from infected human hosts by the bite of *Simulium* black flies. Female worms produce microfilariae, which migrate in the skin and into the eyes. The host immune response to living, dead and dying microfilariae is thought to cause the cutaneous and ocular pathology [20, 43].

Clinical manifestations

The World Health Organization (WHO) classification and grading system of the dermatological manifestations of onchocerciasis include the following.

1 Acute papular onchodermatitis — pruritic papules typically located on the upper trunk and arms (Fig. 6.20).

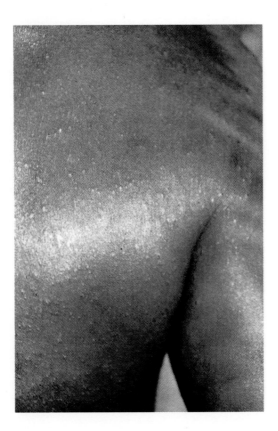

Fig. 6.20 Acute papular onchodermatitis (from reference [44]).

2 Chronic papular onchodermatitis — flat-topped, pruritic, hyperpigmented papules on the buttocks and lower back (Fig. 6.21).

3 Lichenified onchodermatitis — discrete or confluent hyperpigmented nodules or plaques on one or both legs (Fig. 6.22).

4 Atrophy—typically seen on the lower back and buttocks (Fig. 6.23).

5 Depigmentation ('leopard skin') — areas of complete pigment loss surrounding follicularly based islands of normally pigmented skin. This finding is characteristically located on the shins (Fig. 6.24).

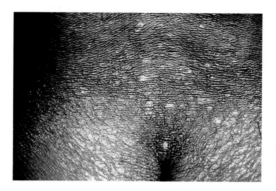

Fig. 6.21 Chronic papular onchodermatitis (from reference [44]).

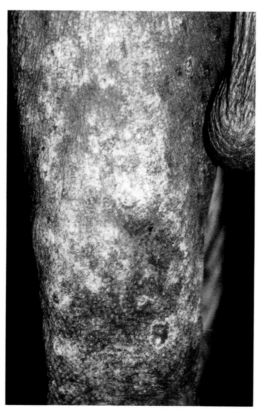

Fig. 6.22 Lichenified onchodermatitis (from reference [44]).

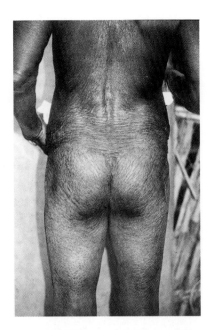

Fig. 6.23 Onchocercal atrophy on the buttocks and lower back (from reference [44]).

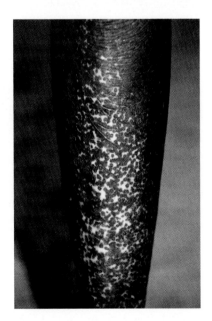

Fig. 6.24 Onchocercal depigmentation (from reference [44]).

6   Onchocercal nodules — contain adult worms, are firm and non-tender and typically located on the head and upper trunk in Latin America and on the trunk, arms and thighs in Africa.

7   Hanging groin — manifested initially as prominent inguinal or femoral lymph nodes and later as atrophic folds of skin in the inguinal region [44].

Diagnosis

The diagnosis of onchocerciasis requires the demonstration of microfilariae in the skin or eyes. Skin snips should be obtained from each scapular area, iliac crest and calf. There is no periodicity of the microfilariae in the skin, so samples may be taken at any time. The specimens are placed in normal saline on a glass slide under a cover slip and observed over several hours for the emergence of microfilariae. When microfilariae are noted, the preparation is allowed to air-dry, fixed with methanol and stained with Giemsa stain. The microfilariae of *O. volvulus* are distinguished on the basis of morphological features [20, 45, 46]. New serological assays using recombinant *O. volvulus* antigens appear to be highly sensitive and specific [47].

Treatment

Ivermectin (150 µg/kg p.o. once, repeated every 6–12 months) is the recommended treatment for onchocerciasis. It causes a signficant and prolonged decrease in the microfilarial load. Adverse reactions to ivermectin (pruritus, headache, myalgias, arthralgias, fever) occur in approximately 10% of patients and are usually self-limited [9, 20, 48].

The former standard therapy, diethylcarbamazine (DEC), is also an effective microfilaricide but causes worsening of ocular pathology. Suramin, which is macrofilaricidal, is indicated for heavy infections. Nodules on the head should be surgically removed to decrease microfilarial invasion of the eyes [20, 49].

Lymphatic filariasis

Definition

Lymphatic filariasis is a chronic infection caused by *Wuchereria bancrofti*, *Brugia malayi* and *Brugia timori*.

Epidemiology

Approximatley 90 million people worldwide are affected, with about 90% of cases due to *W. bancrofti*. Bancroftian filariasis occurs in Africa, Asia, the South Pacific, the Caribbean and Latin America. Infection due to *B. malayi* is seen in southern China, India, Indonesia, Korea and South-East Asia and that caused by *B. timori* is limited to eastern Indonesia. [11, 50, 51].

Aetiology

Wuchereria bancrofti, *B. malayi* and *B. timori* are transmitted from infected human hosts by species of mosquitoes belonging to the genera *Culex*,

Anopheles, *Aëdes* and *Mansonia*. Adult worms preferentially inhabit the lymphatics of the legs, groin, epididymis and labia and produce microfilariae that enter the bloodstream via the thoracic duct or by direct invasion. The clinical manifestations of lymphatic filariasis are believed to be due to recurrent inflammatory reactions to the adult worms [20, 50].

Clinical manifestations

The clinical stages of lymphatic filariasis include: (i) an asymptomatic stage, during which microfilariae are found in the circulation; (ii) an inflammatory phase, characterized by recurrent episodes of fever, lymphangitis, lymphadenitis, oedema, orchitis, epididymitis and funiculitis; and (iii) an obstructive stage, which results from scarring within the lymphatics. Elephantiasis of the legs, genitalia or breasts occurs in about 10% of patients (Fig. 6.25). Affected areas are firm and non-pitting. Obstruction and rupture of lymphatics may result in hydrocoele (Fig. 6.26) or chylocoele of the scrotum as well as chyluria and chylous ascites [20, 50].

Diagnosis

The diagnosis of lymphatic filariasis may be made by finding microfilariae in blood smears collected at night (nocturnal periodicity) and stained with Giemsa stain. Microfilariae may also be found in chylous urine or chylocoele fluid. Because circulating microfilariae may not be present in the early and late stages of infection, serological tests may be required to confirm the diagnosis [20, 45].

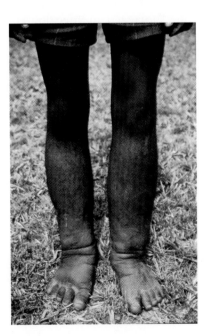

Fig. 6.25 Lymphatic filariasis: elephantiasis (courtesy of Professor Dietrich Büttner, Hamburg, Germany).

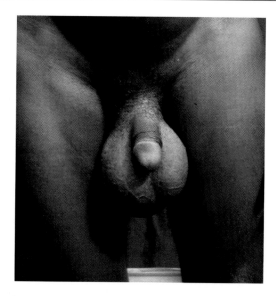

Fig. 6.26 Lymphatic filariasis: hydrocoele (from: Schaller KF (ed.) *Colour Atlas of Tropical Dermatology and Venereology*. Springer-Verlag, Berlin, 1994. Published with permission of Professor Dietrich Büttner, Bernhard-Nocht-Institut für Tropenmedicin, Hamburg, Germany).

Treatment

The drug of choice for lymphatic filariasis is DEC. It is usually administered as 50 mg p.o. on day 1, 50 mg p.o. tid on day 2, 100 mg p.o. tid on day 3 and 6 mg/kg/day p.o. in three doses on days 4–21. Recent studies suggest that single-dose regimens (6 mg/kg) are also effective in causing a prolonged, significant decrease in the microfilarial load. Side-effects occur in 50–90% of patients and consist of fever, chills, malaise and arthralgias, as well as worsening of oedema and lymphatic reactions. Ivermectin also appears to be effective [9, 20, 52].

Loiasis

Definition

Loiasis is a chronic infection caused by *Loa loa*, which is characterized by soft-tissue swellings and involvement of the ocular conjunctivae.

Epidemiology and aetiology

Loiasis occurs throughout the rain forests of equatorial Africa and is transmitted by flies of the genus *Chrysops*. Once inoculated into human hosts, the worms mature and migrate within the subcutaneous tissues [20].

Clinical manifestations

Recurrent erythematous, pruritic and painful 'Calabar swellings' may occur, typically on the hands and forearms and around the eyes. Migration of the worm across the bulbar conjunctivae causes pain, injection and oedema. Peripheral eosinophilia is often present. Microfilaraemia is common after prolonged infection [20, 53].

Diagnosis

The diagnosis of loiasis is often based on a history of exposure in an endemic area, recurrent oedematous swellings and eosinophilia. Serological tests and identification of the worm in a blood smear are helpful in confirming the diagnosis [20].

Treatment

The treatment of choice is DEC 50 mg p.o. on day 1, 50 mg p.o. tid on day 2, 100 mg p.o. tid on day 3 and 9 mg/kg/day p.o. in three doses on days 4–21. Surgical removal of worms as they traverse the eye is recommended when possible [9, 20].

Dracunculiasis

Definition

Dracunculiasis (guinea-worm disease) is a chronic debilitating infection caused by *Dracunculus medinensis*.

Epidemiology

Dracunculiasis affects an estimated 140 million people in Africa, the Indian subcontinent, the Middle East, the Caribbean and northern South America [54, 55].

Aetiology

The disease is transmitted by drinking water contaminated with *Cyclops* crustaceans that harbour *D. medinensis*. The adult female worm, which usually lives in the subcutaneous tissues of the lower extremities, discharges its larvae through a toxin-mediated ulcer in the skin when the ulcer comes into contact with water [20, 54].

Clinical manifestations

Patients are usually asymptomatic while worms mature to adulthood. A visible, serpiginous tract may be noted in the subcutaneous tissues [56]. When the adult female worm prepares to discharge its larvae, it releases a toxin that causes a papule to form, which vesiculates and ruptures to create an ulcer. The toxin also triggers a systemic allergic reaction, with urticaria, dyspnoea, nausea and vomiting. Patients often develop secondary bacterial infections (abscess, cellulitis) at the ulcer or within the subcutaneous tract [20, 55].

Diagnosis

The diagnosis is based on the clinical features or the identification of an adult worm at the discharge site or along a subcutaneous tract or is suggested by the presence of a calcified worm on X-ray [20].

Treatment

Metronidazole (250 mg p.o. tid for 7–10 days) or thiabendazole (50–75 mg/kg/day p.o. in two doses for 3 days) is helpful for its anti-inflammatory properties and because it may cause the adult worm to be spontaneously extruded. Neither medication kills the adult worm. The adult worm may be mechanically extracted through an incision along a subcutaneous path or by slowly winding the worm on a stick at the ulcer site [9, 20, 54–56].

Strongyloidiasis

Definition

Strongyloidiasis, caused by the soil nematode *Strongyloides stercoralis*, ranges from a mild, nearly asymptomatic infection to a severe systemic illness [20].

Epidemiology

Strongyloidiasis affects an estimated 100 million people worldwide, especially in tropical and subtropical regions [20, 57].

Aetiology

Infective filariform larvae in the soil penetrate human skin, are carried by the venous circulation to the lungs, migrate up the airways, are swallowed and mature into adults in the small intestine. Female worms deposit eggs, which hatch into non-infective rhabditiform larvae, which are usually passed in the faeces. Occasionally, rhabditiform larvae mature into filariform larvae within the bowel; such larvae are capable of penetrating the bowel wall or anogenital skin and entering the circulatory system, thereby establishing a cycle of autoinfection [20].

Clinical manifestations

Cutaneous signs of strongyloidiasis include larva currens and periumbilical 'thumbprint' purpura. Larva currens is a pruritic, serpiginous, urticarial plaque, which is usually located in the perianal area, buttocks, thighs or lower back. It characteristically migrates several centimetres a day. Abdominal purpuric lesions (Fig. 6.27) are seen in immunocompromised patients with a disseminated hyperinfection syndrome [20, 57–59].

Diagnosis

The diagnosis of strongyloidiasis is usually made by finding rhabditiform larvae in fresh faeces or duodenal fluid. The diagnosis can also be established by identifying filariform larvae in skin-biopsy specimens from purpuric lesions [20, 58].

Treatment

The standard treatment is thiabendazole 25 mg/kg p.o. bid for 2–3 days, although disseminated infection should be treated for 5–7 days. Ivermectin 200 µg/kg/day p.o. for 1–2 days or albendazole 400 mg/day p.o. for 3–5 days are accepted alternatives [9, 20].

Cutaneous larva migrans

Definition

Cutaneous larva migrans ('creeping eruption') is a self-limiting, pruritic

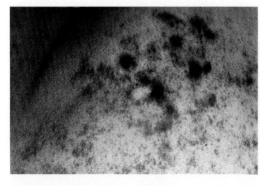

Fig. 6.27 Abdominal purpura in a patient with disseminated strongyloidiasis (from reference [58]. Published with permission of Mosby-Year Book, Inc, St Louis, Missouri, and Marc E. Grossman, MD, New York).

infection caused by the larvae of animal hookworms, most commonly *Ancylostoma braziliensis* [60, 61].

Epidemiology

The disease occurs in warm climates worldwide, especially Africa, South America, the Caribbean, South-East Asia and the south-eastern part of the USA [60].

Aetiology

The eggs of animal hookworms (*A. braziliensis, Ancylostoma caninum, Uncinaria stenocephala* and *Bunostomum phlebotomus*) are passed in faeces, mature into infective larvae in warm sandy soil and then penetrate intact human skin or enter through hair follicles, eccrine sweat ducts or abrasions. The larvae lack the enzymes needed to cross the basement membrane of human skin and therefore usually remain in the epidermis [60, 61].

Clinical manifestations

The most common lesion is a pruritic, red, linear or serpiginous track (2–3 mm wide) (Fig. 6.28), although vesicles, bullae and papules are sometimes seen. The tracks advance 1–3 cm a day. Cutaneous larva migrans usually occurs on the feet but may affect other parts of the extremities, as well as the buttocks and trunk. Multiple lesions and secondary bacterial infection are common. The symptoms and signs subside with the death of the larvae, which usually occurs in weeks to months [60, 61].

Diagnosis

The diagnosis of cutaneous larva migrans is based on clinical findings.

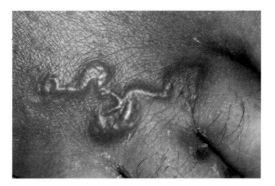

Fig. 6.28 Cutaneous larva migrans (from: Schaller KF (ed.) *Colour Atlas of Tropical Dermatology and Venerology.* Springer-Verlag, Berlin, 1994. Published with permission of Professor Dietrich Büttner, Bernhard-Nocht-Institut für Tropenmedicin, Hamburg, Germany).

Treatment

Cutaneous larva migrans may be treated with topical thiabendazole 15% cream applied two to three times daily for 2–5 days or oral thiabendazole 25–50 mg/kg/day in two doses for 2–5 days. Adverse reactions to oral thiabendazole include nausea, diarrhoea, dizziness, drowsiness and haematuria. Single oral doses of albendazole (400 mg) or ivermectin (12 mg) have also been shown to be efficacious. Liquid-nitrogen cryotherapy is not effective [9, 60–62].

Gnathostomiasis

Definition

Gnathostomiasis, caused by *Gnathostoma spinigerum*, is a chronic infection characterized by pruritic, painful, migratory, soft-tissue swellings [63].

Epidemiology and aetiology

The disease occurs principally in Asia. It is acquired by eating raw freshwater fish, poultry or pork [63].

Clinical manifestations

Patients develop fever, nausea, vomiting and abdominal pain within 1–2 days of ingesting contaminated food. Weeks to months later, intermittent episodes of localized pruritic, painful, non-pitting oedema begin to occur. Individual bouts of oedema last 1–2 weeks and can recur for years. Less often, a serpiginous track, abscess or nodule may be seen. Peripheral eosinophilia is common. Occasionally, involvement of the lungs, gastrointestinal tract, eyes or CNS occurs [63].

Diagnosis

The diagnosis is often based on appropriate clinical signs in a patient who has spent time in an endemic area and who has eaten food that may have been contaminated. Isolation of the worm in the skin or other sites is difficult. Serological tests may be required to confirm the diagnosis [63].

Treatment

The treatment of choice is surgical removal of the worm, if possible (from the eye, in an abdominal mass or cutaneous nodule or on a digit) and the administration of albendazole 400–800 mg/day p.o. for 21 days [9, 63].

Helminth infections: cestodes (tapeworms)

Sparganosis

Definition

Sparganosis refers to infection caused by pleurocercid larvae (spargana) of several species of *Spirometra* tapeworms [20].

Epidemiology and aetiology

Sparganosis occurs primarily in Asia, but may be seen elsewhere. Humans become infected by drinking contaminated water, eating raw fish or frogs or applying a poultice of raw fish or frog flesh to an open wound [20].

Clinical manifestations

A tender or non-tender subcutaneous nodule or mass is the typical manifestation of sparganosis. The noduel may be migratory. Patients often develop fever, chills and urticaria, and peripheral eosinophilia is usually present [20, 64].

Diagnosis

The diagnosis is made by the microscopic identification of the spargana in an excised lesion.

Treatment

The recommended treatment is surgical excision of the worm from affected sites [20].

Cysticercosis

Definition

Cysticercosis refers to the accidental human infection with the larval stage of the pork tapeworm, *Taenia solium* [65].

Epidemiology and aetiology

Cysticercosis occurs throughout Latin America, Africa, Eastern Europe, China and India. The adult worms produce eggs, which are shed in the faeces of the human host. Eggs ingested by humans (or pigs) hatch into larvae, which penetrate the intestinal wall, enter the circulation and are spread to the soft tissues and other organs, where they encyst to form cysticerci. The adult tapeworm is acquired by ingesting raw pork containing encysted larvae [65].

Clinical manifestations

Subcutaneous nodules containing cysticerci range from a few millimetres to several centimentres in diameter, are firm and mobile and may be tender or non-tender. Multiple lesions are typical. Involvement of the CNS and eyes is common [65].

Diagnosis

The diagnosis of subcutaneous cysticercosis is made by identifying the larva in a biopsy specimen of a nodule. Immunological and radiographic studies are helpful in confirming the diagnosis and determining the extent of disease [65].

Treatment

Surgical excision of subcutaneous nodules and cysts in the CNS (especially in the ventricles) and eyes is recommended. Albendazole 15 mg/kg/day p.o. in three doses for 28 days or praziquantel 50 mg/kg/day p.o. in three doses for 15 days is indicated for infection of the cerebral parenchyma, widespread subcutaneous infection and other systemic infections [9, 65].

Helminth infections: trematodes (flukes)

Schistosomiasis

Definition

Schistosomiasis refers to disease caused by *Schistosoma mansoni, S. japonicum* or *S. haematobium*.

Epidemiology

It is estimated that 200 million people worldwide have schistosomiasis. Infection due to *S. mansoni* occurs in the Caribbean, northern South America, central and southern Africa, Madagascar and areas of the Middle East. *Schistosoma japonicum* infection is limited to Asia and India. Disease caused by *S. haematobium* is seen in the Middle East, Africa and Madagascar [11, 66].

Aetiology

Signs and symptoms of chronic infection occur when *Schistosoma* eggs trigger granulomatous inflammatory reactions in the bowel, urinary tract, liver or skin. Adult flukes live in the terminal venules of the large intestine (*S. mansoni*), small intestine (*S. japonicum*) and urinary bladder and pelvis (*S. haematobium*). Eggs produced may travel via the portal circulation to the liver or via anastamoses to the dermal vasculature or remain in the venules and be passed in the stool or urine. On contact with water, miracidia hatch from the eggs and enter intermediate snail hosts. Cercariae eventually emerge from the snails and penetrate human skin while people swim, bathe or wash clothes in contaminated water [20, 66].

Clinical manifestations

A 'cercarial dermatitis', characterized by pruritic erythematous maculae and papules, may occur at the sites of cutaneous penetration. Infection with *S. mansoni* and *S. japonicum* causes gastrointestinal symptoms and periportal hepatic fibrosis. *Schistosoma haematobium* causes inflammation, fibrosis and calcification in the genitourinary tract. Lesions of late cutaneous schistosomiasis occur mainly in the anogenital and periumbilical regions. Papules, nodules and polypoid masses are most common, but ulcers and sinus tracts also occur [20, 66].

Diagnosis

The diagnosis rests on identifying the characteristic eggs of the three *Schistosoma* species in the urine, the stool or a skin-biopsy specimen [20, 66].

Treatment

The treatment for schistosomiasis due to *S. mansoni* or *S. haematobium* is praziquantel 40 mg/kg/day p.o. in two doses for 1 day and 60 mg/kg/day p.o. in three doses for 1 day for infection due to *S. japonicum* [9, 20, 66].

References

1 Ravdin JI. Amebiasis. *Clin Infect Dis* 1995; **20**: 1453–1466.
2 Proctor EM. Laboratory diagnosis of amebiasis. *Clin Lab Med* 1991; **11**: 829–859.
3 Reitano M, Masci JR, Bottone EJ. Amebiasis: clinical and laboratory perspectives. *Crit Rev Clin Lab Sci* 1991; **28**: 357–385.
4 Reed SL. Amebiasis: an update. *Clin Infect Dis* 1992; **14**: 385–393.
5 Adams EB, MacLeod IN. Invasive amebiasis. I. Amebic dysentery and its complications. *Medicine* 1977; **56**: 315–323.
6 Fujita WH, Barr RJ, Gottschalk HR. Cutaneous amebiasis. *Arch Dermatol* 1981; **117**: 309–310.

7 Veliath AJ, Bansal R, Sankaran V, Rajaram P, Parkash S. Genital amebiasis. *Int J Gynaecol Obstetr* 1987; **25**: 249–256.

8 Sattar A. An unusual cutaneous amoebic ulcer. *J Trop Med Hyg* 1979; **82**: 201–202.

9 Anon. Drugs for parasitic infections. *Med Lett Drugs Ther* 1993; **35**: 111–122.

10 World Health Organization. *Epidemiology and Control of African Trypanosomiasis.* World Health Organization Technical Report Series 739, World Health Organization, Geneva, 1986.

11 World Health Organization. *Tropical Diseases 1990.* WHO Division of Control of Tropical Diseases and UNDP/World Bank/WHO Special Programme for Research and Training in Tropical Diseases, World Health Organization, Geneva, 1990.

12 Cochran R, Rosen T. African trypanosomiasis in the United States. *Arch Dermatol* 1983; **119**: 670–674.

13 Greenwood BM, Whittle HC. The pathogenesis of sleeping sickness. *Trans Roy Soc Trop Med Hyg* 1980; **74**: 716–725.

14 Poltera AA. Pathology of human African trypanosomiasis with reference to experimental African trypanosomiasis and infections of the central nervous system. *Br Med Bull* 1985; **41**: 169–174.

15 Cattand P, de Raadt P. Laboratory diagnosis of trypanosomiasis. *Clin Lab Med* 1991; **11**: 899–908.

16 Van Meirvenne N, Le Ray D. Diagnosis of African and American trypanosomiasis. *Br Med Bull* 1985; **41**: 156–161.

17 Boersma A, Noireau F, Hublart M *et al.* Gonadotropic axis and *Trypanosoma brucei gambiense* infection. *Ann Soc Belg Med Trop* 1989; **69**: 127–135.

18 Kuzoe FAS. Current situation of African trypanosomiasis. *Acta Trop* 1993; **54**: 153–162.

19 Kirchoff LV. Trypanosoma species (American trypanosomiasis, Chagas' disease): biology of trypanosomes. In: Mandell GL, Douglas RG Jr, Bennett JE (eds) *Principles and Practice of Infectious Diseases*, 3rd edn. Churchill Livingstone, New York, 1990, pp. 2077–2084.

20 Neva FA, Brown HW. *Basic Clinical Parasitology*, 6th edn. Appleton and Lange, Norwalk, Connecticut, 1994.

21 Wendel S, Gonzaga AL. Chagas' disease and blood transfusion: a New World problem? *Vox Sang* 1993; **64**: 1–12.

22 Kirchoff LV. American trypanosomiasis (Chagas' disease)—a tropical disease now in the United States. *N. Engl J Med* 1993; **329**: 639–644.

23 Libow LF, Beltrani VP, Silvers DN, Grossman ME. Post-cardiac transplant reactivation of Chagas' disease diagnosed by skin biopsy. *Cutis* 1991; **48**: 37–40.

24 Stolf NAG, Higushi L, Bocchi E *et al.* Heart transplantation in patients with Chagas' disease cardiomyopathy. *J Heart Transplant* 1987; **6**: 307–312.

25 Pearson RD, de Queiroz Sousa A. *Leishmania* species: visceral (kala-azar), cutaneous, and mucosal leishmaniasis. In: Mandell GL, Bennett JE, Dolin R (eds) *Principles and Practice of Infectious Diseases*, 4th edn. Churchill Livingstone, New York, 1995, pp. 2428–2442.

26 World Health Organization. *The Leishmaniases: Report of a WHO Expert Committee.* Technical Report Series 701, World Health Organization, Geneva, 1984.

27 Dutta AK. Kala-azar and post-kala-azar dermal leishmaniasis. In: Canizares O, Harman RRM (eds) *Clinical Tropical Dermatology*, 2nd edn. Blackwell Scientific Publications, Boston, 1992, pp. 313–322.

28 Rees PH, Kager PA. Visceral leishmaniasis and post-kala-azar dermal leishmaniasis. In: Peters W, Killick-Kendrick R (eds) *The Leishmaniases in Biology and Medicine.* Academic Press, London, 1987, pp. 583–615.

29 Harman R. Oriental sore—Old World cutaneous leishmaniasis. In: Canizares O, Harman RRM (eds) *Clinical Tropical Dermatology*, 2nd edn. Blackwell Scientific Publications, Boston, 1992, pp. 298–300.

30 Griffiths WAD. Old World cutaneous leishmaniasis. In: Peters W, Killick-Kendrick R

(eds) *The Leishmaniases in Biology and Medicine*. Academic Press, London, 1987, pp. 617–636.

31 Pettit JHS. Chronic (lupoid) leishmaniasis. *Br J Dermatol* 1962; **74**: 127–131.

32 Kerdel-Vegas F, Kerdel F. American leishmaniasis. In: Canizares O, Harman RRM (eds) *Clinical Tropical Dermatology*, 2nd edn. Blackwell Scientific Publications, Boston, 1992, pp. 301–312.

33 Walton BC. American cutaneous and mucocutaneous leishmaniasis. In: Peters W, Killick-Kendrick R (eds) *The Leishmaniases in Biology and Medicine*. Academic Press, London, 1987, pp. 637–664.

34 Marsden PD. Mucosal leishmaniasis ('espundia' Escomel, 1911). *Trans Roy Soc Trop Med Hyg* 1986; **80**: 859–876.

35 World Health Organization. *Control of the Leishmaniases: Report of a WHO Expert Committee*. Technical Report Series 793, World Health Organization, Geneva, 1990.

36 Harman R. Diffuse cutaneous leishmaniasis (DCL). In: Canizares O, Harman RRM (eds) *Clinical Tropical Dermatology*, 2nd edn. Blackwell Scientific Publications, Boston, 1992, pp. 312–313.

37 Palma G, Gutierrez Y. Laboratory diagnosis of *Leishmania*. *Clin Lab Med* 1991; **11**: 909–922.

38 Kalter DC. Laboratory tests for the diagnosis and evaluation of leishmaniasis. *Dermatol Clin* 1994; **12**: 37–50.

39 Kubba R, Al-Gindan Y. Leishmaniasis. *Dermatol Clin* 1989; **7**: 331–351.

40 Koff AB, Rosen T. Treatment of cutaneous leishmaniasis. *J Am Acad Dermatol* 1994; **31**: 693–708.

41 Herwaldt BL, Berman JD. Recommendations for treating leishmaniasis with sodium stibogluconate (Pentostam) and review of pertinent clinical studies. *Am J Trop Med Hyg* 1992; **46**: 296–306.

42 World Health Organization. *WHO Expert Committee on Onchocerciasis: Third Report*. Technical Report Series 752, World Health Organization, Geneva, 1987.

43 Greene BM. Modern medicine versus an ancient scourge: progress toward control of onchocerciasis. *J Infect Dis* 1992; **166**: 15–21.

44 Murdoch ME, Hay RJ, MacKenzie CD *et al*. A clinical classification and grading system of the cutaneous changes in onchocerciasis. *Br J Dermatol* 1993; **129**: 260–269.

45 Eberhard ML, Lammie PJ. Laboratory diagnosis of filariasis. *Clin Lab Med* 1911; **11**: 977–1010.

46 Buck AA (ed.). *Onchocerciasis: Symptomatology, Pathology, Diagnosis*. World Health Organization, Geneva, 1974.

47 Bradley JE, Trenholme KR, Gillespie AJ *et al*. A sensitive serodiagnostic test for onchocerciasis using a cocktail of recombinant antigens. *Am J Trop Med Hyg* 1993; **48**: 198–204.

48 De Sole G, Remme J, Awadzi K *et al*. Adverse reactions after large-scale treatment of onchocerciasis with ivermectin: combined results from eight community trials. *WHO Bull OMS* 1989; **67**: 707–719.

49 Greene BM, Taylor HR, Cupp EW *et al*. Comparison of ivermectin and diethylcarbamazine in the treatment of onchocerciasis. *N Engl J Med* 1985; **313**: 133–138.

50 World Health Organization. *Control of Lymphatic Filariasis: A Manual for Health Personnel*. World Health Organization, Geneva, 1987.

51 Davis BR. Filariases. *Dermatol Clin* 1989; **7**: 313–321.

52 Kazura J, Greenberg J, Perry R *et al*. Comparison of single-dose diethylcarbamazine and ivermectin for treatment of Bancroftian filariasis in Papua New Guinea. *Am J Trop Med Hyg* 1993; **49**: 804–811.

53 Carme B, Mamboueni JP, Copin N, Noireau F. Clinical and biological study of *Loa loa* filariasis in Congolese. *Am J Trop Med Hyg* 1989; **41**: 331–337.

54 Harman R. Dracunculosis. In: Canizares O, Harman RRM (eds) *Clinical Tropical Dermatology*, 2nd edn. Blackwell Scientific Publications, Boston, 1992, pp. 356–359.

55 Grove DI. Tissue nematodes (trichinosis, dracunculiasis, filariasis). In: Mandell GL, Bennett JE, Dolin R (eds) *Principles and Practice of Infectious Diseases*, 4th edn. Churchill Livingstone, New York, 1995, pp. 2531–2537.

56 Rohde JE, Sharma BL, Patton H, Deegan C, Sherry JM. Surgical extraction of guinea worm: disability reduction and contribution to disease control. *Am J Trop Med Hyg* 1993; **48**: 71–76.

57 Gordon SM, Gal AA, Solomon AR, Bryan JA. Disseminated strongyloidiasis with cutaneous manifestations in an immunocompromised host. *J Am Acad Dermatol* 1994; **31**: 255–259.

58 Bank DE, Grossman ME, Kohn SR, Rabinowitz AD. The thumbprint sign: rapid diagnosis of disseminated strongyloidiasis. *J Am Acad Dermatol* 1990; **23**: 324–326.

59 Ronan SG, Reddy RL, Manaligod JR, Alexander J, Fu T. Disseminated strongyloidiasis presenting as purpura. *J Am Acad Dermatol* 1989; **21**: 1123–1125.

60 Davies HD, Sakuls P, Keystone JS. Creeping eruption: a review of clinical presentation and management of 60 cases presenting to a tropical disease unit. *Arch Dermatol* 1993; **129**: 588–591.

61 Jones WB II. Cutaneous larva migrans. *South Med J* 1993; **86**: 1311–1313.

62 Caumes E, Carriere J, Datry A *et al*. A randomized trial of ivermectin versus albendazole for the treatment of cutaneous larva migrans. *Am J Trop Med Hyg* 1993; **49**: 641–644.

63 Rusnak JM, Lucey DR. Clinical gnathostomiasis: case report and review of the English-language literature. *Clin Infect Dis* 1993; **16**: 33–50.

64 Sarma DP, Weilbaecher TG, Human sparganosis. *J Am Acad Dermatol* 1986; **15**: 1145–1148.

65 Wortman PD. Subcutaneous cysticercosis. *J Am Acad Dermatol* 1991; **25**: 409–414.

66 Gonzalez E. Schistosomiasis, cercarial dermatitis, and marine dermatitis. *Dermatol Clin* 1989; **7**: 291–300.

Chapter 7
Skin Infections in AIDS and HIV-immunocompromised Patients

Warren J. Winkelman

Immunosuppression affords a unique opportunity for the physician to observe the power and influence the immune system has on cutaneous function. The immune barrier, when lost, leaves the unprotected human body as vulnerable as an open culture disc in the laboratory. Many pathogens, formerly regarded as harmless colonists, become virulent opportunists, staking their claim and exhausting precious resources necessary for the life and functioning of the individual. In the acquired immune deficiency syndrome (AIDS), for example, the wide range of peculiar infections testifies to the cascade of devastation brought upon the immune system following the precise decimation of its key arm, initiated by infection with the human immunodeficiency virus (HIV). In this chapter, an examination of both the common and the rare infections seen in HIV-infected immunocompromised patients will be presented.

Infections by viruses in AIDS and HIV

Herpesviruses

Herpesviruses are by far one of the most common viral families to play a role in the morbidity of patients infected with the HIV. All human herpesvirus species are known to cause significant disease in these patients. Herpes simplex viruses 1 and 2 cause disease that may be both banal and significantly problematic. Herpes varicella zoster virus manifestations may be significant markers for impending immunological compromise and may contribute to both morbidity and mortality of HIV-infected individuals. Cytomegalovirus (CMV), although rarely involving the skin, is a significant cause of central nervous system and ocular complications. Epstein–Barr virus is responsible for an important marker for progression to AIDS, oral hairy leucoplakia (OHL) and has been implicated in the pathogenesis of leiomyomas and leiomyosarcomas in AIDS patients [1]. Human Herpesvirus 6 may be a cofactor, along with CMV, in the development of AIDS-associated Kaposi's sarcoma [2]. Human herpesvirus 7, a cause of exanthem subitum in children, is believed to cause immunological complications in AIDS patients and, finally human herpesvirus 8 is purported to be the aetiological agent of Kaposi's sarcoma, an important cutaneous manifestation of AIDS and a source of a great deal of morbidity in these patients.

Herpes simplex viruses 1 and 2

Herpes simplex infection of the skin and mucosa is a prevalent problem in the immunocompromised. Both adults and children may be affected [3].

Although the disease may present with typical grouped, herpetiform vesicles on an erythematous base, with neuritic pain and tenderness, the clinical presentation is often atypical, demonstrating persistent, non-healing or bizarre cutaneous and mucosal ulceration [4], verrucous hyperplastic keratotic plaques (Fig. 7.1) [5], generalized vesicular eruption [6] and stomatitis. In the oral cavity, for example, lesions may appear as depapillated areas of the tongue, often in association with classical vesicular lesions periorally.

In HIV infection, the clinical presentation and severity of herpes simplex lesions are often inversely related to the CD4 count [7]. In addition, many patients with advanced HIV disease have acyclovir-resistant strains of virus, leading to further bizarre clinical lesion presentation.

Diagnosis may be quite challenging, and significant clinical suspicion is necessary. History will probably reveal a painful, chronic lesion, often with significant complaints of burning, itching and neuritic symptoms. As the lesional morphology is often bizarre, confirmatory tests are required. Viral culture, skin biopsy, Tzanck smear and monoclonal-antibody direct-immunofluorescence analysis are all helpful [8].

The basic treatment for herpes simplex is acyclovir [9]. In HIV-infected patients with a CD4 count of 200 cells/mm³ or higher, 200 mg orally five times a day for 5–7 days is usually adequate. As the presentation becomes more chronic and symptomatic with lower immunological potential, higher doses for longer periods of time are required. Acyclovir, 400–800 mg

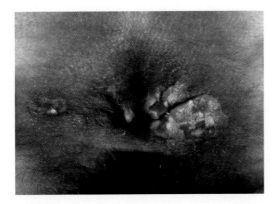

Fig. 7.1 Chronic verrucous perianal herpes simplex virus infection, resistant to acyclovir and foscarnet.

orally five times a day may be necessary for from 1 week to possibly up to 1 month, depending on response. In chronic recurrent cases, acyclovir may be given for suppression at doses of 400 mg orally twice a day (bid) indefinitely. Although well tolerated, rare secondary effects of acyclovir include headache, nausea and skin eruption. Patients with significant allergic reaction and angio-oedema due to acyclovir may be desensitized [10].

Famciclovir, a new acyclovir analogue, may be used in patients who cannot take medication five times a day, as this medication is given thrice daily (tid) at doses of 500 mg each for herpes zoster. However, this utilization is not approved in the USA at this time. Valaciclovir, another new acyclovir analogue, is currently contraindicated in severely immuno-suppressed patients due to reports of AIDS patients developing haemolytic uraemic syndrome with thrombotic thrombocytopenic purpura during therapy.

The development of acyclovir and acyclovir-analogue resistance in patients who are profoundly immunosuppressed has become a problem of note recently [11]. Thymidine kinase-negative herpesvirus species have been isolated in HIV-infected and AIDS patients treated with acyclovir repetitively and chronically. Foscarnet is the treatment of choice for these patients. Foscarnet, or phosphonoformic acid, is an antiherpesvirus chemical that inhibits viral deoxyribonucleic acid (DNA) polymerase, as opposed to the viral thymidine kinase-inhibiting effect of acyclovir [12]. The drug is given intravenously (i.v.), slowly over at least an hour with adequate hydration, as the drug is nephrotoxic. The dosage in AIDS patients is 40–60 mg/kg tid, with duration largely related to the clinical response. Commonly recognized side-effects of this medication include anaemia, nausea, vomiting and painful erosion at the urethral meatus, the latter probably due to a chemical urethritis or mucosal irritation following inadequate hydration during foscarnet administration (Fig. 7.2). In addition, as foscarnet binds to divalent metal ions, such as calcium and magnesium, a patient should be periodically monitored for hypocalcaemia and hypomagnesaemia, as well as other electrolyte abnormalities. There is some evidence that, after a prolonged period of treatment with foscarnet, the thymidine kinase-negative herpesvirus mutants may revert to acyclovir-sensitive strains, once again allowing oral therapy.

In poorly responding patients, as well as patients whose viral strains are apparently both acyclovir- and foscarnet-resistant, topical antiviral agents may be helpful [13]. Trifluridine ophthalmic ointment may be applied to skin lesions up to six times a day [14]. Cidofovir, or (S)-1-(3-hydroxy-2-phosphonylmethoxypropyl)-cytosine (HPMPC), is a new nucleotide analogue that does not require viral enzymes to become activated, therefore potentially allowing for lower incidence of resistant strains [15]. This drug appears to be active against most members of the herpesvirus family, as well as some strains of human papillomavirus (HPV) [16].

Other therapeutic modalities include intralesional interferon, surgical

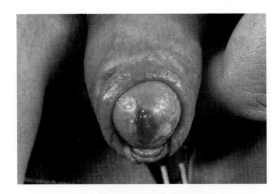

Fig. 7.2 Erosion around the urethral meatus in a patient on intravenous foscarnet.

excision, excision by curettage and electrodesiccation and immunomodulator therapy.

Herpes zoster

Herpes zoster is one of the most frequently recognized early presentations of HIV infection [17], as well as in other forms of immunosuppression [18]. Its presence in these patients may be a foreboding sign of disease progression [19]. Classically, the disease presents as a bandlike collection of painful vesicles on an erythematous base appearing in the distribution of a sensory-nerve dermatome.

What distinguishes herpes zoster in the immunocompromised from the same disease in patients of intact immunity is the severity of the clinical presentation. In HIV patients, for example, the disease is often severe (Fig. 7.3), multidermatomal (Fig. 7.4), disseminated and recurrent, with prolonged acute pain, persistent chronic ulcerative and/or verrucous lesions [20, 21], multiple keratotic papules [22] and a higher incidence of postherpetic neuralgia.

Histopathological examination may demonstrate classic findings of herpes zoster (multinucleated giant cells, necrotic keratinocytes and Cowdry type A nuclear inclusions) with atypical findings corroborating with the often bizarre clinical presentations (verrucous epidermal hyperplasia, pseudocarcinomatous hyperplasia, hyperkeratosis) [23].

Five per cent of patients with herpes zoster are HIV-infected and 6% have cancer. Early recurrences of the disease may be a sign of attendant immunosuppression [24]. Herpes zoster may be seen frequently in both HIV-infected adults and children [25].

Sequelae of herpes zoster are ophthalmic (visual-acuity loss, kerato-uveitis, corneal perforation [26], acute retinal necrosis [27]), neurological (meningoencephalitis [28], syndrome of inappropriate antidiuretic secretion [29], transverse myelitis [30], ventriculitis, acute myeloradiculitis [31] and cerebral infarcts [32]) and dermatological (scarring, dissemination).

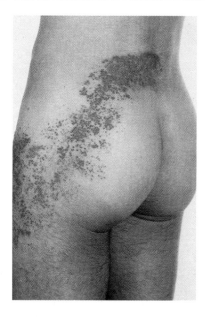

Fig. 7.3 Severe haemorrhagic herpes zoster in a 21-year-old man with HIV.

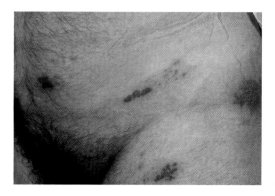

Fig. 7.4 Multidermatomal herpes zoster in a man with AIDS.

Treatment is acyclovir, typically at a dose a 800 mg orally five times daily, for 7–10 days, if the zoster is without complication, or for a longer duration, as the clinical response warrants. Famciclovir, at a dose of 500 mg orally tid is apparently similar to acyclovir in both antiviral efficacy and reduction of zoster-related acute pain, although famciclovir, being a prodrug (propenciclovir), is much more bioavailable.

Intravenous acyclovir is indicated for recurrent, severe and disseminated herpes zoster, at doses of 10 mg/kg every 8 hours. Acyclovir-resistant herpes zoster is treated with intravenous foscarnet at doses of 40–60 mg/kg bid until healing of vesicles.

Other herpesvirus infections

Cytomegalovirus, an encapsulated DNA-genomic virus, causes little disease in the skin of the HIV-infected population, excepting notably the rare reports of diffuse papules, vesicles, ulcers (especially perianal and oral [33]), haemorrhagic vasculitis or morbilliform eruptions seen with disseminated disease. Cytomegalovirus may be a cause of salivary gland dysfunction and xerostomia in severely immunocompromised AIDS patients [34]. In addition, the phenomenon of coinfection of CMV in other skin diseases, such as Kaposi's sarcoma, is well known.

Varicella can be very severe and significantly life-threatening in the immunocompromised, with a high incidence of chronic recurrent and persistent disease, as well as visceral dissemination (e.g. pneumonia), especially with lower CD4 cell counts. Unusual cutaneous lesions, such as hyperkeratotic papules, are seen. Patients may or may not have concurrent dermatomal lesions of herpes zoster. Treatment is intravenous acyclovir, although treatment failures may be seen [35].

Epstein–Barr virus infection on the oral mucosa may produce a lesion well known to clinicians, OHL. This lesion is characterized as velvety-white and corrugated plaques, classically occurring on the sides of the tongue (although they may occur anywhere within the oropharyngeal cavity) which do not scrape off as do the lesions of candidiasis (Fig. 7.5). Oral hairy leucoplakia is an important marker for advancing HIV-related immunodeficiency. Treatment is not often necessary, although oral acyclovir may result in a temporary regression of these lesions. Topical treatments, such as tretinoin gel and 25% podophyllum resin [36], although not palatable, may provide short-term cosmetic efficacy.

Molluscum contagiosum

Molluscum contagiosum virus infection is a common and cosmetically disfiguring infectious dermatosis affecting advanced HIV-infected patients. The lesions, characterized classically by pearly to skin-coloured indurated papules with umbilication, are often morphologically bizarre in these patients. They appear as papules, confluent plaques and nodules [37] with multiple surface umbilications, and may be polypoidal or 'giant'-sized, resembling sessile condylomata or the sebaceous naevus of Jadassohn [38].

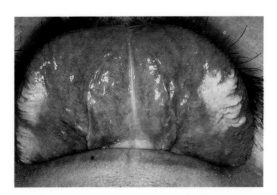

Fig. 7.5 Bilateral lingual oral hairy leucoplakia.

They may additionally appear as cutaneous horns [39] and can be confused with basal-cell carcinoma [40]. Unlike classical molluscum contagiosum in adults, which is a sexually transmitted disease seen largely in the groin, the HIV-infected patient demonstrates infection commonly in the head and neck region as well as the groin, although the lesions may be generalized. Similar findings are seen in HIV-infected children [41]. Unusual involvement of the perioral region [42], eyelids [43], conjunctiva [44], and limbus corneae [45] has also been reported. Secondary bacterial infection of the large nodular lesions, with abscess formation, is common and may necessitate systemic antibiotic therapy [46].

Molluscum contagiosum often occurs as a late manifestation of HIV infection, with the number of lesions increasing significantly as the CD4+ cell count falls below 100 cells/mm³ [47]. The disease is probably acquired in adulthood by contact with other infected individuals, rather than reactivation of a childhood infection [48].

Lesions of systemic fungal infections, such as cryptococcocis [49] and histoplasmosis, may mimic molluscum contagiosum. In fact, both *Cryptococcus neoformans* and molluscum contagiosum may coexist within the same lesions [50]. Thus, any patient known or suspected as being HIV-seropositive who presents with unexplained fever and headache, with or without respiratory dysfunction, with molluscum contagiosum-like lesions should be expeditiously evaluated, with skin biopsy, touch preparation of the skin lesion, radiological examination of the chest, cerebrospinal fluid (CSF) Indian-ink analysis and blood culture, to rule out these often fatal complications [51].

Therapy is difficult and frustrating; resistance and frequent and rapid recurrence [52] may be in part attributed to molluscum-contagiosum DNA virus present in clinically uninvolved skin adjacent to lesions [53]. Thus, a combination approach to treatment is advised. Destructive modalities, such as liquid-nitrogen cryosurgery, electrodesiccation, surgical ablation, curettage and laser excision, provide the first line in most cases. Chemical destruction with topical cantharone, tretinoin, glycolic acid, trichloroacetic acid [54], podophyllotoxin, 5-fluorouracil or salicylic acid should probably be use adjunctively. Multiple molluscum lesions on the eyelids have been treated with excision and retroauricular skin graft [55]. Certainly, adequate concurrent antiretroviral treatment is mandatory, as this may help maximalize therapeutic response [56]. Intralesional vinblastine and bleomycin may be helpful, although subcutaneous interferon-α has proved to be disappointing.

Human papillomavirus infection

The HPV is a frequent cause of morbidity in patients infected with HIV, as well as in patients with AIDS. Many patients are members of epidemiological groups at high risk for both these infection; thus coinfection is likely. Human papillomavirus infections in these patients tend to be chronic,

large, multiple, quite resistant to treatment and, in some cases, oncogenic
[57].

The incidence of venereal warts in HIV-positive women is significantly
higher than in HIV-negative counterparts [58], probably due to a more
rapid progression from initially subclinical infection to clinically apparent
infection seen in the HIV-seropositive female.

In HIV-positive men, anal infection with HPV is quite common, with a
prevalence significantly increasing with dropping CD4 cell count [59]. The
subtypes most prevalent in this population are HPV-16 and 18, those most
significantly associated with subsequent development of anal carcinoma
(Fig. 7.6). Early anal carcinoma may present insidiously as pruritus,
burning, pain, chronic tumour masses, abscesses or leucoplakia. Bowen's
disease, or squamous-cell carcinoma *in situ*, may present perianally as
either a wart-like or eczema-like plaque refractory to treatment. In addition, anal carcinoma may appear in these patients with no history of previous anal HPV infection or despite adequate therapeutic response. Thus, all
HIV patients with a history of anal warts or patients at risk of acquiring anal
warts should have regular examinations externally by observation and palpation, as well as internally by anoscopy. If perianal warts do not clear with
adequate therapy, an anoscopic search for intra-anal warts or carcinomas is

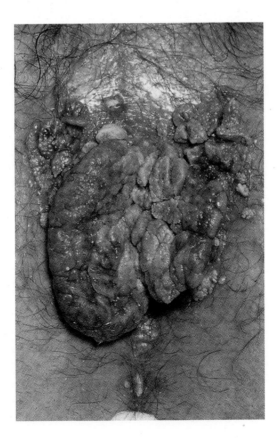

Fig. 7.6 Chronic perianal
and anal condylomata
acuminata, with biopsy
positive for squamous-cell
carcinoma.

indicated. If anal or perianal warts have proved refractory to treatment, biopsy of these lesions is indicated.

Other bizarre infections with HPV may be seen in the HIV-positive patient, including disseminated verruca plana, resembling, in some cases, epidermodysplasia verruciformis, diffuse oral verruca, resembling oral florid papillomatosis, and infections of glabrous skin with HPV types typically seen in condylomas. It is important to remember that biopsy may be indicated in verrucous lesions not responding to therapy, as chronic herpes simplex or zoster may present with verrucous plaques, even in the perianal area and the mouth, especially in patients with very low CD4 counts.

Therapy to eradicate verruca is unsuccessful in most HIV-positive patients. It is best to encourage patients to treat their warts early in HIV disease, when the CD4 cell count is well over 200. Patients may require destructive therapy with liquid nitrogen, topical keratolytics (salicylic acid, lactic acid, retinoic acid, trichloroacetic acid), topical vesicants (podophyllin, cantharone), topical chemotherapy (5-fluorouracil), intralesional injection with bleomycin, vinblastine or interferon, hyperthermia, surgical ablation and oral retinoids. Laser therapy and electrodesiccation are not advised, in light of possible HPV and HIV DNA appearing in the plume. Acitretin and other retinoids, useful in epidermodysplasia verruciformis, may be helpful in the management of patients with innumerable flat warts.

Infections by bacteria in AIDS and HIV

Staphylococcal skin infections

Botryomycosis

Botryomycosis is an infrequent manifestation of skin infection with *Staphylococcus aureus* seen in patients who are immunocompromised. The disease is very difficult to characterize clinically, due to the relatively wide non-specific clinical presentation spectrum. One may see pustules, crusted papules, violaceous plaques with superimposed pustule formation, inflammatory nodules, cysts, ulcerations and erosions. The disease may occur anywhere on the skin, as well as the oral mucosa. In addition, there are reports of internal-organ disease, which may in fact be disseminated [60].

Histopathological examination is often the most important tool towards reaching a diagnosis in cases of botryomycosis. One may see granules with a granulomatous inflammatory reaction, which, on closer examination, actually represents an agglomeration of bacteria surrounded by poorly defined eosinophilic amorphous material.

The unusual presentation of botryomycosis may occur following trauma or prolonged and/or inadequate antibiotic therapy. Furthermore, a reduction in the immune system's capability to kill *S. aureus* adequately may be the reason botryomycosis is seen in AIDS [61]. There is compromised B-cell activation and proliferation, leading to a derangement in the production of antistaphylococcal immunoglobulin. Additionally, disintegration of the T-helper cell and macrophage functional units results in inadequate production of lymphokines necessary for the appropriate killing of bacteria.

Other bacteria may present with the clinical picture of botryomycosis, including *Pseudomonas aeruginosa*, *Escherichia coli*, *Proteus* spp. and *Serratia marcescens*, among others.

Treatment includes prolonged antibiotic therapy with appropriate antistaphylococcal medications, topical antibiotics and astringents, including clindamycin [62], cephalosporins and oxacillin derivatives [63]. In certain cases, surgical excision or laser ablation with débridement and drainage of wounds may be an adjunctive treatment.

Carriage of Staphylococcus aureus

There is an increased incidence of cutaneous colonization with *S. aureus* HIV-seropositive patients, and this may explain the increased incidence of sepsis, pneumonia and skin and soft-tissue infections in these patients [64]. This has been attributed in part to a reduction of secretory immunoglobulin A (IgA) seen in HIV-1-positive individuals, frequent antibiotic therapy, intravenous catheters and concurrent skin disease, such as asteatosis and psoriasis [65]. This HIV-related carriage of *S. aureus* becomes more clinically significant as immunosuppression worsens, with a greater incidence of recurrent infections seen.

Treatment includes mupirocin ointment intranasally to reduce nasal carriage, with the addition of rifampicin 600 mg daily with a cephalosporin or clindamycin.

Staphylococcal scalded-skin syndrome and toxic-shock syndrome

Exotoxin-producing *S. aureus* has been reported in patients of all risk groups for HIV infection. This phenomenon of toxic-shock syndrome (TSS) may not necessarily be related to the menstrual cycle of female patients with HIV disease [66]. Characterized by generalized erythema and desquamation, with hypotension, tachycardia and liver problems, leading to multiorgan failure, TSS in these patients may often be recurrent and resistant to therapy, leading precipitously to renal failure, central nervous system abnormalities, respiratory failure and coagulation disorders [67].

Group II *S. aureus* transfected with phage type 71 may release the toxin responsible for staphylococcal scalded-skin syndrome (SSSS) [68]. It has been reported in adult patients with HIV infection [69, 70].

Other Staphylococcus aureus *infections*

Bullous impetigo has been reported in significant numbers in HIV-1-positive subjects [71]. In addition, some authors believe that certain cases of HIV-related pruritus may be due to the colonization of skin by *S. aureus* [72, 73]. Furthermore, abscess formation around molluscum-contagiosum lesions, pyoderma and recurrent furunculosis [74] have been reported.

Gram-negative and other bacterial skin infections

Pseudomonas aeruginosa *infection*

These infections are becoming more common as more children with HIV disease are living longer and many patients have indwelling catheters to administer medications. Previously banal infections, such as 'hot-tub' folliculitis, may progress to cellulitis in the immunocompromised. Furthermore, with the panoply of neutropenia-inducing medications used in the management of HIV disease increasing and with patients living longer with fewer and fewer white blood cells, it seems likely that clinicians will be seeing more Gram-negative bacterial infections in the future.

Syphilis

Syphilis, when appearing in patients infected with HIV, in unlikely to vary in clinical or serological course, although some reports suggest a more rapid progression or more severe and/or atypical clinical manifestations [75]. Overall, current methods of serological testing for syphilis in HIV to monitor clinical response are considered adequate [76], although exceptions to this rule are found throughout the literature [77], in particular, HIV-positive women with a history of i.v. drug usage may have a significantly greater risk of biological false-positive rapid plasma reagin (RPR) (Venereal Diseases Reference Laboratory (VDRL)) than HIV-seronegative women [78].

None the less, the general consensus is to be aware that the risk of neurosyphilis, serological relapse [79] and late complications remains even after appropriate therapy has been given. In fact, high clinical suspicion is warranted, as CSF VDRL levels consistent with neurosyphilis may be present despite lack of symptomatology, apparent adequate therapeutic response or negative serological titres [80]. Furthermore, a patient may have clinical syphilis and symptoms suggestive of neurosyphilis without consistent CSF changes [81]. Thus, early aggressive therapy, supplemented with prolonged and frequent monitoring of these patients, is required [82].

However, syphilis in patients infected with HIV may present with severe dermatological manifestations, uncommonly seen in the general population. Lues maligna, a rare form of secondary syphilis, characterized by widespread noduloulcerative and vesiculonecrotic lesions, with fever, meningismus and frequent relapses, has been reported many times in HIV patients in the recent literature [83]. Interestingly, this particular form has been reported with both high and low titres on serological testing, suggesting in some cases a 'latent' form of syphilis [84]. These patients may have constitutional symptoms severe enough to require hospitalization. Often, standard protocols of parenteral treatments fail, warranting aggressive treatment with third-generation cephalosporins. Patients who are penicillin-allergic may require desensitization, as i.v. erythromycin may not be adequate to cure lues maligna [83].

Primary syphilis may present in bizarre fashion as well, such as with multiple chancres and erosions [85]. Secondary syphilis in HIV infection is often severe and bizarre as well [86]. In addition to extreme presentations of typical syphilis lesions, sclerodermoid-like changes have been reported [87]. Tertiary syphilis may appear earlier than previously thought [88]. Furthermore, refractory infections [89] and early relapses may be seen in treated cases [90].

The histopathological changes in syphilis complicating HIV disease may be similar to those in the non-HIV population, with the possible exception of endothelial proliferation, which has been reported as being seen less frequently in the HIV-infected [91].

As of this writing, there are no changes in the current recommendations of the Centers for Disease Control (CDC) for treatment guidelines for syphilis in relation to concurrent HIV infection, although many authors advocate a more aggressive primary therapy such as amoxycillin 6 g/day with probenecid or ceftriaxone 1–2 g/day for 10–14 days [92]. Giving additional doses of the gold standards, that is, benzathine penicillin total dose of 4.8–7.2 µg given over 2–3 weeks and penicillin G 18–24 million units i.v. daily for 10–14 days, has been suggested, although even this regimen may be complicated by relapse or progression of neurosyphilis [93]. Reports of erythromycin failures for syphilis in HIV infection are found throughout the literature, thus implicating this drug as a poor choice in these patients.

Bacillary angiomatosis

This unusual and rapidly fatal [94] bacterial infection has been seen mostly in HIV-related immunosuppressed patients [95], but has been reported in patients with B-cell lymphocytic leukaemia [96] or systemic malignancy [97, 98], in patients with normal immune systems [99] and in patients post-organ transplantation on immunosuppressive medication [100]. In HIV-positive patients with bacillary angiomatosis, the patients are often profoundly immunosuppressed, with a mean CD4+ cell count of less than 100 cells/mm³ [101].

Bartonella henselae and *Bartonella quintana*, the causative organisms, originally known as members of the genus *Rochalimaea*, are weakly Gram-negative rod-shaped bacilli [102]. They are of the same genus as *Bartonella bacilliformis*, the causative agent of verruga peruana, a late cutaneous manifestation of Oroya fever, or bartonellosis, seen predominantly in South American mountainous regions. *Bartonella quintana* is also the cause of trench fever. The cat-scratch disease bacillus, formerly believed to be identical to the aetiological agent of bacillary angiomatosis, is now known as *Afipia felis* [103].

Skin lesions manifest most classically as multiple red to violaceous exophytic papulonodules, which resemble pyogenic granulomas (Fig. 7.7); they are often tender and friable. Other variants include subcutaneous nodules, hyperpigmented indurated plaques and furuncle-like masses [104]. The oral mucosa, conjunctiva [105] and genitalia may be affected as well [106]. Differential diagnosis includes Kaposi's sarcoma and pyogenic granuloma [107].

The disease may be complicated by systemic involvement, including fever, pulmonary infiltrates and pleural effusions, lymphadenopathy [108], hepatosplenomegaly, osteolytic lesions [109], peliosis hepatis [110], psychiatric disturbances [111] and gastrointestinal lesions, leading to haemorrhage. Diagnosis is made by clinical examination and history, with skin biopsy demonstrating multiple endothelial vascular channels lined with plump endothelial cells and a heavy neutrophilic infiltrate [112]. Warthin–Starry silver stain exhibits pleomorphic bacilli adjacent to vascular channels. Polymerase chain reaction-mediated genetic amplification for the bacillus may provide additional diagnostic confirmatory evidence.

Treatment of choice is oral erythromycin, 500 mg four times a day (qid), until clearing of lesions, although the high potential risk for relapse may necessitate indefinite treatment [113]. Intravenous therapy is advocated in cases of internal-organ involvement. Other choices include systemic tetracycline, doxycycline, azithromycin (1 g daily as a single dose) [114] and clarithromycin [115]. Although rifampicin and gentamicin may play some role in therapy, penicillins and cephalosporins are ineffective.

Cats appear to be a significant reservoir for the bacillus, occurring in up

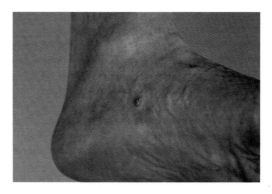

Fig. 7.7 Acute-onset pyogenic granuloma-like lesion of bacillary angiomatosis.

to 40–50% of animals examined in selected urban areas, particularly in kittens [116]. Immunocompromised patients at risk should protect themselves against bites and scratches from cats [117], as well as provide adequate flea control to decrease risk of exposure and infection.

Mycobacterial skin infections

Mycobacteria, a common cause of morbidity and mortality in patients with AIDS and HIV infection, may less frequently cause cutaneous disease in these patients.

Although there is a theoretical supposition that leprosy should be worse when an individual is coinfected with HIV, there is little evidence to confirm this. Cellular immune response, histological presentation and clinical progression of leprosy are unchanged. There may be some lack of lepromin skin testing in normally positive borderline lepromatous-leprosy patients.

Disseminated infection due to atypical mycobacteria, with cutaneous manifestations, may be seen more frequently in HIV-immunosuppressed patients than in immunocompetent controls. Lesions may appear as papules, plaques, pustules, nodules, ulcers, abscesses or cellulitis. *Mycobacterium kansasii* may cause multiple scalp abscesses in association with disseminated systemic infection [118]. *Mycobacterium haemophilum* may present with ulcerated fluctuant nodules, particularly over joints and at injection sites in i.v. drug users. These lesions may be accompanied by fever, arthritis and osteomyelitis.

Cutaneous lesions of *Mycobacterium tuberculosis* may include scrofuloderma, or draining sinuses overlying severe, suppurative tuberculous lymphadenopathy, widespread keratotic papules and nodules, palmoplantar keratoderma and acute miliary or follicular papules.

Infections caused by fungi

Superficial fungal infections and onychomycosis

Cutaneous infection with dermatophytes is a prevalent problem in HIV and AIDS, occurring in at least one-fifth of these patients [119]. These infections are seen both early in the clinical course of HIV infection, with relatively high CD4 counts, and later in progression of disease, when tinea infections may become generalized and refractory to treatment [119]. Onychomycosis presents typically with a CD4 count of 450 cells/mm^3 [120]. Dermatophytes may in fact be found subclinically on the feet in up to 37% of HIV-seropositive men [121].

Tinea pedis and/or tinea unguium are commonly seen in HIV disease; they are caused most frequently by *Tricophyton rubrum* [122].

Tinea capitis is seen in both children and adults with HIV infection. It may present in all the classical ways, inflammatory and/or non-inflammatory, and may be caused not only by dermatophytes but also by *Aspergillus, Rhizopus* and other fungal organisms [123].

Tinea faciale may be seen in adults and children, is commonly caused by *T. rubrum* and may appear centrofacially, imitating seborrhoeic dermatitis [124].

Onychomycosis may present as typical yellow thickening with onycholysis, but may also appear as the proximal white subungual morphology and/or the superficial white infection of the nail plate; the most common organism in these clinical presentations is *T. rubrum*, which is similar to the non-HIV infected population, although white superficial onychomycosis in the non-HIV-infected is most often caused by *Trichophyton mentagrophytes* [125].

Tinea corporis may present typically, as oval or round erythematous plaques, or may appear as non-inflammatory diffuse scaling or as folliculitis [126]. Scutular or favus-like presentations of tinea cruris and tinea pedis due to *Microsporum gypseum* has been reported in AIDS [127].

Diagnosis is achieved by adequate history and physical examination, paying particular attention to the morphology of the lesions, as, in many cases, unusual presentations of tinea infections (e.g. white superficial onychomycosis, extensive fungal folliculitis, tinea incognito, proximal white subungual onychomycosis) may provide an important diagnostic clue to identify previously undiagnosed HIV-infected individuals [128]. In-office diagnostic tools, such as potassium hydroxide examination of skin scrapings, are quite helpful, although, in the immunosuppressed, culture is vital to identify an unusual organism and will help guide the clinician to the adequate systemic therapy, should that be necessary.

Treatment of the morbidity caused by these infections is important in the immunosuppressed. In addition, as tinea infections of the skin provide a portal of entry for potentially life-threatening microorganisms, treatment is mandatory for guarding the overall quality of life and health of these patients. In most cases, treatment of superficial dermatophytosis is largely topical, utilizing one of the many topical antifungals, such as terbinafine, ketoconazole or cicliprox olamine, usually in combination with excellent basic foot care, including appropriate cleansing with antibacterial–antifungal soaps and adequate drying. Antifungal powders provide adjunctive epidemiological control and may help, in the long run, to reduce the risk of recurrence.

In severe or extensive cases of cutaneous tinea infection, as well as for adequate control of nail infection, systemic antifungals are necessary. Oral terbinafine, at a dose of 250 mg daily, may be used for 1 month to treat glabrous skin infection, 6 weeks for tinea capitis, 3 months for fingernail infection and 4 months for toenail infection. The major drawback of this medication is the cost. Baseline monitoring of transaminase levels and white blood-cell counts is important to diagnose potential early toxicity. In addition, urticarial eruptions and typical drug eruptions, generally seen more frequently in HIV patients, may often be prolonged due to the depot effect of terbinafine in keratin. Furthermore, unrealistic patient expectations as to the safety and efficacy of terbinafine may in part be fuelled by the current, aggressive marketing techniques of its manufacturer.

Systemic azoles (ketoconazole, itraconazole, fluconazole) provide a mainstay of treatment for these infections. Unfortunately, hepatic toxicity limits the use of ketoconazole in many HIV patients. In addition, achlorhydria or hypochlorhydria, common in HIV-infected patients, may reduce the gastric absorption of ketoconazole and itraconazole; this is not a problem with fluconazole [129]. Ketoconazole also interacts with many other medications, a fact which may cause increased risk of toxicity or decreased efficacy. None the less, dermatophyte-infected nails may be treated with oral ketoconazole for prolonged periods with good results, and itraconazole may be used either daily for periods of 3–4 months or in 'pulse' or intermittent doses for 1 week for 3–4 consecutive months, with seemingly equivalent results. The risk of recurrence may be higher, despite adequate therapeutic duration, for HIV-infected patients, and therefore long-term maintenance treatment with antifungal creams and powders is important.

Deep fungal infections

Human immunodeficiency virus-seropositive patients with systemic fungal infections, such as cryptococcosis and histoplasmosis, are often acutely ill, with fever, pulmonary distress, acute changes in mental status and skin lesions. Molluscum contagiosum-like lesions seen in some patients with systemic cryptococcosis and histoplasmosis have been discussed earlier in the chapter. Cryptococcosis may also present with skin ulcers, pustules, subcutaneous nodules and granulomas, draining sinuses or cellulitis. Histoplasmosis may present with oral and cutaneous ulcers (Fig. 7.8), verrucous plaques, acneform lesions and vesicles, papules and patches. In addition, both these infections may present concurrently in the same patient [130]. Long-term chronic therapy with fluconazole, 200 mg/day, for prophylaxis against systemic fungal infection, as well as against the development of invasive candidiasis, in patients with significantly depressed numbers of CD4+ lymphocytes is well accepted [131].

Dermatophytes may cause systemic infections in the immunosuppressed. Invasion has been reported by *T. rubrum* in transplant recipients [132], as well as patients with leukaemia [133], lymphoma [134] and myelodysplastic syndrome [135]. In AIDS, skin nodules on the lower legs due to invasion by *T. rubrum* has been reported and effectively treated with oral fluconazole, 100 mg daily, with clearing in 3 weeks [136].

Candidiasis

Oropharyngeal candidiasis is one of the most common mucosal manifesta-

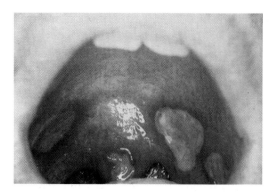

Fig. 7.8 Multiple, deep oral ulcerations in an AIDS patient with systemic histoplasmosis.

tions of significant immunosuppression secondary to HIV infection [137]. The disease is characterized classically by white patches throughout the oral cavity and pharynx, which may, in most cases, be removed, at least partially, leaving a hyperaemic or friable mucosa underneath. Of course, all of the well-described clinical variants of oral candidiasis are seen in these patients, including pseudomembranous candidiasis, ulcers, lingual atrophy and erythematous and gingival hyperplasia, as well as unusual variants, such as hyperplastic papillae of the hard and soft palate [138].

Treatment largely depends on symptomatology and immunological status. Oral clotrimazole troches are effective in treating the disease, although patients may remain persistently subclinically colonized with *Candida albicans* or other *Candida* spp. [139]. Fluconazole at 100 mg/day orally may be effective to eradicate infection in patients with CD4 cell counts of greater than 400 cells/mm³ but relapse and treatment failures are the norm when cells drop below 50 [140]. Many of these treatment failures may be due to the development of fluconazole resistance [141].

Eosinophilic folliculitis of HIV disease (eosinophilic dermatosis)

Although not formally recognized as an infection, there is indirect evidence to suggest that eosinophilic folliculitis (EF) of HIV disease may be initiated, at least in part, by a microorganism [142], although to date none has been definitively found [73]. This pruritic dermatosis, characterized by perifollicular and non-perifollicular erythematous to skin-coloured and oedematous or urticarial papules and nodules, distributed on the face, upper trunk and upper arms, is seen predominantly in advanced HIV-infected patients, most with a CD4 count of less than 250 cells/mm³ [143].

The panoply of reported treatments reflects the often frustrating resistance the disease manifests to therapeutic intervention. Systemic hydroxyzine, often in extremely high doses of 25–50 mg orally qid, is the mainstay of treatment. Itraconazole, a systemic antifungal, is effective in control of pruritus at doses of 200 mg twice daily, often indefinitely [144]. Ultraviolet B phototherapy has a similar suppressive effect on symptomatology, but the long duration of treatment, coupled with possible activation of HIV virus replication by the exposure, renders this therapy less attractive. Cetirizine, a systemic, relatively non-sedating antihistamine, with possible specific antieosinophilic action, appears uniquely effective in reducing the itch and lesion progression [145]. The optimal dose appears to be 10–20 mg daily.

Isotretinoin, in doses from 0.5 to 1.2 mg/kg, is quite effective in controlling symptomatology, although optimal dosage is unclear and patients may require long-term suppressive therapy or repeat courses for frequent relapses [146]. However, baseline and careful concurrent measurement of serum triglycerides during isotretinoin therapy is vital, as many patients with AIDS and severely immunocompromised have elevated triglycerides, thus increasing the risk of fatal pancreatitis. In addition, medications such as protease inhibitors (e.g. ritonavir) may increase serum triglyceride levels, and certain antiretroviral drugs, such as didanosine (ddI), have a reported increased risk of pancreatitis.

Other remedial choices include systemic metronidazole [147], minocycline, tetracycline, dicloxacillin, doxepin, thalidomide and astemizole. The latter should be used with caution in the HIV-infected, as many of these patients will be taking ketoconazole, and the purported association of ketoconazole–astemizole with torsade-des-pointes cardiac dysrhythmia should not be forgotten. In addition, reports of ketoconazole efficacy in EF attests of a possible role for yeast in pathogenesis, possibly *Pityrosporum orbiculare* [148].

Topical intervention provides many patients with relief from the incessant pruritus so devastatingly characteristic of this dermatosis. Topical corticosteroid emollient creams, usually of high potency, such as clobetasol diproprionate 0.05%, are helpful, often compounded with antipruritic counterirritants, such as camphor, menthol or phenol. 'Shake' lotions, such as calamine, are very soothing. Topical doxepin, pramoxine, prilocaine–lidocaine, permethrin [149], sulphur and disodium chromoglycate 4% [150] offer varying degrees of relief. Topical anti-infective agents, such as clindamycin, ketoconazole and metronidazole, are used frequently as adjunctive therapy with variable results.

Seborrhoeic dermatitis

One of the most common dermatoses seen in HIV-infected patients, seborrhoeic dermatitis, is probably caused by a yeast, *Pityrosporum ovale (orbiculare)* or *Malassezia furfur*. A distinguishing feature in its presentation in the immunosuppressed is its severity: the lesions are significantly erythematous and crusted, with involvement extending beyond the 'classic' seborrhoeic areas of the face, scalp, chest, back and groin.

Unusual changes on histopathological examination of seborrhoeic dermatitis in HIV disease attest to the unique nature of the condition. Unlike typical seborrhoea, one sees an interface dermatitis (vacuolar degeneration at the dermal–epidermal junction), with necrotic-appearing keratinocytes in the epidermis and a significant inflammatory infiltrate. Often, special stains for microorganisms are negative.

The patients may be quite symptomatic, with pruritus and 'burning' sensation and a relative intolerance to topical treatments. None the less, most patients are well controlled with topical antifungals, such as clotrimazole or ketoconazole, usually compounded with a mild anti-inflammatory agent, such as hydrocortisone 1%.

Infections caused by parasites

Crusted scabies

Norwegian, or crusted, scabies presents clinically as reactive hyperkeratotic plaques or an eczema-like eruption over distal joints and bony prominences and in body folds. Although classically pruritic, it may not be so in the immunosuppressed. The pruritus is often reported by family members infested by contact with this extremely contagious individual. Morphology may range from classic erythematous vesicles and papules with burrows in web spaces of the hand to psoriasiform plaques to verrucous hyperkeratoses in body folds, reminiscent of Darier's disease. Scraping or biopsy reveals innumerable *Sarcoptes scabei* mites infesting within the lesions.

Treatment must be scabecidal and often repetitive. Topical lindane lotion to the entire cutaneous surface, including face and scalp, at weekly intervals, is curative. However, one must be aware of the potential risk of neurotoxicity in these often relatively cachectic patients. Topical permethrin 5% cream offers a potentially less toxic, though more expensive, alternative. Adjunctive daily treatment with topical 5% sulphur in petrolatum is helpful in both infestation control and crust removal. Topical crotamiton cream may assist in reinfestation control, as may scabene spray.

Systemic ivermectin, not readily available in North America, shows promise as a relatively safe, simple treatment. An oral antihelminthic medication, it is given as a single oral dose of 200 µg/kg body weight in patients with scabies, and may be used in combination with topical scabicides for eradication of disease [151].

Fomite deinfestation is vitally important for epidemiological control.

Other parasitic infections of the skin

Cutaneous infection with mites of the *Demodex* spp. has been reported in patients with AIDS, as well as other forms of immunosuppression. Two organisms are often implicated: *Demodex folliculorum*, seen in folliculitis-type eruptions, otherwise known as 'papular demodiciosis', and *Demodex brevis*, seen in a seborrhoeic dermatitis-like eruption, which affects children with lymphoblastic leukaemia. The treatment is daily antiscabetic topical creams, such as permethrin or crotamiton, until clearing, usually after 5–8 weeks.

Acanthamoeba can present with pustules, oral ulcers (hard palate) and perianal ulcers, as well as disseminated, painful, erythematous, cutaneous nodules with secondary ulceration and fever [152]. Prognosis is guarded, despite aggressive therapy with various combinations of intravenous pentamidine, fluconazole, flucytosine, itraconazole or sulphadiazine. *Pneumocystis carinii* infection of the skin, or cutaneous pneumocystosis, has been reported as polypoid lesions occurring in the external auditory meatus in association with systemic infection. *Strongyloides stercoralis* may present with its classic oval purpura or 'thumbprint' sign.

References

1 McClain KL, Leach CT, Jenson HB *et al.* Association of Epstein–Barr virus with leiomyosarcomas in young people with AIDS. *N Engl J Med* 1995; **332**: 12–18.
2 Kempf W, Adams V, Pfaltz M *et al.* Human herpesvirus type 6 and cytomegalovirus in AIDS-associated Kaposi's sarcoma: no evidence for an etiological association. *Hum Pathol* 1995; **26**: 914–919.
3 Choudhury SA, Hodes DS, Peters VB, Bottone EJ. Cutaneous herpes simplex virus infection in a child with acquired immunodeficiency syndrome. *Clin Pediatr* 1994; **33** (11): 698–700.
4 LaGuardia KD, White MH, Saigo PE, Hoda S, McGuinness K, Ledger WJ. Genital ulcer disease in women infected with human immunodeficiency virus. *Am J Obstetr Gynecol* 1995; **172** (2, Part 1): 553–562.
5 Military Medical Consortium of Applied Retroviral Research Washington, DC. Verrucous lesions secondary to DNA viruses in patients infected with the human immunodeficiency virus in association with increased factor XIIIa-positive dermal dendritic cells. *J Am Acad Dermatol* 1992; **27** (6, Part 1): 943–950.
6 Langtry JA, Ostlere LS, Hawkins DA, Staughton RC. The difficulty in diagnosis of cutaneous herpes simplex virus infection in patients with AIDS. *Clin Exp Dermatol* 1994; **19** (3): 224–226.
7 Bagdades EK, Pillay D, Squire SB, O'Neil C, Johnson MA, Griffiths PD. Relationship between herpes simplex virus ulceration and CD4+ cell counts in patients with HIV infection. *AIDS* 1992; **6** (11): 1317–1320.
8 Cohen SM, Schmitt SL, Lucas FV, Wexner SD. The diagnosis of anal ulcers in AIDS patients. *Int J Colorectal Dis* 1994; **9** (4): 169–173.
9 Montauk SL, Mandell K. Update on durg therapy for HIV and related infections in adults. *Am Fam Physician* 1992; **46** (6): 1772–1781.
10 Henry RE, Wegmann JA, Hartle JE *et al.* Successful oral acyclovir desensitization. *Ann Allergy* 1993; **70**: 386–388.
11 Balfour HH, Benson C, Braun J *et al.* Management of acyclovir-resistant herpes simplex and varicella-zoster virus infections. *J Acquired Immun Defic Syndr* 1994; **7**: 254–260.
12 Wagstaff AJ, Bryson HM. Foscarnet: a reappraisal of its antiviral activity, pharmacokinetic properties and therapeutic use in immunocompromised patients with viral infections. *Drugs* 1994; **48** (2): 199–226.
13 McGrath BJ, Newman CL. Genital herpes simplex infections in patients with the acquired immunodeficiency syndrome. *Pharmacotherapy* 1994; **14** (5): 529–542.

14 Murphy M, Morley A, Eglin RP, Monteiro E. Topical trifluridine for mucocutaneous acyclovir-resistant herpes simplex II in AIDS patient. *Lancet* 1992; **340** (8226): 1040.

15 Lazelari JP, Drew WL, Glutzer E *et al.* Treatment with intravenous (S)-1-[3-hydroxy-2-(phosphonylmethoxy)propyl]-cytosine of acyclovir-resistant mucocutaneous infection with herpes simplex virus in a patient with AIDS. *J Infect Dis* 1994; **170** (3): 570–572.

16 Snoeck R, Andrei G, Silverman A *et al.* Successful treatment of progressive mucocutanoeus infection due to acyclovir and foscarnet-resistant herpes simplex virus with (S)-1-(3-hydroxy-2-phosphonylmethoxypropyl)-cytosine (HPMPC). *Clin Infect Dis* 1994; **18**: 570–578.

17 Wong KJ, Lee SS, Lo YC *et al.* Profile of opportunistic infections among HIV-1 infected people in Hong Kong. *Chung Hua I Hsueh Tsa Chih—Chinese Med J* 1995; **55** (2): 127–136.

18 Nakayama H, Okamura J, Ohga S *et al.* Herpes zoster in children with bone marrow transplantation: report from a single institution. *Acta Paediatr Japon* 1995; **37** (3): 302–307.

19 Smith KJ, Skelton HG, Yeager J *et al.* Cutaneous findings in HIV-1-positive patients: a 42-month prospective study. Military Medical Consortium for the Advancement of Retroviral Research (MMCARR). *J Am Acad Dermatol* 1994; **31** (5, Part 1): 746–754.

20 Vaughan Jones SA, McGibbon DH, Bradbeer CS. Chronic verrucous varicella-zoster infection in a patient with AIDS. *Clin Exp Dermatol* 1994; **19** (4): 327–329.

21 Grossman MC, Grossman ME. Chronic hyperkeratotic herpes zoster and human immunodeficiency virus infection. *J Am Acad Dermatol* 1993; **28** (2, Part 2): 306–308.

22 Lokke Jensen B, Weismann K, Mathiesen L, Klem Thomsen H. Atypical varicella-zoster infection in AIDS. *Acta Dermatol Venereol* 1993; **73** (2): 123–125.

23 LeBoit PE, Limova M, Yen TS, Palefsky JM, White CR Jr, Berger TG. Chronic verrucous varicella-zoster virus infection in patients with the acquired immunodeficiency syndrome (AIDS): histologic and molecular biologic findings. *Am J Dermatopathol* 1992; **14** (1): 1–7.

24 Donahue JG, Choo PW, Manson JE, Platt R. The incidence of herpes zoster. *Arch Intern Med* 1995; **155** (15): 1605–1609.

25 Prose NS. Cutaneous manifestations of pediatric HIV infection. *Pediatr Dermatol* 1992; **9** (4): 326–328.

26 Lewallen S. Herpes zoster ophthalmicus in Malawi. *Ophthalmology* 1994; **101** (11): 1801–1804.

27 Sellitti TP, Huang AJ, Schiffman J, Davis JL. Association of herpes zoster ophthalmicus with acquired immunodeficiency syndrome and acute retinal necrosis. *Am J Ophthalmol* 1993; **116** (3): 297–301.

28 Poscher ME. Successful treatment of varicella zoster virus meningoencephalitis in patients with AIDS: report of four cases and review. *AIDS* 1994; **8** (8): 1115–1117.

29 Arzuaga JA, Estirado E, Roman F, Perez-Maestu R, Masa C, de Letona JM. Syndrome of inappropriate antidiuretic hormone secretion and herpes zoster infection: 1. Report of this association in a patient suffering from AIDS. *Nephron* 1994; **68** (2): 262–264.

30 Grant AD, Fox JD, Brink NS, Miller RF. Detection of varicella-zoster virus DNA using the polymerase chain reaction in an immunocompromised patient with transverse myelitis secondary to herpes zoster. *Genitourin Med* 1993; **69** (4): 273–275.

31 Glesby MJ, Moore RD, Chiasson RE. Clinical spectrum of herpes zoster in adults infected with human immunodeficiency virus. *Clin Infect Dis* 1995; **21**: 370–375.

32 Gray F, Belec L, Lescs MC *et al.* Varicella-zoster virus infection of the central nervous

system in the acquired immunodeficiency syndrome. *Brain* 1994; **117** (5): 987–999.

33 Schubert MM, Epstein JB, Lloid ME *et al.* Oral infections due to cytomegalovirus in immunocompromised patients. *J Oral Pathol Med* 1993; **22**: 268–273.

34 Greenberg M, Dubin G, Stewart J *et al.* The relationship of oral disease to the presence of cytomegalovirus DNA in the saliva of AIDS patients. *Oral Surg Oral Med Oral Pathol* 1995; **79**: 175–179.

35 Srugo I, Israele V, Wittek A *et al.* Clinical manifestations of varicella-zoster virus infections in human immunodeficiency virus-infected children. *Am J Dis Child* 1993; **147**: 742–745.

36 Gowdey G, Lee PK, Carpenter WM. Treatment of HIV-related hairy leukoplakia with podophyllum resin 25% solution. *Oral Surg Oral Med Oral Pathol* 1995; **79**: 64–67.

37 Petersen CS, Gerstoft J. Molluscum contagiosum in HIV-infected patients. *Dermatology* 1992; **184** (1): 19–21.

38 Itin PH, Gilli L. Molluscum contagiosum mimicking sebaceous nevus of Jadassohn, ecthyma and giant condyloma accuminata in HIV-infected patients. *Dermatology* 1994; **189** (4): 396–398.

39 Schwartz JJ, Myskowski PL. HIV-related molluscum contagiosum presenting as a cutaneous horn (letter). *Int J Dermatol* 1992; **31** (2): 142–144.

40 Fivenson DP, Weltman RE, Gibson SH. Giant molluscum contagiosum presenting as basal cell carcinoma in an acquired immunodeficiency syndrome patient. *J Am Acad Dermatol* 1988; **19** (5, Part 1): 912–914.

41 Fejes L. [Incidence of molluscum contagiosum in children with AIDS at the Cervanoda Orphanage, District of Constanta, Romania]. *Bull Soc Pathol Exot* 1993; **86** (5): 327–328.

42 Ficarra G, Cortes S, Rubino I, Romagnoli P. Facial and perioral molluscum contagiosum in patients with HIV infection: a report of eight cases. *Oral Surg Oral Med Oral Pathol* 1994; **78** (5): 621–626.

43 Robinson MR, Udell IJ, Garber PF, Perry HD, Streeten BW. Molluscum contagiosum of the eyelids in patients with acquired immunodeficiency syndrome. *Ophthalmology* 1992; **99** (11): 1745–1747.

44 Charles NC, Friedberg DN. Epibulbar molluscum contagiosum in acquired immunodeficiency syndrome: case report and review of the literature. *Ophthalmology* 1992; **99** (7): 1123–1126.

45 Merisier H, Cochereau I, Hoang-Xuan T, Toublanc M, Ruggeri C. Multiple molluscum contagiosum lesions of the limbus in a patient with HIV infection (letter). *Br J Ophthalmol* 1995; **79** (4): 393–394.

46 Dhar J, Carey PB, Hart A. Molluscum contagiosum—a novel presentation. *Int Conf AIDS* 1993; **9** (1): 354 (abstract PoB 081311).

47 Schwartz JJ, Myskowski PL. Molluscum contagiosum in patients with human immunodeficiency virus infection: a review of twenty-seven patients. *J Am Acad Dermatol* 1992; **27** (4): 583–588.

48 Thompson CH, de Zwart-Steffe RT, Donovan B. Clinical and molecular aspects of molluscum contagiosum infection in HIV-1 positive patients. *Int J STD AIDS* 1992; **3** (2): 101–106.

49 Picon L, Vaillant L, Duong T *et al.* Cutaneous cryptococcosis resembling molluscum contagiosum: a first manifestation of AIDS. *Acta Dermatol Venereol* 1989; **69** (4): 365–367.

50 Sulica RL, Kelly J, Berberian BJ, Glaun R. Cutaneous cryptococcosis with molluscum contagiosum coinfection in a patient with acquired immunodeficiency syndrome. *Cutis* 1994; **53** (2): 88–90.

51 Ghigliotti G, Carrega G, Farris A *et al.* Cutaneous cryptococcosis resembling molluscum contagiosum in a homosexual man with AIDS: report of a case and review of the literature. *Acta Dermatol Venereol* 1992; **72** (3): 182–184.

52 Ficarra G, Gaglioti D. Facial molluscum contagiosum in HIV-infected patients. *Int J Oral Maxillofac Surg* 1989; **18** (4): 200–201.

53 Smith KJ, Skelton HG III, Yeager J, James WD, Wagner KF. Molluscum contagiosum: ultrastructural evidence for its presence in skin adjacent to clinical lesions in patients infected with human immunodeficiency type 1. *Arch Dermatol* 1992; **128** (2): 223–227.

54 Garrett SJ, Robinson JK, Roenigk HH Jr. Trichloroacetic acid peel of molluscum contagiosum in immunocompromised patients. *J Dermatol Surg Oncol* 1992; **18** (10): 855–858.

55 Pope-Pegram LD, Micheletti G, Stool E, Gathe H III, Garland J. Management of molluscum contagiosum of the eyelids by retroauricular skin graft in a patient with acquired immune deficiency syndrome. *Int Conf AIDS* 1993; **9** (1): 346 (abstract PO-B08-1262).

56 Betlloch I, Pinazo I, Mestre F, Altes J, Villalonga C. Molluscum contagiosum in human immunodeficiency virus infection: response to zidovudine (letter). *Int J Dermatol* 1989; **28** (5): 351–352.

57 Wang CY, Brodland DG, Su WP. Skin cancers associated with acquired immunodeficiency syndrome. *Mayo Clin Proc* 1995; **70** (8): 766–772.

58 Chirgwin KD, Feldman J, Augenbraun M, Landesman S, Minkoff H. Incidence of venereal warts in human immunodeficiency virus-infected and uninfected women. *J Infect Dis* 1995; **172** (1): 235–238.

59 Breese PL, Judson FN, Penley KA, Douglas JM Jr. Anal human papillomavirus infection among homosexual and bisexual men: prevalence of type-specific infection and association with human immunodeficiency virus. *Sex Transm Dis* 1995; **22** (1): 7–14.

60 Ahdoot D, Rickman LS, Haghighi P, Heard WU. Botryomycosis in the acquired immunodeficiency syndrome. *Cutis* 1995; **55** (3): 149–152.

61 Murphy PM, Lane C, Fauci AS. Impairment of neutrophil bactericidal capacity in patients with AIDS. *J Infect Dis* 1988; **158**: 1268–1276.

62 Rolston KV. Clindamycin for staphylococcal skin infections in AIDS. *JAMA* 1989; **261** (10): 1444–1445.

63 Weitzner JM, Dhawan SS, Rosen LB *et al.* Successful treatment of botryomycosis in a patient with acquired immunodeficiency syndrome. *J Am Acad Dermatol* 1989; **21**: 1312–1314.

64 Smith KJ, Wagner KF, Yeager J, Skelton HG, Ledsky R. *Staphylococcus aureus* carriage and HIV-1 disease: association with increased mucocutaneous infections as well as deep soft-tissue infections and sepsis. *Arch Dermatol* 1994; **130** (4): 521–522.

65 Jaffe D, May LP, Sanchez M, Moy J. Staphylococcal sepsis in HIV antibody seropositive psoriasis patients. *J Am Acad Dermatol* 1991; **24** (6, Part 1): 970–972.

66 Woods SL, Jackson B. The human immunodeficiency virus and nonmenstrual toxic shock syndrome: a female case presentation. *Nurse Pract* 1994; **19** (1): 68–71.

67 Cone LA, Woodard DR, Byrd RG, Schulz K, Kopp SM, Schlievert PM. A recalcitrant, erythematous, desquamating disorder associated with toxin-producing staphylococci in patients with AIDS. *J Infect Dis* 1992; **165** (4): 638–643.

68 Strumia R, Bedetti A, Cavazzini L. Staphylococcal scalded-skin syndrome in corso di AIDS. *Giornale Ital Dermatol Venereol* 1990; **125** (10): 461–464.

69 Donohue D, Robinson B, Goldberg NS. Staphylococcal scalded skin syndrome in a woman with chronic renal failure exposed to human immunodeficiency virus. *Cutis* 1991; **47** (5): 317–318.

70 Richard M, Mathieu-Serra A. Staphylococcal scalded skin syndrome in a homosexual adult. *J Am Acad Dermatol* 1986; **15** (2, Part 2): 385–389.

71 Donovan B, Rohrsheim R, Bassett I, Mulhall BP. Bullous impetigo in homosexual men—a risk marker for HIV-1 infection? *Genitourin Med* 1992; **68** (3): 159–161.

72 Duvic M. Staphylococcal infections and the pruritus of AIDS-related complex. *Arch Dermatol* 1987; **123**: 1599.

73 Scully M, Berger TG. Pruritus, *Staphylococcus aureus,* and human immunodeficiency virus infection. *Arch Dermatol* 1990; **126** (5): 684–685.

74 Thoma-Greber E, Froschl M, Stolz W, Landthaler M, Plewig G. Interferon-Gamma. Therapie von rezidivierenden Furunkulosen bei HIV Infektion. *Hautarzt* 1993; **44** (9): 587–589.

75 Caumes E, Janier M, Janssen F, Feyeux C, Vignon-Pennamen MD, Morel P. Syphilis acquise au cours de l'infection par le virus de l'immunodéficience humaine: six cas. *Presse Med* 1990; **19** (8): 369–371.

76 Johnson PC, Farnie MA. Testing for syphilis. *Dermatol Clin* 1994; **12** (1): 9–17.

77 Tikjob G, Russel M, Petersen CS, Gerstoft J, Kobayasi T. Seronegative secondary syphilis in a patient with AIDS: identification of *Treponema pallidum* in biopsy specimen. *J Am Acad Dermatol* 1991; **24** (3): 506–508.

78 Augenbraun MH, DeHovitz JA, Feldman J *et al.* Biological false-positive syphilis test results for women infected with human immunodeficiency virus. *Clin Infect Dis* 1994; **19**: 1040–1044.

79 Malone JL, Wallace MR, Hendrick BB *et al.* Syphilis and neurosyphilis in a human immunodeficiency virus type-1 seropositive population: evidence for frequent serologic relapse after therapy. *Am J Med* 1995; **99**: 55–63.

80 Plettenberg A, Bahlmann W, Stoehr A, Meigel W. Klinische und serologische Befunde der Lues bei HIV-infizierten Patienten. *Deutsche Med Wochenschr* 1991; **116** (25): 968–972.

81 Drobacheff C, Moulin T, Van Landuyt H, Merle C, Vigan M, Laurent R. Syphilis cutanée tertiaire avec symptomes neurologiques. *Ann Dermatol Venereol* 1994; **121** (1): 34–36.

82 Hicks CB. Syphilis and HIV infection. *Dermatol Clin* 1991; **9** (3): 493–501.

83 Sands M, Markus A. Lues maligna, or ulceronodular syphilis, in a man infected with human immunodeficiency virus: case report and review. *Clin Infect Dis* 1995; **20** (2): 387–390.

84 Don PC, Rubinstein R, Christie S. Malignant syphilis (lues maligna) and concurrent infection with HIV. *Int J Dermatol* 1995; **34** (6): 403–407.

85 Garcia-Silva J, Velasco-Benito JA, Pena-Penabad C. Primary syphilis with multiple chancres and porphyria cutanea tarda in an HIV-infected patient. *Dermatology* 1994; **188** (2): 163–165.

86 Rodriguez-Diaz E, Moran-Estefania M, Lopez-Avila A *et al.* Clinical expression of secondary syphilis in a patient with HIV infection. *J Dermatol* 1994; **21** (2): 111–116.

87 Glover RA, Piaquadio DJ, Kern S, Cockerell CJ. An unusual presentation of secondary syphilis in a patient with human immunodeficiency virus infection: a case report and review of the literature. *Arch Dermatol* 1992; **128** (4): 530–534.

88 Bari MM, Shulkin DJ, Abell E. Ulcerative syphilis in acquired immunodeficiency syndrome: a case of precocious tertiary syphilis in a patient infected with human immunodeficiency virus. *J Am Acad Dermatol* 1989; **21** (6): 1310–1312.

89 Duncan WC. Failure of erythromycin to cure secondary syphilis in a patient infected with the human immunodeficiency virus. *Arch Dermatol* 1989; **125** (1): 82–84.

90 Mahrle G, Rasokat H, Kurz K, Steigleder GK. Abnormer Verlauf der Syphilis bei HIV-Infektion. *Zeitschr Hautkrankheit* 1989; **64** (5): 393–394.

91 Pandhi PK, Singh N, Ramam M. Secondary syphilis: a clinicopathologic study. *Int J Dermatol* 1995; **34** (4): 240–243.

92 Rolfs RT. Treatment of syphilis, 1993. *Clin Infect Dis* 1995; **20** (Suppl): 523–538.

93 Gordon SM, Eaton ME, George R *et al.* The response of symptomatic neurosyphilis to high-dose intravenous penicillin G in patients with human immunodeficiency virus infections. *N Engl J Med* 1994; **331**: 1469–1473.

94 Cockerell CJ, Whitlow MA, Webster GF *et al.* Epitheloid angiomatosis: a distinct vascular disorder in patients with acquired immunodeficiency syndrome or AIDS-related complex. *Lancet* 1987; **ii**: 654–656.

95 Webster GF, Cockerell CJ, Friedman-Kien AE. The clinical spectrum of bacillary angiomatosis. *Br J Dermatol* 1991; **126**: 535–541.

96 Milde P, Brunner M, Borchard F *et al.* Cutaneous bacillary angiomatosis in a patient with chronic lymphocytic leukemia. *Arch Dermatol* 1995; **131** (8): 933–936.

97 Pembroke AC, Grice K, Levantine AV, Warin AP. Eruptive angiomata in malignant disease. *Clin Exp Dermatol* 1978; **3**: 147–156.

98 Mulvany NJ, Billson VR. Bacillary angiomatosis of the spleen. *Pathology* 1993; **25** (4): 398–401.

99 Paul MA, Fleischer AB Jr, Wieselthier JS, White WL. Bacillary angiomatosis in an immunocompetent child: the first reported case. *Pediatr Dermatol* 1994; **11** (4): 338–341.

100 Kemper CA, Lombard CM, Deresinski SC *et al.* Visceral bacillary epithelioid angiomatosis: possible manifestations of disseminated cat-scratch disease in the immunocompromised host: a report of two cases. *Am J Med* 1990; **89**: 216–222.

101 Koehler JE, Tappero JW. Bacillary angiomatosis and bacillary peliosis in patients infected with human immunodeficiency virus. *Clin Infect Dis* 1993; **17**: 612–624.

102 Koehler JE, Quinn FD, Berger TG *et al.* Isolation of *Rochalimaea* species from cutaneous and osseous lesions of bacillary angiomatosis. *N Engl J Med* 1992; **327**: 1625–1631.

103 Brenner DJ, Hollis DG, Moss CW *et al.* Proposal of *Afipia* gen. nov., with *Afipia felis* sp. nov. (formerly the cat scratch disease bacillus), *Afipia clevelandensis* sp. nov. (formerly the Cleveland Clinic Foundation strain), *Afipia broomeae* sp. nov., and three unnamed genospecies. *J Clin Microbiol* 1991; **29** 2450–2460.

104 Lipa J, Peters W, Fornasier V, Fisher B. Bacillary angiomatosis: a unique cutaneous complication of HIV infection. *Can J Plast Surg* 1995; **3** (2): 96–101.

105 Lee WR, Chawla JC, Reid R. Bacillary angiomatosis of the conjunctiva. *Am J Ophthalmol* 1994; **118** (2): 152–157.

106 Levell NJ, Bewley AP, Chopra S *et al.* Bacillary angiomatosis with cutaneous and oral lesions in an HIV-infected patient from the UK. *Br J Dermatol* 1995; **132** (1): 113–115.

107 Cotell SL, Noskin GA. Bacillary angiomatosis: clinical and histologic features, diagnosis, and treatment. *Arch Intern Med* 1994; **154** (5): 524–528.

108 Haught WH, Steinbach J, Zander DS, Wingo CS. Case report: bacillary angiomatosis with massive visceral lymphadenopathy. *Am J Med Sci* 1993; **306** (4): 236–240.

109 LeBoit PE. Bacillary angiomatosis: a systemic opportunistic infection with prominent cutaneous manifestations. *Semin Dermatol* 1991; **10** (3): 194–198.

110 Slater LN, Welch DF, Min KW. *Rochalimaea henselae* causes bacillary angiomatosis and peliosis hepatis. *Arch Intern Med* 1992; **152** (3): 602–606.

111 Baker J, Ruiz-Rodriguez R, Whitfield M, Heon V, Berger TG. Bacillary angiomatosis: a treatable cause of acute psychiatric symptoms in human immunodeficiency virus infection. *J Clin Psychiatr* 1995; **56** (4): 161–166.

112 Tsang WY, Chan JK. Bacillary angiomatosis: a 'new' disease with a broadening clinicopathologic spectrum. *Histol Histopathol* 1992; **7** (1): 143–152.

113 Berger TG, Koehler JE. Bacillary angiomatosis. *AIDS Clin Rev* 1993–94: 43–60.

114 Guerra LG, Neira CJ, Boman D *et al.* Rapid response of AIDS-related bacillary angiomatosis to azithromycin. *Clin Infect Dis* 1993; **17** (2): 264–266.

115 Foltzer MA, Guiney WB Jr, Wager GC, Alpem HD. Bronchopulmonary bacillary angiomatosis. *Chest* 1993; **104** (3): 973–975.

116 Koehler JE, Glaser CA, Tappero JW. *Rochalimaea henselae* infection: a new zoonosis with the domestic cat as reservoir. *JAMA* 1994; **271** (7): 531–535.

117 Tappero JW, Mohle-Boetani J, Koehler JE *et al.* The epidemiology of bacillary angiomatosis and bacillary peliosis. *JAMA* 1993; **296** (3): 770–775.

118 Nandwani R, Shanson DC, Fisher M *et al. Mycobacterium kansasii* scalp abscesses in an AIDS patient. *J Infect* 1995; **31**: 79–86.

119 Sindrup JH, Weismann K, Sand Petersen C *et al.* Skin and oral mucosal changes in patients infected with human immunodeficiency virus. *Acta Dermatol Venereol* 1988; **68** (5) 440–443.

120 Conant MA. The AIDS epidemic. *J Am Acad Dermatol* 1994; **31** (3, Part 2): S47–S50.

121 Torssander J, Karlsson A, Morfeldt-Manson L, Putkonen PO, Wasserman J. Dermatophytosis and HIV infection: a study in homosexual men. *Acta Dermatol Venereol* 1988; **68** (1): 53–56.

122 Berger TG. Treatment of bacterial, fungal, and parasitic infections in the HIV-infected host. *Semin Dermatol* 1993; **12** (4): 296–300.

123 Diamond HJ, Phelps RG, Gordon ML, Lambroza E, Namdari H, Bottone EJ. Combined *Aspergillus* and zygomatic (*Rhizopus*) infection in a patient with acquired immunodeficiency syndrome: presentation as inflammatory tinea capitis. *J Am Acad Dermatol* 1992; **26** (6): 1017–1018.

124 Perniciaro C, Peters MS. Tinea faciale mimicking seborrheic dermatitis in a patient with AIDS. *N Engl J Med* 1986; **314** (5): 315–316.

125 Elmets CA. Management of common superficial fungal infections in patients with AIDS. *J Am Acad Dermatol* 1994; **31**: S60–S63.

126 Staughton R. Skin manifestations in AIDS patients. *Br J Clin Pract* 1990; **71**: 109–113.

127 Bakos L, Bonamigo RR, Pisani AC, Mariante JC, Mallmann R. Scutular favus-like tinea cruris and pedis in a patient with AIDS. *J Am Acad Dermatol* 1996; **34**: 1086–1087.

128 Odom RB. Common superficial fungal infections in immunosuppressed patients. *J Am Acad Dermatol* 1994; **31** S56–S59.

129 Lake-Bakaar G, Tom W, Lake-Bakaar D *et al.* Gastropathy and ketoconazole malabsorption in the acquired immunodeficiency syndrome (AIDS). *Ann Intern Med* 1998; **109**: 471–473.

130 Myers SA, Kamino H. Cutaneous cryptococcosis and histoplasmosis coinfection in a patient with AIDS. *J Am Acad Dermatol* 1996; **34**: 898–900.

131 Powderly WG, Finkelstein DM, Feinberg J *et al.* A randomized trial comparing fluconazole with clotrimazole troches for the prevention of fungal infections in patients with advanced human immunodeficiency virus infection. *N Engl J Med* 1995; **332**: 700–705.

132 Novick NL, Tapia L, Bottone EJ. Invasive *Trichophyton rubrum* infection in an immunocompromised host. *Am J Med* 1987; **82**: 321–325.

133 Baker RL, Para MF. Successful use of ketoconazole for invasive *T. rubrum* infection. *Arch Intern Med* 1984; **144**: 615–617.

134 Lestringent GG, Lindley SK, Hillsdon-Smith J *et al.* Deep dermatophytosis to *T. rubrum* and *T. verrucosum* in an immunosuppressed patient. *Int J Dermatol* 1988; **27**: 707–709.

135 Faergemann J, Gisslen H, Dahlberg E *et al. Trichophyton rubrum* abscesses in immunocompromised patients: a case report. *Acta Dermatol Venereol (Stockh)* 1989; **69**: 244–247.

136 Tsang P, Hopkins T, Jimenez-Lucho V. Deep dermatophytosis caused by *Trichophyton rubrum* in a patient with AIDS. *J Am Acad Dermatol* 1996; **34**: 1090–1091.

137 Katz MH, Mastrucci MT, Leggott PJ *et al.* Prognostic significance of oral lesions in children with perinatally acquired human immunodeficiency virus infection. *Am J Dis Child* 1993; **147**: 45–48.

138 Reichart P, Schmidt-Westhausen A, Samaranayake L *et al. Oral Pathol Med* 1994; **23**: 403–405.

139 Sangeorzan J, Bradley S, He X *et al.* Epidemiology of oral candidiasis in HIV-infected patients: colonization, infection, treatment, and emergence of fluconazole resistance. *Am J Med* 1994; **97**: 339–346.

140 Dios P, Alvarez A, Feijoo J *et al.* Fluconazole response patterns in HIV-infected patients with oropharyngeal candidiasis. *Oral Surg Oral Med Oral Pathol* 1995; **79**: 170–174.

141 White A, Goetz M. Azole-resistant *Candida albicans*: report of two cases of resistance and review. *Clin Infect Dis* 1994; **19**: 687–692.

142 Brenner S, Wolf R, Ophir J. Eosinophilic pustular folliculitis: a sterile folliculitis of unknown cause? *J Am Acad Dermatol* 1994; **31** (2, Part 1): 210–212.

143 Rosenthal D, LeBoit PE, Klumpp L, Berger TG. Human immunodeficiency virus-associated eosinophilic folliculitis: a unique dermatosis associated with advanced human immunodeficiency virus infection. *Arch Dermatol* 1991; **127** (2): 206–209.

144 Berger TG, Heon V, King C, Schulze K, Conant MA. Itraconazole therapy for human immunodeficiency virus-associated eosinophilic folliculitis (letter). *Arch Dermatol* 1995; **131** (3): 358–360.

145 Harris DW, Ostlere L, Buckley C, Johnson M, Rustin MH. Eosinophilic pustular folliculitis in an HIV-positive man: response to cetirizine. *Br J Dermatol* 1992; **126** (4): 392–394.

146 Otley CC, Avram MR, Johnson RA. Isotretinoin treatment of human immunodeficiency virus-associated eosinophilic folliculitis. *Arch Dermatol* 1995; **131** (9): 1047–1050.

147 Smith KJ, Skelton HG, Yeager J, Ruiz N, Wagner KF. Metronidazole for eosinophilic pustular folliculitis in human immunodeficiency virus type 1-positive patients (letter). *Arch Dermatol* 1995; **131** (9): 1089–1091.

148 Ferrandiz C, Ribera M, Barranco JC, Clotet B, Lorenzo JC. Eosinophilic pustular folliculitis in patients with acquired immunodeficiency syndrome. *Int J Dermatol* 1992; **31** (3): 193–195.

149 Blauvelt A, Plott RT, Spooner K, Stearn B, Davey RT, Turner ML. Eosinophilic folliculitis associated with the acquired immunodeficiency syndrome responds well to permethrin (letter). *Arch Dermatol* 1995; **131** (3): 360–361.

150 Ferrer S, Baselga E, Domingo P *et al.* [Eosinophilic pustular folliculitis in acquired immunodeficiency syndrome: report of 6 cases.] *Rev Clin Esp* 1995; **195** (2): 92–96.

151 Meinking TL, Taplin D, Hermida JL, *et al.* The treatment of scabies with ivermectin. *N Engl J Med* 1995; **333**: 26–30.

152 Sison J, Kemper C, Loveless M *et al.* Disseminated acanthamoeba infection in patients with AIDS: case reports and review. *Clin Infect Dis* 1995; **20**: 1207–1216.

Chapter 8
Fungal Infection

David T. Roberts

Introduction

Well over 100 000 species of fungi have been described and are widely distributed in nature in many differing environmental conditions. Fungi are thus very successful microorganisms, which comprise a diverse group of eukaryotes that have definite cell walls but contain no chlorophyll and are therefore incapable of producing their own means of nutrition. Fungi exist as either parasites or saprophytes and are dependent on living or dead organic material for nutrition. The majority are moulds, which are composed of a network of branching filaments, known has hyphae, which look rather like cotton wool when cultured. Primitive moulds have no crosswalls or septa within the hyphae, whereas the more advanced groups are septate. In these groups, additional septa may form, which then fragment into chains of spores, termed arthrospores. Yeasts, unlike moulds, exist as single cells, which divide by budding, and have a different appearance, colonies being smooth-surfaced and compact. In culture, they look much more like bacteria than do moulds. Although fungi can be identified by their appearance, they are classified on the basis of their method of sexual reproduction. They are divided into five groups or phyla, namely chytridiomycetes, zygomycetes, ascomycetes and basidiomycetes; the fifth group, which contains many human pathogens, is known as fungi imperfecti, which have no known method of sexual reproduction. Some fungi are dimorphic, in that they are able to exist at different stages of the life cycle in both mould and yeast forms.

Fungi are ubiquitous in a wide range of habitats and are commonly found in soil, on leaves and around the roots of trees and other plants. Some fungi are commensals of the skin or gastrointestinal tracts of animals and some exist in water. Fungal spores are often airborne and the density of fungal spores found in the air varies with the location. Fungi may impinge upon humans in various ways. The ability of yeasts to ferment sugars, thus producing gas and alcohol, is well known to bakers and brewers, and many varieties of mushroom are a popular foodstuff worldwide. Some moulds, notably *Penicillium*, have the ability to produce antibiotics, notably penicillin and griseofulvin, itself an antifungal specific to dermatophyte species. Fungal diseases are known as mycoses or mycotic infections. Such disease may be caused by direct invasion, which may be confined to the skin and mucous membranes, such diseases being known as superficial mycoses. Subcutaneous mycoses are also relatively localized but invade tissues just deep to the skin. Deep or systemic mycoses can involve any of the internal organs.

Some fungi are poisonous and cases of both accidental and deliberate poisoning have been recorded following ingestion of toxic mushrooms. In fact, most mushrooms are non-poisonous, but a few are fatal and unusual mushrooms deserve to be treated with considerable suspicion.

Fungi may also produce toxins capable of causing disease. Many of these have only been identified relatively recently; they include aflatoxins, ochratoxins and trichothecenes, most of which are found in contaminated grain. Older fungal toxins are well known in medicine, including the ergot alkaloids and muscarine.

Finally, airborne fungi are capable of producing allergic reactions and a significant minority of cases of asthma are related to inhalation of fungal spores. Occasionally, contact allergy to lichens occurs.

Fungi may also be indirectly but significantly detrimental to human well-being because of an ability to render foodstuffs inedible. Grain crops and potatoes are the most vulnerable and the potato famine of the mid-nineteenth century caused by the fungus *Phytophthora infestans* produced disastrous consequences with many deaths.

Pathogenic fungi

Although many thousands of species of fungi have been described, fewer than 200 have been recognized as human pathogens and many of these are only pathogenic in circumstances of diminished host defence. In relatively new diseases, such as acquired immune deficiency syndrome (AIDS), fungi previously unsuspected of being pathogenic may cause significant infection. The emotive statement that AIDS patients are 'walking culture plates' is not entirely misplaced. Most fungal infections are exogenous, in that they originate in the environment, and are either inhaled, ingested or implanted in some way into the skin. However, the commonest are caused by those species of dermatophtye which inhabit only the keratin layer of the epidermis, the hair or the nail. In some countries, around 15% of the population have a fungal infection of the toe clefts, and antifungal drugs of various sorts are the most commonly prescribed pharmacological agents in dermatology.

Cutaneous manifestations of fungal infection are seen in superficial and subcutaneous mycoses. Systemic mycoses will not be considered further in this chapter, although, in immunocompromised patients, the presence of cutaneous infection should alert one to the possible existence of more serious systemic disease secondary to the same organism.

Superficial mycoses

Infection of the skin and mucous membranes are predominantly caused by dermatophyte moulds, *Candida* yeasts and *Pityrosporum* yeasts. Superficial infections are limited to the topmost layers of the skin, usually the keratin layer, and the mucous membranes. Dermatophytes are primary pathogens in that they do not have a symbiotic or commensal relationship with the host. However, clinical manifestations vary significantly in degree, related to both environmental and physical factors, together with variations in host defence. Conversely, *Candida* and *Pityrosporum* yeasts are known commensals of mucous membranes and skin, respectively, and are nearly always secondary pathogens to intercurrent disease or to specific environmental factors.

Host–parasite interaction in superficial infection

Dermatophytes

There is no doubt that cell-mediated immune response eliminates dermatophytes from the skin surface, although *Trichophyton rubrum* in particular has adapted especially well to survival on human skin and *T. rubrum* infections are notably recalcitrant. It may be that this is because *T. rubrum* rarely produces a significant inflammatory response, as is the case with *Trichophyton mentagrophytes* infection. In the acute phase, the proliferation of keratinocytes secondary to the inflammatory process is likely to be responsible for resolution of dermatophyte infection. There are, however, a number of non-specific defence mechanisms unrelated to immunity which prevent invasion by dermatophytes. The dry intact epidermis is less susceptible to invasion than moist areas, as illustrated by the prevalence of infection of the toe clefts. Dermatophytes inhabit the stratum corneum and dermatophytosis is more common in those diseases where there is inhibition of cell turnover of the stratum corneum, as seen in congenital tylosis. Spontaneous resolution of scalp infection in puberty, when it is known that the constituents of sebum change, suggest that unsaturated fatty acids found in sebum have an inhibitory effect on dermatophytes. There is a serum inhibitory factor recognized which denies fungi iron, an essential fungal nutrient. Complement may be activated by fungal cell wells via the alternative pathway, thus inhibiting growth. Phagocytosis inhibits dermatophyte growth by adherence to hyphae. The production of mannan, a sugar, by the fungal cell wall is known to inhibit both cell-mediated immunity and proliferation of keratinocytes [1].

Candida *infections*

Candida yeasts are commensal organisms and their relationship with the host is rather more complex than is the case with dermatophytes. Epidermal proliferation and T-lymphocyte immune responses are important factors in host defence, but the inflammatory response and non-specific inhibitors are also likely to play a role. Cellular adhesion is the first stage in establishment of infection and the yeast is capable of producing surface-adhesion molecules to aid this process, along with proteinase, which facilitates penetration of cells. Hyphae then form, which allows for deeper penetration. Vacation of adhesion sites by bacterial flora, such as occurs in antibiotic therapy, is important in establishment of yeast infection [2].

Pityrosporum *infection*

Pityrosporum yeasts are also part of the commensal skin flora, particularly of the scalp. Increased moisture on the skin surface, as seen in hot sweaty conditions, is an important factor in stimulating the yeast mycelial shift seen in pityriasis versicolor. The fungus is capable of invasion of hair follicles, producing an inflammatory response in normal individuals, but this becomes more severe in AIDS patients, indicating that T-lymphocyte function plays an important role in prevention of infection.

The relationship between fungi, both moulds and yeasts, and the host is therefore a complex one and establishment of infection depends upon a number of factors, many of them unrelated. Clearly, exposure to fungal load is important in dermatophyte infection, whereas diminution of host defence is perhaps the crucial factor in yeast infections.

Dermatophytosis

Dermatophytes may be anthropophilic, having humans as the primary host; zoophilic, where animals are the primary hosts; or geophilic, where the fungus exists primarily in the soil. All three varieties of dermatophyte are capable of causing disease in humans, but anthropophilic dermatophytes produce the bulk of infection. Examples of various types of the more important dermatophytes are shown in Table 8.1. *Trichophyton rubrum* is the commonest cause of dermatophyte infection, mainly causing disease in the toe clefts, nails and groin area, as well as disease of the trunk and lower extremeties [3]. Zoophilic dermatophytes most often produce infection in exposed sites, such as the scalp, face, hands and arms [4].

Dermatophyte infections are often known as 'ringworm' or 'tinea'. Both these terms refer to the active edge and central clearing which occur in skin lesions, producing a ring-like appearance. Dermatophytosis is usually classified anatomically, using the prefix tinea. There is some logic to this classification, partly because of the differing clinical appearances and partly because of the various dermatophytes involved. Hence dermatophytosis is classified as tinea capitis (scalp infection), tinea corporis (body infection), tinea cruris (groin infection), tinea pedis (foot infection) and tinea

Table 8.1 Dermatophytes of medical importance.

Anthropophilic species*	Zoophilic species†	Geophilic species
Epidermophyton floccosum	*Microsporum canis* (cat, dog)	*Epidermophyton stockdaleae*
Microsporum audouinii (Africa)	*Microsporum equinum* (horse)	*Microsporum gypseum*
Microsporum ferrugineum	*Microsporum gallinae* (fowl)	(complex of three species)
(eastern Asia, eastern Europe)	*Trichophyton equinum* (horse)	*Microsporum nanum*
Trichophyton concentricum	*Trichophyton mentagrophytes*	*Microsporum praecox*
(South-East Asia, Melanesia	(rodents, rabbit)	
Amazon area, Central	*Trichophyton simii* (monkey)	
America, Mexico)	*Trichophyton verrucosum*	
Trichophyton gourvilii	(cattle, sheep)	
(central Africa)		
Trichophyton megnenii		
(Portugal, Sardinia)		
Trichophyton mentagrophytes		
(complex of two species)		
Trichophyton rubrum		
Trichophyton schoenleinii		
Trichophyton soudanense		
(sub-Saharan Africa)		
Trichophyton tonsurans		
Trichophyton violaceum		
(North Africa, Middle East,		
Mediterranean)		

* Endemic areas in parentheses.
† Primary hosts in parentheses.

unguium (nail infection); sometimes subtypes, such as tinea faciei (face), tinea barbae (beard area) and tinea manuum (hands), are added.

Tinea capitis

The size of fungal arthrospores and method of hair invasion are important in classification of scalp infections. The spore size may vary from two to four μm up to ten μm and may remain outside the hair (ectothrix) or invade the hair shaft itself (endothrix). *Microsporum canis, Microsporum audouinii* and the less common *Microsporum ferrugineum* produce small-spored ectothrix infections, whereas *T. mentagrophytes, Trichophyton verrucosum* and *Microsporum gypseum* cause large-spored ectothrix infections. *Trichophyton tonsurans, Trichophyton violaceum* and *Trichophyton soudanense* are all endothrix. Favus, caused by *Trichophyton schoenleinii*, is classified separately. Organisms responsible for tinea capitis tend to occur in specific geographical locations and these are shown, together with primary hosts and clinical features, in Table 8.2.

Lesions may appear as a dry scaling patch of alopecia (Fig. 8.1), which is characteristic of anthropophilic infection secondary to *M. audouinii* or zoophilic infection caused by *M. canis*, which has cats and dogs as its

Table 8.2 Varieties of tinea capitis.

Organism	Type	Primary host	Wood's rays	Endemic areas
Microsporum canis	Ectothrix	Cat, dog	+ve	Europe
Microsporum audouinii	Ectothrix	Human	+ve	Africa
Microsporum ferrugineum	Ectothrix	Human	+ve	SE Asia
Trichophyton verrucosum	Ectothrix	Cattle	−ve	Europe
Trichophyton violaceum	Endothrix	Human	−ve	India, Middle East, Africa
Trichophyton soudanense	Endothrix	Human	−ve	Africa
Trichophyton tonsurans	Endothrix	Human	−ve	USA, Central America
Trichophyton schoenleinii	Favus	Human	+ve	Worldwide

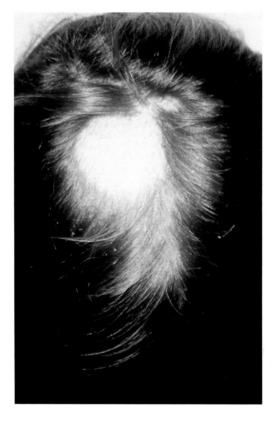

Fig. 8.1 Tinea capitis secondary to *Microsporum canis* infection.

primary host. The cattle ringworm fungus *T. verrucosum* causes a boggy inflammatory swelling, known as a kerion (Fig. 8.2), and is usually seen in rural communities. *Trichophyton tonsurans* is a dermatophyte producing diffuse alopecia, whereby the hair breaks off, producing a characteristic 'black-dot' appearance.

Tinea capitis is mainly a disease of children, which is now, with certain exceptions, uncommon in the Western world, largely due to improved social conditions and the advent of effective drugs which are both available

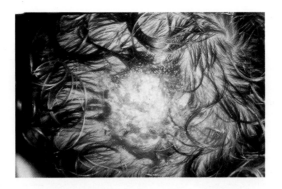

Fig. 8.2 Kerion of scalp secondary to *Trichophyton verrucosum*.

and affordable. However, tinea capitis remains extremely prevalent in the developing world, where it still exists in endemic proportions. In the Western world, zoophilic infection is commonest, presumably because of the difficulties in eradicating infection from animals. In the developing world, anthropophilic infection is predominant and varies somewhat according to geographical location. *Trichophyton violaceum* infection predominates in Asia, whereas *T. tonsurans* is most common in Afro-Caribbean populations. Very recently, the incidence of *T. tonsurans* infection in such populations has been much on the increase in both the UK and the USA. Presumably, such patients' hair type precludes early detection and eradication of disease, although economic factors may also play some part [5].

Favus is a specific clinical type of infection, caused by *T. schoenleinii*, characterized by crusting and inflammation. The crust, which consists of a mixture of mycelium, neutrophils and epidermal cells, is typically cup-shaped and is known as a scutulum (Fig. 8.3). Large numbers of such crusts may develop and cover the whole of the scalp, which assumes a whitish-yellow appearance. Although favus induces a significant degree of inflammatory change, the infection is not self-limiting and follows a protracted course, which may rarely involve other body sites, including the nails. The hair shafts are invaded by small amounts of mycelium, but the hair tends not to fracture and alopecia, when it does occur, is related to inflammatory change in and around the follicle. It is often permanent thereafter, due to follicular scarring. *Trichophyton schoenleinii* infection fluoresces under Wood's rays. Favus tends to occur in long-stay institutions, such as mental hospitals, although it is now rare in the developed world. In some parts of Africa, Asia and Latin America, the disease remains prevalent, which produces widespread infection.

The degree of inflammation seen in scalp infection is variable and sometimes related to individual host response. However, animal *Trichophyton* species, together with the geophilic *M. gypseum*, are more prone to induce a significant inflammatory response, which often develops into a kerion. This large boggy inflammatory swelling is often misdiagnosed as an abscess, and surgeons have a tendency to drain such lesions and treat with antibiotics,

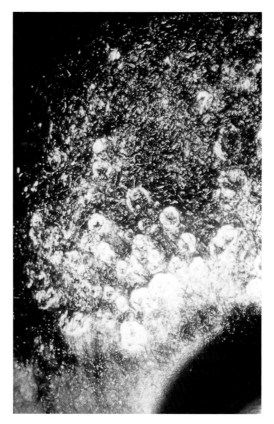

Fig. 8.3 Favus showing typical scutula.

which simply delays ultimate resolution. A history of contact with cattle (*T. verrucosum*) or rodents (*T. mentagrophytes*) is helpful in diagnosis. Laboratory diagnosis is not difficult, but infected hairs must be examined microscopically and the kerion should be suspected in all abscesses where infection is multifocal and centred around hair follicles. Early diagnosis is important in such lesions in order to prevent, as far as possible, the development of permanent scarring alopecia.

Tinea capitis in all its forms is a contagious disease, which may reach epidemic proportions in some communities [6]. Prior to the introduction of effective antifungal drugs, the only method of treatment was epilation of the scalp, either by shaving or by the ingestion of thallium acetate. This rather draconian method of treatment was rendered unnecessary by the introduction of the drug griseofulvin in the late 1950s. Although this drug is only weakly fungistatic, it proved highly effective in the control of tinea capitis and virtually eradicated many anthropophilic infections in the Western world. Now newer fungicidal agents are becoming available, which are likely to significantly shorten treatment periods. However, new drugs are, of necessity, expensive and are not likely to be readily available in the developing world, where even an inexpensive agent, such as griseofulvin, is often beyond the scope of either patients or medical authorities in terms of its cost. Tinea capitis is therefore likely to remain a problem for the foreseeable future in developing countries unless they obtain some assistance in terms of drug costs. It would seem unfortunate that a widespread and contagious but relatively easily treated disease remains prevalent purely because of economic factors.

Differential diagnosis. Tinea capitis may produce well-demarcated or diffuse areas of scarring or non-scarring alopecia and therefore may be confused with other diseases producing similar lesions. These include alopecia areata, trichotillomania, seborrhoeic dermatitis, psoriasis, discoid lupus erythematosus, lichen planus, syphilis and bacterial infection producing boils and carbuncles.

Tinea corporis

Tinea corporis refers to infection of the glabrous skin of the body and limbs and is usually caused by either anthropophilic or zoophilic species. Typically, lesions are ring-like, with a raised scaling edge and healing centre (Fig. 8.4). Hair follicles are often prominently involved. The edge may be irregular and lesions can vary in size from small to very large and may be multiple (Fig. 8.5). Zoophilic species tend to produce rather more inflammatory lesions than anthropophilic fungi and occasionally the healing centre is less prominent, leading to more difficulty in clinical diagnosis (Fig. 8.6). Untreated disease may become very widespread and in some circumstances can assume an almost granulomatous appearance.

Almost all dermatophytes can cause tinea corporis but, in general, zoophilic infection is most commonly seen on the hands, arms and face, which are more likely to be in contact with an infected animal than are the legs and trunk, which are more often affected by anthropophilic species.

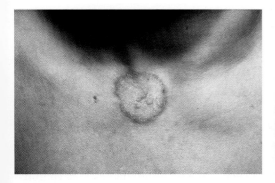

Fig. 8.4 Tinea corporis showing typical ring-like configuration.

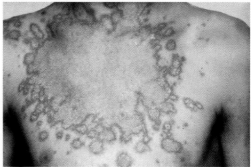

Fig. 8.5 Widespread tinea corporis with satellite lesions.

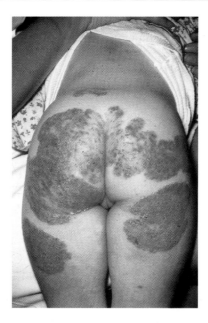

Fig. 8.6 Tinea corporis exhibiting psoriasiform lesions.

Differential diagnosis. All skin diseases producing discoid or annular lesions may be confused with tinea corporis. These include psoriasis, discoid eczema, pityriasis rosea, granuloma annulare and annular erythemas. In the Western world, tinea corporis is overdiagnosed by non-specialist practitioners, many of the above diseases being much commoner. However, it is not a cardinal sin to treat an inflammatory dermatosis with a topical antifungal agent initially. It is certainly preferable to treating a fungal infection with a topical steroid, which will be discussed further below.

Tinea imbricata

This variety of tinea corporis merits separate consideration, because it produces such a specific clinical appearance. It is caused by a single dermatophyte, *Trichophyton concentricum,* and is entirely a tropical disease, being widespread in Asia, the Pacific islands [7] and South and Central America. The infection generally occurs in early life and runs a prolonged course, during which time the disease becomes very widespread. It is thought that the fungus requires average temperatures of 40°C or above to proliferate. The disease starts on the trunk and has a classic and very typical clinical appearance, wherein concentric rings develop in each lesion. Scaling is more pronounced at the periphery, and each ring is slightly infiltrated, such that the whole lesion appears to be ridged. Rings become multiple and spread insidiously, until eventually the whole body is covered by this bizarre eruption, which is very typical. However, chronic disease can become much more diffuse or even exfoliative and then may be confused with diseases such as ichthyosis vulgaris, exfoliative dermatitis or even pemphigus foliaceus.

Although the disease responds to antifungal drugs, it becomes prevalent and widespread because it occurs in communities where drug therapy is not readily available, in rather the same way as tinea capitis in the tropics.

Tinea barbae

Tinea barbae refers to infection of the beard area of the face and merits separate consideration simply because the organisms involved are often different from those affecting the glabrous skin of the face, which are similar to those causing tinea corporis. Tinea barbae is usually of animal origin, and *T. verrucosum* and *T. mentagrophytes* are responsible for many cases, although *T. violaceum* can occur in Africa. Kerion-like lesions, which may be localized or diffuse, are most common (Fig. 8.7).

Tinea cruris

Tinea cruris, as the name implies, affects the groin area, although the axillae may also be involved. In the Western world, it is a disease confined almost entirely to males and is delineated by the anatomical landmarks of

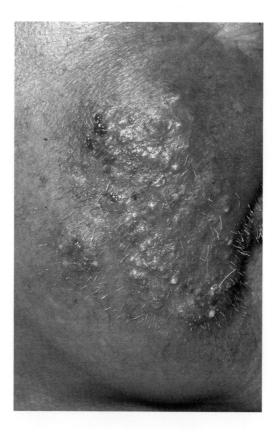

Fig. 8.7 Tinea barbae: kerion type.

the scrotum and adjacent thigh area. However, in the tropics, it is much more readily recognized in females also. The anthropophilic dermatophytes *T. rubrum, T. mentagrophytes* var. *interdigitale* and *Epidermophyton floccosum* are usually causal, and spread takes place from infected toe clefts and feet. It is unusual for a patient with tinea cruris not to have tinea pedis. It is most likely that the disease spreads via towels used to dry both feet and groin area. The disease has the same basic configuration as all dermatophyte infections, there being a raised scaly edge and a healing centre (Fig. 8.8). Undiagnosed and untreated cases slowly spread to the area below the scrotum and into the perianal region. Spread to the axillae may also occur for the same reason. Although the disease is common in the Western world, it is more likely, because of climatic conditions, to be more florid in the tropics.

Differential diagnosis. Flexural infected eczema, intertrigo, psoriasis and ery-thrasma may all be confused with tinea cruris and again it is likely to be an overdiagnosed disease, as is the case with tinea corporis.

Tinea pedis

This is by far the commonest variety of dermatophyte infection in the developed world and is most often referred to as athlete's foot. The disease is contracted in communal bathing places, where small pieces of infected keratin are deposited on the floors of changing rooms, shower cubicles and swimming-baths. It is recognized that fungal elements may survive in such small pieces of keratin for many months, so it is also possible for infection to spread via dry carpeted floors. However, it is recognized that incidence of disease mirrors exposure in terms of both time and infected material, so most infections are in fact contracted in communal bathing places, which are much more heavily contaminated with infected material.

    The disease nearly always begins in the fourth toe cleft initially, with a minor degree of maceration and scaling, which eventually develop into a small fissure, which at this stage may become itchy or even painful (Fig. 8.9). In some patients, disease may remain confined to the fourth toe cleft for many years and be relatively unsymptomatic. It is likely that such patients, who do not always seek treatment, are most likely to deposit

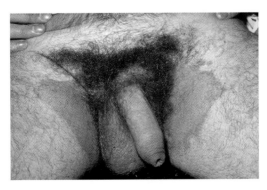

Fig. 8.8 Tinea cruris.

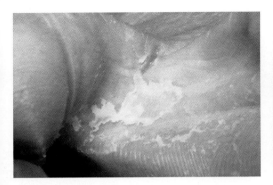

Fig. 8.9 Interdigital tinea pedis showing fissure.

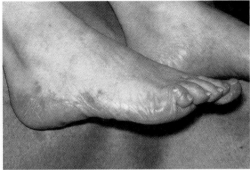

Fig. 8.10 'Moccasin' tinea pedis.

infected material and thus cause spread of infection. All of the toe clefts may become involved, and ultimately disease may spread on to the soles and sides of the foot, where it is known as 'moccasin' tinea pedis (Fig. 8.10). When infection becomes established on the soles, a dry-type scaling rather than maceration develops. Secondary infection with bacteria and yeasts can occur and occasionally, especially in *T. mentagrophytes* infection, a brisk inflammatory response is elicited, which regularly causes the most complaint but is in fact much less recalcitrant than the low-grade *T. rubrum* infection, which thus remains by far the commonest pathogen.

Allergic reactions to tinea pedis are well recognized. They are known as dermatophytid reactions. Two forms are recognized. The commonest is desquamation of the skin of the palms, which simply peels off with no associated dermatitis reaction or itch. Treatment should be directed at the toe cleft, and the hands only require emollients. A blistering reaction on the soles (podopompholyx), hands (cheiropompholyx) (Fig. 8.11) or both (cheiropodopompholyx) is also sometimes seen. When it is confined to the soles, it is difficult to separate from direct spread of the infection to the centre of the sole, which may also occur. In any event, systemic treatment is usually indicated and, if the reaction is severe, a short course of systemic steroids along with an antifungal drug is most helpful.

The incidence of tinea pedis is, as stated, directly related to exposure. It is reckoned to occur in 10–15% of the general population in Western [8] society but various surveys have revealed the incidence to be over 20% in regular users of swimming-baths [9], over 30% in children attending boarding-school [10], 50% in inmates of long-stay mental institutions [11] and over 80% in coalminers [12], who have the highest incidence of any occupational group, which is not surprising in that they have a communal shower every working day. Surveys of the number of infected pieces of keratin or colony-forming units have been carried out and the results are variable. The highest recorded figure is 1500 colony-forming units/m^2 communal bathing space. It is predictable that the degree of cross-infection in the users of such communal bathing facilities is high; hence the high prevalance of disease in these users. The eradication of infected material

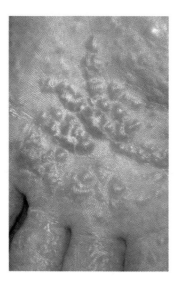

Fig. 8.11 Cheiropompholyx secondary to tinea pedis.

from communal bathing places is not easy. While suitably potent disinfectants are available to kill off the fungus, they have to penetrate the keratin and are thus likely to be very irritant to the feet and are therefore not feasible for general use. There is often present a trough containing disinfectant, which users of swimming-baths are expected to walk through on their way from the changing room to the bathing pool. This is unlikely to contain disinfectant potent enough to be useful and indeed may preferentially collect hyphal fragments protected within small pieces of keratin. It may well be that such troughs of disinfectant do more harm than good in terms of spread of infection.

Antifungal powders are not useful as therapeutic agents but have been shown to reduce the incidence of foot infection in communal bathing places when used prophylactically. Similarly, the constant use of plastic socks would prevent both contraction and spread of infection, but both of these preventive methods are costly if the material is to be supplied by the communal bathing place and it is not possible to force users to comply in any event. It is therefore likely that significant decrease in the incidence of tinea pedis in regular users of communal bathing places is only going to be achieved by the use of effective therapy providing high cure and low relapse rates.

Differential diagnosis. Bacterial infection, usually Gram-negative (Fig. 8.12), of the toe clefts, *Candida* infection or erythrasma may be confused with interdigital tinea pedis. Pustular psoriasis, various varieties of dermatitis, podopompholyx, tylosis and pitted keratolysis may all be confused with fungal infection of the soles.

If the fourth toe cleft is normal and the eruption is bilateral and symmetrical, fungal infection is much less likely. Conversely, fungal infections should certainly be excluded in any unilateral rash of the feet.

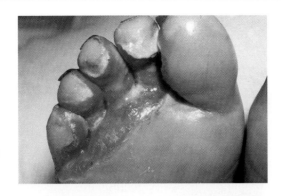

Fig. 8.12 Bacterial infection of toe clefts secondary to tinea pedis.

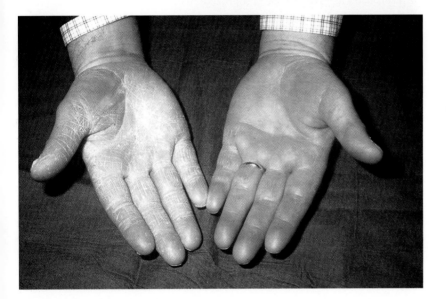

Fig. 8.13 Tinea manuum.

Tinea manuum

Tinea manuum is analogous to a dry-type eruption of the soles and almost always secondary to *T. rubrum* infection. It is usually unilateral and one palm is covered with dry scaling, the skin folds being particularly involved (Fig. 8.13). Tinea manuum is often accompanied by fingernail infection of the same hand.

Patients with the genodermatosis tylosis palmaris are particularly prone to secondary dermatophyte infection.

Differential diagnosis. Psoriasis, dermatitis and tylosis may all be confused with fungal infection, but most of these conditions are bilateral and, as in the case of foot infection, a unilateral eruption should always be treated as likely to be secondary to fungus.

Tinea unguium

Fungal nail infection may be caused by dermatophytes. yeasts or non-dermatophyte moulds. While the incidence of causal pathogens varies somewhat geographically, it is generally accepted that dermatophytes are by far the predominant pathogens of nails. Surveys in several countries have revealed the prevalence of tinea unguium to be around 3% and toenails are affected four times as frequently as fingernails. *Trichophyton rubrum* is the commonest pathogen and the disease is nearly always secondary to toe-cleft infection, although it may take many years to develop and is a disease of insidious onset but relentless progression.

Four clinical varieties are recognized: distal and lateral subungual onychomycosis (DLSO); superficial white onychomycosis (SWO); proximal subungual onychomycosis (PSO); and total dystrophic onychomycosis (TDO) [13]. In order to make the aetiology clearer, it is important to add a fifth variety, namely *Candida* onychomycosis, which is, of course, a description of the causal agent rather than the clinical appearance. However, this does lead to less confusion.

Distal and lateral subungual onychomycosis. This is the commonest variety of tinea unguium or onychomycosis and is the type most often seen in dermatophyte infection. Dermatophyte infection is initially a disease of the hyponychium, which produces hyperkeratosis of the distal nail bed, thus causing onycholysis. The disease then spreads proximally along the nail bed and onycholysis progresses. Ultimately the underside of the nail is involved and, as the nail plate becomes more and more infected, it becomes friable and begins to crumble away. The nail plate is progressively destroyed from the distal end (Fig. 8.14). Sometimes, a densely packed area of fungus spreads as a narrow band below the nail bed but does not destroy the nail. In this variety, which appears as a creamy white streak or line down the nail, the mycelium appears to be packed into a cylindrical formation, and this form is often especially resistant to treatment.

Non-dermatophyte moulds are occasionally recognized as causal pathogens of DLSO. The role of these moulds as pathogens is controversial.

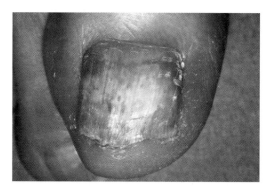

Fig. 8.14 Distal and lateral subungual onychomycosis showing proximal spread.

Such moulds are well recognized to grow saprophytically on damaged keratin, but there is precious little evidence that they are able to act as parasites and actually destroy normal keratin. *Scopulariopsis brevicaulis* is regularly quoted as a nail pathogen and there is no doubt that it can invade damaged nails (Fig. 8.15); whether or not it has the ability to further damage the nail once it has entered the nail plate remains open to question, and ultrastructural studies using electron microscopy have thus far failed to reveal any convincing parasitic tendency. The non-dermatophyte mould *Scytalidium dimidiatum*, commonly known as *Hendersonula toruloidea*, is without question a nail pathogen (Fig. 8.16), and it is revealing to note that it is the only non-dermatophyte mould capable of producing toe-cleft disease. Indeed, in some parts of the tropics, it is the commonest cause of tinea pedis in certain groups. *Aspergillus* species are sometimes isolated from nails, but their role as true pathogens is again unproved. The question of pathogenicity of non-dermatophyte moulds is of some importance, although they are uncommon. Some antifungal drugs may be more active against such moulds than others, but, if these moulds are secondary invaders of a previously damaged nail, even successful eradication of the fungus will not lead to clinical cure, as the original damage remains.

Superficial white onychomycosis. This variety is much less common than DLSO and the most common pathogen is *T. mentagrophytes* (Fig. 8.17). Some moulds, such as *Acremonium* and *Fusarium*, may also cause SWO (Fig. 8.18) and it is the only variety of tinea unguium which affects the dorsal surface of the nail. A powdery white deposit, which can readily be scraped off, is seen on the surface of the nail, although it will ultimately begin to destroy the nail plate and an especially dense white variety of SWO is seen in patients with AIDS. Although rare, infection with *Fusarium* species is relevant in patients who develop neoplastic disease and who require to be rendered neutropenic as part of their treatment. In such patients, *Fusarium* may become systematized and is regularly fatal in such circumstances.

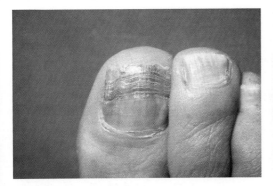

Fig. 8.15 *Scopulariopsis brevicaulis* infection showing typical grey/green discoloration.

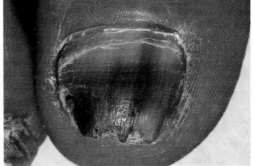

Fig. 8.16 *Scytalidium dimidiatum* infection showing black discoloration.

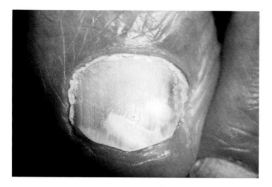

Fig. 8.17 Superficial white onychomycosis secondary to *Tricophyton mentagrophytes*.

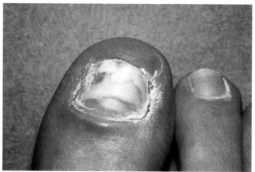

Fig. 8.18 Superficial white onychomycosis secondary to *Fusarium* infection.

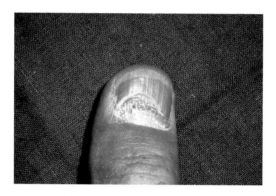

Fig. 8.19 Proximal subungual onychomycosis secondary to *Trichophyton rubrum* infection in AIDS patient.

Although it is likely to be a very uncommon coincidence that SWO secondary to *Fusarium* should occur in such individuals, it should always be remembered and the nails removed, or at least effectively treated, before cytotoxic therapy is commenced.

Proximal subungual onychomycosis. In the absence of paronychia, this is a very unusual type of onychomycosis. *Trichophyton rubrum* occasionally enters the nail at the proximal end (Fig. 8.19), and again this is more commonly seen in patients with AIDS or peripheral vascular disease, where the host defence mechanism is in some way compromised.

Total dystrophic onychomycosis. All of the above varieties of onychomycosis may ultimately destroy the nail plate and are then properly described as TDO.

Candida *onychomycosis.* Chronic mucocutaneous candidiasis (CMCC) is an inborn defect of T-cell-mediated immunity. There are various subtypes of CMCC, but they are ultimately capable of resulting in primary *Candida* nail dystrophy, which produces gross thickening and hyperkeratosis of the nail bed, often accompanied by *Candida* infection of the surrounding skin and mucous membranes. Chronic paronychia is most often seen in patients with 'wet' occupations, especially food handlers. It is a disease that affects the fingernails and is most common in females. It begins with swelling of the posterior nail fold, which ultimately results in elevation of the cuticle off the nail plate (Fig. 8.20). This allows moisture often containing both yeasts and bacteria to penetrate the space below the posterior nail fold thus increasing the degree of inflammation which results in further swelling and cuticle separation and thus a vicious circle is set up. It remains a matter of controversy whether or not the primary inflammation is a result of the irritant effect of water or whether it is a food allergy which some authorities believe. Ultimately the nail becomes proximally dystrophic because of inflammation in and around the nail matrix and it is likely that both yeast and bacteria contribute to this (Fig. 8.21). The yeast isolated is usually

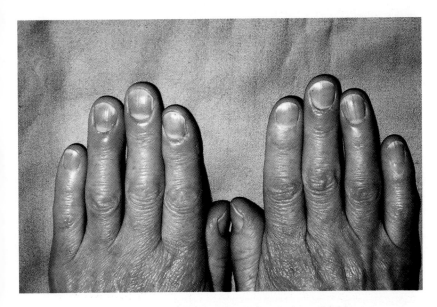

Fig. 8.20 Chronic paronychia showing swelling of posterior nail folds.

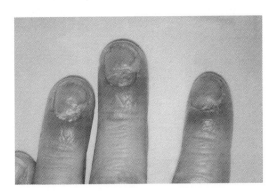

Fig. 8.21 Proximal nail dystrophy secondary to chronic paronychia.

Candida albicans, but *Candida parapsilosis* occurs frequently. Sometimes, frank pus can be obtained by squeezing the posterior nail fold, and this should be submitted for microscopy and culture. Successful treatment is likely to be multifactorial, aimed at yeasts, bacteria and the inflammatory process.

Patients with peripheral vascular disease, usually Raynaud's disease, affecting the hands can develop onycholysis and hyperkeratosis of the nail bed (Fig. 8.22). *Candida* is often cultured from such nails and sometimes these patients respond to antifungal therapy. It remains unclear whether vascular insufficiency directly precipitates onycholysis or whether diminished blood supply encourages growth of yeasts, which then produce the nail changes. There is no direct evidence that yeasts are keratolytic and, indeed, the nail plate itself often remains intact in such cases, despite the presence of onycholysis and subungual hyperkeratosis [14].

Significance of yeast isolation from nails. Yeasts of the *Candida* species, usually *C. albicans* but quite often *C. parapsilosis*, are regularly isolated from dystrophic fingernails and occasionally from dystrophic toenails. The decision to treat such patients with antifungal agents active against yeasts depends upon whether or not the yeasts are the causal agents of nail dystrophy in such patients. Generally speaking, it is most likely that yeasts are secondary pathogens of previously damaged nails, and treatment is unlikely to effect a clinical improvement in these cases. Even then, it is not possible to predict a detrimental effect of yeast colonization in dystrophic nails. It is generally accepted that nails should be positive for yeasts on microscopy of nail clippings; in other words, the yeasts should be demonstrated to have invaded the nail substance and a significant number of inocula should be positive on culture. When reporting yeast growth in culture, some laboratories state the number of positive inocula and this is to be encouraged. It is always likely that, say, 80% of positive inocula is more significant than 20% of positive inocula. It remains impossible, however, to predict the beneficial

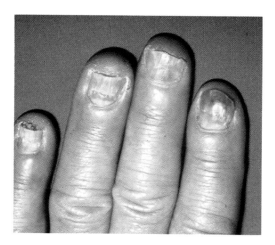

Fig. 8.22 Distal onycholysis and *Candida* infection in patient with Raynaud's disease.

effects of antifungal therapy in such cases, and this should always be discussed with the patient before initiation of treatment. This is particularly so in cases where a lengthy course of systemic therapy is likely to be costly. The only situation where systemic antifungal treatment of yeast infection in nails is of proved benefit is in cases of CMCC.

Differential diagnosis. Almost all causes of nail dystrophy are sometimes confused with fungal infection. Onychogryphosis and psoriasis are the commonest of these, but lichen planus, traumatic onychodystrophy and ischaemic changes in nails may all be confused with fungal infection; hence the importance of confirmation of the diagnosis before initiation with therapy.

Scytalidium dimidiatum *infection*

This saprophytic mould is found in vegetation in tropical regions, such as India, Africa, South-East Asia and the West Indies, and is a recognized plant pathogen. It is capable of producing foot, hand and nail infection very similar to those produced by dermatophytes. All recorded cases have been in immigrants from tropical regions or have been visitors to such regions. It is not known, therefore, whether it is capable of spread from human to human in communal bathing places or whether it can only be contracted directly with contact from vegetation. It produces black discoloration in nails and, when this appearance is seen in appropriate patients, the laboratory should be alerted to the possibility of *Scytalidium* infection. This is because the fungus does not grow in the presence of cycloheximide, which is regularly included in media used to grow fungi. The appearances on direct microscopy are very similar to those seen in dermatophyte infection, although the hyphae are slightly nodular and pigmented [15].

This infection, particularly when it occurs in nails, appears to be resistant to all available antifungal agents and is thus important in that prolonged courses of costly systemic therapy are likely to prove ineffective.

Tinea profunda

This is an exceptionally rare circumstance where dermatophytes invade the living epidermis, the dermis and subcutaneous tissues. In such cases, the clinical appearances look rather like a mycetoma. This disease is likely to occur in the presence of impaired host defence, although very few dermatophyte infections exhibit this tendency, even in the presence of immunosuppression.

Tinea incognito

This term is used to describe changes which occur in the clinical appearance of dermatophyte infections following treatment with topical steroids, which are often inappropriately used in all skin diseases. It is not a good term, in that it does not represent a disease entity at all but rather a misdiagnosis and inappropriate therapy.

In such cases, the inflammatory response to dermatophytes is suppressed and the integrity of the original ring is lost (Fig. 8.23). Scaling is much reduced and sometimes small nodules develop within and at the edge of the lesion. To the inexperienced eye, it looks less and less like a dermatophyte infection, so correct diagnosis is likely to be further delayed.

Laboratory diagnosis of dermatophyte infection

A specimen should be submitted to a laboratory experienced in the diagnosis of fungal infection. The specimen should be accompanied by information recording the site of infection and history of animal contact, together with information as to the patient's occupation and evidence of recent travel and any underlying disease.

All suspected lesions should be cleaned with 70% alcohol prior to sampling, in order to reduce the likelihood of bacterial overgrowth and especially to remove any topical medicaments previously applied. Ideally, skin, hair and nail specimens should be collected on to black paper for ease of visualization, and this will also enable the specimen to dry out.

Specimens from the scalp should include plucked hairs, so that the root can be examined, and skin scales, especially those from around hair follicles. Specimens can also be obtained from the scalp using a brush or comb technique. The brush or comb is pulled through the scalp and then pressed directly on to a culture plate. This does not allow for microscopic examination but is certainly a useful method when screening large numbers of patients. Of course, each brush or comb has to be sterilized after use, so large numbers require to be available for screening purposes. Specimens from the skin, groins and toe clefts should be obtained from the edge of the lesion by scraping outwards with a blunt scalpel blade. Generally, a small area of healthy-looking skin will peel off during the procedure and this should be included, because fungus is most abundant in this area. Where

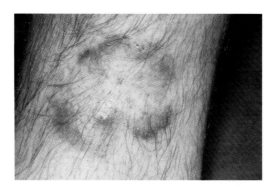

Fig. 8.23 Tinea incognito.

skin scrapings are impossible to obtain, as, for example, in children, a Sellotape strip represents an alternative method of collection. The adhesive tape is pressed against the edge of the lesion, peeled off and placed face down on a glass microscope slide. This method, however, is not as good as skin scrapings, because it does not allow for direct microscopic examination as well as culture.

Particular care should be taken in obtaining nail specimens. Even in the best of laboratories, 30–40% of all positive nail samples fail to grow in culture, and this is almost certainly due to a defect in the sampling procedure rather than in laboratory methods. In dermatophyte nail infection, disease spreads slowly proximally and the fungus is most abundant in the hyperkeratotic material found on the nail bed and on the underside of the nail. Fungus in the very distal part of the nail may be visualized microscopically, but these hyphae are often dead and will not grow in culture. Good pincer-type nail-clippers should be used and a wedge removed from the nail which extends as far proximally as possible. This is generally not too difficult because the nail is onycholytic. The wedge should be sent to the laboratory, along with scrapings taken from the nail bed. A dental scraper or small blunt curette is especially useful for this purpose. In this way, a positive culture is most likely to be obtained and this is always helpful. However, positive microscopy alone is sufficient evidence to commence therapy. Although hyphae may be dead, dermatophytes are not commensal organisms and the disease does not resolve spontaneously. Thus, in untreated patients, even dead hyphae provide virtually certain evidence of active infection.

Dermatophytes are known to survive for some weeks within small pieces of keratin, so specimens can safely be sent to the laboratory by post and certainly do not have to be processed with undue haste.

Upon arrival at the laboratory, scalp specimens are submitted to Wood's rays examination, which shows a green fluorescence in some dermatophyte infections. A positive Wood's rays test is helpful in isolating those hairs to be submitted for microscopy and culture. Material from hair and skin specimens is cleared in 5–10% potassium hydroxide (KOH), which softens the surrounding keratin. The specimen is then viewed directly, when, in positive cases, dermatophyte hyphae will be seen. Sometimes, these hyphae are pretty scanty and time should be taken to examine the whole of the specimen. Keratinocyte cell walls may be confused with hyphae to the inexperienced eye, and the microscopist should have adequate experience in examination of such specimens. Calcofluor white is a fluorescent brightener, which makes visualization of dermatophytes much easier, but unfortunately it requires a fluorescent microscope. Specimens are cultured on a medium containing an organic source of nitrogen, and 4% malt-extract agar and Sabouraud's dextrose agar are most commonly used. Chloramphenicol or cyclohex-imide is often added to the medium to reduce contamination by bacteria and saprophytes. The culture is incubated at 25–30°C, and this incubation must be continued for several weeks, as dermatophytes grow slowly [16].

Interpretation of results. The laboratory workers should not simply report every organism growing on a culture plate to the clinician. They should interpret the laboratory results in the context of the clinical description and disregard organisms that are commensals or those known to grow as saprophytes. This is a particular problem in nail infections, where many non-dermatophyte moulds and some yeasts find dystrophic nail a congenial growth environment. However, these organisms are not parasitic in such nails and do not contribute to nail dystrophy; thus, treatment of such organisms is likely to be futile and it is the laboratory's responsibility to point this out to the clinician, who may not be expert in such matters. Only dermatophytes and *S. dimidiatum* are certain primary pathogens of nail. *Scopulariopsis brevicaulis, Fusarium* species, *Acremonium* and some species of *Aspergillus* may occasionally be pathogenic, but even then do not respond well to antifungal drugs, and nail removal should be contemplated in such cases, as well as in those nails that grow any other non-dermatophyte mould in culture.

Pityrosporum **yeast infections**

Pityrosporum yeasts are lipophilic organisms which are skin commensals. They are associated with pityriasis versicolor, *Pityrosporum* folliculitis and seborrhoeic dermatitis. Very rarely, they can cause systemic infection in neonates who are receiving parenteral nutrition with intravenous lipids. The yeast exists in a round form (*Pityrosporum orbiculare*) and an oval form (*Pityrosporum ovale*). *Pityrosporum ovale* occurs most commonly on the scalp and *P. orbiculare* is usually found on the trunk. It is likely that the yeast is dimorphic and these two forms are simply variants of the same species. Under certain conditions, a yeast–mycelial shift occurs and hyphae are formed, when the fungus is often known as *Malassezia furfur.* This yeast–mycelial shift occurs in pityriasis versicolor [17].

Pityriasis versicolor

This is a mild superficial infection, which is common worldwide. It develops under hot sweaty conditions and is thus more frequent in the tropics. It is sometimes known as tinea versicolor, but this is inappropriate name, which confuses the disease with a dermatophyte infection. It consists of well-demarcated, pale brown, scaly patches, which begin on the upper trunk and slowly spread to involve the whole of the trunk and upper parts of the limbs (Fig. 8.24). It does not commonly affect the lower parts of the limbs or the face. The colour of the lesions is consistent, regardless of skin type. Thus the lesions initially appear darker than surrounding white skin but paler

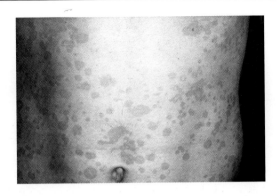

Fig. 8.24 Pityriasis versicolor.

then surrounding dark skin. In addition, the yeast produces dicarboxylic acids, notably azeleic acid, which inhibits melanin formation. Therefore, progressive whitening of the lesions occurs, which is even more obvious in dark-skinned individuals. This hypopigmentation persists for some time even after successful treatment, and this must be explained to the patient. However, repigmentation will eventually occur and there is no fear of a permanent piebald appearance developing. None the less, such depigmentation causes considerable distress in dark-skinned people and carries the stigma of vitiligo or even leprosy. Pityriasis versicolor is not an itchy disease and the patient will tend only to complain of the cosmetic appearance. The lesions produce a yellowish fluorescence under Wood's rays, but this is not always diagnostic and scrapings should be sent to the laboratory.

Differential diagnosis. Vitiligo, erythrasma, pityriasis alba and large naevi may all be confused with pityriasis versicolor, but there is of course no notable scaling in such lesions.

Pityrosporum *folliculitis*

This condition is regularly seen in young adults on the upper trunk. It is usually most prominent on the back, and consists of a low-grade folliculitis with some degree of perifollicular erythema (Fig. 8.25). Small pustules do occur, but they are not as large as those seen in bacterial infection nor is there the same degree of inflammation. In addition, the pus is a pale cream colour rather than the deeper yellow associated with bacteria. This is an itchy disease and can become very pronounced in AIDS patients. Indeed, severe *Pityrosporum* folliculitis is often an early indicator of conversion from human immunodeficiency virus (HIV) positivity to AIDS. Again, the condition is associated with hot sweaty conditions. Scrapings are much less likely to yield a fungus than in pityriasis versicolor, but biopsy will often reveal yeasts deep within the hair follicle (Fig. 8.26).

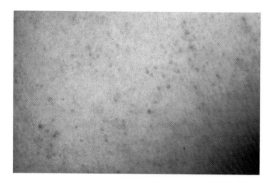

Fig. 8.25 *Pityrosporum* folliculitis.

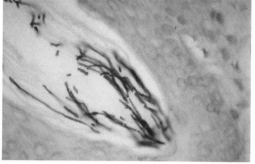

Fig. 8.26 Histology of *Pityrosporum* folliculitis.

Differential diagnosis. Acne and staphylococcal folliculitis must be differentiated from this condition.

Seborrhoeic dermatitis

It is likely that seborrhoeic dermatitis is a multifactorial disease. Infantile seborrhoea is almost certainly not the same disease as adult seborrhoeic dermatitis and there is no strong evidence that *Pityrosporum* yeasts are associated with infantile seborrhoea, which is sometimes a precursor of atopic dermatitis or psoriasis. The simplest form of seborrhoea in adults is dandruff. *Pityrosporum* yeasts are found in larger quantities in scalp scales and in patients with significant dandruff, and the problem responds well in most cases to shampoos containing agents toxic to yeasts. These include ketoconazole, zinc pyrithione and selenium sulphide. These agents cause temporary diminution of yeasts and coincide with clinical improvement. There is thus circumstancial evidence that *Pityrosporum* yeasts are implicated in severe dandruff.

Similarly, patients with seborrhoeic dermatitis of the face, trunk and flexures often respond to washing with such shampoos, together with topical antifungal agents, in combination with topical steroids. Facial seborrhoeic dermatitis consists of greasy scaling, concentrated in the eyebrows and nasolabial folds (Fig. 8.27). Sometimes, the surrounding areas on the cheeks and forehead are involved. The disease may spread, as well-demarcated patches, on to the central chest in males, which it is known as petaloid seborrhoeic dermatitis. Occasionally, axillary lesions are present and, even less often, groin lesions.

Induction of seborrhoeic dermatitis in experimental animals following inoculation with *Pityrosporum* yeasts, plus raised antibody levels to *Pityrosporum* yeasts in patients with seborrhoea, tends to confirm the connection between *Pityrosporum* yeasts and seborrhoea. Finally, seborrhoeic dermatitis, as well as *Pityrosporum* folliculitis, occurs in its most severe form

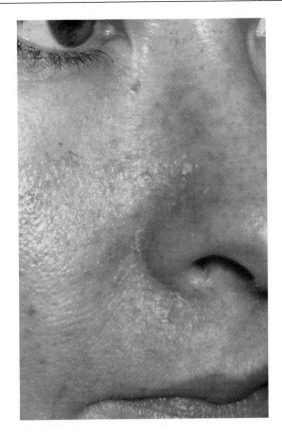

Fig. 8.27 Nasolabial scaling in seborrhoeic dermatitis.

in patients with AIDS, which again supports the contention that it is infective in origin.

Differential diagnosis. All forms of dermatitis, psoriasis and dermatophyte infection can be misdiagnosed as seborrhoea.

Laboratory diagnosis of Pityrosporum *yeast infection*

Pityriasis versicolor. Skin scrapings taken with a scalpel blade from the surface of lesions yield profuse quantities of fine white scale. The specimen is sent to the laboratory in folded black paper, as in dermatophyte infection. The scales are cleared with KOH and round or oval spores, accompanied by multiple fragmented non-branching hyphae, are clearly seen. The appearance is diagnostic and most laboratories do not proceed to culture. If culture is considered necessary, it should be carried out on Sabouraud's agar, with an overlying layer of oil, such as olive oil, and incubated at 27–30°C. Typical cream-coloured colonies appear within 1 week.

Pityrosporum *folliculitis and seborrhoea.* Pityrosporum folliculitis and seborrhoeic dermatitis are nearly always diagnosed clinically; given that the organism is a skin commensal, it is very difficult to interpret qualitative evidence of yeast presence as the causal agent of disease. There is no doubt that the yeast is present in much more abundant quantity in dandruff and seborrhoeic dermatitis, but such quantitative assessment is really only useful in comparative rather than absolute terms. Histology of *Pityrosporum* folliculitis does show yeast within the hair follicle and this is sometimes helpful in diagnosis, but of course the appearances are sometimes also seen in normal skin.

Superficial candidiasis

A number of *Candida* species are known to cause disease of the skin or mucous membranes. *Candida albicans*, a commensal of the mouth and gut, is the commonest of these, but other species, such as *Candida parapsilosis*, *Candida tropicalis*, *Candida glabrata* and *Candida krusei* can also cause infection. Pathogenicity appears to be associated with a yeast–mycelial shift and this begins with adherence and thereafter production of hyphae, which penetrate cells. *Candida* yeasts are rarely, if ever, primary pathogens of skin. They require interference with host defence mechanisms in order to become established. These factors include antibiotic therapy, which alters the commensal flora, pre-existing skin disease, which allows for a better substrate, intercurrent disease, such as diabetes, which reduces phagocyte activity, and various forms of immunosuppression, all of which can lead to secondary candidiasis. The same considerations apply to all forms of candidiasis, but vaginal candidiasis does appear to arise *de novo* and furthermore can be recalcitrant and notably recurrent in otherwise healthy women.

Systemic candidiasis, which can affect many internal organs in susceptible patients, is a serious and often fatal disease, which is difficult to diagnose early enough for effective treatment to be instituted. This chapter will not deal with vaginal or systemic *Candida* infection, which is outside the scope of a dermatology text.

Oral candidiasis

The mouth is a common site for *Candida* infection, because the yeast is a normal commensal of this area. It occurs predominantly in infants, elderly denture wearers, patients receiving antibiotic therapy and those who are immunocompromised. It is the commonest superficial infection in patients with AIDS. Several clinical subtypes are recognized.

Acute pseudomembranous candidiasis. Acute pseudomembranous candidiasis appears as white plaques on a background of inflamed epithelium (Fig. 8.28). Sometimes, the white plaques are not prominent and the mucosal surface appears to be red and swollen, and the condition is then referred to as acute erythematous candidiasis. It occurs in denture wearers who either

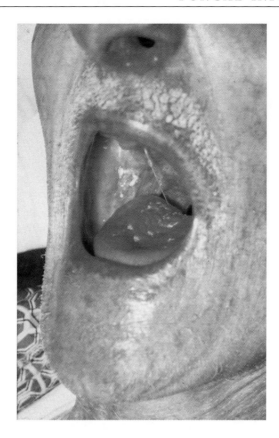

Fig. 8.28 Acute pseudomembranous oral candidiasis.

do not remove their false teeth or fail to sterilize them when they are removed. The pink acrylic material in which the teeth are embedded is porous to the yeast and acts as a focus of infection. Antibiotic therapy temporarily destroys the bacterial flora of the mouth, thus leading to an overgrowth of yeasts and also freeing far more sites for yeast adherence. Acute oral candidiasis, often known as thrush, is regularly seen in infants and, along with other acute varieties, responds to antifungal therapy, together with correction of the source of infection. Dentures require to be sterilized and antibiotic therapy discontinued in order for treatment to be wholly effective. In AIDS patients, the underlying problem is not remediable and the condition then becomes resistant and refractory and is known as chronic pseudomembranous candidiasis.

Chronic oral candidiasis. This can occur in non-AIDS patients who are, usually, smokers. The plaques become adherent, often to the tongue, and sometimes take on a granulomatous appearance, when it is known as chronic nodular candidosis. These chronic forms are sometimes associated with carcinoma of the tongue. This chronic variety can sometimes spread to involve the angles of the mouth (cheilitis) and this is the first visible sign of infection. When *Candida* infection is confined to an oval area in the centre of the tongue, it is often referred to as median rhomboid glossitis. In AIDS patients, infection can spread down the oesophagus as the CD4 count falls.

Differential diagnosis. Lichen planus, leucoplakia or carcinoma *in situ* may be confused with oral candidiasis, but in these conditions the white plaque is much more adherent to the mucosal surface. However, in cases of doubt, a biopsy should be carried out.

Cutaneous candidiasis *or* Candida *intertrigo*

This condition occurs in the groin area, vulva, axillae, submammary folds or within abdominal fat folds in obese individuals. The condition is most often seen in diabetics or in patients receiving antibiotic therapy, although obese patients who perhaps pay less attention than they should to personal hygiene can develop yeast infection with no underlying factor. Flexural skin disease, such as psoriasis or eczema, may also develop secondary *Candida* infection.

Acute *Candida* vulvitis (Fig. 8.29) may accompany vaginal infection, although it is by no means invariable. Factors that encourage vulvitis in patients with vaginal infection include inappropriate antibiotic therapy, the wearing of tights and tight nylon underwear (as opposed to loose cotton) or profuse sweating or friction, as may occur in hobbies such as bicycle riding.

Napkin dermatitis

This condition is secondary to an irritant dermatitis reaction to ammonia, resulting from the failure to change wet dirty nappies often enough. Yeasts are present in faeces and overgrow on inflamed skin. Treatment requires to be directed at the cause as well as the effect of the problem.

Interdigital candidiasis

This condition was formerly known as erosio interdigitalae blastomycetica.

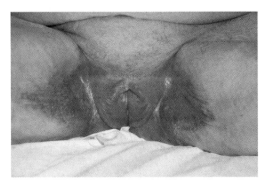

Fig. 8.29 Acute *Candida* vulvitis.

Typical white plaques with fissuring are seen in the interdigitial folds (Fig. 8.30) and is seen in patients such as cooks and hairdressers between the finger and sometimes between the toes in hot climates, particularly in patients such as soldiers who may keep their boots on for prolonged periods. It is occasionally seen in patients on long-term topical steroids especially where there is fluid retention and swelling of the digits.

Generalized infantile candidiasis

This unusual condition is occasionally seen in infants recently delivered of a mother who has vaginal candidiasis. It looks alarming, in that the baby's skin is erythematous and covered in small pustules. However, it responds well enough to therapy, providing it is recognized.

Chronic mucocutaneous candidiasis

This rare condition results from a number of syndromes associated with a defect in cell-mediated immunity. It generally presents in infancy or childhood, and the nails, mucous membranes and skin are variously and variably involved. It is sometimes associated with cutaneous viral and dermatophyte infections. When the disease presents in adults, it is usually associated with thymoma or systemic lupus erythematosus. Chronic pseudomembranous oral candidiasis occurs, along with crusted plaques on the skin, often referred to as *Candida* granuloma. Nail changes are most commonly seen in the fingers and the nail plates become very thickened and dystrophic. The nail folds and surrounding skin are usually involved as well (Fig. 8.31).

In children, there are two inherited forms, an autosomal recessive and an autosomal dominant type, as well as an idiopathic variety and a type associated with endocrinopathy syndromes, usually affecting the thyroid, parathyroids and adrenal glands. The severity of the cutaneous lesions is variable, according to type, and the lesions are sometimes associated with chest infection, leading to bronchiectasis. Some cases improve with age,

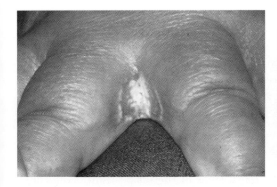

Fig. 8.30 Interdigital candidiasis.

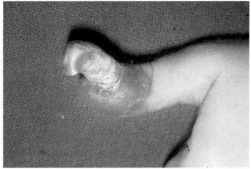

Fig. 8.31 Chronic mucocutaneous candidiasis.

while other deteriorate, and there is no certain way to correct the underlying immunological defects. Infusions of transfer factor have been used in the past but with no real lasting benefit. The advent of oral agents active against yeasts has undoubtedly improved the quality of life of these patients significantly.

Differential diagnosis. Chronic mucocutaneous candidiasis is a disease that produces unique signs and symptoms, and diagnosis only presents difficulty because of the its rarity. Even a dermatologist with a large practice would expect to see only a few cases in a professional lifetime.

Laboratory diagnosis of candidiasis

Scrapings should be taken from white plaques in the mouth or from the edge of skin lesions. After clearing with KOH, mycelium and pseudomycelium may be seen on direct microscopy, but these are accompanied by clusters of yeast cells, which are diagnostic. Sometimes, swabs taken from very active lesions yield enough yeast to be visualized on a Gram film.

Candida yeasts may be cultured on Sabouraud's dextrose agar, but a positive culture in the absence of positive microscopy is of doubtful significance, as the organism is a commensal. Certainly, a few colonies grown from a skin scraping or mouth swab should probably be disregarded as indicative of active infection. Identification of the specific *Candida* species is becoming more important with the advent of yeast resistance to some antifungal drugs, particularly in AIDS patients. Assimilation or fermentation tests are necessary for this purpose [18].

Histological evidence of yeast invasion is important in systemic candidiasis. However, it is not usually necessary in superficial disease, other than in the occasional chronic mouth lesion, where it could be associated with carcinoma.

Tropical superficial fungal infection

Tinea nigra

This condition occurs predominantly in the tropics, but may present in Europe, the USA and Australia. Clinically, it appears as a flat, well-demarcated area of pigmentation on the palms or soles. Scraping reveals the lesion to be scaly, thus differentiating it from acral melanoma. The causal organism is a black yeast, *Exophiala werneckii*. It responds to keratolytics and topical and systemic antifungal agents.

Piedra

Piedra is an infection of the hairy areas of the scalp, beard, axillae and pubic area. It is an infection of the hair shafts, where small nodules develop.

There are two clinical varieties: black piedra and white piedra. The causal organism of black piedra, which occurs mainly on the scalp, is *Piedraia hortae*. White piedra, which is mainly seen in the genital area but can affect the axilla and scalp, is the yeast *Trichosporon beigelii*. Microscopic examination of the hair shaft and culture, if necessary, confirm the fungal nature of the disease.

Clinically, it can be confused with trichorrhexis nodosa, monilethrix and trichonodosis.

Traditionally, treatment consists of cutting the hair short, which may be unacceptable. Rinsing with a 2% formalin solution is usually effective, as are topical antifungals, and an amphotericin lotion has been found useful in white piedra [19].

Allergic reactions to fungi

Secondary sensitization rashes, known as dermatophyteid reactions, are recognized. The dry peeling of the hands and fingers associated with tinea pedis has been previously mentioned. Sometimes, a generalized lichenoid rash can occur, and urticarial, pityriasis rosea-like and morbilliform eruptions have all been described. Occasionally, erythema nodosum and annular erythemas are associated with dermatophytosis. Allergic reactions to the carriage of *Candida* in the gut are thought by some to account for numerous non-specific symptoms, such as general malaise, joint pains and depression, but there is no convincing evidence whatsoever that this is the case. Certainly, no benefit is likely to ensue by eradication of *Candida* from such patients. There is some work indicating that persistent adult atopic dermatitis, particularly when it affects the head and neck, is related to a type 1 hypersensitivity reaction to *P. ovale*. Such patients have specific immunoglobulin E (IgE) antibodies to *P. ovale* and a positive *P. ovale* prick test [20]. By no means all adult atopics have this association, but antifungal agents active against yeasts may be worth trying in such patients who prove recalcitrant to conventional therapy and have positive antibody and prick tests.

Fungal infection in AIDS

Around 90% of HIV-positive patients who develop AIDS are likely to suffer from cutaneous and/or mucous-membrane infection. Oral, pharyngeal and oesophageal candidiasis is the commonest fungal infection and these patients may also develop flexural candidiasis. Seborrhoeic dermatitis and *Pityrosporum* folliculitis is common and usually severe in AIDS patients, although it is not easy to distinguish from the varieties occuring in those who are not HIV-positive.

Dermatophytosis of the glabrous skin is thought to occur in about 40%

of HIV-positive patients, and tinea pedis is the most frequent type. Tinea corporis, tinea cruris and dermatophyte infection of the face are also quite common. The organisms and clinical appearances are similar to those in non-HIV-positive patients, but the disease may be more widespread and is certainly more frequent. Onychomycosis secondary to *T. rubrum* is the most common fungal nail infection and is again more frequent than the prevalence in the general population. It is interesting to note that isolation of dermatophytes from clinically normal nails is almost unheard of in the normal population but rises to almost 40% in HIV-positive patients, strongly suggesting that a diminished cell-mediated immune response is implicated in the establishment of dermatophyte infection in nails.

Fungal infection in AIDS patients presents a real treatment challenge but also provides some indication as to the stage of disease. Acquired immune deficiency syndrome patients are generally monitored by measuring the CD4 lymphocyte count. Oral pharyngeal candidiasis and seborrhoeic dermatitis occur at CD4 counts around or below 500, whereas it is said that generalized dermatophyte infection occurs when the CD4 count is below 200 and onychomycosis presents at CD4 counts below 100. It must be pointed out, however, that the CD4 count associated with superficial fungal infection varies in different series, but certainly evidence of such infection identifies conversion from HIV positivity to AIDS [21].

Treatment of superficial fungal infections

Therapy of superficial fungal infections has improved more significantly in recent years than in most other therapeutic areas. A number of new agents are now available in both topical and oral formulations which are much more effective than their immediate predecessors. These drugs act in different ways and have a differing spectrum of activity, so drug selection based upon accurate diagnosis is of great importance.

Topical therapy is generally very effective in infections of the glabrous skin and mucous membranes; however, when disease is widespread, patient compliance and cost efficacy may be enhanced by selection of a systemic agent. In those areas where the keratin layer is thickest, namely the scalp, palms, soles and nails, systemic treatment is nearly always necessary because of its significantly greater efficacy. Antifungal drugs are divided into four groups: the polyenes, the azoles, the allylamines and others, such as griseofulvin and the undecenoates, which do not fall into any of the above groups. Drugs in these groups are illustrated in Table 8.3.

The azoles and the allylamines are the most important agents in the treatment of superficial infection. Both of these groups of drugs act by inhibition of ergosterol biosynthesis in the fungal cell wall. The allylamines interfere with the enzyme squalene epoxidase, thus inhibiting the conversion of squalene to squalene epoxide, which occurs at any early stage in the biosynthesis of ergosterol. Azoles interfere with the enzyme 14-α-demethylase, which allows conversion of lanosterol to ergosterol. Azoles

Table 8.3 Systemic treatment of superficial infection.

Disease	Drug	Dose (daily)	Duration
Tinea capitis	Griseofulvin	1–1.5 g (adults)	8–12 weeks
		10 mg/kg (children)	8–12 weeks
	Terbinafine	250 mg (adults)	2–4 weeks
		62.5 mg (<20 kg)	2–4 weeks
		125 mg (20–40 kg)	2–4 weeks
		250 mg (>40 kg)	2–4 weeks
Tinea corporis/cruris	Griseofulvin	500 mg	4 weeks
	Terbinafine	250 mg	1 week
	Itraconazole	100 mg	4 weeks
		200 mg	? 2 weeks
Tinea pedis/manuum	Griseofulvin	1 g	8 weeks
	Terbinafine	250 mg	2 weeks
	Itraconazole	400 mg	1 week
Tinea unguium	Griseofulvin	1 g	6–9 months (fingernails)
			12–18 months (toenails)
	Terbinafine	250 mg	6 weeks (fingernails)
			12 weeks (toenails)
	Itraconazole	200 mg	12 weeks
		400 mg	For 1 week × 3 (fingernails)
		400 mg	For 1 week × 4 (toenails)
Pityriasis versicolor	Itraconazole	200 mg	5–7 days
Candidiasis/nails	Itraconazole	200 mg	6–12 weeks depending upon underlying condition

thus inhibit production of ergosterol. 14-α-Demethylase is a cytochrome P450 enzyme, whereas squalene epoxidase is not, and it is thus immediately more likely that there will be fewer drug interactions related to drugs of the allylamine group than with azoles. Furthermore, accumulation of squalene is thought to result in cell death, providing the allylamines with a fungicidal mode of action. Azole drugs, on the other hand, by producing ergosterol depletion are thought to be fungistatic. This effect is apparently dose-dependent and it is possible to produce a cidal effect with increased concentration of azole drugs. Fungicidal and fungistatic activity as demonstrated *in vitro* provides only a guide to *in vivo* activity, which remains the acid test of antifungal agents. Similarly, the measurement of the minimal inhibitory concentration (MIC), which is the starting-point in the measurement of activity of all antimicrobial agents, also only provides a guide to *in vivo* acitivity. The allylamines have a very low MIC against dermatophytes and, furthermore, the MIC level is the same as the minimal fungicidal concentration (MFC), and this, together with its mode of action, provides important initial *in vitro* evidence that the allylamines are the best drugs against dermatophytes.

Dermatophytosis

Topical therapy. There are numerous topical azole preparations available worldwide. Notable examples include clotrimazole, miconazole, econazole and sulconazole. There are two topical allylamines: naftifine and terbinafine. Amorolfine is the only member of the morpholine group of drugs and is available as a cream and nail lacquer. Older agents, such as Whitfield's ointment and topical undecenoates, have largely been supplanted by these newer agents. Terbinafine 1% cream appears to be the best topical agent for dermatophyte infections. A notable study revealed it to be more effective in tinea pedis following 1 week's therapy applied twice daily than clotrizamole applied twice daily for 4 weeks, in terms of both cure and relapse rates. It is likely to be effective over 1 week's treatment duration in tinea corporis, tinea cruris and interdigital tinea pedis, where topical therapy is indicated. Although more costly than azole creams, its better cure rates, lower relapse rates and likely better patient compliance, given the shorter treatment duration, suggest that it is the more cost-effective option.

Systemic therapy. Griseofulvin, the azoles ketoconazole, itraconazole and fluconazole and the allylamine terbinafine are all available for systemic treatment of dermatophyte infections. Griseofulvin, introduced in the late 1950s, is a weakly fungistatic agent, which works well in tinea capitis, tinea corporis and tinea cruris when given for an adequate period. It is not so effective in the more recalcitrant infections involving the palms, soles and nails. The bioavailability of the original formulation of griseofulvin was poor because of inadequate absorption. Since that time, a small-particle or micronized type was introduced, followed by the very small-particle or ultramicronized variety, which allowed for reduction in dosage. Treatment durations remain comparatively lengthy and are equivalent to the epidermal turnover at the site involved. Current dosage regimens range from 500 mg daily in adults up to 1 g daily in nail infection. In children, the drug should be administered in dosages of between 10 and 20 mg/kg body weight.

Ketoconazole is an imidazole used in a dose of 200 mg daily. It is a broader-spectrum agent than griseofulvin but not very much more effective in dermatophyte infections, although treatment durations may be slightly shorter. Fatal hepatotoxicity has occurred and, although such cases are uncommon, the drug has been supplanted by better alternatives in dermatophyte infections.

Fluconazole is hydrophilic and has the highest bioavailability of all oral antifungal agents. It is an expensive drug, originally licensed and priced for single-dose treatment of vaginal candidiasis and serious systemic infections. Its continuous use in superficial dermatophyte infection is therefore likely to be prohibitively costly, although there are some studies showing good efficacy.

Itraconazole, a triazole like fluconazole, is much less toxic than ketoconazole and has a similar broad spectrum. It was originally licensed in a dose of 100 mg daily, but this is probably suboptimal in terms of dose/duration for dermatophyte infections, and doses of up to 400 mg daily have been used for recalcitrant foot infections for only 1 week with good results. In nail infections, the drug is given either continuously for 6 or 12 weeks for fingernail and toenail infections, respectively, in a dose of 200 mg daily, or in a pulse regimen of 400 mg daily for 1 week each month, repeated three, four or more times, depending upon response. Three pulses are likely to be adequate for fingernail infection, whereas four pulses are probably necessary for toenail disease. It is as yet unclear whether this is as effective as continuous therapy, but it certainly reduces cost and the drug would appear to remain in the nail in consistent concentrations during the outgrowth phase in both continuous and pulsed regimens [22].

Terbinafine, like its topical variant, is probably the most effective anti-dermatophyte agent. It is effective in a dose of 250 mg daily when given for only 1 week in tinea corporis and tinea cruris, while 2 weeks' therapy produced good cure rates in infections of the palms and soles. Cure rates of 90% have been found after 6 weeks' therapy in fingernail infections and around 80% following 3 months' treatment of toenail infections. Early studies using terbinafine in tinea capitis reveal that 4 weeks' therapy is as effective as 8 weeks' treatment with griseofulvin, and there is one study which shows that the treatment duration can be reduced to 2 weeks with similar efficacy. The patients included in these studies have mostly had *T. violaceum* infection of the scalp, and studies on zoophilic infections are awaited. Terbinafine is not active when given systemically against *C. albicans* infection, although it does work topically in cutaneous candidiasis. Use of systemic terbinafine is therefore concentrated on dermatophyte infections [23].

A summary of the dose and duration of various systemic treatments in dermatophyte infection is shown in Table 8.3.

Thus far, adverse events with these newer drugs appear to be few and significant adverse events are very rare. They would appear to be safe drugs for use in non-life-threatening disease and certainly an advance over older drugs, such as griseofulvin and ketoconazole, in terms of both efficacy and safety.

Pityrosporum *yeast infections*

Pityriasis versicolor. Pityriasis versicolor responds well to many forms of topical therapy. However, the whole of the trunk, neck, arms and legs down to the knees should always be treated, even when overt disease appears to affect only small areas. Propylene glycol 50% in water applied twice daily for 2 weeks is very inexpensive and effective. Topical azoles require to be used over the same area for 2–4 weeks, but this will require large quantities of cream and is therefore expensive. Topical selenium sulphide can be applied less frequently and there are numerous suggested regimens. Once-weekly application repeated three times is probably as good as any, although the drug is available only in a soap base, as it is mainly used as a shampoo. It is therefore not a very comfortable product to apply. Systemic azoles are likely to be effective over very short treatment durations. Again numerous regimens have been suggested. A single dose of ketoconazole or fluconazole 400 mg daily may be effective. The mode of delivery of these drugs is quite probably via the sweat. Itraconazole 200 mg daily for 5 days also provides cure rates of greater than 90%. The patient must be warned that depigmentation may persist for some time even after successful treatment.

There are therefore numerous therapeutic regimens available for the treatment of pityriasis versicolor and all are effective, although clearly some are more convenient than others. Treatment choice is therefore dependent upon local drug availability and cost.

Pityrosporum *folliculitis*. This is a more difficult condition to treat than pityriasis versicolor and relapses are common. Some authorities believe that the inflammatory reaction should be reduced by a topical steroid initially and thereafter a topical antifungal agent applied. It is likely that treatment will require to be repeated with a topical antifungal from time to time to prevent relapse. There are few studies proving efficacy of systemic antifungal drugs in *Pityrosporum* folliculitis and their use should probably be reserved for patients with AIDS.

Seborrhoeic dermatitis. Again, the place of antifungal therapy alone in this condition is unproved. Combinations of shampoo containing either ketoconazole, selenium sulphide or zinc pyrithione, used at least once weekly for washing both the hair and other affected areas, along with a combination of antifungal drugs and hydrocortisone, are often useful and keep the condition in check. Thus far, there does not appear to be a significant role for systemic antifungal agents in this disease, although patients with AIDS may well be the exception [3].

Cutaneous candidiasis

Control or eradication of the underlying disease or precipitating factor is an important first step in the treatment of cutaneous *Candida* infections, which are usually secondary. Topical azole preparations, as well as topical terbinafine, have been shown to be effective, and combination products containing an antifungal drug along with a topical steroid are probably the most useful in this condition where flexural infected eczema or atopic dermatitis is the precipitating factor. Uncomplicated oral candidiasis will respond to amphotericin lozenges, nystatin pastilles or drops or miconazole oral gel. Again, removal of the precipitating factor is most important and attention should be paid to sterilization of dentures. The advent of oral agents active against yeasts has much improved the prognosis of patients with CMCC. Ketoconazole, fluconazole and itraconazole are all effective and dosages and treatment regimens vary with disease severity.

Patients who have *Candida* nail infection with associated paronychia should be advised to keep the hands as dry as possible when cooking and washing. As the infection is mixed, both an antifungal and an antibacterial topical agent should be applied. An azole lotion should be dropped on to the proximal nail plate and allowed to wash under the cuticle once daily, alternating with antibacterial solution, such as 15% sulphacetamide in 70% alcohol or 4% thymol in chloroform. Some authorities advocate the application of clear nail varnish to the cuticular area in order to provide a watertight seal, but this should only be done after the initial infection has been eradicated. Systemic antifungal agents active against *Candida* do appear to effect an improvement in chronic paronychia with secondary nail changes, but there is no definite evidence that they are superior to much cheaper topical preparations. In either case, treatment requires to be continued for a lengthy period until the nail has grown out and the cuticle is reattached to the nail plate, thus providing a natural watertight seal. Selection of treatment for patients with distal *Candida* nail infection is initially complicated by the question as to whether or not the yeast is the primary pathogen or merely secondary to pre-existing nail dystrophy, which would not, of course, respond to antifungal drugs. If antifungal agents are to be used systemically, itraconazole or fluconazole are the drugs of choice, in that terbinafine is ineffective in candidiasis and ketoconazole is much less safe for long-term use. It is impossible to recommend a dosage/duration regimen for fluconazole, because of lack of proper studies, but it is likely that 300 mg weekly for at least 6 months would be necessary. Itraconazole should be given in a dose of 200 mg daily for 6 weeks in fingernails and 12 weeks in the unlikely event of a toenail infection.

The advent of new and more effective antifungal agents has certainly led to more rewarding treatment of dermatophyte and *Pityrosporum* yeast infection. Antifungal agents active against *Candida* are good drugs but the underlying cause of disease often leads to continuing high relapse rates.

Subcutaneous mycoses

This group of conditions affects subcutaneous tissues, including bones, as well as the skin. The three most important diseases in this group are mycetoma; chromoblastomycosis and phaeohyphomycosis; and sporotrichosis, plus less common infections, which include lobomycosis and zygomycosis.

Mycetoma

This condition is also known as Madura foot, after an Indian province, although the disease is by no means confined to the Indian subcontinent. The disease may be caused by fungi (eumycetoma) or filamentous bacteria (actinomycetoma). Large abscesses develop at the site of inoculation of the organism, which follows local injury from thorns or branches. Hence the lesions are most common on a lower limb but may occur on any site. Abscesses are filled with grains, which consist of filaments of the microorganisms. These grains are of varying colour, depending upon the organims involved. Black grains are seen secondary to infection with *Madurella mycetomatis* and *Madurella grisea*. Whitish-yellow grains are seen in infections due to *Pseudallacheria boydii*, *Actinomadura madurae* and *Streptomyces somaliensis*. *Nocardia* species produce much smaller grains, not visible to the naked eye. Clinically, these present with a chronically swollen area, often a limb, with draining sinuses. The condition is often painful and bone involvement occurs late and often causes considerable pain and disability. Late-stage disease often requires extensive and mutilating surgery, and eumycetomas are recognized to be more recalcitrant to therapy than actinomycetomas.

Chromoblastomycosis

The most important organisms responsible for this infection are *Fonsecaea pedrosoi*, *Fonsecaea compacta* and *Cladosporium carrionii*. Verrucose lesions develop on the hands and lower legs and spread relentlessly. These may be flat and plaque-like (Fig. 8.32) or large and cauliflower-like. It is not a common disease and occurs sporadically in Central and South America, Africa, South-East Asia and occasionally Japan. Characteristic thick-walled or sclerotic cells are seen histologically (Fig. 8.33).

A variant of this condition is phaeohyphomycosis, which presents as a subcutaneous cyst containing hyphae on histological examination.

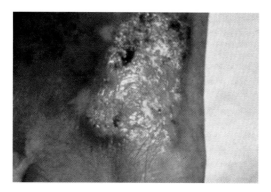

Fig. 8.32 Characteristic tumours of chromomycosis (courtesy of Upjohn Company, Kalamazoo, Michigan).

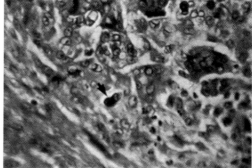

Fig. 8.33 Fungal spores that cause chromomycosis (courtesy of Upjohn Company, Kalamazoo, Michigan).

Sporotrichosis

This infection is quite widespread in the tropics and subtropics but may occur in the USA and Japan. The infection is caused by *Sporothrix schenckii* and follows injury from plant materials. The lesions may be fixed and solitary, occurring on the face or trunk (Fig. 8.34), or sporotrichoid, where spread occurs up the lymphatics in the limbs. Characteristic chains of nodular lesions develop up the limb (Fig. 8.35). Histology shows a characteristic single fungal cell surrounded by eosinophils (Fig. 8.36).

Lobomycosis and zygomycosis

Lobomycosis, secondary to *Loboa loboi*, is confined to the Amazon region of South America. The lesions are keloid-like and many occur on the ear. The disease runs a chronic course and is generally not fatal, but it causes considerable cosmetic disability. Yeast cells are seen within Langerhans cells and the appearance is characteristic. It is interesting that this organism has never been cultured.

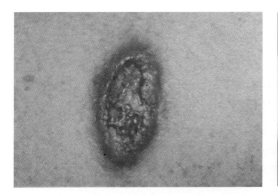

Fig. 8.34 Fixed form of sporotrichosis (courtesy of Upjohn Company, Kalamazoo, Michigan).

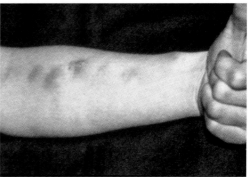

Fig. 8.35 Sporotrichosis nodules along lymph channels (courtesy of Upjohn Company, Kalamazoo, Michigan).

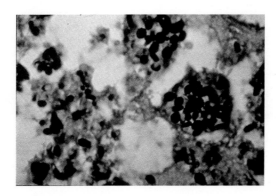

Fig. 8.36 Yeast sometimes associated with sporotrichosis (courtesy of Upjohn Company, Kalamazoo, Michigan).

Zygomycosis occurs in Africa, South-East Asia and Indonesia. It is caused by *Basidiobolus ranarum* and produces a hard rubbery swelling of the involved site, often buttocks. Histologically, an eosinophilic granuloma is seen containing numerous hyphae.

Coccidioidomycosis

This disease is primarily a respiratory infection, caused by *Coccidioides immitis*. It is endemic in the south-western USA and in parts of Central and South America. Some cases have been reported in the southern areas of Europe and the Middle East. Infection begins with the inhalation of arthrospores of the saprophytic phase of fungal growth. These spores develop in the lung tissue to form spherules, and this primary lesion is associated with lymphadenopathy but generally does not spread further. The disease at this stage is often asymptomatic but may produce mild symptoms akin to influenza. From the third to seventh week of infection, erythema multiforme or erythema nodosum (Fig. 8.37) develops in 3–25% of cases, most of which are females. The disease is recognized as the commonest cause of erythema nodosum in endemic areas. Primary skin lesions are extremely rare and consist of firm indurated nodules, usually as a result of local trauma (Fig. 8.38). In less that 0.5% of cases, disseminated disease occurs, which can affect the skin, subcutaneous tissues, bones, joints and, indeed, all other organs. The skin lesions can take the form of abscesses, granulomas, ulcers or discharging sinuses. Such patients are often immunosuppressed, and AIDS must be excluded.

The diagnosis may be made by visualization of spherules on KOH mounts of sputum or pus, and the fungus can be grown in culture (Fig. 8.39). It is highly infectious and cultures must be handled with great care in the laboratory. Precipitin tests are positive in 90% of individuals after 2–4 weeks of infection, but complement-fixation tests are more useful

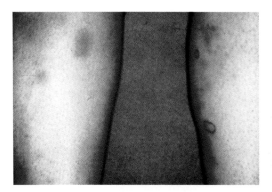

Fig. 8.37 Erythema nodosum of coccidioidomycosis (courtesy of Upjohn Company, Kalamazoo, Michigan).

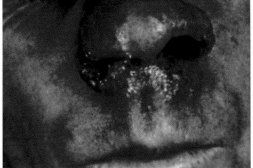

Fig. 8.38 Typical cutaneous plaque of coccidioidomycosis (courtesy of Upjohn Company, Kalamazoo, Michigan).

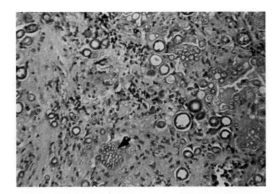

Fig. 8.39 *Coccidioides immitis* endospores (courtesy of Upjohn Company, Kalamazoo, Michigan).

in the diagnosis of severe disease and increase to a maximum after 6 months [24].

Paracoccidioidomycosis

This chronic granulomatous disease affects the skin, mucous membranes, lymph nodes and sometimes the internal organs. It is caused by *Paracoccidioides brasiliensis*. The disease is found in Latin America but is most common in the state of São Paulo in Brazil.

Pulmonary infection most commonly occurs, although mucocutaneous and lymphatic forms are well recognized, which involve the skin and mucous membranes and the lymph nodes, respectively. Mucocutaneous lesions are sometimes present in patients with pulmonary disease but may occur without lung involvement. Lesions often affect the gums, nose, conjuctivae and perianal region and take the form of superficial ulceration, which becomes progressively erosive and granulomatous. The disease may spread by the haematogenous or lymphatic routes and subcutaneous abscesses occur. Painful regional lymphadenopathy is common [25].

The diagnosis depends upon visualization of fungal cells on KOH mounts and culture of *P. brasiliensis*.

Histoplasmosis

This is a highly infectious disease, caused by *Histoplasma capsulatum*, and is usually a pulmonary infection. This disease is widely distributed world-wide, occurring in both temperate and tropical zones in North and South America, Africa and Australia. The fungus exists as a saprophyte in nature and is regularly isolated from the soil, particularly that which has been contaminated by chicken and bat droppings. The disease is only contracted by the inhalation of airborne spores [26].

In its benign form, the lung lesions heal by calcification and appear on X-ray to be very similar to the lesions of tuberculosis. Skin lesions most commonly occur secondary to infection with *Histoplasma duboisii*, which is closely related to *H. capsulatum*. This variety is usually found in Africa, and skin lesions consist of papules, ulcers and nodules, together with granuloma abscesses, which heal with scarring. A cellulitis may occur in patients who are immunosuppressed. The diagnosis is made by identifying small intracellular yeast-like cells in the sputum, peripheral blood, marrow or skin-biopsy specimens. Sometimes lymph-node aspiration is helpful. Typical colonies are seen on culture. An increasing titre on complement-fixation testing indicates progressing dissemination.

Actinomycosis

This chronic granulomatous disease is nearly always caused by *Actinomyces israelii* [27]. *Actinomyces bovis* is usually found in cattle and may well be an identical organism to *A. israelii*. Rarely, *Actinomyces naeslundii*, *Arachnia propionica* and *Bifidobacterium eriksonii* can cause human disease, but they are generally found as commensals in the mouth and nose. Following trauma or dental extraction, granulomatous lesions occur in the jaw area but can affect all other organs. The facial variety presents as an indurated nodule on the cheek or maxillary region and multiple sinuses, with secondary scarring regularly developing. The lesions may extend widely into the surrounding tissues and can involve the bones of the skull as well as the brain. Thoracic, abdominal and pelvic types of actinomycosis are recognized, where the disease affects lungs, intra-abdominal organs and gynaecological organs, respectively. Draining sinuses reveal characteristic 'sulphur' granules, which are seen as quite large yellow granules 1–2 mm in diameter. Microscopic examination reveals both bacillus and hyphal forms. Typical colonies are seen after anaerobic incubation at 37°C.

Nocardiasis

Nocardia species are aerobic actinomycetes. Primary infection occurs through inhalation of contaminated dust, and *Nocardia brasiliensis* and *Nocardia asteroides* are the commonest pathogens [27]. *Nocardia brasiliensis* is a cause of localized mycetoma.

Primary pulmonary or meningeal disease is much commoner than skin infection. However, the latter can occur and presents as multiple abscesses.

Diagnosis depends upon the visualization of characteristic organisms by Gram staining or acid-fast techniques. Culture will identify the specific organism.

Cryptococcosis

This disease may be an acute, subacute or chronic infection, caused by the yeast *Cryptococcus neoformans*. It is most often a disease of the brain and meninges, but occasionally the skin can be involved. *Cryptococcus neoformans* is a saprophyte of soil and is often found in pigeon droppings. The disease usually presents as a meningitis or as a focal brain lesion that resembles a tumour. Untreated, the disease progresses slowly, with a low-grade fever followed by coma and death. The organism is not highly pathogenic but is a common cause of death of AIDS patients in all parts of the world [28]. Small solitary skin lesions can occur, which have a typical gelatinous-looking edge and may be mistaken for a basal-cell carcinoma.

Large budding yeast cells are seen on direct microscopy when the specimen is mounted in Indian ink. The organism grows in culture and produces typical colonies. Antigen tests are especially useful in detecting subclinical infection.

Aspergillosis

This infection only produces skin lesions in patients who are immunosuppressed or who have end-stage malignant disease; even then, they are extremely rare. Fungal infections of the external ear or otomycosis may be caused by *Aspergillus fumigatus* or *Aspergillus niger*, when typical fungal elements can be seen macroscopically. Very rarely, aspergillomas are recognized in the oral cavity and the rhinocerebral type may cause necrosis of the palate.

Typical fungal elements are seen on microscopic examination and grow readily in culture.

Treatment of subcutaneous mycosis

Mycetoma

Eumycetomas usually require surgery and the treatment may be worse than the disease. About half the cases of eumycetoma secondary to *M. mycetomatis* respond to ketoconazole in a dose of 200–400 mg daily. Itraconazole may prove to be superior in terms of both efficacy and safety, but there are few reports of its use available currently.

Actinomycetomas respond better to treatment. Dapsone 100–150 mg daily or co-trimoxazole is useful, and rifampicin and streptomycin are also sometimes used.

Chromomycosis

Itraconazole 100–200 mg daily, together with flucytosine 30–35 mg/kg four times a day (qid), is often effective. Alternative regimens include a combination of amphotericin B and flucytosine or thiabendazole.

Sporotrichosis

This condition responds to potassium iodide in a saturated solution of 1 ml three times a day (tid), increasing to 4–6 ml tid. The dose must be increased slowly to prevent iodism. Both itraconazole and terbinafine have been reported as effective and may eventually supplant potassium iodide in the treatment of this condition.

Lobomycosis and zygomycosis

Because the organism responsible for lobomycosis cannot be cultured, drug sensitivities cannot be examined *in vitro*. Thus far, no therapeutic regimen has produced satisfactory cure rates [29].

Zygomycosis, on the other hand, responds well to potassium iodide, using a similar regimen to that prescribed for sporotrichosis.

Coccidioidomycosis

In primary pulmonary disease, no specific therapy is necessary, apart from rest, and spontaneous resolution usually occurs. Intravenous amphotericin B remains useful, but the oral azoles ketoconazole and itraconazole may be given orally and are likely to be less toxic. Itraconazole is a safer drug than ketoconazole and is given in doses of 100–200 mg daily [30].

Paracoccidioidomycosis

Both itraconazole and ketoconazole have been shown to be effective, and itraconazole is the drug of choice, given in doses of 100–200 mg daily for 3–6 months, although relapses are common [31].

Actinomycosis

The organism is sensitive to sulphonamides, streptomycin, penicillin, chloramphenicol, tetracyclines, erythromycin and rifampicin. Long-term penicillin therapy in very high doses is usually the treatment of choice, and 10–12 million units a day are necessary intravenously, often for up to 45 days. Wide surgical excision of the involved area should follow, and long-term treatment with intramuscular penicillin in a dose of 2–5 million units daily should be given for 12–18 months.

Nocardiasis

Co-trimoxazole is the treatment of choice, but sulphonamides may also be useful, as may ampicillin, minocycline, amikacin and imipenem. Therapy should be modified or continued, dependent upon clinical response.

Histoplasmosis

Oral ketoconazole has been shown to be very effective in both disseminated and localized forms of disease. This drug may be replaced by itraconazole, which has fewer side-effects, especially in patients who are immunosuppressed and may require long-term treatment [31]. The fungus also responds to amphotericin B, which should be given when the infection is widespread and severe.

Cryptococcosis

This disease is now most frequently seen in AIDS patients and is usually treated using either fluconazole or itraconazole, which requires to be given long-term. Amphotericin B, in combination with flucytosine, is useful in non-AIDS cases, who are less likely to develop complications of therapy and do not require such long-term treatment.

Aspergillosis

Aspergillosis responds to amphotericin B and this may be given locally in both oral and ear infections. It is unlikely to be justified systemically in such cases, given its toxic effects, and itraconazole may become the treatment of choice, although the results of convincing studies are awaited.

References

1 Dahl MV. Dermatophytosis and the immune reponse. *J Am Acad Dermatol* 1994; **31** (3, Part 2): S34–S41.
2 Odds FC. Pathogenesis of *Candida* infections. *J Am Acad Dermatol* 1994; **31** (3, Part 2): S2–S5.
3 Weitzman I, Summerbell RC. The dermatophytes. *Clin Microbiol Rev* 1995; **8**, No. 2: 240–259.
4 Faergemann J. *Pityrosporum* infections. *J Am Acad Dermatol* 1994; **31** (3, Part 2): S18–S20.
5 Bronson DM, Desai DR, Bharsky S. An epidemic of infection with *Trichophyton tonsurans* reviewed in a 20 year survey of fungal infections in Chicago. *J Am Acad Dermatol* 1983; **8**: 322–330.
6 Neil G, Hanslo D. Control of the carrier state of scalp dermatophytes. *Paediatr Infect Dis J* 1990; **9**: 57–58.
7 MacLennan R, O'Keefe M. Altitude and prevalence of tinea imbricata in New Guinea. *Trans Roy Soc Trop Med Hyg* 1975; **69**: 91–93.
8 Howell SA, Clayton YM, Pham QC. Tinea pedis, the relationship between symptoms, organisms and host characteristics. *Microbiol Ecol Health Dis* 1988; **1**: 131–135.
9 Gentles JC, Evans EGV. Foot infections in swimming baths. *Br Med J* 1973; **3**: 260–262.
10 English MP, Gibson MD, Warin RP. Studies in the epidemiology of tinea pedis in a boys' boarding school. *Br Med J* 1961; **1**: 1083–1086.
11 English MP, Wethered RR, Duncan EHL. Studies in the epidemiology of tinea pedis: fungal infection in a longstay hospital. *Br Med J* 1967; **3**: 136–139.

12 Gotz H, Hantschke D. Einblicke in die Epidemiologie der Dermatomykosen. *Kohlenbergbau Hautarzt* 1965; **16**: 543–548.

13 Zaias N. Onychomycosis. *Arch Dermatol* 1972; **105**: 263–274.

14 Hay RJ, Baran R, Moore MK, Wilkinson JD. *Candida* onychomycosis—an evaluation of the role of *Candida* in nail disease. *Br J Dermatol* 1988; **118**: 47–58.

15 Gentles JC, Evans EGV. Infection of feet and nails with *Hendersonula toruloidea*. *Sabouraudia* 1970; **9**: 72–75.

16 Evans EGV, Richardson MD (eds). *Medical Mycology: Practical Approach*. IRL Press at Oxford University Press, Oxford, 1989.

17 Faergemann J. *Pityrosporum* infections. In: Elewski BE (ed.) *Cutaneous Fungal Infections*. Igaku-Shoin, Tokyo, 1992, pp. 69–83.

18 Odds FC. Candida *and Candidosis*. Baillière Tindall, London, 1988.

19 Canizares O. Tropical superficial fungal infections. In: Canizares O, Harman R (eds) *Clinical Dermatology*. Blackwell Scientific Publications, Oxford, 1992, pp. 16–17.

20 Hjorth N, Clemensen OH. Treatment of dermatitis of the head and neck with ketoconazole in patients with type 1 hypersensitivity to *Pityrosporum orbiculare*. *Semin Dermatol* 1983; **2**: 26–29.

21 Odom RB. Common superficial fungal infections in immunosuppressed patients. *J Am Acad Dermatol* 1994; **31**: S56–S59.

22 Degreef HJ, DeDoncker PRG. Current therapy of dermatophytosis. *J Am Acad Dermatol* 1994; **31**: S25–S30.

23 Roberts DT. Oral therapeutic agents in fungal nail disease. *J Am Acad Dermatol* 1974; **31**: S78–S81.

24 Drutz DJ, Catanzako A. Coccidioidomycosis. Parts I and II. *Am Rev Respir Dis* 1978; **117**: 559–585, 727–771.

25 Del Negro G, Lacaz CS, Fiorillo AM (eds). *Paracoccidioidomicose*. Sarvier Editora, São Paulo, 1982.

26 Schwartz J. *Histoplasmosis*. Praeger, New York, 1981.

27 Peabody JW, Seabury JH. Actinomycosis and nocardiosis. *Am J Med* 1960; **28**: 99–115.

28 Dismukes WE. Cryptococcal meningitis in patients with AIDS. *J Infect Dis* 1988; **157**: 5624–5627.

29 Lavalle P, Goncalves AP, Jerdim ML, Hay RJ, Canizares O, Harman R. Tropical deep fungal infections. In: Canizares O, Harman R (eds) *Clinical Tropical Dermatology*. Blackwell Scientific Publications, Oxford, 1992, pp. 41–87.

30 Ganer A, Arathoone Stevens DA. Initial experience in therapy for progressive mycoses with itraconazole: the first clinically studied triazole. *Rev Infect Dis* 1987; **9** (Suppl 1): 577–586.

31 Negroni R, Palmieri O, Karen K *et al.* Oral treatment of paracoccidioidomycosis and histoplasmosis with itraconazole. *Rev Infect Dis* 1987; Suppl 1: 47–50.

Chapter 9
Leprosy

A. Colin McDougall

Definition

Leprosy may be briefly defined as a chronic, potentially disabling disease of humans, caused by infection by *Mycobacterium leprae*, mainly affecting the nerves and skin. However, as with all complex diseases, such brevity is misleading and a complete definition of leprosy calls for attention to a much wider range of characteristics, including the following: (i) its remarkable range of clinical findings, apparently related to the level of cell-mediated immune (CMI) response in different individuals; (ii) the long incubation period between infection and disease, commonly 2–5 years; (iii) the frequent occurrence of adverse immunological reactions, based on either cell-mediated or immune-complex mechanisms, leading to tissue damage and neuritis; (iv) the social and psychological consequences of developing leprosy, including stigmatization, loss of family support, employment status and, in some circumstances, outright rejection; and (v) the excellent results of early treatment with multiple drug therapy (MDT), the increasingly wide use of which has led to the development of an elimination programme by the World Health Organization (WHO), aimed at reducing prevalence to less than one case per 10 000 of the population by the year 2000.

In addition to this general definition of leprosy as a disease, another more specific one concerning case definition, proposed by WHO in 1988 [1], calls for attention. For many years, a patient diagnosed and registered as having leprosy carried the 'label' on an almost indefinite basis, no doubt partly due to the long, or even lifelong, periods of treatment advised during the dapsone monotherapy era. In 1988, however, the WHO Expert Committee on Leprosy drew attention to the confusion, notably with regard to obtaining prevalence and other statistics, which had resulted from the custom of grouping patients needing or undergoing treatment with those who had completed treatment or who were under surveillance or continuing care because of disabilities. They proposed that 'a case of leprosy' should be defined as 'a person showing clinical signs of leprosy, with or without bacteriological confirmation of the diagnosis, and requiring chemotherapy', and continued: 'It is recommended that this definition be adopted by all countries so that information on prevalence can be meaningfully interpreted. It is also recommended that separate lists of the other two categories (patients who have completed their treatment but require, or are under, surveillance, and those who have deformities and disabilities due to past leprosy) be maintained.' The increasingly wide adoption of this definition has contributed greatly to improvement in the accuracy of prevalence figures worldwide, while at the same time releasing many thousands of patients from the burden of a potentially stigmatizing diagnosis.

Epidemiology

Estimated prevalence

There have been remarkable changes to the WHO estimate for the number of cases worldwide in recent years. From a previous figure of 11.5 million, the estimate was reduced to 5.5 million in 1991, to 2.4 million in 1995, and is now (late 1996) 1.3 million [2, 3]. These changes are to a large extent due to the progressive implementation of regimens of MDT as advised by WHO in 1982 [4]. Seventy-nine countries now have significant numbers of cases, and the main areas affected are Central and South America, the African continent, South-East Asia (particularly India) and the Far East.

Registered prevalence

From the total of 79 countries mentioned above, the top 25 contribute nearly 95% of all registered cases worldwide and, of these, the top five (India, Brazil, Bangladesh, Indonesia and Myanmar) contribute 82%. India is in a leading class of its own, with 560 000 registered cases and a prevalence rate of 6.1 per 10 000 of the population [3]. It is, however, important to recognize, especially when calculating the number of patients still in need of chemotherapy (see below), that, of the world total of 926 259 cases currently registered, large numbers are still in need of assessment with regard to clinical status and the possible need for chemotherapy. Experience from many leprosy-endemic countries has revealed that large numbers of cases are removed from the registers during the 'screening' process, prior to the implementation of MDT.

New-case detection rate

Worldwide, approximately 560 000 new cases are being detected each year, 456 000 of them in South-East Asia. There was a reduction in the rate in 1993, but this has to be interpreted with caution since fluctuations may occur due to factors which do not reflect the underlying epidemiological situation. These include the intensity of control-programme activities, the enthusiasm and ability of staff, the extension of control services to previously uncovered areas, changes in the criteria for new-case diagnosis and the extent to which active case-finding (contact, school or other sections of the community), as opposed to passive (voluntary) approaches, is used. Currently, there is no consensus view among experts as to whether or not incidence (at least as revealed by the new-case detection rate) is declining, notably in relation to the implementation of MDT. Although there are indications of a decline from some programmes in which MDT has been implemented for 5 years or more, this is as yet by no means a general observation worldwide.

Child rate

Leprosy is rarely reported in infants. Incidence figures usually rise to a peak between 10 and 20 years of age and then fall. The child rate (0–14 years) has previously been considered to be a useful indicator of the likely prevalence of leprosy in the community generally [5], but it is now clear, particularly from observations in India, that this indicator is highly influenced by the quality and intensity of case-detection activities directed at this age-group, including school examinations, and it is now generally regarded to be of limited significance, unless assessed over a period of years during which other conditions have not varied significantly.

Sex ratios

Incidence and prevalence rates are almost universally higher in adult males than in females, the ratio commonly being about 2:1, but in children the ratio is equal [6]. The sex difference in adults is also greater for the lepromatous, compared with the tuberculoid, form of the disease. Whether the difference between figures for males and females is to be regarded as an inherent (biological) feature of leprosy or simply due to differences in lifestyle and the limited facilities available for the examination of women by female staff is unknown — and clearly calls for further investigation.

Genetic factors

Despite a number of studies revealing a genetic influence on the type of leprosy developed, there is no evidence that basic susceptibility to this disease is genetically determined. Twin studies also support a genetic influence on the type of disease developed after infection. The subject has been reviewed in detail by Van Eden and De Vries [7] and by Harboe [8]. The familial nature of leprosy has been known for a long time, but it remains difficult to assess the relevant importance of genetic and other factors in relation to the sequence of events after infection. The extent to which genetic factors operate through immunological mechanisms is discussed by Convit and Ulrich [9]. Although it would seem unlikely that further information on the genetic control of susceptibility will contribute to case-finding and treatment, it might be of considerable value in the selection of subjects for vaccination, if an effective vaccine is forthcoming in the future.

Transmission

Despite the possibility of reservoirs of *M. leprae* in certain animals (nine-banded armadillos and some primates [10]) and in the environment in soil [11] or moss [12], there is no evidence that these sources are of epidemiological importance in the spread of leprosy in humans. The disease is essentially transmitted from untreated patients with the lepromatous form to susceptible hosts, mainly by the shedding of organisms from the nose and upper respiratory tract. Patients with paucibacillary (PB) forms of the disease, including indeterminate, tuberculoid and most borderline-tuberculoid cases, do not excrete bacilli in this way and are not generally regarded as sources of infection. However, the role of individuals with tuberculoid forms as sources of infection is still not entirely clear and

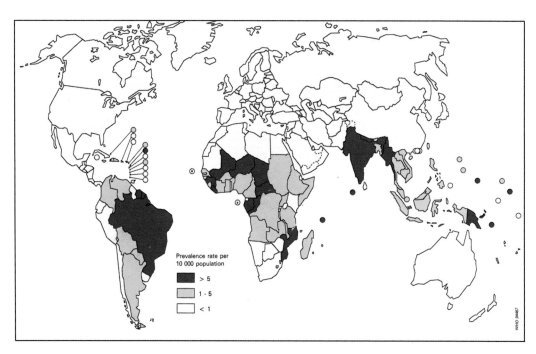

Fig. 9.1 Prevalence of registered leprosy cases in the world as at 1994. The figure of 10 000 population (rather than 1000 as in previous years) relates to the decision of the World Health Assembly in 1991 to set a goal of elimination of leprosy as a public-health problem, reducing the prevalence to below 1 per 10 000 of the population by the year 2000. Currently (late 1996), WHO estimates that there are 1.3 million cases worldwide. Approximately 560 000 new cases are detected yearly, nearly 400 000 of them from India alone. The designations employed and the presentation of the material on this map do not imply the expression of any opinion whatsoever on the part of the secretariat of the World Health Organization concerning the legal status of any country, territory, city or area or of its authorities, or concerning the delimitation of its frontiers or boundaries. Dotted lines on maps represent approximate border lines for which there may not yet be full agreement.

merits further study, if only because they constitute the majority of all cases in most endemic communities. In untreated lepromatous cases, broken skin or ulcerating lesions may lead to spread of organisms into the environment, but this is a relatively uncommon portal of exit. The way in which shed organisms enter a susceptible host is unknown; ingestion in food or drink, inoculation into the skin via scratches, abrasions, wounds, insect bites or inhalation with deposit and entry of organisms in the upper respiratory tract are all possibilities. There is both clinical and experimental evidence to favour the respiratory route as being the most likely portal of entry.

Environmental factors

A glance at the map in Fig. 9.1 may suggest that the present-day distribution of leprosy is somewhat equatorial and it has been suggested that the development and spread of leprosy is favoured by hot and humid climatic conditions. However, leprosy was previously common in countries such as Siberia, North Korea, Scandinavia and other cold regions, and the observed distribution, at least as seen at the present time, is much more likely to be associated with poverty, overcrowding, poor hygiene, illiteracy, poor diet, inadequate water-supplies and deficient general health services. The importance of these factors in favouring the spread and maintaining the endemicity of leprosy is supported by the observation that the problem tends to regress, even in the absence of an organized programme for case detection and chemotherapy, in countries which experience a steady improvement in socioeconomic conditions over a period of decades.

Aetiology

Despite the fact that it is still impossible to grow the leprosy bacillus *in vitro*, there is now overwhelming evidence that the organism identified by Armauer Hansen in 1873 is the cause of leprosy. In 1960, Shepard [13] demonstrated that consistent growth could be achieved in the mouse footpad and, in 1971, Kirchheimer and Storrs [14] showed that the nine-banded armadillo is naturally susceptible to infection with leprosy bacilli of human origin and that it develops a heavy and systemic infection, thus making available vast numbers of organisms for various forms of research. *Mycobacterium leprae* is classified in the order Actinomycetales and is a member of the family Mycobacteriaceae. It is Gram-positive and strongly acid-fast following staining with carbol fuchsine. The latter property is characteristically lost following extraction with pyridine. *Mycobacterium leprae* is typically an obligate intracellular organism, multiplication within the cytoplasm of macrophages and some other host cells producing clumps or 'globi' (Fig. 9.2), some of which may contain several hundred bacilli. It has also been shown by Brennan and Barrow [15] to contain a phenolic

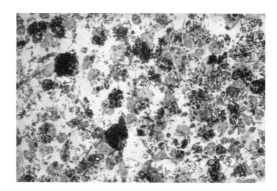

Fig. 9.2 *Mycobacterium leprae*. Nasal mucous smear from a patient with untreated lepromatous leprosy. Modified Ziehl–Neelsen stain. Original magnification × 1200. Bacilli are seen in large clumps or masses ('globi'), also in small groups and singly. Bacilli: red. Nuclei of macrophages: blue.

glycolipid (PGL) which is unique to this organism, and the use of this highly specific antigen in an enzyme-linked immunosorbent assay (ELISA) test has confirmed earlier work, which strongly suggested that *M. leprae* infection, given suitable exposure, is very much more common than is suggested by the number of clinical cases (overt disease).

Clinical manifestations

Although leprosy, particularly in its lepromatous form, may attack a wide range of body systems (with the exception of the brain and spinal cord), its main manifestations in clinical practice are seen in skin and peripheral nerves. The frequent involvement of peripheral and dermal nerves of sensory, motor and/or autonomic type has given rise to the statement that leprosy is essentially a disease of neural origin. While this may well be true and while it is certainly true that damage to nerves is vastly more important than damage to skin, many cases, and probably the majority in practice, present with dermatological rather than neural symptoms and signs. From the point of view of the primary or peripheral health-care worker, their most valuable contribution is the recognition and referral of patients with skin lesions which could be due to leprosy, particularly if there is loss or impairment of sensation. At the referral level, whether it be district hospital, dermatology department or specialized clinic, the important element is a medical or paramedical worker who has sufficient knowledge and clinical experience to recognize leprosy, confirm the diagnosis and classify for the purpose of chemotherapy. It bears emphasis that such expertise can best be obtained by seeing a considerable number of cases of different classification, before, during and after treatment, preferably with the help of an experienced observer. The generally declining prevalence of leprosy in many parts of the world will, in due course, inevitably lead to a reduction in the number of cases, both in the field and in training centres, which are available for teaching and demonstration, and there is already a need to develop strategies, including illustrated teaching material, to aid recognition and diagnosis following the main phase of MDT implementation, when an elimination level has been achieved (less than one case per 10 000 of the population).

The following section refers to a large extent to classification, a subject which has attracted a great deal of interest within the speciality, even before the discovery of the bacillus by Hansen in 1873. The historical development of various systems of classification has been described by Cochrane and Smyly [16], leading up to the Madrid Congress of 1953, which attempted to bring together prevailing viewpoints at that time into one common classification: lepromatous (L), including macular, diffuse, infiltrated, nodular and pure neuritic forms; tuberculoid (T), including macular, major and minor tuberculoid; borderline (B), including infiltrated forms; and indeterminate (I) including macular and pure neuritic forms. This brought a welcome ray of light to what was becoming a confusing and at times almost incomprehensible subject, and the 'Madrid classification' was soon adopted by clinicians and control programmes and used widely. A further advance, and one of far-reaching importance, came with the publication by Ridley and Jopling in 1962 of 'A classification of leprosy for

Table 9.1 Main features of the Ridley–Jopling classification of leprosy (from reference [29]).

| Observation or test | Type of leprosy | | | | |
	TT	BT	BB	BL	LL
Number of lesions	Single usually	Single or few	Several	Many	Very many
Size of lesions	Variable	Variable	Variable	Variable	Small
Surface of lesions	Very dry, sometimes scaly	Dry	Slightly shiny	Shiny	Shiny
Sensation in lesions (not face)	Absent	Moderately–markedly diminished	Slightly–moderately diminished	Slightly diminished	Not affected
Hair growth in lesions	Absent	Markedly diminished	Moderately diminished	Slightly diminished	Not affected
AFB in lesions	Nil	Nil or scanty	Moderate numbers	Many	Very many (plus globi)
AFB in nasal scrapings or in nose blows	Nil	Nil	Nil	Usually nil	Very many (plus globi)
Lepromin test	Strongly positive (+++)	Weakly positive (+ or ++)	Negative	Negative	Negative

TT, tuberculoid; BT, borderline-tuberculoid; BB, mid-borderline; BL, borderline-lepromatous; LL, lepromatous; AFB, acid-fast bacilli.

research purposes' [17], expanded in 1966 by 'Classification of leprosy according to immunity—a five-group system' [18], the main characteristics of which are shown in Table 9.1. Originally intended for research purposes and seen by some as too detailed for use in control programmes, the Ridley–Jopling classification has in fact become increasingly popular through the years and is now often used as a basis for the allocation of cases to either paucibacillary (PB) or multibacillary (MB) regimens of MDT, as recommended by WHO in 1982 [4].

Tuberculoid leprosy

Tuberculoid (TT) leprosy (Fig. 9.3) occurs on the skin as either maculae or well-defined plaques, usually single or few in number. The surface is typically dry, rough, irregular in texture and hypopigmented, coppery or erythematous in colour. Hair growth is lost or impaired, and there is reduction or loss of sensation to light touch, temperature or pain. A thickened peripheral nerve may be palpated in the vicinity of a TT skin lesion, or a thickened cutaneous nerve may be found entering, crossing or leaving the lesion. The low total of combined skin and nerve lesions is an important characteristic of this form of leprosy. Skin smears are negative for *M. leprae* and the lepromin test is invariably strongly positive.

Borderline-tuberculoid leprosy

Borderline-tuberculoid (BT) leprosy has skin lesions that resemble those of TT leprosy but which are: (i) more numerous; (ii) less well-defined at the edges; (iii) often larger, sometimes involving a whole limb or other body area; and (iv) more likely to vary in size, shape or texture within the same patient (Fig. 9.4). The distribution of maculae or plaques tends to be asym-

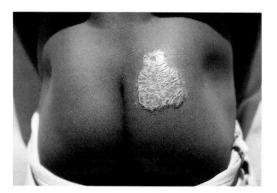

Fig. 9.3 Tuberculoid (TT) leprosy on the buttock of a 14-year-old boy in Zambia. Tuberculoid lesions are single or few in number, well defined, dry or scaly, hairless, non-sweating and show loss or diminution of sensation to pinprick or light touch. Skin smears are negative for *M. leprae* and the lepromin test is strongly positive.

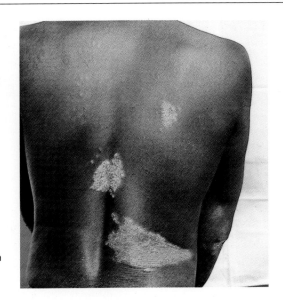

Fig. 9.4 Borderline-tuberculoid (BT) leprosy. Lesions are few in number, asymmetric in distribution. Individually they resemble those of TT leprosy but tend to be less well defined and other TT characteristics, such as loss of sensation and hair growth, are less marked.

metric. Nerves are frequently involved, also asymmetrically; nerve damage in this form of leprosy tends to be severe and includes a propensity to develop reversal (syn. upgrading, type 1) reactions (see below). Sensation in skin lesions is moderately or markedly reduced. Skin smears are either weakly positive or negative. The lepromin test is usually only weakly positive.

Mid-borderline leprosy

Skin lesions in mid-borderline (BB) leprosy show a range of polymorphic forms with a tendency to symmetry, their numbers being greater than in BT and fewer than in borderline-lepromatous (BL) leprosy. Maculae or plaques with curious 'geographical' patterns and 'punched-out' or 'hole-in-cheese' centres are seen, the edges often being poorly defined (Fig. 9.5). Sensation on the lesions may be slightly or moderately diminished. Damage to peripheral nerves is variable, possible because BB leprosy is an unstable form of disease which may represent a 'transition state' from either a BT or BL classification. Deterioration (downgrading) from the BT may be associated with fairly widespread, symmetric involvement of nerves, as described above. Improvement (upgrading) from BL, perhaps as a result of chemotherapy, may be accompanied by a more symmetrical involvement of a larger number of nerves, but without much evidence of damage to sensory or motor elements, unless the situation has been complicated by a reversal (syn. upgrading, type 1) reaction (see below). Skin smears from lesions show moderate numbers of bacilli and the lepromin test is negative.

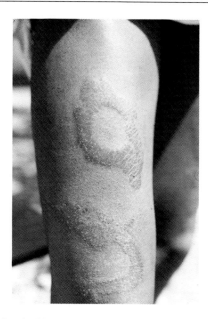

Fig. 9.5 Mid-borderline (BB) leprosy. Several lesions of variable size occur, showing slight or moderate diminution of sensation. The typical 'punched-out' or 'hole-in-cheese' appearance, as seen here, is probably one of the most curious forms of leprosy from a dermatological point of view and has not been fully explained. The finding of moderate numbers of bacilli in lesions and a negative lepromin test account for the inclusion of BB leprosy in the multibacillary (MB) group for the purposes of chemotherapy.

Borderline-lepromatous leprosy

There are many lesions, widely distributed, macular in the early stages, but later developing into papules, nodules and plaques, with a tendency to symmetry. In general, the lesions of BL leprosy tend to show central, rather than peripheral infiltration, with indefinite 'streaming' or 'amoeboid' edges (Fig. 9.6). Peripheral-nerve involvement may be widespread, with a tendency to bilateral symmetry; nerve damage may be marked, especially if there has been reversal (syn. upgrading, type 1) reactions. Although not so common as in lepromatous (LL) leprosy (see below), episodes of erythema nodosum leprosum (ENL) may occur in patients with BL leprosy.

Lepromatous leprosy

This is a generalized, systemic disease with a continuous bacteraemia, in which bacilli may be found in a wide range of tissues, including skin, nerves, nose, eyes, kidneys, liver, spleen, lymph nodes and bone marrow. The early lesions consist of widespread numerous maculae, symmetrically distributed over the skin surface, with subtle alterations of skin texture but often minimal disturbance of pigmentation. These can be difficult to see and can be missed in their early stages, even by experienced observers, unless the whole body surface is examined in a good light—oblique illumination from sunlight being vastly better than artificial light for this purpose. As LL leprosy progresses, these maculae tend to coalesce and involve all parts of the body except the so-called 'immune areas'—axillae, groins, perineum, midline of the back and scalp.

Papules and nodules may be of normal skin colour, erythematous or coppery, and they are intradermal, not subdermal, on palpation. The fully developed nodular picture particularly affects the face, ears and limbs and is often accompanied by broadening of the nose, loss of eyebrows ('madarosis') and general thickening of the facial skin, with deepening of the furrows, producing a 'leonine' appearance (Fig. 9.7). In the still more advanced stages (much less commonly seen nowadays), the voice becomes hoarse due to laryngeal involvement, upper incisor teeth loosen and may fall out, the nasal bridge collapses and, in the male, there may be testicular atrophy and gynaecomastia. Despite the traditional emphasis given to loss of sensation in skin lesions as one of the cardinal signs of leprosy, it is important to note that neither the early stages nor the later nodules of LL leprosy typically show this change. Particularly in those parts of the world where LL leprosy forms a high percentage of all cases (Mexico, Central and South America), the diagnosis of LL leprosy, especially in the early stages, must lean heavily on clinical appearances and the use of multiple-site slit-skin smears, examined in a reliable laboratory. Peripheral nerves harbour many bacilli, but evidence of change to sensory or motor elements is not typically found in the early stages of this form of leprosy, mainly because of

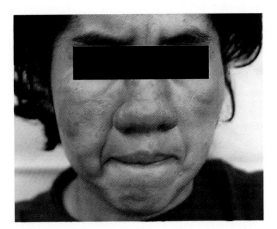

Fig. 9.6 Borderline-lepromatous (BL) leprosy. There are many lesions with 'streaming' or 'amoeboid' edges and they tend to be high in the middle, sloping to a lower level at the periphery, in contrast to those of tuberculoid leprosy in which the centre of the lesions may be flattened and the edge raised. There is a tendency towards bilateral symmetry and there are many bacilli in lesions, though not invariably in the intervening normal skin.

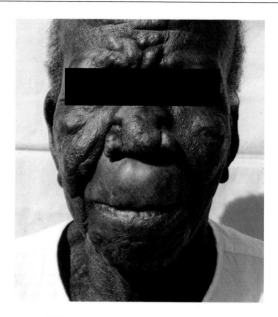

Fig. 9.7 Lepromatous (LL) leprosy. There are numerous lesions, bilaterally symmetrical, manifesting as maculae papules or nodules, according to the stage of development. This patient shows fully developed, nodular leprosy with heavy involvement of the face and ears. There was nasal blockage and a complaint of epistaxis. All lesions in every part of the body are strongly positive for *M. leprae* and the lepromin test is invariably negative.

the absence of a CMI response. In the later stages, however, clinical examination may reveal symmetric enlargement of many nerves, with sensory and motor deficit in their area of supply. At a variable point in the development of LL leprosy, it is possible to demonstrate an interesting and unusual form of sensory loss in the upper and lower limbs peculiar to LL leprosy, in which there is a 'glove-and-stocking' anaesthesia closely related to areas of skin with relatively low temperature.

Clinically, it is not uncommon for patients to remain virtually symptom-free until the later stages of LL leprosy, when clinical signs may be obvious; or to report first to a special department with symptoms affecting parts of the body other than skin or nerves, including eyes, nose, testes or joints. Skin smears, taken either from lesions or from routine sites, are strongly positive and the lepromin test is invariably negative.

Indeterminate leprosy

Although included in other classifications. I leprosy does not appear in the five-group Ridley–Jopling system, mainly because it is not a 'determined' form of leprosy. Its definition and criteria for diagnosis have created considerable argument among experts for several decades, but it is now generally recognized as an early form of leprosy, with one or a few maculae on the skin, hypopigmented, coppery or erythematous in colour, and with edges which are either hazy or clear-cut (Fig. 9.8). If multiple, the distribution is asymmetric. Opinions differ from one country to another on the most common sites; the frequent observation that I lesions are most often seen on the face or on a limb may reflect the ease with which these areas are examined, especially in countries where female workers are not available for the thorough inspection of the skin surface in female patients. Slight anaesthesia may be demonstrated, but it is usually absent. Because it is so well innervated, it is notoriously difficult to demonstrate loss of sensation in suspected lesions on the face. Skin smears are negative and the result of the lepromin test unpredictable, but usually negative. In some cases, a thickened nerve may be palpable in the vicinity of an I lesion. Biopsy of a skin lesion, especially if of sufficient depth and if many well-stained sections are examined by an expert, may reveal a single bacillus in a lower or subdermal nerve, but this is unusual; in most cases, the histopathological findings are non-specific and unhelpful. Furthermore, the routine use of biopsies in this context, especially in control programmes, is likely to be unpopular, especially for suspected lesions on the face and in female patients.

From the above description, it will readily be seen that this form of the

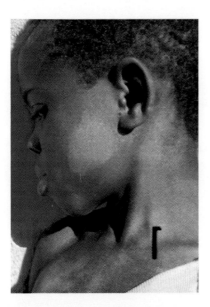

Fig. 9.8 Indeterminate (I) leprosy. There are typically one or a few maculae (any lesion which is infiltrated and raised above the surface of the surrounding normal skin is not to be included in this classification), hypopigmented, coppery (as here) or erythematous in colour and with edges which are either hazy or clear-cut. Slight loss of sensation may be demonstrated, but sensation is usually normal. Skin smears are almost invariably normal and biopsy is often undiagnostic. Despite the difficulties of testing for loss or diminution of sensation on the face, and of obtaining conclusive replies, especially in children, I leprosy should not be diagnosed unless the lesions show loss or diminution of sensation.

disease presents a considerable problem with regard to over- and wrong diagnosis. Especially for control-programme purposes, it is now strongly recommended, for instance in India (currently reporting nearly 400 000 new cases yearly), that the diagnosis of leprosy should not be made in suspect cases unless definite loss or impairment of sensation has been demonstrated. It is advised in India that suspect cases are to be entered in a 'suspect register' and re-examined at 3-, 4- or 6-monthly intervals — a policy that could well be adopted elsewhere, in view of the importance of avoiding misdiagnosis in a disease that still attracts considerable social stigma.

Histoid leprosy

This interesting form of leprosy (Fig. 9.9) consists of firm, erythematous

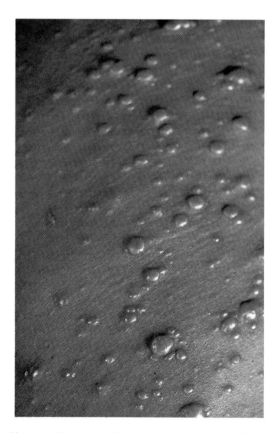

Fig. 9.9 Histoid leprosy. This unusual form of leprosy consists of firm, erythematous nodules, round or oval in shape, which arise in lepromatous patients who are relapsing either because they have stopped treatment or because they have become dapsone-resistant. Although occasional cases may present with histoid leprosy at the outset, before treatment, the link between histoid lesions and dapsone resistance is well established. (With acknowledgements to Dr T. Fajardo, Leonard Wood Memorial, Cebu City, The Philippines.)

nodules, round or oval in shape, which arise in lepromatous patients who are relapsing, either because they have stopped treatment or because they have become drug-resistant. The association of such nodules, occurring in unusual body sites, such as the surface of the eye, midline of the chin or antecubital fossa, is well established clinically as an indication of the development of bacillary resistance to *M. leprae*. The differential diagnosis includes cutaneous leishmaniasis and many other dermatologically nodular conditions. The histological appearances in routine sections stained with haematoxylin and eosin have often been reported as dermato-fibroma, because of the predominant spindle-shaped cells—a reminder of the importance of performing a suitable stain for acid-fast bacilli in sections [19], which in the case of histoid leprosy will reveal very large numbers of *M. leprae*. Skin smears from histoid nodules are also highly positive.

Pure neural leprosy

A form of leprosy with one or more enlarged peripheral nerves, but without any evidence, on total body-area inspection, of past or present skin lesions, is well described in India and occurs less frequently in other parts of the world. It is, however, important to note that the diagnosis of this form of leprosy calls for expert assessment; it is not uncommon for this label to be applied to cases who have in fact had skin lesions in the past but they are no longer visible at the time of presentation, sometimes because of treatment. Skin smears should be taken from routine sites, but they are almost invariably negative. A nerve biopsy may be necessary in order to establish the diagnosis of leprosy and to exclude the other (rare) causes of peripheral-nerve thickening, but this should be undertaken only by an experienced operator, taking a shallow segment of nerve and selecting sensory nerves only, not those carrying motor or combined sensory and motor fibres. Classification of pure neural cases, especially if nerve biopsy is not feasible, may be difficult, but a lepromin test is of considerable value, being strongly positive in TT, weakly positive in BT and negative in BB, BL and LL, as already indicated in Table 9.1. If in doubt, it is usually wise to offer pure neural cases the benefit of 2 years' treatment with the three-drug MB regimen advised by WHO [4].

Lucio leprosy

This is a diffuse, non-nodular form of LL leprosy, which occurs mainly (some say exclusively) in the American continent, notably in Mexico. There is a diffuse infiltration of the face and trunk, with loss of body hair, including eyebrows and eyelashes (but not scalp hair). Additional features, such as laryngeal involvement, oedematous legs and anaemia, may strongly support myxoedema, but an examination of skin smears will reveal large numbers of bacilli from all routine sites. These patients are prone to develop a peculiar form of immunological reaction, known as

Lucio's phenomenon, seen only in untreated patients, characterized by painful, tender, red patches on the skin, some with jagged edges, with a tendency to become purpuric.

Leprosy and tuberculosis

The two conditions not infrequently coexist (Fig. 9.10) and it is possible that this association will increase with the continuing rise in tuberculosis rates worldwide, much of it associated with human immunodeficiency virus (HIV) coinfection [20] and occurring in countries where leprosy is endemic. The important practical point is to appreciate that the drugs used for the treatment of leprosy, including the three-drug regimen for MB patients, is inadequate for the treatment of tuberculosis. Antituberculosis drugs must be given according to the patient's category and continued for the recommended periods [21], in addition to MDT for leprosy. At present, only rifampicin is common to the two regimens and it must be given in the doses indicated for tuberculosis. It is thus possible that a patient with combined tuberculosis and leprosy will be taking six or possibly seven drugs, several of which require careful observation and supervision on account of

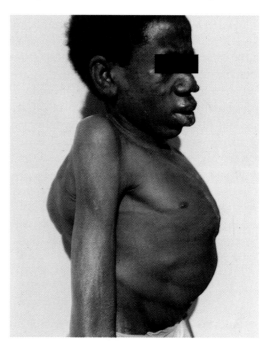

Fig. 9.10 Coexistent leprosy and tuberculosis. This patient has active lepromatous leprosy with nodules on the ears and face, together with active tuberculosis of the spine with a gibbus (vertebral body collapse). Even the three-drug regimen used for MB leprosy is not adequate for the treatment of tuberculosis, the only drug common to the treatment of both diseases being rifampicin. Effective treatment calls for the simultaneous administration of drugs for both diseases, together with expert clinical management and, preferably, a period of admission to hospital.

toxicity. Whether under control-programme or other conditions, the management of such patients clearly calls for considerable ability and experience and often for admission to a special unit or hospital.

Leprosy and HIV infection/AIDS

Human immunodeficiency virus infection has already been shown to be strongly linked to the development of active tuberculosis, and many countries where both diseases are prevalent have already seen a significant increase in both pulmonary and extrapulmonary disease [20]. Although a few cases of coexistent leprosy and HIV/AIDS have been reported in the literature, as also an association between the two diseases in a hospital-based study from Zambia [22], this has not been confirmed in other countries in Africa and no significant association was reported in a detailed community-based study from Malawi [23]. However, a recent publication based on patients in Tanzania [24] found that HIV infection was significantly associated with MB but not PB leprosy and the authors concluded that HIV is indeed a risk factor for leprosy. The subject of HIV/AIDS and mycobacterial infections was reviewed in detail by Nunn and McAdam in 1988 [25] and by Miller in 1991 [26]. Despite the above reports, and keeping in mind the need to continually monitor clinical and epidemiological trends, it has to be concluded that leprosy is, so far, remarkably fortunate in that the extremely adverse effect of HIV infection on the course of tuberculosis has not been observed.

Leprosy and pregnancy

The potentially adverse effects of pregnancy and the puerperium on leprosy have been well recognized for many years, but it is only recently that the subject has been extensively studied, mainly by Elizabeth Duncan and her colleagues in Ethiopia [27, 28]. They have described the appearance of new lesions during pregnancy, also relapse in apparently 'cured' patients and a tendency to downgrading of clinical and immune status, with emphasis on: (i) clinical deterioration, especially in the third trimester; (ii) type 1 reaction, especially during the first 6 months of lactation, probably related to the regaining of CMI suppression during pregnancy; and (iii) type 2 reaction, particularly in the third trimester and the first 6 months of lactation. They have also described the occurrence of insidious 'silent' neuritis in a considerable number of patients during pregnancy. Babies born to mothers with leprosy weighed less than those of healthy mothers and grew more slowly.

Adverse immunological reactions

Apart from the basic clinical forms of leprosy described above, it has to be recognized that the varied manifestations of this disease include several types of adverse immunological reaction, based on ether cell-mediated or immune-complex mechanisms, often calling for skilled clinical management. Although there is some overlap, reactions due to CMI factors tend to occur mainly in non-LL forms of leprosy, while those due to immune complexes and involving humoral immunity (HI) occur in LL and, to a lesser extent, in BL forms. The terminology of reactions in leprosy has been confusing through the years, no doubt mainly due to our somewhat limited knowledge of their pathogenesis. In 1959, Jopling [29] proposed the terms type 1 and type 2 for the two major types of reaction occurring in clinical practice. Type 1 covers those called 'upgrading' (syn. reversal) and 'downgrading' and type 2 those called 'lepromatous' or ENL [30].

Type 1 reaction

The type 1 reaction (Fig. 9.11) is a delayed-type hypersensitivity (DTH) reaction corresponding to Coombs and Gell type IV hypersensitivity reaction. It does not occur in TT and is unusual in LL leprosy, being most

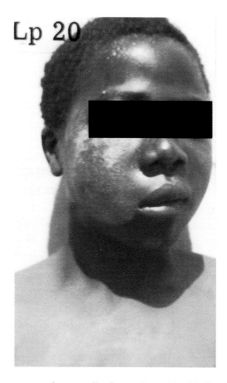

Fig. 9.11 Type 1 (syn. reversal, upgrading) reaction. This child had borderline-tuberculoid (BT) leprosy, with asymmetrically distributed skin and nerve lesions to other parts of the body. Three months after starting dapsone monotherapy, he developed a reaction in a plaque on the right side of the face, with swelling, redness, pain and tenderness, accompanied by paralysis of the facial nerve. Both elements responded well to treatment with (oral) prednisolone.

common in BT, BB or BL patients. If the reaction occurs in the absence of treatment and with a reduction in the patient's immune status, it is called 'downgrading', in contrast to that form of type 1 reaction called 'upgrading' (syn. reversal), which is associated with a rapid increase in CMI and usually occurs during the first 6 months of treatment in BT and BB, but after longer intervals in BL patients. Downgrading reactions have not been well documented, possibly because they are said to occur in patients who are not on treatment and are therefore less well observed than those who are on treatment, and it is perhaps for this reason that the term type 1 is often used to refer only to 'upgrading' (syn. reversal) reactions. From a practical point of view, this is certainly the most frequently occurring and important form of type 1 reaction. Clinically, there are rapidly developing changes in some or all skin lesions, which become red, more raised, shiny, warm and occasionally necrotic. New skin lesions may develop. In contrast to type 2 reactions, systemic features, such as fever and malaise, are unusual. A curious (and unexplained) manifestation is oedema of the face, hands or feet (rarely of one hand or foot), which is not associated with reactional changes in a lesion or lesions at these sites. Even more important than the above skin changes are those which commonly occur in peripheral nerves, which may rapidly become swollen, painful and tender. Intraneural oedema and cellular infiltration may rapidly lead to damage to sensory and/or motor axons, with resultant loss of sensation and/or paralysis, unless treatment (see below) is instituted promptly. Type 1 reversal reaction is an extremely important cause of nerve damage and disability in leprosy. Although long recognized, remarkably little is known about its natural history, and a recent publication by Lienhardt and Fine [31], reviewing the epidemiological situation with regard to type 1 reaction, neuritis and disability, included the statement that 'we still lack the means to predict reactions confidently enough to prevent them'. Risk factors listed through the years include BCG vaccination, pregnancy, puerperium, antileprosy chemotherapy, intercurrent infection, trauma and psychological stress.

The clinical manifestations of reversal reaction are often difficult to distinguish from those of relapse, a matter of concern because of their totally different significance and management. Specialized texts should be consulted for details, but some of the most important points of difference are listed in Table 9.2.

Type 2 reaction

This is an immune-complex syndrome, involving antigen, antibody and complement. The underlying mechanism is thus HI; there is no alteration in CMI. Type 2 leprosy reaction corresponds to type III hypersensitivity reaction (Coombs and Gell). It occurs typically in LL and less frequently in BL patients. In contrast to type 1, there is no clinical change in existing lesions. The term ENL, frequently used to describe this reaction, refers to the characteristic crops of erythematous nodules or plaques, mainly

Table 9.2 Differences between reversal reaction and relapse (reproduced, by permission of WHO, from: *A Guide to Leprosy Control*, 2nd edn. World Health Organization, Geneva, 1988).

Feature	Reversal reaction	Relapse
Time interval	Generally occurs during chemotherapy or within 6 months of stopping treatment	Usually occurs long after chemotherapy is discontinued, generally after an interval of 1 year
Onset	Abrupt and sudden	Slow and insidious
Systemic disturbances	May be accompanied by fever and malaise	Never accompanied by fever and malaise
Old lesions	Some or all become erythematous, shiny and considerably swollen, with infiltration	The margins of some may show erythema
New lesions	Usually several	Few
Ulceration	Lesions often break down and ulcerate	Ulceration is unusual
Subsidence	With desquamation	Desquamation does not occur
Nerve involvement	Many nerves may be involved, with pain, tenderness and motor disturbances occurring rapidly	May occur only in a single nerve; motor disturbances develop very slowly
Response to steroids	Excellent	Not distinctive

small, lasting 2–3 days and then regressing (Fig. 9.12). The distribution tends to be bilateral and symmetrical; in contrast to erythema nodosum of other causes, the lesions appear on face, arms and legs, but may be seen on almost any part of the body, with the exception of the warmer areas (scalp, axillae, groins, perineum). Erythema nodosum leprosum lesions are warm and tender on pressure; on fading, they leave a dusky-blue stain on the skin.

In many cases, type 2 reaction is accompanied by fever, malaise, leuco-cytosis, raised erythrocyte sedimentation rate (ESR), albuminuria and anaemia, and a wide range of body systems may be affected, giving rise to neuritis, iritis, epididymo-orchitis, bone pain, arthritis, lymphadenitis and epistaxis. Sometimes the skin lesions may become pustular or ulcerate. Again in contrast to type 1, type 2 reactions are uncommon during the first 6 months of treatment; they tend to occur considerably later during the course of treatment, when the original lesions are quiescent and bacilli in smears or biopsies are all granular or fragmented. Furthermore, type 2 reactions, at least in the past, have tended to be recurrent over a long period of time and, in some cases, unresponsive to treatment. It is encouraging to note that the increasingly wide implementation of MDT has not, as feared by some experts at the outset, produced an increase in type 2 (or type 1) reactions and that in recent years there has in fact been a notable reduction

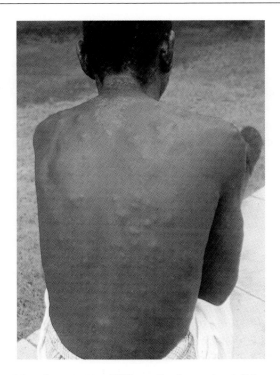

Fig. 9.12 Type 2 (syn. lepromatous, ENL) reaction in a male adult 3 years after initial diagnosis and the start of treatment. Extensive lesions of erythema nodosum leprosum (ENL) are shown on the back. They are typically red, raised nodules or small plaques, with a tendency to bilateral symmetrical distribution. They are often tender and warmer than surrounding skin. In contrast to the erythema nodosum associated with tuberculosis, sarcoidosis or rheumatism, their distribution may be widespread, with heavy involvement of face, flexor aspects of the forearms and medial aspects of the thighs. This patient had fever, weight loss, malaise and joint pain—all evidence of the systemic nature of this form of reaction. (With acknowledgements to the German Leprosy Relief Association, Würzburg, Germany.)

in the number of type 2 reactions, both in the field and in hospital practice. Whether this is due to generally improved standards of diagnosis and treatment or to the inclusion of clofazimine (which has not only chemotherapeutic but also anti-inflammatory and immunomodulatory properties) in the three-drug regimen for the treatment of MB cases is not clear.

The above brief description may be adequate to indicate that this form of reaction may involve many body systems and is potentially damaging to the nerves, kidneys, eyes and other organs. While mild ENL may in some cases be treated in the field, more severe or recurrent cases should be admitted to hospital for investigation and treatment, especially if eyes, nerves, joints or testicles are involved. To the above list of risk or precipitating factors given for type 1 reaction may be added a strongly positive Mantoux test and the ingestion of potassium iodide.

In summary, the two main types of adverse immunological reaction described above continue to account for a major part of the overall morbidity of this disease. In particular, type 1 reversal reactions are a major cause of nerve damage, leading to disability and deformity. It is a matter of concern that there has been little progress in recent years in our knowledge of the immunological processes involved and of the risk or precipitating factors. In addition, there is a need for antireaction drugs that are safer and more suitable for use under field conditions than those currently available.

Diagnosis

It is traditionally advised that the diagnosis of leprosy should only be made if one or more of the following 'cardinal signs' are present: (i) skin lesions of a type characteristic of leprosy, with diminution or loss of sensation; (ii) enlarged peripheral nerves in typical situations; and (iii) the finding of *M. leprae*, usually in skin smears, less commonly in other sites. However, each of these findings calls for qualification if over- or wrong diagnosis is to be avoided. Single lesions due to leprosy and those forms of the disease towards the TT end of the spectrum almost invariably show diminution or loss of sensation. However, in forms of the disease near the LL pole, this does not apply. In LL leprosy, the early maculae do not show loss of sensation (although there may be diminished sweating due to autonomic-nerve involvement), and it is only in the later stages that definite sensory loss develops, including that due to fibrosis in peripheral nerves and a unique pattern of sensory loss in relatively low-temperature areas of skin, which, if carefully established, is virtually diagnostic. The diagnosis of LL leprosy at an early stage will thus lean heavily on: (i) a high level of clinical suspicion; and (ii) the taking of slit-skin smears and their examination by a reliable technician or doctor.

The finding of an enlarged peripheral nerve or nerves, either in a leprosy-endemic country or in a patient presenting from such a country, may well point strongly to a diagnosis of leprosy, but, if this is the only sign and there are absolutely no skin lesions, the case should be referred to an experienced observer for careful assessment. Pure neural leprosy (see above) is not a common condition and may call for consideration, preferably by a neurologist, of some of the rarer conditions causing enlargement of peripheral nerves. It has also to be acknowledged that the examination of peripheral nerves in leprosy, including a careful comparison between the findings on the right and left side of the body, is not a skill that can be acquired quickly and easily; doubtful cases should certainly be referred for an expert opinion.

The finding of *M. leprae* in smears, provided that attention has been paid to the selection of sites, taking of smears, fixation, labelling, staining and interpretation by trained and reliable, staff may indeed be diagnostic in some cases. However, as an isolated finding, without any clinical evidence of leprosy, a positive report of *M. leprae* in the skin at one or more sites should be interpreted with considerable caution, particularly if there is any doubt about the reliability of the technical steps involved [32]. Doubtful cases, including those in whom the bacteriological and clinical findings are incompatible, should certainly be referred for further assessment.

Provided the above cardinal signs are carefully established and interpreted with care, they are nevertheless valuable as a basis for diagnosis, but in more general terms it may be said that a high level of clinical suspicion, notably for any skin or nerve lesion which is atypical and which occurs in an endemic country or in a patient from an endemic country, is equally important. Early forms of leprosy may be difficult to diagnose with confidence, but most of the established forms are relatively easy to distinguish from other dermatological and neurological conditions. Cases that give rise to difficulty, even for the experienced observer, include those with early macular lesions, especially on the face, where loss or diminution of sensation is not easy to demonstrate, as also early LL leprosy with either smooth, diffuse infiltration or faint maculae and minimal changes in skin texture, which are easily missed unless the patient is examined in good light. It also has to be kept in mind that by no means all patients admit previous treatment and that this may considerably modify the typical clinical findings in various forms of leprosy, particularly if highly effective bactericidal drugs have been used.

Special tests and procedures

Slit-skin smears

It has, for a number of years, been generally recommended that slit-skin smears should be taken from lesions and/or a number of 'routine sites' (ears, the back of each forearm, the front of each thigh, just above the knee) and the finding of acid-fast bacilli has been included, as described above, as one of the cardinal signs of leprosy. While the value of smears for certain specific purposes remains undisputed, a number of reservations, particularly about their routine use in control programmes, have now to be recorded.

1 Experience through the years, especially under field conditions, has indicated that there are often serious defects in the quality and supervision of laboratory work for this purpose and it has been suggested that the continued use of unreliable peripheral units and personnel should be either curtailed or abandoned in favour of the retention of a few high-quality central units [32]. Unreliable smear examination are not only useless, but potentially misleading, especially to health staff with limited clinical experience.

2 Current WHO advice [33] is that smear services should be retained as part of the strategy of leprosy control and clinical work, but that their existence should not be a prerequisite for the implementation of MDT.

3 The WHO definition of 'a case of leprosy' [1] (see above, under 'Definition') specifically states that the definition can be established 'with or without bacteriological confirmation of the diagnosis.'

4 The WHO further advises that, in view of the known and, in some situations, increasing risks of any skin-piercing procedures in the spreading of hepatitis B virus or HIV, the number of skin smears taken in leprosy work should be reduced to the minimum [34].

For details of technique and laboratory procedures, specialized texts should be consulted [30, 35, 36].

Biopsies

Skin biopsy of a typical lesion may be helpful in confirming the diagnosis and classification and in the interpretation and management of adverse immunological reactions. Biopsies are essential in most research studies concerned with chemotherapy or vaccines, in which precise diagnosis and classification at the outset are essential, but they are neither essential nor advisable in routine leprosy-control programmes, where they may in fact prove counterproductive, due to their unpopularity, particularly with women and children. Technical aspects and interpretation of skin biopsies have been described in detail by Ridley [19]. Nerve biopsies may rarely be indicated, either for the investigation of suspected cases of pure neural leprosy or for nerve enlargement, suspicious for leprosy but possibly due to some other (rare) cause. Only sensory nerves should be biopsied, not mixed or motor nerves, and the procedure should be carried out by a neurosurgeon or a qualified doctor with appropriate training. As with skin biopsies, an essential prerequisite is that there should be available someone with the ability and experience to ensure that the material is properly processed, including techniques for the demonstration of *M. leprae* in sections, and then carry out the necessary histopathological examination.

Lepromin test

This involves the intradermal injection of a small quantity of an autoclaved preparation of lepromatous tissue, standardized with regard to its content of killed *M. leprae*. It is not (as often supposed) a diagnostic test for leprosy, but it is of value, in some situations, for the more accurate classification of patients, once the diagnosis has been made. It is typically negative in LL and BL cases, usually negative in BB cases and positive in TT and BT cases. In I leprosy, the results are variable but usually negative or weakly positive. The use of this test may be appropriate in dealing with small numbers of patients in well-equipped centres or for research purposes, but it has no application in control-programme situations.

Pilocarpine and histamine tests

Pilocarpine has been used in the past to test the integrity of sweating in a patch suspected to be due to leprosy, in which the parasympathetic fibres may be damaged, and an intradermal injection of histamine chlorohydrate or phosphate may be used to elicit the histamine flare. Specialized texts should be consulted for further details of technique and interpretation [30]. Most clinical leprologists have abandoned the use of these tests on the grounds that they are impractical under most circumstances and even likely to be misleading.

Polymerase chain reaction

The polymerase chain reaction (PCR) is a powerful tool for the amplification of specific sequences of deoxyribonucleic acid (DNA). Deoxyribonucleic acid hybridization of these products permits the detection of incredibly small quantities of the original DNA, and preliminary reports suggest that this procedure will provide an exceptionally sensitive and specific method for the detection of very small numbers of *M. leprae* in biological samples. The advantages, disadvantages and potential research applications for *M. leprae* detection and disease control have been reviewed by WHO experts in relation to problems in the early diagnosis of leprosy [37]. Future applications may include the diagnosis of early leprosy, the detection of very small numbers of persisting bacilli after treatment and epidemiological studies related to infection rates and subclinical infection. An interesting epidemiological study of leprosy infection, in two adjacent villages of southern Sulawesi, Indonesia, which includes the use of PCR in the examination of nasal swabs, has recently been published [38], indicating that *M. leprae* was widespread in the population and suggesting that, in endemic areas, many individuals may carry *M. leprae* in their nasal cavities without having obvious symptoms of leprosy.

Phenolic glycolipid

In 1980, Brennan and Barrow described a species-specific antigen in *M. leprae*, PGL-1 [15], giving rise to the possibility that it would be valuable in cases of suspected leprosy and subclinical infection and as an indicator of the likely outcome in individuals already infected. Unfortunately, these hopes have not been realized. This is partly because the diagnosis of leprosy can be established in most cases, with a considerable degree of certainty, by clinical examination alone, with or without skin smears or biopsy, but also because of its lack of sensitivity and specificity. It has about 30% sensitivity (70% false negatives) for PB leprosy, thus limiting its usefulness in the early stages of this form of leprosy, in which diagnosis can be difficult. It has a specificity of 98% and thus 2% false negatives, so that, even in a population of 1000 with a prevalence rate as high as 1%, a PGL-1 test would identify only three out of 10 leprosy cases, while at the same time incorrectly identifying no fewer than 20 people without leprosy as being affected [39].

In summary, the diagnosis of leprosy, not only in control programmes under field conditions but also in situations where smaller numbers of patients are seen with readily available laboratory and other facilities for investigation, still relies heavily on clinical expertise. Many leprologists consider that the development of tests based on either serological or immunological findings has been disappointing in recent years. Despite their continuing potential and research interest, it does indeed seem evident that none has so far attained the level of sensitivity and specificity needed for practical application, particularly in control programmes. Meanwhile, diagnosis (and classification) relies heavily on a high level of clinical suspicion, careful examination of the whole body surface in a good light, palpation of peripheral nerves and careful testing for loss or diminution of sensation.

Differential diagnosis

The number of dermatological, neural or other system diseases which can be confused with leprosy is very considerable, but, if attention is given to those which occur or do not occur in various leprosy-endemic countries or regions, the list may be greatly reduced. It is also helpful to group the dermatological conditions according to the main type of lesion (maculae, nodule, etc.) and the presence or absence of pigmentation and the neural conditions with regard to the occurrence of sensory or motor (or combined) disturbance and whether or not peripheral nerves are palpably thickened. Dermatological conditions that have been confused with leprosy include the following: morphoea, vitiligo, yaws, onchocerciasis, pityriasis alba, pityriasis versicolor, post-kala-azar dermal leishmaniasis, fungal infections, sebhorrhoeic dermatitis, nutritional dyschromia (all macular), ringworm, granuloma annulare, granuloma multiforme (Mkar disease), gyrate erythemas, Wegener's granulomatosis, tinea corporis, acquired syphilis, sarcoidosis, tuberculosis, lupus erythematosus, cutaneous leishmaniasis, neurofibromatosis, necrobiosis lipoidica, atypical necrobiosis of the face, mycosis fungoides, Kaposi's sarcoma and infection with *Mycobacterium marinum*. This somewhat lengthy list of dermatological conditions should not present a problem to anyone with dermatological training, and the chances of misdiagnosis by those without such specialized knowledge would be reduced by careful testing for loss or diminution of sensation. Although some loss of sensation has been described in the lesions of necrobiosis lipoidica [40], psoriasis, morphoea and vitiligo [41], definite loss of sensation is remarkably rare in dermatological conditions other than leprosy.

Neurological conditions causing confusion are less common and several are also rare in the field of neurology. They include: peroneal muscular atrophy (Charcot–Marie–Tooth disease). Déjerine–Sottas disease (familial hypertrophic interstitial neuritis), amyloidosis, syringomelia, tabes dorsalis, sensory radicular neuropathy, congenital indifference to pain and peripheral neuropathies of varied aetiology. Clearly, the finding of loss of sensation or muscle power in association with palpably enlarged peripheral nerve(s) is a potential source of confusion, but such cases are rare and, in general, it can be stated that any patient in a leprosy-endemic area who presents with definite peripheral-nerve enlargement should be regarded as having leprosy until proved otherwise.

Finally, neither the dermatological nor the neural conditions described above take account of a number of mundane and commonly occurring conditions that may relate to local practices or lifestyle, which may also cause confusion. These include scars, wounds, postinflammatory dyschromia and deformity following trauma or fractures. Attention to local lifestyle, skin colouring and established pattern or tropical and dermatological disease is essential if diagnostic mistakes are to be avoided.

Treatment

Chemotherapy of the bacterial infection

Dapsone (diaminodiphenylsulphone (DDS)) first became available in the 1940s and was soon used extensively for the treatment of all forms of leprosy in regimens of varying duration, as a single drug (monotherapy). It was successful in the arrest or cure of many hundreds of thousands of patients during the next few decades in all leprosy-endemic countries worldwide, but in the 1970s and 1980s it became increasingly apparent that dapsone resistance was developing on an alarming scale and likely to undermine the whole basis of leprosy control. The long periods of treatment needed for LL and some borderline cases, together with the poor level of development of many national control programmes and the shortage of trained staff, all contributed to the failure of dapsone to achieve a significant level of control, including reduction in transmission. Although not difficult to assess in retrospect, it is possible that this was due as much to operational factors, including the use of dapsone in low doses or irregularly, as to inherent defects in dapsone as an antileprosy drug. It has also to be recognized that dapsone contributed significantly to the decline of prevalence and incidence in many leprosy-endemic countries, before the advent of MDT. However, the potential threat of dapsone resistance to the strategy of leprosy control was rightly judged to be of great importance. In 1981 WHO convened a meeting of experts to consider the best possible use of the available antileprosy drugs, and in 1982 published its recommendations for regimens of MDT for all cases, consisting of three drugs (dapsone, rifampicin and clofazimine) for MB cases and two drugs (dapsone and rifampicin) for PB cases [4] (see Fig. 9.13). It recommended that MB cases should be treated for a minimum of 2 years, but whenever possible until skin smears had become negative, but this has recently been modified to a fixed treatment of 2 years, in view of the accumulating evidence that this period is highly satisfactory for control-programme purposes. A period of 6 months' treatment was recommended in PB cases, treatment then being stopped. The details of these regimens are shown in Table 9.3.

From a control-programme point of view, these regimens have proved outstandingly successful. From the outset, they proved acceptable and popular with health staff, patients, voluntary agencies and ministries of health: not unreasonably expensive, clinically effective and not accompanied by unacceptable levels of toxicity or reactions due to adverse immunological reactions, based on either cell-mediated or immune-complex mechanisms. After a somewhat hesitant start, MDT has been steadily implemented in virtually all countries, worldwide, where leprosy is endemic, resulting in highly significant reductions in prevalence rates, prevention of disability and — at least in those programmes where MDT has been steadily used for a period of 5 years or more — early indications of reductions in incidence as measured by new-case detection rates. The out-

Table 9.3 Multiple drug therapy (MDT) regimens for pauci- and multibacillary leprosy as recommended by WHO in 1982 [4]. Adult doses.

Group	Regimen	Duration	Compliance	Cost
Multibacillary (MB)	*Monthly, supervised* Rifampicin 600 mg Clofazimine 300 mg Dapsone 100 mg *Daily, unsupervised* Clofazimine 50 mg Dapsone 100 mg	Originally (1982) advised for a period of at least 2 years and to be continued, wherever possible, up to smear negativity. However, in view of the highly successful results, including very low relapse rates (for both PB and MB regimens), a WHO Study Group on the Chemotherapy of Leprosy has recently (1994) advised a fixed period of 2 years only	Preferably 24 doses in 24 months, but if this is not possible, 24 doses within a period of 36 months is acceptable	Difficult to assess in view of varying operational conditions, but a figure of US$100 per patient (PB and MB combined) may be a fair estimate. On average about 40% of this will be needed for drugs, the remainder for staff training, implementation, transport education of patients and the public, etc.
Paucibacillary (PB)	*Monthly, supervised* Rifampicin 600 mg Dapsone 100 mg *Daily, unsupervised* Dapsone 100 mg	6 months	Preferably six doses in 6 months, but if this is not possible, six doses within a period of 9 months is acceptable	

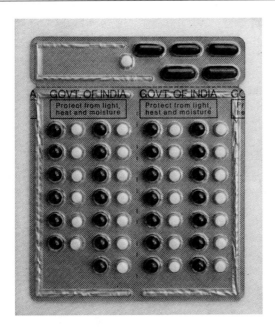

Fig. 9.13 Blister calendar packs have been used extensively, particularly in India, Sri Lanka and the Philippines, for the dispensing of multiple drug therapy (MDT) on an out-patient basis. The pack shown here carries 1 month's supply of drugs for the treatment of multibacillary (MB) leprosy. It was produced by Pharmanova (later Scanpharm), Copenhagen, Denmark, for use in India; similar packs are available for the treatment of paucibacillary (PB) leprosy and also for appropriately lower doses of MDT for children. The top line carries clofazimine (three capsules, each of 100 mg), rifampicin (two capsules, each of 300 mg) and one white tablet of dapsone 100 mg—all for supervised, monthly treatment. The remainder carries 27 daily doses of dapsone 100 mg and clofazimine 50 mg for unsupervised, daily treatment. Although adding to the cost of medication, blister calendar packs are judged by many programmes to be cost-effective, compared with the handling and administration of loose drugs, and they are likely to be even more widely used in the near future, notably in the national leprosy eradication programme in India.

standing success of MDT has transformed the entire picture with regard to world leprosy in recent years, giving rise to the possibility (many would say likelihood) that this disease can be reduced to an elimination level, as defined by WHO, of less than one case per 10 000 of the population by the year 2000. In July 1994, the director-general of WHO announced the formation of the WHO Special Programme for the Elimination of Leprosy [42], with three major components: (i) country support and special action project; (ii) monitoring and evaluation of elimination of leprosy; and (iii) capacity building and health-systems research. These exciting developments, which are to some extent linked to the WHO definition of a case of leprosy (see above), should not divert attention from two important aspects of the present situation: (i) the need to maintain and, in some cases, intensify efforts to identify all cases in leprosy-endemic countries or regions and to ensure that they are started on MDT as soon as possible, modifying the operational approach if necessary, to overcome impediments with regard to supervision of monthly dosage, attendance at clinics, etc.; and (ii) the need to fundamentally improve current strategies for disability prevention, management and rehabilitation. The WHO estimates that there are currently between 1.3 and 1.5 million people with significant degrees of disability in various parts of the world and it is widely recognized that the involvement of both specialized and general health staff in the prevention and management of disability due to leprosy is unsatisfactory. Facilities for physical and social rehabilitation, even when available, are generally inadequate, even in countries with well-developed programmes for case detection and chemotherapy.

Alternative regimens of chemotherapy

As the title of the original WHO publication indicates, the recommendations were originally intended for control programmes and there was no intention that they should be binding on clinicians dealing with patients in smaller numbers, perhaps in non-endemic countries, including private practice or situations where dapsone resistance might not necessarily be an important factor. The crucially important elements are: (i) the use of combined drug regimens, stringently avoiding the use of any antileprosy drug as monotherapy; and (ii) the inclusion and proper use of bactericidal drugs, such as rifampicin. A number of alternative regimens were in use considerably before the WHO recommendations of 1982, including those devised by Freerksen and colleagues in Germany, consisting of isoniazid, dapsone and prothionamide, to which rifampicin was later added [43]. These appear to have been outstandingly successful in the control and probable eradication of leprosy in Malta and in the national leprosy control programme in Tanzania and some parts of South America. In recent years, a number of new drugs have been produced with impressive activity against *M. leprae*, the most important of which are minocycline, ofloxacin and clarithromycin. The main properties and dosage of these drugs are shown in Table 9.4. It is inevitable that one or more of these highly active compounds will be used in drug combinations in the near future, and WHO has recently advised on the use of these drugs in instances of rifampicin resistance or toxicity, severe dapsone toxicity or refusal to accept clofazimine [33]. However, WHO has also emphasized that the standard PB and MB regimens described above should continue to be used for all cases in routine leprosy control programmes.

Immunotherapy

The concept of immunotherapy for leprosy is based essentially on the search for measures to overcome or reverse the characteristic antigen-specific non-responsiveness seen in lepromatous patients. Only limited data are so far available on the effect of agents such as transfer factor or

Table 9.4 New drugs for the treatment of leprosy.

Name	Group	Mode of action	Half-life (hours)	Dose (adult)	Main side-effects	Cost
Ofloxacin*	Fluoroquinolones	Bactericidal: interferes with bacterial DNA replication by inhibiting the A subunit of the enzyme DNA gyrase	7	400 mg daily	Nausea, diarrhoea and other GI tract complaints, insomnia, headache, dizziness, nervousness and hallucinations. Serious problems are infrequent	£2.05
Minocycline	Tetracyclines	Bactericidal: inhibits protein synthesis via a reversible binding at the 30S ribosomal subunit	11–23	100 mg daily	Discoloration of teeth in infants and children, occasional pigmentation of skin and mucous membranes, various GI tract and central nervous system complaints, including dizziness. Widely used for acne vulgaris and well tolerated	£0.64
Clarythromycin	Macrolides	Bactericidal: inhibits bacterial protein synthesis by linking to the 50S ribosomal subunit	6–7	500 mg daily	GI tract irritation, nausea, vomiting and diarrhoea. Relatively non-toxic	£1.61

* Other members of this group, including nor-, cipro-, pe- and sparfloxacin, have been investigated for their action against mycobacteria, including *M. leprae*.
DNA, deoxyribonucleic acid; GI, gastrointestinal.

interferon-γ, but the use of a preparation of heat-killed *M. leprae* plus viable BCG by Convit and colleagues in Venezuela has attracted considerable attention for this purpose, while at the same time suggesting that it could be used as a vaccine for prevention [44]. For immunotherapy, the preparation is given intradermally into three sites across the upper back and repeated, if required, at intervals over a period of 2–3 months, during which chemotherapy may be continued. It has been shown that non-responsiveness can indeed be overcome in a high percentage of lepromatous patients by this procedure and that it is even more effective in patients with lepromin-negative, indeterminate leprosy and in patients whose bacterial load has been reduced by chemotherapy. Although described in 1982 and subsequently used as the basis of vaccine trials (for the prevention of leprosy) in different parts of the world, the value of these important and interesting observations for the treatment of leprosy or as an adjunct to chemotherapy has still to be established in controlled clinical trials. As is the case with the continuing search for a vaccine, the value and likely cost-effectiveness of such trials would call for careful assessment, in view of the remarkable progress which is currently being made by case detection and the implementation of MDT.

The treatment of adverse immunological reactions

The early recognition and treatment of reactions in leprosy constitute an aspect of the total management of patients which is at least as important as (and in many ways more difficult than) diagnosis, classification and the administration of appropriate chemotherapy. Whether type 1 (syn. reversal, upgrading) or type 2 (syn. lepromatous, ENL, immune complex), reactions call for expert attention and management and under ideal circumstances a high percentage of all patients, especially those with painful involvement of peripheral nerves or involvement of the eyes, should be admitted to hospital, if only because nerve damage may occur so rapidly and lead to serious sensory and/or motor deprivation, which is in some cases irreversible. In practice, however, and especially in control-programme situations where patients live far from the nearest hospital of special centre, it is recommended that treatment should be given on an out-patient basis, including the use, where indicated, of steroids, as described below.

Mild type 1 reactions may respond to general measures, including rest of an affected limb, eye protection and analgesics. Contrary to previous practice, it is strongly recommended that antileprosy drugs should be continued, without modification of dosage. More severe cases, especially those with nerve pain, tenderness or loss of nerve function, should be referred to hospital or a special centre, but, even if this is not possible, steroids should be started without delay. Opinion is still divided on dosage and duration. The WHO Expert Committee on Leprosy (1988) [1] advised that dosage should depend on the severity of the reaction and on the patient's body weight and response to treatment, but should be sufficient to relieve both nerve pain and tenderness, and that the duration should be for several months, depending on individual circumstances. Others have drawn attention to the need for clinical caution in the use of steroids, especially under field conditions, in patients with tuberculosis, and also in those with a positive urine test for sugar or albumin, pregnancy, dysentery or intestinal worm infestations [45].

Although both lower and higher dosages have been recommended, a course of prednisolone, which has been found effective and reasonably safe under most circumstances, is as follows:

40 mg once a day for the first 2 weeks, then
30 mg once a day for weeks 3 and 4,
20 mg once a day for weeks 5 and 6,

15 mg once a day for weeks 7 and 8,

10 mg once a day for weeks 9 and 10, and

5 mg once a day for weeks 11 and 12.

In cases of severe nerve pain and/or sudden motor paralysis and provided that experienced staff are available, a maximum dose of 60 mg/day may be given, followed by progressive reduction of dosage as shown above (5–10 mg every 2 weeks).

In the case of type 2 (syn. lepromatous, ENL, immune complex) reactions, mild cases may be handled safely in the field but severe cases should be referred to hospital. Steroids are widely used and there is a consensus view that shorter courses of treatment, in terms of weeks rather than months, should be used in type 2 (as opposed to type 1) reactions, mainly because the episodes may be recurrent and there is a greater danger of steroid complications. Clofazimine in an adult dose of 300 mg daily for not more than 3 months is also effective, but it is slow in achieving clinical effect and doses of this order are often highly pigmenting to the skin and may also produce gastrointestinal side-effects. Thalidomide is highly effective and rapid in the treatment of type 2 reaction, but it is useless, and

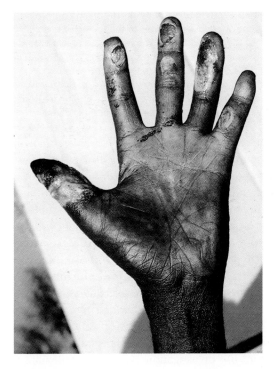

Fig. 9.14 Extensive loss of sensation due to peripheral neuropathy in a patient with previously treated leprosy, inactive at the time of this phototraph. Due either to late presentation or to the mismanagement of reactive episodes causing nerve damage, the ulnar, median and terminal radial nerves are all affected, resulting in extensive (and irreversible) loss of sensation. Small muscles of the hand, supplied by median and ulnar nerves, are also weak.

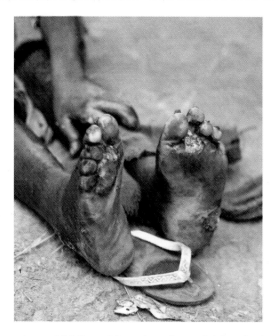

Fig. 9.15 This patient, with bilateral foot ulceration and deformity, had been treated with dapsone, inadequately, prior to the taking of this photograph. Severe bilateral damage to the posterior tibial nerves has led to loss of sensation in the soles of both feet and muscle weakness. Chronic ulceration is accompanied by bone infection and a vicious circle of events leading, if untreated, to progressive loss of tissue. Apart from surgical and general medical care, patients with sole sensory loss of the kind shown here require constant education in self-care, together with suitable protective footwear on a permanent basis.

should never be used, for type 1 reaction. It is given in an adult dose in the order of 100 mg, four times daily, tapering down as soon as the reaction is controlled. Some cases require 100 mg every other day or daily to control chronic reaction, but attempts should be made to discontinue, at least every 6 months. Thalidomide is highly teratogenic and should never be given to females of child-bearing age, even under in-patient conditions.

The difficulty of recording clear-cut advice on the treatment of reactions, especially type 1, is partly related to our continuing ignorance about precipitating factors and the detailed nature of the underlying immunological disturbance, but also to the need to select measures which are appropriate, safe and effective under widely varying circumstances. With declining prevalence, it is to be hoped that it may be possible in the future to admit a higher percentage of all reaction cases to hospitals or special centres, so that they benefit from full investigation and the best possible regimens available. Meanwhile, it is of some consolation to record that type 2 reactions are now much less commonly seen, possibly due to the inclusion of clofazimine in the three-drug MDT regimen for MB cases, and that the widespread implementation of MDT has not, as some experts predicted, resulted in an increase in the number or severity of type 1 reactions.

The treatment of disability and deformity in leprosy

A detailed description of this aspect is beyond the range of the present chapter, but no account of leprosy would be complete without at least drawing attention to the large and increasing number of patients world-wide with significant levels of disability due to leprosy (Figs 9.14, 9.15). By this is usually meant obvious or visible disability (grade 2 on a scale used by WHO), such as claw hand, lagophthalmus, drop foot or trophic ulceration. The WHO estimates that there are between 1.3 and 1.5 million patients in this category worldwide, but this does not take account of a large number with loss of sensation only (grade 1), who may deteriorate into states of obvious and visible deformity if not repeatedly instructed in self-care. Specialist texts should be consulted on procedures which have already been extensively described with regard to self-care, physiotherapy, plastic and orthopaedic surgery, the provision and use of protective footwear and care of the eyes [46–48]. The extent to which primary health-care services and community-based or integrated rehabilitation programmes, dealing with leprosy alongside all other forms of disability, can contribute to this problem has yet to be established.

References

1   WHO. *Expert Committee on Leprosy: Sixth Report*. Technical Report Series 768, World Health Organization, Geneva, 1988.
2   WHO. Progress towards elimination of leprosy as a public health problem *WHO Weekly Epidem Rec* 1994; **20**: 145–151; **21**: 153–157.
3   WHO. Progress towards the elimination of leprosy as a public health problem. *WHO Weekly Epidem Rec* 1996; **71**: 149–156.
4   WHO. *Chemotherapy of Leprosy for Control Programmes: Report of a WHO Study Group*. Technical Report Series 675, World Health Organization, Geneva, 1982.
5   Bechelli LM, Garbajosa PG, Mg Mg Gyi *et al*. Proposed method for estimating leprosy prevalence based on rates in children. *Bull World Health Org* 1973; **48**: 502–503.
6   WHO. *Epidemiology of Leprosy in Relation to Control: Report of a WHO Study Group*. Technical Report Series 716, World Health Organization, Geneva, 1985.
7   Van Eden W, De Vries RRP. Occasional review—HLA and leprosy: a re-evaluation. *Lepr Rev* 1984; **55**: 89–104.
8   Harboe H. The immunology of leprosy. In: Hastings RC (ed.) *Leprosy*. Medicine in the Tropics, Churchill Livingstone, Edinburgh, London, Melbourne, New York, 1985.
9   Convit J, Ulrich MI. Leprosy: bacterial, pathological, immunological and immunopathological aspects. In: Harahap M (ed.) *Mycobacterial Skin Diseases*. Kluwer Academic Publishers, Dordrecht, Boston, London, 1989.
10 Walsh GP, Meyers WM, Binford CH, Gerone PJ, Wolff RH, Leininger JR. Leprosy, a zoonosis. *Lepr Rev* 1981; **52** (Suppl 1): 77–83.
11 Kazda J, Ganapati R, Revankar C, Buchanan TM, Young DB, Irgens LM. Isolation of environment-derived *M. leprae* from soil in Bombay. *Lepr Rev* 1986; **57** (Suppl 3): 201–208.
12 Kazda J, Irgens LM, Kolk A. Acid-fast bacilli found in sphagnum vegetation of coastal Norway, containing *M. leprae*-specific phenolic glycolipid-1. *Int J Lepr* 1990; **58**: 353–357.
13 Shepard CC. The experimental disease that follows the injection of human leprosy bacilli into foot-pads of mice. *J Exp Med* 1960; **112**: 445–454.

14 Kirchheimer WF, Storrs EE. Attempts to establish the armadillo (*Dasypus novemcinctus* Linn.) as a model for the study of leprosy. I. Report of lepromatoid leprosy in an experimentally infected armadillo. *Int J Lepr* 1971; **39**: 693–702.

15 Brennan PJ, Barrow WW. Evidence for species-specific lipid antigens in *Mycobacterium leprae. Int J Lepr* 1980; **48**: 382–387.

16 Cochrane RG, Smyly HJ. Classification. In: Cochrane RG, Davey TF (eds) *Leprosy in Theory and Practice*. John Wright and Sons, Bristol, 1964.

17 Ridley DS, Jopling WH. A classification of leprosy for research purposes. *Lepr Rev* 1962; **33**: 119–128.

18 Ridley DS, Jopling WH. Classification of leprosy according to immunity—a five-group system. *Int J Lepr* 1966; **34**: 255–273.

19 Ridley DS. *Skin Biopsy in Leprosy*, 3rd edn. Documenta Geigy, Ciba-Geigy, Basle, 1990.

20 WHO. *Report on the Tuberculosis Epidemic 1995*. WHO/TB/95.183, Tuberculosis Programme, World Health Organization, Geneva, 1995.

21 WHO. *Treatment of Tuberculosis: Guidelines for National Programmes*. World Health Organization, Geneva, 1993.

22 Meeran K. Prevalence of HIV infection among patients with leprosy and tuberculosis in rural Zambia. *Br Med J* 1989; **298**: 364–365.

23 Ponnighaus JM, Mwanjasi LJ, Fine PE *et al*. Is HIV infection a risk factor for leprosy? *Int J Lepr* 1991; **59**: 221–228.

24 Borgdorff MW, van den Broek J, Chum HJ *et al*. HIV-1 infection as a risk factor for leprosy: a case–control study in Tanzania. *Int J Lepr* 1993; **61**: 556–562.

25 Nunn PP, McAdam KPWJ. Mycobacterial infections and AIDS. *Br Med Bull Tubercul Lepr* 1988; **44** (3): 801–813.

26 Miller RA. Leprosy and AIDS: a review of the literature and speculation on the impact of CD4+ lymphocyte depletion on immunity to *Mycobacterium leprae. Int J Lepr* 1991; **59**: 639–644.

27 Duncan ME, Melsom R, Pearson JMH, Ridley DS. The association of pregnancy and leprosy, 1. New cases, relapse of cured patients and deterioration in patients on treatment during pregnancy and lactation—results of a prospective study of 154 pregnancies in 147 Ethiopian women. *Lepr Rev* 1981; **52**: 245–262.

28 Duncan ME, Pearson JMH, Ridley DS, Melsom R, Bjune G. Pregnancy and leprosy: the consequences of alterations of cell-mediated and humoral immunity during pregnancy and lactation. *Int J Lepr* 1982; **50**: 425–435.

29 Jopling WH. Reactional leprosy or leprosy in reaction. *Lepr Rev* 1959; **30**: 194–196.

30 Jopling WH, McDougall AC. *Handbook of Leprosy*, 5th edn. CBS Publishers, New Delhi, 1996.

31 Lienhardt C, Fine PEM. Type 1 reaction, neuritis and disability in leprosy: what is the current epidemiological situation? *Lepr Rev* 1994; **65**: 9–30.

32 Georgiev GD, McDougall AC. Skin smears and the bacterial index (BI) in multiple drug therapy control programmes: an unsatisfactory and potentially hazardous state of affairs. *Int J Lepr* 1988; **56**: 101–103.

33 WHO. *Chemotherapy of Leprosy: Report of a WHO Study Group*. Technical Report Series 847, World Health Organization, Geneva, 1994.

34 WHO. *Guidelines for Personnel Involved in Collection of Skin Smears in Leprosy Control Programmes for the Prevention and Control of Possible Infection with HIV*. WHO/CDS/LEP/87.1, World Health Organization, Geneva, 1987.

35 Leiker DL, McDougall AC. *Technical Guide for Smear Examination for Leprosy*, 2nd revised edn. German Leprosy Relief Association, Würzburg 1987.

36 Hastings RC (ed.). *Leprosy*. Medicine in the Tropics, Churchill Livingstone, Edinburgh, London, Melbourne, New York, 1985.

37 WHO. *Report of the Consultation on the Early Diagnosis of Leprosy*. WHO/CDT/LEP/90.2, World Health Organization, Geneva, 1990.

38 Van Beers SM, Izumi S, Madjid B, Maeda Y, Day R, Klatser PR. An epidemiological study of leprosy infection by serology and polymerase chain reaction. *Int J Lepr* 1994,

62: 1–9.

39 TDR (Special Programme for Research and Training in Tropical Diseases) Techniques for leprosy diagnosis; 'exciting' but still experimental. *TDR News* 1990; **34**: 3 and 7. (Published by UNDP/World Bank/WHO, Geneva.)

40 Mann RJ, Harman RRM. Cutaneous anaesthesia in necrobiosis lipoidica. *Br J Dermatol* 1984; **110**: 323–325.

41 Ghosh S, Haldar B. Quantitative evaluation of cutaneous thermal sensitivity in psoriasis, morphoea and vitiligo. *Ind J Dermatol Venereol Lepr* 1989; **55**: 30–33.

42 International Conference on the Elimination of Leprosy. Hanoi, Vietnam, July, 1994. WHO and the Sasakawa Memorial Health Foundation, Tokyo, Japan.

43 Freerksen E, Rosenfeld M. Leprosy eradication programme of Malta. *Chemotherapy* 1977; **23**: 356–386.

44 Convit J, Aranzazu N, Ulrich M, Pinardi ME, Reyes O, Alvarado J. Immunotherapy with a mixture of *Mycobacterium leprae* and BCG in different forms of leprosy and in Mitsuda-negative contacts. *Int J Lepr* 1982; **50**: 415–424.

45 Becx-Bleumink M, Mannetje WT, Berhe D. The management of nerve damage in the leprosy control services (editorial). *Lepr Rev* 1990; **61**: 1–11.

46 Srinivasan H. *Prevention of Disabilities in Patients with Leprosy: A Practical Guide*. World Health Organization, Geneva, 1993.

47 Watson JM. *Essential Action to Minimise Disability in Leprosy Patients*. Leprosy Mission International, Brentford, Revised 2nd ed., 1994.

48 Brand MB. *Care of the Eye in Hansen's Disease*, 2nd edn. Teaching and Learning Materials in Leprosy (Talmilep), Leprosy Mission International, Brentford, 1987.

Chapter 10
Infections in Dermatological Surgery

Treatment
Eckart Haneke

Definition

Infections are the most serious local disturbance of wound healing. They are defined as bacterial densities of more than 10 000 pathogens/g tissue [1]. However, the definition of wound infection in dermatological surgery is not clear: Are erythema, swelling, warming and purulent changes true infections even when cultures remain negative, whereas, in contrast, bacteria may be grown from wounds that do not show clinical signs of an infection? Skin ulcerations may be colonized by pathogenic bacteria and still heal without antibiotics. Pathogens may also colonize normal skin [2].

Unfortunately, the classification of wound infections has therefore to rely on clinical criteria. A pragmatic approach is to classify a wound as non-infected when it heals primarily or secondarily without inflammatory criteria, such as reddening, localized heat, swelling and pus formation.

Infections in dermatological surgery may be defined as acute infections, developing within 3 days to a week after operation, and latent infections, developing after a symptom-free interval. They are usually bacterial infections, but viral infections may also develop, whereas mycobacterial and mycotic infections are rare.

Epidemiology

Skin is never sterile and always harbours pathogens. Bacteria are found in about 90% of all surgical incisions [3]. Certain body areas, especially those rich in sebaceous glands, contain high numbers of potentially virulent pathogens [4]. Initially, the number of these microorganisms is low. It may, however, increase considerably under conditions that are favourable for the pathogens or in immunocompromised hosts and give rise to a wound infection or even sepsis. Of 149 immunocompetent patients with non-infected sites of skin surgery, bacteria were cultured in 127, mostly coagulase-negative staphylococci (68.5%), but only one developed postoperative

416

bacteraemia for 1 day [5]. Endocarditis associated with skin surgery and acupuncture was reported in four patients for each [5].

The overall rate of wound infections in dermatological surgery is very low [2, 6, 7] as compared with organ surgery. Most modern textbooks of dermatological surgery do not even mention infection in their index. In accordance with general surgery, a wound classification was given by Haas and Grekin [8]. Most skin wounds are considered clean (class I) and those in the genitoanal area, perineum, groins, axillae and nails as well as the oral mucosa are clean-contaminated (class II). The frequency of wound infections ranges from less than 5% to approximately 10%, respectively. However, acute non-purulent inflammation indicates a contaminated wound (class III), with an infection rate of 20–30%. Infected wounds (class IV) are seen in tumours with putrid secretions and crusts or necrotic material, as well as in inflamed and ruptured cysts, hidradenitis, furuncles, pyodermia fistulans sinifica, etc. Their infection rate is said to be 30–40%. Furthermore, the infection rate has been observed to double with each hour of operation [8].

The infection rate of surgical skin wounds depends on the contamination of the surgical field. Therefore, four groups of dermatological operations were proposed [2] that correspond to the wound classification cited above.

1 Aseptic dermatological operations: primary surgical treatment of skin lesions with intact skin surface and immediate covering of defect on trunk, neck and extremities, e.g. excision of naevi, melanomas, tattoos, precancerous lesions, etc.

2 Relatively aseptic dermatological operations: primary surgical treatment of lesions with immediate closure of defect on scalp, nails and around orifices (nose, mouth, genitals, anus), e.g. removal of melanomas and naevi on mucous membranes and on the scalp, nail operations.

3 Contaminated dermatological operations: surgical treatment of skin lesions colonized with pathogenic organisms, but without clinical signs of inflammation, with primary or secondary wound closure, e.g. delayed defect closure with grafts or flaps, vein surgery in the presence of an ulcer, ulcerated tumours, operations in the presence of a concurrent infection elsewhere.

4 Septic dermatological operations: surgical treatment of skin lesions with clinical signs of inflammation and presence of pathogens, e.g. extirpation of necrotic and ulcerated tumours, abscesses and fistulas.

A comparison of wound infections in general surgery and dermatological surgery confirms the low incidence of wound infections in dermatological surgery (Table 10.1) [2, 9].

Diabetic patients have many complications, causing delayed wound repair and chronic skin ulcers (Table 10.2) [8, 10]. Their impaired host defence against infections renders them highly susceptible also to postoperative infection after skin surgery, and both peripheral vascular disease and autonomic and sensory neuropathy add to this problem.

Table 10.1 Frequency of wound infections, depending on type of operation.

	General surgery (Hartel and Steinmann [9])	Dermatological surgery (Steinert et al. [2])
Aseptic operations	1.8% ($n = 23\,362$)	0.74% ($n = 673$)
Relatively aseptic operations	9.0% ($n = 4983$)	1.47% ($n = 273$)
Contaminated operations	19.0% ($n = 1183$)	2.75% ($n = 109$)
Septic operations	39.5% ($n = 965$)	— ($n = 14$)

Table 10.2 Risk factors for wound infections [8, 10].

Risk factor	Reason of risk
High risk	
Preoperative stay in hospital	May acquire hospitalization and multiresistant bacteria
Razor-shaving 1 day prior to surgery	Minute wounds may harbour pathogens
Length of operation	Drying of wounds causes cell death, impairs blood supply, allows bacteria to enter
Drains and other foreign material, including sutures	Foreign material interferes with wound healing
Presence of remote infections	Asepsis may not be achieved, latent bacteraemia may cause wound infection
Old age, malnutrition, obesity, anaemia, protein deficiency, diabetes mellitus, chronic renal failure, alcoholism, vitamin C deficiency, X-irradiation	Wound healing slowed down, allowing infections to become manifest
Smoking	Decreased wound healing, delayed scar formation
Corticosteroids, immunosuppressive drugs, HIV infection	Impaired or absent host defence
Low risk	
Out-patient	No virulent and multiresistant hospital pathogens
Preoperative showering with an antiseptic soap	Reduction of pathogens on skin surface
Young, healthy, immunocompetent	Normal wound healing, normal host defence

HIV, human immunodeficiency virus.

Infections after dermatological surgery are also more frequent in immunosuppressed and immunocompromised subjects, elderly persons, vitamin C deficiency, protein deficiency, anaemia, alcoholics [11], and X-irradiated skin and during certain drug therapies. Delayed wound healing in debilitated persons is another serious risk factor. Recently, it was observed that punch defects take considerably longer to heal in persons under stress.

Certain areas are particularly prone to develop wound infections: tip of the nose, nail apparatus, genitoanal region, lower legs and feet. An antibiotic perioperative prophylaxis might be considered, particularly if the infection rate is over 5%.

The most common cause for the loss of skin grafts is infection at the recipient site [12].

Any wound infection ought to be documented in order to have a quality control of prophylactic measures and surgical techniques.

About 7% of 10038 patients from 1417 intensive-care units had wound infections [13]; however, these were probably not from dermatological surgery.

Aetiology

Most wound infections are caused by *Staphylococcus aureus*, less frequently by *Streptococcus pyogenes*, enterococci, *Pseudomonas aeruginosa* and other Gram-negative bacteria. Anaerobic bacteria are rarely encountered. If a pathogenic organism is isolated intraoperatively, the probability of its being associated with subsequent wound infection is 100% with *Enterobacter* species, 79% with *Proteus* species, 68% with *Klebsiella*, 65% with *P. aeruginosa*, 55% with *S. aureus* and 31% with *Escherichia coli*. The increasingly important role of *Staphyolococcus epidermidis* in postoperative wound infections has been confirmed [14]. There is a theoretical risk of *Clostridium tetani* infection as well as *Clostridium perfringens*, causing tetanus and gas gangrene, respectively.

Staphylococcus aureus continues to be the most frequent cause of skin and skin-wound infections. Streptococcal infections have become more frequent during the last 10 years, after a period of decline due to improved hygiene, diminished virulence and efficacious antibiotics [15], and both the toxic-shock syndrome and the streptococcal toxic shock-like syndrome have also been observed to be due to wound infections.

Herpes simplex virus may cause widespread disseminated herpes infection in persons with recurrent labial herpes simplex after dermabrasion, chemical peeling or laser skin resurfacing of the face.

Fungal infections are exceptionally seen after skin surgery [16]; they are mainly due to inoculation during surgery. An infection with *Candida* species after full-face dermabrasion is very rare [17].

Wound infections vary in frequency from surgeon to surgeon, depending on the setting where the surgery was performed, on the body region and on the lesion being operated on.

It is not yet clear whether the suture material plays an important role in wound infection. Whereas plain catgut was shown to have the highest wound infection rate [18], this was not shown for other material [19]. Polyfil non-resorbable threads may act as a nidus for pathogenic bacteria and be responsible for longer duration of an infection [20].

Local anaesthesia was suggested to be a risk in potentially infected areas. However, Lidocaine has an intrinsic bactericidal activity, which is even enhanced by adding sodium bicarbonate, which makes injection less painful [21].

Occlusive moist dressings were shown to reduce the infection rate as compared with conventional dressings [22]. Transparent dressings also allow the wound to be inspected regularly.

Clinical manifestations

Before starting the incision, the surgeon should have disinfected a wide area of the skin around the site of surgery. Sterile towels are used to cover the surrounding skin. Any potentially infected lesion is avoided during the surgery (no-touch technique). Crusted or oozing tumours are covered with gauze soaked with a potent disinfective agent, and any gauze that might have come into contact with this lesion is immediately discarded. Disinfective solutions are used to clean surgical instruments during non-aseptic surgery and also to flush the surgical wound. Tissue injury has to be minimized by using an atraumatic technique. Proper disinfection is performed after skin suture. Blood on and around the wound is removed using 3% hydrogen peroxide; this is also a mild disinfectant. Finally, the wound is covered with Steri-strips or other material protecting the wound from exogenous bacteria and supporting the suture. These measures are taken routinely and will decrease the number of postoperative wound infections.

The clinical manifestation of skin wound infections is usually obvious. After 1–3 days, the wound area becomes tender, erythematous and swollen. The stitches tend to cut through the epidermis. Pus may show at the stitches, incision and follicular openings. Throbbing pain may develop and important perilesional oedema may be seen in the orbital and genital area. If not treated, the infection will spread to involve a larger area. The overlying epidermis may blister or dissolve. Eventually, the skin may turn black as a sign of intravascular coagulation and necrosis, and further complications may be encountered (see below). Regional lymphadenitis is often present. Constitutional symptoms are absent or mild.

Intact scalp skin is only relatively aseptic. Most patients do not want to get their hair shaved and, quite often, single hairs get into the incision wound. Modern suture material is not much thicker than hair shafts, and it may be difficult to distinguish hair from monofil threads. Careful and intensive disinfection of the scalp and hair is therefore necessary before operating on the scalp. Meticulous haemostasis and wide undermining of the wound margins to avoid suture under tension will reduce the risk of infection. After suture, the wound has to be cleaned of blood and dried. A dressing is often not necessary provided the patient is able to avoid dust and dirt. Inspection of the wound is recommended after 2–3 days; it is cleaned again, if necessary, and disinfected. Stitches are usually removed after 7–9 days. Wound infection is commonly seen as circumscribed festering of the stitch marks. The wound margins may become necrotic. Widespread suppuration of the scalp is rare but may have catastrophic consequences.

The pinna is also at risk of infection. Often, there is an acute postoperative erythema in the concha as a direct sequel of the surgical trauma, especially after electrosurgery. Infections are frequently due to *P. aeruginosa*. They are painful and difficult to treat since the cartilage is a bradytrophic tissue without its own blood-vessels.

Infections from surgery of the forehead tend to give marked oedema of the orbits, quite often associated with extensive haematoma. Necrotizing eyelid infections can complicate simple forehead epidermal cyst extirpation [23].

The skin of the tip of the nose and the alae nasi is different from that of most other facial areas. It is very thick, contains a huge number of densely arranged, very large sebaceous glands and adheres firmly to the underlying cartilage structures and arterial blood-vessels enter it vertically. Bleeding is intense during incision and undermining. For buried sutures, the stiff skin has to be firmly grasped with the pincer, causing considerable trauma to the wound margins. Sutures are often under tension. The sebaceous glands contain large numbers of potentially pathogenic microorganisms. Thus infection of surgical wounds after tumour removal is rather frequent. It is characterized by intense localized erythema, small pustules in the stitches and the follicular openings around the wound and, eventually, suppuration from the incision. Small tissue necroses are common.

The lips are very well supplied with blood-vessels and even large defects can be closed without the risk of necrosis and wound infection.

Axillary skin is rich in eccrine sweat glands and apocrine glands. It harbours a rich resident flora, but may also be colonized with staphylococci and other potentially pathogenic bacteria. Axillary hair should be shaved immediately prior to an operation, and thorough disinfection of the region is crucial. Maceration is common after operation, especially when the arm was immobilized, and bacteria will find good conditions to grow. Wound infection was observed in five of 52 patients operated for axillary hyperhidrosis [24].

Nail surgery is usually associated with marked postoperative pain for about 24–36 hours; if pain resumes after 48–72 hours, an infection must be considered. The tip of the finger is tender, red to bluish-red and swollen. Secretion of pus may develop and parts of the nail organ may become necrotic. Lymphangitis and regional lymphadenitis are frequently seen.

Skin surgery of genital skin, especially scrotum, vulva and perineum, has an increased incidence of postoperative infection because of the higher density of potentially pathogenic organisms such as stapholococci, streptococci, *P. aeruginosa*, enterobacteria and *Proteus* species. Quite often, this type of infection is only a minor one due to sutures tied too tautly, with pus formation at the site of the stitches. The skin of the scrotum, labia majora of the vulva and labia minora is extremely sensitive to ischaemia from circumscribed pressure and will rapidly undergo limited necrosis, which may become secondarily infected. Circumscribed swelling between the stitches is the earliest sign of this type of tissue injury. More severe wound infections will produce genital oedema, tender inguinal lymph nodes and pain.

Wound infections and dehiscence are also the most frequent complications of radical vulvectomy [25].

Perineal surgical procedures, particularly in subjects suffering from diabetes mellitus, may rarely lead to necrotizing infections of the vulva [26, 27] or of the scrotum (Fournier's gangrene). These regional variants of necrotizing fasciitis may be due to a single pathogen, such as group A streptococci or *Vibrio* species, exceptionally to Zygomycetes, or to a synergistic infection by aerobic streptococci and enterobacteria plus anaerobic *Bacteroides* and *Peptostreptococcus* gas-forming organisms. This infection rapidly destroys deep soft tissue along fascial planes with relative sparing of the overlying skin. Early clinical signs are local erythema, marked oedema and tenderness, whereas lymphadenitis is often absent. Systemic toxicity is moderate to severe. Within hours or a few days, extensive necroses develop, spreading to the perineum, penis and abdominal wall. Vulvar necrotizing fasciitis has been observed to be followed by the staphylococcal toxic-shock syndrome [28].

Wound infections after operations on the trunk, arms and thighs are rare.

The lower leg and the foot are delicate areas to operate on. The vascular supply is poor, especially in the elderly, smokers, diabetic subjects and persons with impaired peripheral arterial circulation. The skin is tight and firm. Infections usually result from delayed healing, from wound margin necroses from suture tension and from both arterial and venous insufficiency, as well as from lymphatic obstruction. Compression bandages are therefore a must even for small defects. It has to be kept in mind that the sole of the foot has a unique cushion-like subcutaneous tissue, which should never be wantonly sacrificed because even the most sophisticated plastic repair cannot restore this tissue. Antibiotic prophylaxis should be considered if there is the slightest hint of an infection of the foot or lower leg.

Infection of electrosurgical wounds is infrequent because these wounds are usually left open for secondary-intention healing. However, excessive crust formation may be indicative of an infection. Upon removing such a crust, a purulent base can often be seen. It is also not correct to assume that the heat generated by the electrical current will kill pathogenic bacteria; rather, the heat will produce necrotic tissue, which may become a good medium for bacterial growth.

Infection after cryosurgery is very rare. It is only seen in delayed epithelialization or under thick crusts [17].

Grafts are at an increased risk of infection because it takes about 5 days for the graft to get revascularized. If the wound is left to granulate in its bed, it is always colonized with bacteria, which are potentially harmful. Pathogens in the space between the wound bed and the graft are relatively inaccessible for the host's immune system and the overlying graft does not have an active defence at all. Infection of the graft may reveal itself by slight fever, malodour and a purulent secretion. The peripheral skin is congested. Pus may sometimes be expressed from under the graft. Full-thickness skin grafts are mainly at risk in poorly vascularized areas. The most common infectious agents responsible for graft failure are coagulase-positive staphylococci, β-haemolytic streptococci and *P. aeruginosa*. The latter is frequently seen in auricular skin grafts [29].

Infection of the donor site of a split-thickness skin graft is infrequent; however, when it occurs it may destroy the remnants of the follicular structures that are responsible for the re-epithelialization and cause scarring. Oozing and secretion after 2–3 days usually indicate infection or too deep a defect. The pathogens are mainly *P. aeruginosa*, *Proteus* spp., *S. aureus*, *E. coli* and, rarely, *Serratia marcescens* [30]. Group A β-haemolytic streptococci, once very frequent, have become rather rare [25].

Infections in skin flaps are infrequently observed. However, they are a considerable threat to the survival of the flap because they greatly enhance the metabolic activity of the inflamed tissue, causing a greater demand for oxygen. Since the flap has only a reduced blood supply, a breakdown of the flap metabolism may occur, resulting in flap necrosis [31].

The infection rate of skin expanders is less that 1% when they are placed under completely intact skin. Delayed infections may be seen from the repeated puncture of the port when antisepsis is neglected [32–34]. Infection often requires removal of the expander.

Chemical peeling, dermabrasion and laser skin resurfacing are techniques to ablate superficial layers of the skin, usually of the face. The infection risk is very low in superficial procedures but increases with depth. An inherent risk of all of these procedures is the reactivation of (recurrent labial) herpes simplex, causing an outbreak of disseminated facial herpes simplex that is very similar to eczema herpeticum. With more and more procedures done, there have been reports of patients in whom there was no history of preceding labial herpes simplex but who nevertheless developed disseminated facial herpes simplex.

Chemical peels, laser ablation and dermabrasion cause necrosis or remove a superficial portion of the skin to a certain depth over a wide area.

Wound care after these cosmetic procedures determines the cosmetic results. Peeling agents usually induce important inflammation, slowing down healing [1]. Bacterial infection after full-face chemical peels, dermabrasion or laser resurfacing is rare and should be avoided by abundant use of moist compresses, removing serous exudate and preventing crust formation. If the patients do not perform adequate wound care, secondary impetiginization with crust formation may occur, and maceration and purulent secretion develop, with accumulation of necrotic debris [35, 36]. *Pseudomonas aeruginosa* is not uncommon as the cause for an acute infection, as are pyogenic micrococci, which may even cause toxic-shock syndrome [37]. For laser resurfacing, a broad-spectrum antibiotic cephalexin, 500 mg twice a day for 1 week, is given by some authors [38, 39]. Herpes simplex virus may be reactivated and cause a disseminated facial herpes [38–43]. Infection with *Candida* spp. is exceptional [17].

Liposuction is a very safe technique, and surveys from thousands of patients have shown that infection was hardly ever a complication of this widely used cosmetic surgery modality [44, 45].

Diagnosis

The diagnosis is primarily a clinical one, using the classical signs of inflammation, as outlined above.

Each infection of a surgical wound requires immediate cultivation of the pathogens, permitting their identification and determination of sensitivity to antibiotics. Surgical infections have to be monitored to be able to identify possible sources of infection, such as operation personnel, surgeons' nares and hands, cleansing staff, housekeepers, etc.

Necrotizing skin infections, characterized by undermining and dissection of the subcutaneous tissue at the fascial planes, show destruction and liquefaction of the subcutaneous fat. They initially spare the dermis and epidermis as well as the deep fasciae and muscles. Gas produced by the anaerobes *Peptococcus* and *Bacteroides*, but also by aerobic bacteria, such as the Gram-negative *E. coli*, *Klebsiella*, *Pseudomonas* spp. and enterobacteria, gives rise to typical crepitation. A biopsy should be performed and frozen sections cut. Histopathology will show subcutaneous necrosis, polymorphonuclear leucocyte infiltration, fibrinous intravascular thrombi and microorganisms within the destroyed fascia and dermis. Histopathology also allows the diagnosis of Zygomycetes infection, requiring amphotericin B (and fluconazole) treatment. Only rapid diagnosis and surgical intervention are able to decrease the appalling mortality rate of this life-threatening infection.

Infections of chemical peels, laser skin resurfacing and dermabrasion become obvious after 2–3 days. Excessive crust formation and malodour are indicative of a bacterial infection; pain and the appearance of small ulcers tending to merge may be the signs of a herpetic infection.

Treatment

Most skin-surgery wound infections are due to *S. aureus*, far less frequently to group A β-haemolytic *S. pyogenes* or other pathogens. Therefore, swabs have to be taken and, until the result of the antibiogramme is ready, a *Staphylococcus*-fast semisynthetic penicillin is advisable. Then an antibiotic is instituted, according to sensitivity testing.

Any infected skin wound should be immobilized. Sutures are usually removed, either all or at least partially, to allow the wound to be drained. Pus and purulent secretion are evacuated. Warm soaks with saline or a mild antiseptic solution are applied to prevent crust formation. If there is a wound cavity, it should be rinsed daily with sterile 1% hydrogen peroxide or saline, and small tablets of local antibiotics may be inserted. Necrotic tissue is removed.

Staphylococcal wound infections are treated with penicillinase-resistant penicillin, 0.5 g orally four times daily, or with a cephalosporin, again 0.5 g every 6 hours; in severe cases or those with particularly delicate wound infections, penicillinase-resistant penicillin is given intravenously 0.5–1.0 g every 4 hours. For patients allergic to penicillin, erythromycin 0.5 g every 6 hours or clindamycin 300 mg orally every 6 hours is an alternative [46]. Multi(methicillin)-resistant *S. aureus* infections are treated with 1.0 g vancomycin intravenously twice a day or clindamycin 600 mg three times daily.

Infections due to *P. aeruginosa* are treated with tetracyclines or gentamicin systemically and soaks with diluted acetic acid solution four times daily.

Necrotizing soft-tissue infections — necrotizing cellulitis, necrotizing fasciitis and myonecrosis—require prompt diagnosis and immediate surgical treatment [47].

Facial herpes simplex requires oral acyclovir, five times 200 mg daily; in severe cases the dose may be doubled or acyclovir administered intravenously every 8 hours 5–10 mg/kg body weight. Valacyclovir, three times 500 mg, and brivudin, four times 125 mg daily, are more recent alternatives.

Surgical treatment of skin infections

A variety of skin infections require surgical treatment. These operations have to be classified as septic (class IV).

Uncomplicated furuncles are treated conservatively with hot compresses, whereas lesions with surrounding cellulitis and fever as well as carbuncles require systemic penicillinase-resistant antibiotics. Surgical draining is adequate for fluctuant lesions. Severely inflamed epidermoid cysts and abscesses should be incised where palpation shows the thinnest skin over the lesion. Incision and drainage of soft-tissue abscesses may also be necessary in chronic granulomatous disease [48].

Pyoderma fistulans significa is not an uncommon disease. It is also called acne tetrad/pentad or chronic hidradenitis (suppurativa). Although its main localization is in areas rich in apocrine glands, it is rather a disease of follicular epithelium than of apocrine glands [49]. Virtually all conservative treatments fail and surgery is the only effective therapy [50]. We use electrosurgery to widely excise the involved area. It is used for convenience because there is much less bleeding than with scalpel excision. Fistulas are probed and filled with sterile 1% methylene-blue solution to demonstrate all lesions, which often extend very widely into the subcutaneous tissue. Indurated dermis, even if not obviously inflamed, must also be removed [51]. Carbon dioxide (CO_2) laser surgery is a modern alternative, but does not give better results [52]. The defects are left for secondary-intention healing, or granulation tissue is waited for until a mesh graft is applied. Despite large defects, healing is usually surprisingly fast with daily baths with povidone-iodine (poly(vinylpyrrolidone)-iodine (PVP-I)) soap and antimicrobial ointments. No systemic antibiotics are necessary. No wound infection other than a colonization of the surface is observed. The results are functionally and cosmetically acceptable to good. Recurrences are seen only at the margin where skin prone to develop this debilitating disease was left.

It has already been stressed that prompt surgical intervention in necrotizing fasciitis is absolutely necessary and may be life-saving [53]. The skin has to be widely incised and necrotic skin removed and débridement of all necrotic fat and fascia has to be extended beyond the area of involvement until normal fascia is seen. This wound is left open and a second-look operation is performed after 24–48 hours if the pathological process has extended further. In addition to surgery, heparin is infused and high-dose antibiotics are given intravenously [46]. Vancomycin, gentamicin and either metronidazole or clindamycin are an effective initial regimen for suspected non-clostridial infections, whereas clostridia are susceptible to high-dose penicillin. Zygomycetes infection is treated with amphotericin B intravenously. Fluconazole, alone or in combination with amphotericin B, may become an alternative. Hyperbaric oxygen may reduce the morbidity and mortality. Débridement defects must never be repaired primarily. Rubber-band wound closure [54] or a dynamic skin suture [55] will considerably decrease the size of the wound after complete resolution of the necrotizing infection.

Pressure sores and ulcers from X-irradiation are always heavily contaminated. Apart from general measures in severely ill patients, local wound care with antiseptic rinses, prevention of exudate accumulation in dead space, dissection of necrotic tissue and systemic antibotics in cases of surrounding cellulitis are necessary. For X-ray ulcers and when the patient's condition in bed sores has improved, myocutaneous flaps are best to cover the defects. They are well vascularized and have an optimal survival rate even in (still) infected areas. Myocutaneous flaps are also widely used for other septic defects [56, 57].

Atypical mycobacterioses, if well circumscribed, may be completely excised. This obviates the need for long-term antibiotic treatment [58]. However, a close follow-up is recommended, and some authors advocate a short course of antibiotic treatment.

Lupus vulgaris (tuberculosis cutis luposa) should always be treated with tuberculostatic drugs even is the lesion is small and appears to be amenable to complete surgical removal.

The plethora of wart treatments is evidence that no one therapy is reliable effective. In general, a conservative or semiconservative approach is advisable, since it has been shown that human papillomavirus deoxyribonucleic acid (DNA) can be demonstrated up to 15 mm around condylomata acuminata. For a surgical operation to be almost 100% effective, this would mean removing viral warts with a safety margin of 15 mm — more than for most malignant skin tumours. This is obviously not an adequate treatment, since almost all warts in immunocompetent persons are self-limited. The most common surgical technique for warts is cryosurgery, giving a success rate of 50–70%. It has to be avoided over superficially located nerves and over the nail matrix, because a deep freeze may cause permanent nerve or matrix damage, respectively. Filiform warts, often seen on eyelids, respond quite well to cutting their base. A single large wart may be excised and the defect sutured. Plantar warts should not be operated on and electrosurgery is contraindicated on plantar (and palmar) skin. Carbon dioxide laser vaporization can be tried but has to be carried out cautiously to avoid scarring. Superficial vaporization of the surrounding epidermis may have the advantage of removing latent papillomaviruses around the warts.

Genital warts — condylomata acuminata, pigmented penile papules, Bowenoid papules and flat condylomas — respond to electrosurgical ablation in about 60%; adjuvant interferon may increase the cure rate. Carbon dioxide laser treatment was reported to have a better success rate.

It has been shown that the plume from CO_2 laser vaporization, and also from electrosurgery, of viral warts contains intact virus particles, which are potentially infectious and may be transmitted to the laser surgeon, operation personnel and patient [59, 60]. This risk may also exist for hepatitis B, herpes simplex [61] and human immunodeficiency virus [62]. Since particles in the laser plume are as small as 0.1 μm, the common surgical mask is of no value for protection [63].

Treatment complications

Depending on the type of wound infected, topical and/or systemic antibiotic and antimicrobial treatments are used. Topical antibiotic therapy carries a relatively high risk of allergic sensitization, especially the aminoglycosides neomycin, kanamycin and gentamicin, as well as chloramphenicol and sulphonamides. Drug rashes are also common with systemic antibiotics. These agents should therefore be used only when indicated.

A number of topically active antimicrobial substances, such as quaternary amines, 0.5% chlorhexidine solution, gentian violet and other traditional dyes, have been shown to slow down wound healing or even cause ulcers [64].

Iodine-containing agents are highly active against most pathogens. Povidone-iodine has a high germicidal activity. The 10% PVP-I solution contains 1% iodine, but the concentration of free iodine is only 0.001%, making this preparation less toxic, irritant and sensitizing. However, prolonged use has been shown to produce an ulceration of the tip of a finger. The relatively poor acral blood supply was thought to be responsible for this rare side-effect [65].

References

1 Moy LS. Management of acute wounds. *Dermatol Clin* 1993; **11**: 759–766.

2 Steinert M, Breuninger H, Heeg P, Rassner G. Die Durchführung infektionsprophylaktischer Maßnahmen und deren Auswirkung auf die Infektionsrate. In: Breuninger H, Rassner G (eds) *Operationsplanung und Erfolgskontrolle*. Fortschritte der operativen Dermatologie 5, Springer, Berlin, Heidelberg, New York, 1989, pp. 53–58.

3 Martin C. Antimicrobial prophylaxis in surgery: general concepts and clinical guidelines. *Infect Control Hosp Epidemiol* 1994; **15**: 463–471.

4 Bencini PL, Galimberti M, Signorini M. Utility of topical benzoyl peroxide for prevention of surgical skin wound infection. *J Dermatol Surg Oncol* 1994; **20**: 538–540.

5 Carmichael AJ, Flanagan PG, Holt PJA, Duerden BI. The occurrence of bacteraemia with skin surgery. *Br J Dermatol* 1996; **134**: 120–122.

6 Duane CW, Donald JG, Sally SJ. Wound infection rate in dermatologic surgery. *J Dermatol Surg Oncol* 1988; **14**: 525–528.

7 Futoryan T, Grande D. Postoperative wound infection rates in dermatologic surgery. *Dermatol Surg* 1995; **21**: 509–514.

8 Haas AF, Grekin RC. Antibiotic prophylaxis in dermatologic surgery. *J Am Acad Dermatol* 1995; **32**: 155–176.

9 Hartel W, Steinmann R. Prioritäten für ein infektionsarmes Operieren aus der Sicht des Chirurgen. *Hyg Med* 1986; **11**: 445–447.

10 Haneke E, Storbeck K. Developments and techniques in general dermatologic surgery. *Curr Opin Dermatol* 1996; **3**: 151–157.

11 Rantala A, Lehtonen O-P, Niinikoski J. Heavy consumption of alcohol increases the risk for wound infections. In: *7th Eur Cong Clin Microbiol Inf Dis, Vienna, Book of Abstracts*. 1995, p. 242 (abstract 1246).

12 Alexander JW, MacMillan BG, Law EJ, Kummel R. Prophylactic antibiotics as an adjunct for skin grafting in clean reconstructive surgery following burn injury. *J Trauma* 1982; **22**: 687–690.

13 Vincent JL. Incidence of infections in the ICU—the EPIC study. In: *7th Eur Cong Clin Microbiol Inf Dis, Vienna, Book of Abstracts*. 1995, p. 309 (abstract 73).

14 Twum Danso K, Grant C, Al-Suleiman SA *et al*. Microbiology of postoperative wound infection: a prospective study of 1770 wounds. *J Hosp Infect* 1992; **21**: 29–37.

15 Aly R, Levit S. The changing spectrum of streptococcal and staphylococcal disease. *Curr Opin Dermatol* 1993; **1**: 290–295.

16 Greenberg RG, Berger TG. Postoperative *Trichosporon beigelii* soft tissue infection. *J Dermatol Surg Oncol* 1989; **15**: 432–434.

17 Serrano G. Criocirugía. Dermoabrasión. In: Camacho F, de Dulanto F (eds) *Cirugía Dermatológica*. Grupo Aula Medica, Madrid, 1995, pp. 275–287, 297–302.

18 Alexander JW, Kaplan JZ, Altermeier WA. Role of suture materials in the development of wound infection. *Ann Surg* 1967; **165**: 192–199.

19 Mouzas GL, Yeadon A. Does the choice of suture material affect the incidence of wound infection? A comparison of dexon (polyglycolic acid) sutures with other commonly used sutures in an accident and emergency department. *Br J Surg* 1975; **62**: 952–955.

20 Nockemann PF. *Die chirurgische Naht*. Thieme, Stuttgart, New York, 1980, p. 16.

21 Thompson KD, Welikyj S, Massa MC. Antibacterial activity of lidocaine in combination with a bicarbonate buffer. *J Dermatol Surg Oncol* 1993; **19**: 216–220.

22 Hutchinson JJ. Prevalence of wound infection under occlusive dressings: a collective survey of reported research. *Wounds* 1989; **1**: 123–133.

23 Overholt EM, Flint PW, Overholt EL, Murakami CS. Necrotizing fasciitis of the eyelids. *Otolaryngol Head Neck Surg* 1992; **106**: 339–344.

24 Blank AA, Eichmann F. Operative Therapie der Hyperhidrosis axillaris: Indikationsabwägung und Komplikationen. In: Konz B, Braun-Falco O (eds) *Komplikationen in der operativen Dermatologie*. Springer, Berlin, Heidelberg, New York, 1984, pp. 73–81.

25 Camacho F, de Dulanto F. *Cirugía Dermatológica*. Grupo Aula Medica, Madrid, 1995.

26 Stephenson H, Dotters DJ, Vatz V, Droegemueller W. Necrotizing fasciitis of the vulva. *Am J Obstetr Gynecol* 1992; **166**: 1324–1327.

27 Nolan TE, King LA, Smith RP, Gallup DC. Necrotizing surgical infection and necrotizing fasciitis in obstetrical and gynecologic patients. *South Med J* 1993; **86**: 1363–1367.

28 Farley DE, Katz VL, Dotters DJ. Toxic shock syndrome associated with vulvar necrotizing fasciitis. *Obstetr Gynecol* 1993; **82**: 660–662.

29 Johnson TM, Ratner D, Nelson BR. Soft tissue reconstruction with skin grafting. *J Am Acad Dermatol* 1992; **27**: 151–165.

30 Camacho Martínez F. Skin grafts. In: Harahap M (ed.) *Principles of Dermatologic Plastic Surgery*. PMA, New York, 1988, pp. 95–134.

31 Haneke E. Indications for skin flaps and mechanism of flap survival. In: Harahap M (ed.) *Principles of Dermatologic Plastic Surgery*. PMA, New York, 1988, pp. 145–155.

32 Argenta LC. Advances in tissue expansion. *Clin Plast Surg* 1985; **12**: 159–171.

33 Austad ED. Tissue expansion techniques. *Arch Dermatol* 1987; **123**: 588–589.

34 Austad ED. Complications in tissue expansion. *Clin Plast Surg* 1987; **14**: 549–550.

35 Fulton JE. The prevention and management of post-dermabrasion complications. *J Dermatol Surg Oncol* 1991; **17**: 431–437.

36 Raab B. A new hydrophilic copolymer membrane for dermabrasion. *J Dermatol Surg Oncol* 1991; **17**: 323–328.

37 Matarasso SL, Glogau RG. Chemical face peels. *Dermatol Clin* 1991; **9**: 131–150.

38 Ho C, Nguyen Q, Lowe NJ, Griffin ME, Lask G. Laser resurfacing in pigmented skin. *Dermatol Surg* 1995; **21**: 1035–1037.

39 Lowe JN, Lask G, Griffin ME. Laser skin resurfacing: pre- and posttreatment guidelines. *Dermatol Surg* 1995; **21**: 1017–1019.

40 Collins PS. The chemical peel. *Clin Dermatol* 1987; **5**: 57–74.

41 Asken S. Unoccluded Baker–Godon phenol peels: review and update. *J Dermatol Surg Oncol* 1989; **15**: 998–1008.

42 Brody HJ. Complications of chemical peeling. *J Dermatol Surg Oncol* 1989; **15**: 1010–1019.

43 Waldorf HA, Kauvar ANB, Geronemus RG. Skin resurfacing of fine to deep rhytides

using a char-free carbon dioxide laser in 47 patients. *Dermatol Surg* 1995; **21**: 940–946.

44 Bernstein G, Hanke CW. Safety of liposuction: a review of 9478 cases performed by dermatologists. *J Dermatol Surg Oncol* 1988; **14**: 1112–1114.

45 Teimourian B, Rogers WB III. A national survey of complications associated with suction lipectomy: a comparative study. *Plast Reconstr Surg* 1989; **84**: 628–631.

46 Swartz MN. Bacterial diseases of the skin. In: Rakel RE (ed.) *Conn's Current Therapy 1994.* Saunders, Philadelphia, 1994, pp. 778–783.

47 Dubin DB, Johnson RA. Necrotizing soft-tissue infections. *Curr Opin Dermatol* 1995; **2**: 235–242.

48 Eckert JW, Abramson SL, Starke J, Brandt ML. The surgical implications of chronic granulomatous disease. *Am J Surg* 1995; **169**: 320–323.

49 Yu CC-W, Cook MG. Hidradenitis suppurativa: a disease of follicular epithelium, rather than apocrine glands. *Br J Dermatol* 1990; **122**: 763–769.

50 Banerjee AK. Surgical treatment of hidradenitis suppurativa. *Br J Surg* 1992; **79**: 863–866.

51 Hilker O. Die klinischen Eigenschaften und die effektive operative Therapie der Pyodermia fistulans sinifica. In: Haneke E (ed.) *Gegenwärtiger Stand der operativen Dermatologie.* Fortschritte der operativen Dermatologie 4, Springer, Berlin, Heidelberg, New York, 1988, pp. 255–261.

52 Lapins J, Marcusson JA, Emtestam L. Surgical treatment of chronic hidradenitis suppurativa: CO_2 laser stripping—secondary intention techique. *Br J Dermatol* 1994; **131**: 551–556.

53 Voros D, Pissiotis C, Georganta D, Katsargakis S, Antoniou S, Papadimitriou J. Role of early and extensive surgery in the treatment of severe necrotising soft tissue infection. *Br J Surg* 1993; **80**: 1191–1192.

54 Fankhauser G, Vereb L, Maurer W. Sekundärverschluss von Hautdefekten unter Anwendung von Gummizügen (dynamische Sekundärnaht). *Chirurg* 1995; **66**: 1154–1157.

55 Strich R, Böhm HJ. Dynamische Hautnaht zum sekundären Hautverschluss und zur Behandlung von Hautdefekten. *Swiss Surg* 1995; **5**: 236–240.

56 Ascherman JA, Hugo NE, Sultan MR, Patsis MC, Smith CR, Rose EA. Single-stage treatment of sternal wound complications in heart transplant recipients in whom pectoralis major myocutaneous advancement flaps were used. *J Thorac Cardiovasc Surg* 1995; **110**: 1030–1036.

57 Maurer F, Müller J, Horst F, Seboldt H. The sternocleidomastoid flap for treatment of a septic sternum defect. *Thorac Cardiovasc Surg* 1995; **43**: 236–238.

58 Glorioso L, Webster GF. The role of surgery in the management of uncommon skin infections. *Dermatol Surg* 1995; **21**: 136–144.

59 Garden JM, O'Banin MK, Shelnitz LS *et al.* Papillomavirus in the vapor of carbon dioxide laser-treated verrucae. *JAMA* 1988; **259**: 1199–1202.

60 Sawchuk WS, Weber PJ, Lowry DR, Dzubow LM. Infectious papillomavirus in the vapor of warts treated with carbon dioxide laser or electrocoagulation: detection and protection. *J Am Acad Dermatol* 1989; **21**: 41–49.

61 Colver GB, Peutherer JF. Herpes simplex virus dispersal by Hyfrecator electrodes. *Br J Dermatol* 1987; **117**: 627–629.

62 Wheeland RG. *Lasers in Skin Disease.* Thieme Med Publ, Stuttgart, New York, 1988.

63 Nezhat C, Winer WK, Nezhat F, Nezhat C, Forrest D, Reeves WG. Smoke from laser surgery: is there a health hazard? *Lasers Surg Med* 1987; **7**: 376–382.

64 Niedner R, Schöpf E. Inhibition of wound healing by antiseptics. *Br J Dermatol* 1986; **115**: 41–44.

65 Mochida K, Hisa T, Yasunaga C, Nishimura T, Nakagawa K, Hamada T. Skin ulceration due to povidone-iodine. *Contact Derm* 1995; **33**: 61–62.

Antibiotic prophylaxis
Ann F. Haas

The subject of antibiotic prophylaxis is controversial for many practitioners in many disciplines, including dermatology. Historically, antibiotics have been given either to prevent wound infection or to prevent the potential for infective endocarditis (IE) in patients or for situations deemed to be 'high-risk'. Even the recommendations for antibiotic prophylaxis for non-dermatological procedures remain controversial and are not uniformly accepted, considered uniformly effective or uniformly adhered to. There have been no large, multivariate studies to help us define what is the actual risk for either wound infection or endocarditis following dermatological surgery procedures. Although there are a few small studies and case reports in the dermatological literature, most of the data that form the basis for defining the 'at-risk' population come from the general surgical or dental literature.

Wound-infection prophylaxis

Surgical-wound classification

The general surgical literature has classified surgical wounds, for the purpose of anticipating risk of infection, into four categories.

Class I (clean) wounds are those performed on non-contaminated skin with sterile technique, and would include such dermatological procedures as excision of non-inflamed cysts and excision of tumours. This class is associated with a <5% postoperative infection rate.

Class II (clean-contaminated) wounds result from procedures performed in contaminated areas, such as the mouth, respiratory tract, axilla or perineum, or which have minor breaks in aseptic technique. Most dermatological surgery procedures fall into either this classification (associated with a 10% infection rate) or the class I group.

Class III (contaminated) wounds include traumatic wounds, inflamed (non-purulent) wounds and procedures with major breaks in sterile technique. Such procedures as removal of intact, inflamed cysts and tumours with inflammation are included in this group, which is associated with a 20–30% infection rate.

Class IV (infected) wounds are those which are grossly contaminated or have devitalized tissue and would include ruptured cysts, hidradenitis and tumours with purulence or with necrotic material. This class has a potential infection rate of 30–40%.

Antibiotics have customarily been given to prevent wound infection when dealing with a significant risk of infection or where there might be severe consequences of infection. The Centers for Disease Control (CDC) state that, 'prophylaxis is most useful for operations associated with a moderate level of contamination' [1]. It is generally accepted that the routine use of systemic antibiotic prophylaxis for class I wounds is of no benefit, as the incidence of wound infection is already very low [2–4]. Although one study suggested that antibiotic prophylaxis might be beneficial for selected superficial, clean procedures, such as breast and hernia operations [5] the study was subject to criticism [6]. The greatest controversy exists for prophylaxis of class III wounds. Although there are studies failing to show a benefit when antibiotics are administered for otological, sinonasal or facial plastic/reconstructive procedures of the head and neck with exposure to mucosa-lined cavities [2], there are a significant number of other studies which do demonstrate the efficacy of perioperative antibiotics in reducing wound infection in clean-contaminated head and neck surgical procedures [3, 7, 8]. Probably the majority of the head and neck literature recommends giving antibiotics perioperatively for clean-contaminated head and neck procedures involving incision through oral or pharyngeal mucosa. Antibiotics are considered therapeutic, not prophylactic, for class III and class IV wounds.

Most dermatological surgery procedures fall into the clean and clean-contaminated classes, and the overall incidence of wound infection is thought to be low, so prophylaxis is not routinely recommended in a recent review [9]. This review does suggest certain circumstances for which antibiotic prophlaxis might be warranted. It has been suggested that those patients undergoing dermatological surgical procedures involving oronasal areas invading mucosa, gastrointestinal and genitourinary areas and axilla (areas considered 'contaminated') should receive prophylactic antibiotics (Table 10.3) [9].

Certain other factors that can contribute to risk of development of wound infection, apart from wound classification, need also to be considered, such as the surgical site, nature and length of the procedure, level of contamination and overall health of the patient. Because the incidence of wound infection in clean or clean-contaminated surgery is so low, estimation of potential success of any given prophylactic regimen to decrease the incidence of infection would require very large numbers of patients to obtain data achieving statistical significance [10]. From a review of the general surgical literature (where, admittedly, most patients undergo procedures involving penetration of a hollow viscus and have operating-room procedures with in-hospital recovery periods), there are some factors which may be significant in affecting the incidence of wound infection.

Environmental risk factors

There are a number of environmental risk factors that may influence development of wound infection. The duration of preoperative hospital stay has been correlated with development of postoperative wound infections [11], as has the length of the operation [12]. With each hour of surgery, the

Table 10.3 Suggestions for wound infection prophylaxis [9].

	Skin	Oral cavity	GI/GU	GI/GU
Organism	*Staphylococcus aureus*	*Streptococcus viridans*	*Escherichia coli*	Enterococcus
Antibiotic/ dose*	1 gen cephalosporin 1 g p.o./500 mg p.o.	1 gen cephalosporin 1 g p.o./500 mg p.o.	1 gen cephalosporin 1 g p.o./500 mg p.o.	Vancomycin 500 mg i.v./ 250 mg i.v.
	Dicloxicillin 1 g p.o./500 mg p.o.	Amoxycillin 3 g p.o./1.5 g p.o.	TMP-SMX (DS) 1 tablet p.o.†	
	Clindamycin‡ 300 mg p.o./150 mg p.o.	Erythromycin‡ 1 g p.o./500 mg p.o.	Ciprofloxacin 500 mg p.o.†	
	Vancomycin§ 500 mg i.v./250 mg i.v.	Clindamycin‡ 300 mg p.o./150 mg p.o.		

* Recommended dose is a single preoperative dose, unless it is a prolonged case in a contaminated area with a significant risk of infection; then consider a second dose 6 hours after the initial dose given.
† Can repeat dose at 12 hours, for long cases in contaminated areas.
‡ Choices for penicillin-allergic patients.
§ If *Staphylococcus epidermidis* is present and considered a true pathogen.
GI/GU, gastrointestinal/genitourinary; p.o., by mouth; i.v., intravenously.

infection rate can almost double, and it has been recommended that an antibiotic dose be repeated during long procedures [11, 13]. When faced with preoperative shaving of a hair-bearing area, the current recommendation is to clip the hair, rather than to shave (actually, best to do neither, if possible), as preoperative shaving a day before surgery is associated with a higher wound infection rate [12]. Preoperative showering with an antiseptic soap has been demonstrated to decrease postoperative wound-infection rates when done the evening prior to surgery. The presence of remote infection has been demonstrated to negatively influence postoperative wound-infection rate and it is recommended that treatment of a urinary-tract, respiratory-tract or remote skin infection be instituted prior to the surgical procedure [14]. Reports of other factors, such as surgical technique, gloving practices and hand-washing techniques, show a variable degree of influence in development of postoperative wound infections [12].

Patient risk factors

Several patient risk factors have been positively identified as contributing to the development of postoperative wound infection. Malnutrition has been associated with the development of a number of postoperative complications, including wound infection, either as a single factor or in combination with anergy [11, 15]. In one study, perioperative short-term prophylactic antibiotics significantly reduced the risk of postoperative wound infection in malnourished, anergic patients [15], although this has not uniformly been the case for anergic patients (without malnutrition), who also are thought to have higher incidences of postoperative wound infection [15–17]. The uraemia associated with chronic renal failure has been associated with a number of decreased immune functions, as well as with postoperative wound infections [18]. Studies have suggested that increased patient age is correlated with an increase in wound infection rate (and a lower incidence of postoperative infections is seen in children) [19].

Diabetes mellitus and obesity have a combined and an independent incidence of increased postoperative wound infection [20]. Diabetes is associated with a number of immune-system abnormalities and the assumption that diabetics are predisposed to infection is controversial [21]. The incidence of postoperative infections in diabetics is variable and some investigators believe that infections may be no more common in well-controlled diabetics than in the general population. Infections in diabetics may be more difficult to treat [21]. Although diabetes and obesity have been implicated as causal factors for increased wound infection rates following cardiac surgery [22], a study of postoperative wound infections following head and neck surgical procedures did not find a statistically significant incidence of postoperative wound infections in the diabetic population [23].

Corticosteroids depress leucocyte function and have been known to increase infectious complications when administered to patients with head trauma [24]. A study of post-transplant patients taking immunosuppressants, such as corticosteroids and cyclosporin, found that there was a significant risk of nosocomial wound infections following post-transplant reconstructive surgical procedures (again, most of these patients had procedures done in the operating-room with in-hospital recovery periods, making extrapolation of these data to the out-patient setting somewhat difficult) [25]. It has been suggested that if steroids are withheld until after the third day after wounding, the deleterious effects on wound healing are significantly reduced [26]. For patients otherwise immunosuppressed because of intrinsic immunological disease, it has been suggested that prophylactic antibiotics be given when 'the insult of the surgical procedure will result in significant bacterial contamination or when the patient's host defences are inadequate to resist a bacterial insult of any size' [27] or 'for patients in whom normal mechanisms for control of bacteremia and septicemia are inadequate' [28]. The *Medical Letter on Drugs and Therapeutics* consultants have suggested that prophylactic antibiotics should be given to patients receiving cytotoxic drugs when the granulocyte count falls below 1000/mm³, while realizing that antibiotics in this situation can cause colonization with resistant organisms [29]. The human immunodeficiency virus (HIV)-positive group of patients represents a unique group of immunocompromised patients in terms of antibiotic prophylaxis for wound infection. Although it would seem otherwise, an increased risk of wound infection following invasive procedures in these patients has not been described [30, 31], except for patients with acquired immune deficiency syndrome (AIDS) undergoing anorectal procedures [32, 33].

There is no standardization of recommendations for antibiotic prophylaxis for patients 'at risk' to develop postoperative wound infection. It is prudent to consult a patient's specific subspecialist (transplant surgeon, oncologist, etc.), who may have protocols for treating those patients who undergo certain types of invasive procedures. Because dermatological surgery tends to have unique characteristics, consultation with a subspecialist also helps educate him/her in terms of the nature of a proposed procedure, so that an educated decision regarding the need for antibiotic prophylaxis can be made. For dermatological-surgery procedures (which are out-patient procedures, usually of short duration and associated with a low risk of significant infection), the recommendation has been made that, unless the 'at-risk' patient is at significant risk for major morbidity from a postoperative wound infection, antibiotics are not suggested for procedures for which non-'at-risk' patients would not be given antibiotics [9]. Clearly, however, each patient needs to be dealt with on an individual basis.

Antibiotics for prophylaxis

The treatment of wound infections is well discussed in another section. For the purposes of prophylaxis, the selection of an appropriate antibiotic is based on the probable microbial causative organism. It is most commonly the case that *Staphylococcus aureus* causes the greater proportion of skin infections, with *Streptococcus viridans* causing most of the oral-cavity infections and *Escherichia coli* or enterococcus causing most of the infections of skin surrounding the gastrointestinal and genitourinary tracts. Although *Staphylococcus epidermidis*, which is usually considered resident flora, is a causal agent for prosthetic-valve endocarditis (PVE) and for vascular-graft infection, it is not a common pathogen in wound infections. There have, however, been reported cases where *S. epidermidis* was considered the pathogen in sternal incisions of cardiothoracic patients who had sternal wires removed prior to the infection. Recent antibiotic-prophylaxis recommendations for wound-infection prophylaxis in dermatological surgery are given in Table 10.3. It should be noted that, for *S. aureus* coverage in the penicillin-allergic patient, erythromycin is no longer considered a good choice because of the significant resistance of the organism to the drug. Vancomycin is also a drug which, although difficult to use in the dermatology setting because it must be given intravenously, is becoming more of an issue due to the emergence of drug resistances. It is considered the drug of choice for *S. epidermidis* when *S. epidermidis* is considered a pathogen, for methicillin-resistant *S. aureus* (MRSA) and for patients with prosthetic cardiac valves less than 60 days old. In addition, emergent strains of enterococci are now being seen, rendering cephalosporins, nafcillin and gentamicin ineffective in treating this organism. The CDC is now reporting rapid emergence of vancomycin-resistant enterococci nationwide, causing many hospital infectious-disease departments to place restrictions on vancomycin use. If vancomycin is truly needed for prophylaxis for wound infection or endocarditis (see next section), contacting the infectious-disease specialist at the nearest referral centre might be wise.

Appropriate timing of antibiotic dose for prophylaxis may be as important as the selection of the antibiotic agent. Most modern surgical literature recommends starting antibiotics prior to the procedure, so that the drug can be incorporated into the wound coagulum. This recommendation is based on studies by Burke, who found that antibiotics are ineffective if given more than 3 hours after the start of wounding, because the coagulum which develops in the wound isolates trapped bacteria from the circulating antibiotic [34, 35]. The duration of antibiotic dosing is less clear. Studies have shown that a single preoperative dose of an antibiotic provides optimal prophylaxis and postoperative doses yield no further benefit [11, 36, 37]. The *Medical Letter on Drugs and Therapeutics* states that: 'a single dose of a parenteral antimicrobial given within 30 minutes of an operation usually provides adequate tissue concentrations throughout the procedure . . . When surgery is delayed or prolonged, a second dose is advisable. Postoperative administration of prophylactic drugs is usually unnecessary and may be harmful' [13]. Although some investigators feel that the preoperative dose should be followed by a second dose 6 hours later for prolonged procedures for up to a 24-hour course of treatment [4, 38, 39], many clinical trials found no reduction in septic complications when a single preoperative dose only of an antibiotic was compared with outcome in cases where a multiple-dose regimen was used [13, 37, 40]. The fact that investigations seem to indicate that an antibiotic agent should be in the tissue until bacterial contamination ceases (usually at wound closure) [37] forms the basis for the recommendations given in Table 10.3, particularly with respect to the addition of a postoperative dose in a prolonged case in a contaminated area, if dealing with significant risk of infection [9].

One other type of wound, the 'granulating wound', should be mentioned. Dermatological surgery is unique in that wounds are often created which are not sutured. Unless the wound is located in an area that is considered contaminated, open wounds, although they do get colonized, rarely get infected if they are properly cared for [41]. Since it appears that postoperative doses of antibiotics would not penetrate the coagulum that seals these wounds, a single preoperative dose of an antibiotic would be the most effective approach for prevention of potential wound infection of open wounds in areas of the body considered to be contaminated.

Endocarditis prophylaxis

There is a great deal of controversy in many specialities regarding appropriate endocarditis prophylaxis for certain patients and certain procedures. The American Heart Association (AHA) guidelines are often used as the basis for decision-making regarding endocarditis prophylaxis; unfortunately, they do not cover most dermatological surgery procedures, and it may be the case that those recommendations may not be effective. It is interesting that the incidence of IE in a general population has not changed since the advent of antibiotic prophylaxis [42, 43]. The reasons for the controversy will be examined, as will the small quantity of data in the dermatology literature and the rationale behind recent suggested guidelines published for dermatological surgery.

The AHA's guidelines are based on several theories, many of which are not well substantiated. It has been postulated that individuals with specific heart anomalies may be 'at risk' for developing IE. It has also been assumed that giving antimicrobial therapy against primarily streptococci (assuming that streptococci cause most cases of endocarditis and that it has predictable antibiotic susceptibility patterns) to those persons 'at risk' undergoing certain 'at-risk' procedures will decrease the risk of subsequent endocarditis development. The 'at-risk' procedures are thought to involve trauma to mucosal surfaces, thought likely to produce bacteraemia. The reality is that the precise risk of endocarditis is not known for any specific type of cardiac lesion or for any specific traumatic procedure. Streptococci may no longer cause most cases of endocarditis and may no longer have predictable antibiotic susceptibility patterns (e.g. enterococci (group D streptococci) are more commonly pathogenic after lower gastrointestinal and genitourinary procedures and do not have a predictable susceptibility pattern). Most important, there have been no adequate, controlled clinical trials of antibiotic regimens to document that antibiotic therapy is even effective in preventing endocarditis in the presence of bacteraemia (and it is likely that such a study will not be carried out, because of the large patient population needed to achieve statistical significance, not to mention the ethical difficulties in dealing with the control group).

Infective endocarditis is an infection of the endocardial surface, most commonly of heart valves, but septal defects, arteriovenous shunts and arterioatrial shunts, as well as mural endocardium and coarctation of the aorta, have also been implicated. Streptococci and staphylococci account for 80–90% of cases, although many organisms have been implicated in IE. Prosthetic-valve endocarditis can occur 'early', when onset is within 60 days of prosthetic-valve placement, or 'late', when onset is beyond 60 days of valve placement. *Staphylococcus epidermidis* is the most common cause of early PVE; however, aerobic Gram-negative bacilli and fungi are becoming more important agents. In terms of microbiology, late PVE resembles native-valve endocarditis, in that non-group D *Streptococcus* is a major causal agent [44].

Examining mitral-valve prolapse (MVP) illustrates some of the problems with endocarditis prophylaxis. Although MVP is commonly seen in the population and reported to have a five to eight times greater risk of endocarditis than the general population (and 13 times greater if regurgitation is present) [45–47], the absolute risk of developing endocarditis is small. In patients with MVP without mitral regurgitation, the risk of penicillin-induced anaphylaxis has been shown to be greater than the risk of death from endocarditis [45]. Because of this, the current recommendations suggest prophylaxis for MVP only for those who have a systolic murmur, particularly men over age 45 [47–52].

Transient bacteraemia is a significant consideration in potential development of endocarditis. Although bacteraemia is common after many invasive procedures (particularly after procedures or instrumentation involving mucosal surfaces or contaminated tissue) [44, 48, 53], it is usually short-lived (approximately 15 minutes) and the actual incidence of endocarditis in humans after bacteraemia is uncertain. In addition, although bacteraemia is common after many invasive procedures, only a few bacterial species are common causes of endocarditis. Random bacteraemias are common and can occur after such routine activities as tooth-brushing, dental-flossing, defecation and mastication (Table 10.4) [54]. Mucosal damage caused by defecation has been thought to be a portal of entry for enterococcal endocarditis and cases of *S. viridans* endocarditis have been reported in edentulous patients, probably as a result of mucosal trauma [55]. Understandably, patients with underlying cardiac disease may always be at some risk for developing endocarditis and it may be impossible to determine with certainty which bacteraemia might have caused any given episode of endocarditis. One large study of 544 episodes of IE in 541 patients found that, in 60% of patients, the portal of entry of the infection could not be identified [56]. In a retrospective study of cases of endocarditis seen in residents of Olmsted County, Minnesota, over a 30-year period, no source of infection could be identified in 41% of cases, including half of those cases with rheumatic or congenital heart disease [57]. Similarly, another study found that only about 15% of all cases of endocarditis have been associated with medical, surgical or dental procedures [58]. Ideally, to determine when to provide antibiotics for prophylaxis of endocarditis, the risk of endocarditis after any given procedure needs to be considered, as does the 'incubation period' for development of endocarditis, and neither of these is known. In examining the dental literature, although it is known that invasive dental procedures do cause bacteraemia, they are generally of low intensity and brief duration, with blood becoming sterile 15–30 minutes following the procedure [37, 54]. The risk of IE following a dental extraction is probably low, because bacteraemia is common after that pro-

Chewing sweets or paraffin
Brushing teeth
Using an oral irrigation device
Using unwaxed dental floss
Defecation

Table 10.4 Selected daily events known to cause transient bacteraemias [54].

cedure and endocarditis is relatively rare. Several reviews have suggested that bacteraemias induced by dental procedures and IE may be associated in fewer than 4% of cases [59–61]. Although there have been studies that suggest that endocarditis occurred relatively soon after an antecedent dental procedure, other studies indicate that less than 15% of patients with IE had dental treatment in the prior 3 months [62, 63]. In examining statistics for the risk of bacteraemia from patient-related vs. dental-related activities, one author concluded that, 'in any situation where dental treatment is judged the cause of IE, the odds are 100 times greater that the IE was patient-caused rather than dentist-induced' [64]. Some authors feel that delivering good oral hygiene in order to decrease daily bacteraemia may be more effective in preventing endocarditis than giving antibiotics prior to specific dental procedures [59, 65, 66].

Not only is it unclear which procedures might be causally related to endocarditis and thus would require prophylaxis, it is also unclear which cardiac lesions are truly a 'risk'. It has been thought that about 50% of patients who get IE do not have a recognized predisposing cardiac lesion for which prophylaxis would be considered [42, 55, 60, 67].

Despite the fact that the AHA guidelines have defined certain procedures and certain cardiac lesions which should be considered for endocarditis prophylaxis (Tables 10.5 and 10.6) [48], as well as suggestions for appropriate antibiotic selections, the efficacy of these regimens has not

Table 10.5 AHA guidelines for endocarditis prophylaxis: cardiac conditions [48].*

Endocarditis prophylaxis recommended
Prosthetic cardiac valves, including bioprosthetic and homograft valves
Previous bacterial endocarditis, even in the absence of heart disease
Most congenital cardiac malformations
Rheumatic and other acquired valvular dysfunction, even after valvular surgery
Hypertrophic cardiomyopathy
Mitral-valve prolapse with valvular regurgitation

Endocarditis prophylaxis not recommended
Isolated secundum atrial septal defect
Surgical repair without residua beyond 6 months of secundum atrial septal defect,
    ventricular septal defect or patent ductus arteriosus
Previous coronary-artery bypass graft surgery
Mitral-valve prolapse without valvular regurgitation†
Physiological functional or innocent heart murmurs
Previous Kawasaki disease without valvular dysfunction
Previous rheumatic fever without valvular dysfunction
Cardiac pacemakers and implanted defibrillators

* This table lists selected conditions and is not meant to be all-inclusive.
† Individuals who have a mitral-valve prolapse associated with thickening and/or redundancy of the valve leaflets may be at increased risk for bacterial endocarditis, particularly men who are 45 years of age or older.
AHA, American Heart Association.

Table 10.6 AHA guidelines for endocarditis prophylaxis: dental or surgical procedures [48].*

Endocarditis prophylaxis recommended
Dental procedures known to induce gingival or mucosal bleeding, including professional cleaning
Tonsillectomy and/or adenoidectomy
Surgical operations that involve intestinal or respiratory mucosa
Bronchoscopy with a rigid bronchoscope
Sclerotherapy for oesophageal varices
Oesophageal dilatation
Gall-bladder surgery
Cystoscopy
Urethral dilatation
Urethral catheterization if UTI present
Urinary-tract surgery if UTI present†
Prostatic surgery
Incision and drainage of infected tissue†
Vaginal hysterectomy
Vaginal delivery in the presence of infection†

Endocarditis prophylaxis not recommended‡
Dental procedures not likely to induce gingival bleeding, such as simple adjustment of orthodontic appliances or fillings above the gum line
Injection of local intraoral anaesthetic (except intraligamentary injections)
Shedding of primary teeth
Tympanostomy-tube insertion
Endotracheal intubation
Bronchoscopy with a flexible bronchoscope, with or without biopsy
Cardiac catheterization
Endoscopy with or without gastrointestinal biopsy
Caesarean section
In the absence of infection for: urethral catheterization, dilatation and curettage, uncomplicated vaginal delivery, therapeutic abortion, sterilization procedures or insertion/removal of intrauterine devices

* This table lists selected procedures and is not meant to be all-inclusive.
† In addition to prophylactic regimen for genitourinary procedures, antibiotic therapy should be directed against the most likely bacterial pathogen.
‡ In patients who have prosthetic heart valves, a previous history of endocarditis or surgically constructed systemic–pulmonary shunts or conduits, physicians may choose to administer prophylactic antibiotics even for low-risk procedures that involve the lower respiratory, genitourinary or gastrointestinal tracts.
AHA, American Heart Association; UTI, urinary-tract infection.

been proved by controlled clinical trials. In a registry of cases of IE following endocarditis prophylaxis which were reported to the AHA, the infecting organism (in cases where sensitivities were known) was sensitive to the antibiotics selected in only 63% of cases and a few of the cases occurred after procedures not recommended for coverage by the AHA [68]. In addition, the incidence of bacterial endocarditis caused by organisms such as *S. aureus,* Gram-negative bacilli and fungi has increased and these organisms would not be covered by the AHA regimens now recommended, which are directed primarily at *S. viridans* or enterococci. In addition to the fact that the complete spectrum of causal organisms is not covered by the current AHA regimen and the fact that all 'at-risk' cardiac patients cannot be accurately identified, the fact that many cases of endocarditis do not necessarily follow procedures and can occur as a result of non-surgical events may further render the AHA guidelines ineffective. Consequently, because of the lack of susceptibility of certain causal organisms to the current AHA regimens, lack of recognized predisposing factors in many patients and the high incidence of daily transient bacteraemias, Kaye has calculated that probably fewer than 10% of cases of endocarditis are theoretically preventable [67].

There have been very few studies which have looked at the cost–benefit ratio of antibiotic prophylaxis for endocarditis. Tzukert *et al.* examined the AHA's recommendations for the prevention of dental-induced IE and concluded that 1.36 persons per million are likely to die from anaphylaxis due to penicillin prophylaxis and that only 0.26 deaths per million persons are caused by dental-related IE [61]. The suggestion from this study and from other similar studies arriving at similar conclusions [45, 64] was that the risk–benefit ratio is favourable only in the highest IE incidence/mortality group and that the value of prophylaxis in moderate or lower-risk patients was doubtful. In addition to the low but present risk of morbidity and death from penicillin anaphylaxis, there is the issue of increasingly resistant strains of *S. aureus*, streptococci and enterococci, which is becoming a significant therapeutic problem and has probably resulted from overuse of antibiotics. Because of these considerations, the AHA recommends antibiotic prophylaxis only to patients with high-risk cardiac lesions undergoing procedures with a high risk of bacteraemia (Table 10.5 and 10.6) [62, 65].

Bacteraemia and dermatological surgery

Except for incision and drainage (I and D) of skin infection, dermatological surgery procedures are notably absent from the AHA guidelines for procedures which should receive antibiotic prophylaxis. There have been a few recent studies and case reports which have attempted to define the incidence of bacteraemia following skin surgery. Unfortunately, these few reports contain very low case numbers, so it is impossible to get good statistical data. Certainly, manipulation of infected skin is associated with a high incidence of bacteraemia with organisms that do cause endocarditis [69–71]. The incidence of bacteraemia following surgery on intact skin or on clinically uninfected but eroded skin (both very common situations in dermatology) is almost unknown. Sabetta and Zitelli studied a group of patients undergoing surgical removal of both intact and eroded (but not infected) skin lesions. Preoperative and postoperative blood cultures obtained in this study showed that only one patient (in the eroded group) had transient bacteraemia and led the authors to recommend prophylatic antibiotics only in patients with eroded cutaneous tumours and a prosthetic valve [72]. When random blood cultures were obtained from healthy volunteers, a 2.1% incidence of bacteraemia was found (the predominant organism was *S. epidermidis*) [73]. Blood cultures obtained 30 minutes after the start of scalpel excision or curettage and electrodesiccation of either eroded (non-infected) or intact skin lesions were found to be negative after 14 days [74]. Halpern *et al.* performed blood cultures preoperatively and at 1, 5 and 15 minutes following the start of a number of different types of dermatological surgery procedures (six of the lesions excised were eroded, but not infected). Three patients (7%) had positive blood cultures at 15 minutes after the procedures, but those cultures grew *Propionibacterium acnes* in two and *Staphylococcus hominis* in the other, neither being a common cause of endocarditis [75]. Another study, which did pre- and postprocedure cultures of benign skin lesions treated with curettage and electrodesiccation, found one positive blood culture prior to, but not after, the procedures [76]. However, a recent report causally relates a blood-sampling finger prick which resulted in PVE by *P. acnes* [77]. In the retrospective study of incidence of IE in Olmsted County, one case was noted which 'followed' a skin biopsy; no mention was made of the resulting organism or the nature of the lesion (?eroded, ulcerated) or the type of 'skin biopsy' performed [57]. A recent series of four case reports discusses patients who developed IE (three had known cardiac-valve abnormalities) 'following skin procedures' [78]. Although three of the cases of endocarditis occurred within a week of the presumed causative procedure (the other occurred at 3 weeks postprocedure), the causative agent (*S. epidermidis*) in one of the cases is not a common skin pathogen. Again, because the incidence of transient bacteraemias resulting simply from daily events is so frequent, it is difficult to implicate a given procedure (i.e. was it the excision or was it some other event in the interim which produced the endocarditis-related bacteraemia?) as the cause of a particular episode of endocarditis.

From these few studies, it appears that the incidence of bacteraemia after surgical manipulation of intact skin is low and may not warrant prophylaxis in all high-risk patients in all situations. The actual incidence of bacteraemia from manipulation of eroded skin and the subsequent implications for antibiotic prophylaxis remain unclear. Even if transient bacteraemia is found routinely when doing procedures on eroded skin, is it a serious enough potential cause of endocarditis to warrant prophylaxis in those 'at risk'?

Despite the fact that no adequate controlled trials of the efficacy of antibiotic regimens for prevention of endocarditis have been done in humans and that it is impossible to predict which patients will develop endocarditis or which particular procedures (or daily events) may cause it, recommendations have recently been published regarding endocarditis prophylaxis for dermatological surgery, which were additionally reviewed by a cardiologist, pharmacologist and infectious-disease specialist (Table

Table 10.7 Suggestions for endocarditis prophylaxis [9].

Consider coverage for patients	Procedures
Classifed by AHA as high risk	Manipulation of eroded, not infected skin
Classified by AHA as high risk Patients with orthopaedic prostheses Patients with ventriculoatrial and ventriculoperitoneal shunts	Manipulation of infected skin or if distant skin infection is present

NB: routine coverage not necessary for manipulation of intact skin; those patients with prosthetic valves undergoing long procedures in contaminated areas may require coverage (see text).

Antibiotic selections			
	Skin	Oral cavity	GI/GU
Organism	*Staphylococcus aureus*	*Streptococcus viridans*	Enterococcus

Antibiotic/
dose*
	1 gen cephalosporin
	1 g p.o./500 mg p.o.
	Dicloxicillin
	1 g p.o./500 mg p.o.
		Amoxycillin
		3 g p.o./1.5 mg p.o.
		Erythromycin†
		1 g p.o./500 mg p.o.
			Low risk Ampicillin
			                3 g p.o./1.5 g p.o.
			High risk
			Preop. Ampicillin 2 g p.o.‡
			            Gentamicin 1.5 mg/kg i.v.

	Clindamycin† 300 mg p.o./150 mg p.o. Vancomycin‡ 500 mg i.v./250 mg i.v.	Clindamycin† 300 mg p.o./150 mg p.o.	Postop. Amoxicillin 1.5 mg p.o. or Preop. Vancomycin 1.0 g i.v.‡ Gentamicin 1.5 mg/kg i.v. or i.m. Postop. Can repeat dose 8 hours later

* Give preoperative dose followed by second dose administered 6 hours later.
† Antibiotic choices for penicillin-allergic patients.
‡ For patients with MRSA or proshetic valves less than 60 days old.
AHA, American Heart Association; GI/GU, gastrointestinal/genitourinary; p.o., by mouth; i.v.,
intravascularly; i.m., intramuscularly; MRSA, methicillin-resistant *S. aureus*.

10.7) [9]. These recommendations were based loosely on those of the AHA and the fact that the incidence of bacteraemia following skin surgery (although based on a few, small studies) appears to be low. The pre- and postoperative dosing regimens used are as recommended by the AHA. Although these recommendations suggest prophylaxis for 'high-risk' patients (as defined by the AHA) for surgical manipulation of eroded, non-infected skin, as well as for manipulation of infected skin or in the presence of distant skin infection, these recommendations do not suggest giving routine prophylaxis for 'high-risk' patients undergoing surgery of intact skin for minor procedures, such as biopsies, shave excisions and small simple excisions in clean areas, which can be closed quickly. There certainly may be situations in which it might be appropriate to give antibiotic prophylaxis to certain 'high-risk' patients for intact skin procedures (such as patients with a prosthetic valve who undergo large excisions requiring more than 20 minutes to close and for procedures performed on areas of the skin considered 'contaminated'). Clearly, any set of recommendations needs to be applied on a case-by-case basis. The authors of these recommendations stipulate that, for 'high-risk' patients who undergo a long procedure taking place over several hours prior to wound closure, consideration may be given to one or two postoperative doses as long as the procedure is ongoing. For 'high-risk' patients with large wounds or wounds in contaminated areas which are allowed to heal by second intention, because of the production of coagulum, which was previously discussed, giving only a preoperative dose should be sufficient.

Other prosthetic devices

The recommendations in Table 10.7 also include recommendations for endocarditis prophylaxis for patients with orthopaedic prostheses and those with ventriculoatrial and ventriculoperitoneal shunts. In general, very little is known about the risks of non-valvular prosthetic devices becoming infected after invasive procedures and causing a transient bacteraemia which might secondarily lead to endocarditis. There is virtually nothing known about whether skin procedures can cause secondary infection of a previously implanted prosthetic device. Orthopaedic devices probably represent the largest group of implanted devices that need to be considered. The predominant microorganism involving orthopaedic joint prostheses is *S. aureus*, followed by *S. epidermidis* [79–81]. In cases where haematogenous infection of orthopaedic (or vascular) prostheses has been convincingly implicated, the site of origin has generally been an established infection, not a procedure-related transient bacteraemia [37, 82]. A recent review of dental procedures concludes that evidence is insufficient to justify antibiotic prophylaxis before all dental procedures likely to cause bacteraemia in patients with orthopaedic prostheses [79]. In hip arthroplasties, the infection is usually a clearly identified distant source, such as an abscess, chronic bacteraemia or septicaemia [83, 84]. Although the recommendations are controversial, it has been suggested that antibiotic prophylaxis is not indicated when elective, clean surgery is done at sites other than the prosthetic joint, but antibiotic prophylaxis is recommended if infected tissues are encountered [83]. If there is any question, the patient's orthopaedic surgeon should at least be consulted regarding whether to use antibiotics and the specific choice of antibiotic.

Because of the reasons stated above, the authors of the recommendations noted in Table 10.7 feel that the incidence of bacteraemia after skin surgery is sufficiently low for antibiotic prophylaxis not to be required for patients undergoing dermatological surgery procedures who have haemodialysis and arteriovenous or arterial grafts after the first month of placement (as they become at least partially endothelialized after the first month of placement), unless excising an eroded or contaminated skin lesion within close proximity to the graft [9]. Because the incidence of bacteraemia following skin surgery is so low, the authors also do not recommend prophylaxis in the case of genitourinary prostheses, breast implants or indwelling pacemakers. The AHA recommendation for endocarditis prophylaxis states that the physician 'may choose' whether or not to use antibiotics prior to certain dental or high-risk surgical procedures in patients with indwelling pacemakers. Because there have been documented cases of bacterial endocarditis developing in patients who received ventriculoatrial shunts for hydrocephalus, the AHA states that endocarditis prophylaxis 'deserves consideration' [49], and the authors of the recent recommendations for dermatological surgery also recommend that these patients receive prophylaxis when dealing with infected skin or in the presence of distant skin infection [9]. Again, it is suggested that the rationale for antibiotic prophylaxis in these patients be discussed with the patient's neurosurgeon whenever possible.

It is understandable that many physicians use a 'shotgun approach' to antibiotic use both for prevention of wound infection and for endocarditis prophylaxis. However, given the increasing incidence of resistant bacteria, the risk–benefit issues of actual need for antibiotics vs. potential anaphylaxis or morbidity and the controversies that have been discussed regarding the effectiveness of such regimens, a careful case-by-case approach to administration of antibiotics would seem to be the most prudent. Further investigation is clearly necessary to help resolve the risk issues for bacteraemia following dermatological surgery and, as more becomes known about the incidence of wound infection, the risks for the development of endocarditis and the incidence of bacteraemia following certain procedures, both the AHA guidelines and any subsequent guidelines that are applied to dermatological surgery will continually need to be redefined.

References

1 Centers for Disease Control. *Guidelines for Prevention of Surgical Wound Infections, 1985.* US Department of Health and Human Services, Atlanta, 1985.
2 Johnson J, Wagner R. Infection following uncontaminated head and neck surgery. *Arch Otolaryngol Head Neck Surg* 1987; **113**: 368–369.
3 Weber R, Callender D. Antibiotic prophylaxis in clean-contaminated head and neck oncologic surgery. *Ann Otol Rhinol Laryngol* 1992; **101**: 16–20.
4 Nichols R. Use of prophylactic antibiotics in surgical practice. *Am J Med* 1981; **70**: 686–692.
5 Platt R, Zaleznik D, Hopkins C, Dellinger EP, Karchmer AW, Bryan CS *et al.* Perioperative antibiotic prophylaxis for herniorraphy and breast surgery. *N Engl J Med* 1990; **332**: 153–160.
6 Ergina PS, Gold S, Meakins J. Antibiotic prophylaxis for herniorraphy and breast surgery (letter). *N Engl J Med* 1990; **332**: 1884.
7 Friberg D, Lundberg C. Antibiotic prophylaxis in major head and neck surgery when clean-contaminated wounds are established. *Scand J Infect Dis* 1990; **70**: 87–90.
8 DiPiro J, Record K, Schanzenback K, Bivins BA. Antimicrobial prophylaxis in surgery: part 1. *Am J Hosp Pharmacol* 1981; **38**: 320–334.
9 Haas A, Grekin R. Antibiotic prophylaxis in dermatologic surgery. *J Am Acad Dermatol* 1995; **32**: 155–176.

10 Classen D, Evans R, Pestotnik S, Horn SD, Menlove RL, Bunke JP. The timing of prophylactic administration of antibiotics and the risk of surgical-wound infection. *N Engl J Med* 1992; **326**: 281–286.

11 Nichols R. Surgical wound infection. *Am J Med* 1991; **91**: 54S–64S.

12 Cruse P, Foord R. A five-year prospective study of 23 649 surgical wounds. *Arch Surg* 1973; **107**: 206–210.

13 Anon. Antibiotic prophylaxis in surgery. *Med Lett Drugs Therapeut* 1985; **26**: 105–108.

14 Valentine R, Weigett J, Dryer D, Rodgers C. Effect of remote infections on clean wound infection rates. *Am J Infect Control* 1986; **14**: 64–67.

15 Braga M, Baccari P, Di Palo S, Radaelli G, Gianotti L, Cristallo M *et al.* Effectiveness of perioperative short-term antibiotic prophylaxis in reducing surgical risk induced by malnutrition and anergy. *Acta Chir Scand* 1990; **156**: 751–757.

16 Cainzos M, Alcalde J, Potel J, Puente JL. Anergy in patients with gastric cancer. *Hepatogastroenterology* 1989; **36**: 36–39.

17 Moesgaard F, Lykkegaard-Nielsen L. Preoperative cell-mediated immunity and duration of antibiotic prophylaxis in relation to postoperative infectious complications. *Acta Chir Scand* 1989; **155**: 281–286.

18 Wilson W, Kirkpatrick C, Talmage D. Suppression of immunologic response in uremia. *Ann Intern Med* 1965; **62**: 1–14.

19 Battacharya N, Kosloske A. Preoperative wound infection in pediatric surgical patients: a study of 676 infants and children. *J Pediatr Surg* 1990; **25**: 125–129.

20 Postlethwait R, Johnson W. Complications following surgery for duodenal ulcer in obese patients. *Arch Surg* 1972; **105**: 348–350.

21 Condon R. Antibiotic prophylaxis in gastrointestinal surgery. In: Davis J, Shires G (eds) *Principles and Management of Surgical Infection*. JB Lippincott, Philadelphia, 1991, pp. 133–134.

22 Lilienfeld D, Vlahov D, Tenney J, McLaughlin JS. Obesity and diabetes as risk factors for postoperative wound infections after cardiac surgery. *Am J Infect Control* 1988; **16**: 3–6.

23 Tabet J, Johnson J. Wound infection in head and neck surgery: prophylaxis, etiology and management. *J Otolaryngol* 1990; **19**: 197–200.

24 DeMaria E, Reichman W, Kenney P, Armitage JM, Gann DS. Septic complications of corticosteroid administration after central nervous system trauma. *Ann Surg* 1985; **202**: 248–252.

25 Cohen M, Pollak R, Garcia J, Mozes MF. Reconstructive surgery for immunosuppressed organ-transplant patients. *Plast Reconstr Surg* 1989; **83**: 291–295.

26 Hunt T. Wound complications. In: Hardy J (ed.) *Complications in Surgery and Their Management*. WB Saunders, Philadelphia, 1981, pp. 20–31.

27 Peterson L. Antibiotic prophylaxis against wound infections in oral and maxillofacial surgery. *J Oral Maxillofac Surg* 1990; **48**: 617–620.

28 Wilson R. *Surgical Problems in Immunodepressed Patients*. WB Saunders, Philadelphia, 1984, p. 188.

29 Anon. Antimicrobial prophylaxis and treatment in patients with granulocytopenia. *Med Lett Drugs Therapeut* 1981; **23**: 55–56.

30 Beuhrer J, Weber D, Meyer A, Becherer PR, Rutala WA, Wilson B. Wound infection rates after invasive procedures in HIV-1 seropositive versus HIV-1 seronegative hemophiliacs. *Ann Surg* 1990; **211**: 492–498.

31 Benotti P, Jenkins R, Cady B, O'Hara C, Groopman JE. Surgical approach to generalized lymphadenopathy in homosexual men. *J Surg Oncol* 1987; **36**: 231–234.

32 Christen D, Buchmann P, Grob R. Anal condylomata acuminata in HIV positive patients. *Langenbecks Arch Chir* 1991; **377**: 207–210.

33 Wexner S, Smithy W, Milsom J, Dailey TH. The surgical management of anorectal diseases in AIDS and pre-AIDS patients. *Dis Colon Rectum* 1986; **29**: 719–723.

34 Burke J. The effective period of preventive antibiotic action in experimental incisions and dermal lesions. *Surgery* 1961; **50**: 161–168.

35 Burke J. Preventing bacterial infection by coordinating antibiotic and host activity: a time dependent relationship. *South Med J* 1977; **70**: 24–26.

36 Ulualp K, Condon R. Antibiotic prophylaxis for scheduled operative procedures. *Infect Dis Clin* 1992; **6**: 613–625.

37 Hirschmann J. Controversies in antimicrobial prophylaxis. *Chemoterapia* 1987; **6**: 202–207.

38 DiPiro J, Record K, Schanzenback K *et al.* Antimicrobial prophylaxis in surgery: part 2. *Am J Hosp Pharmacol* 1981; **38**: 487–494.

39 Sebben J. Prophylactic antibiotics in cutaneous surgery. *J Dermatol Surg Oncol* 1985; **11**: 901–906.

40 Strachan CJ, Black J, Powis S, Waterworth TA, Wise R, Wilkinson AR *et al.* Prophylactic use of cephazolin against wound sepsis after cholecystectomy. *Br Med J* 1977; **1**: 1254–1256.

41 Zitelli J. Secondary intention healing. *Clin Dermatol* 1984; **2**: 92–106.

42 Bayliss R, Clarke C, Oakley C, Somerville W, Whitfield AG. The teeth and infective endocarditis. *Br Heart J* 1983; **50**: 506–512.

43 Oakley C, Sommerville W. Prevention of infective endocarditis. *Br Heart J* 1981; **45**: 233–235.

44 Korzeniowski O, Kaye D. Endocarditis. In: Gorbach S, Bartlett J, Blacklow N (eds) *Infectious Diseases*. WB Saunders, Philadelphia, 1992, pp. 548–557.

45 Clemens J, Ransohoff D. A quantitative assessment of predental antibiotic prophylaxis for patients with mitral valve prolapse. *J Chron Dis* 1983; **37**: 531–543.

46 Kaplan E. Bacterial endocarditis prophylaxis: tradition or necessity? *Am J Cardiol* 1986; **57**: 478–479.

47 MacMahon S, Roberts J, Kramer-Fox R, Zucker DM, Roberts RB, Devereux RB. Mitral valve prolapse and infective endocarditis. *Am Heart J* 1987; **113**: 1291–1298.

48 Dajani A, Bisno A, Chung KJ, Durack DT, Freed M, Gerber MA *et al.* Prevention of bacterial endocarditis. *JAMA* 1990; **264**: 2919–2922.

49 Shulman S, Amren D, Bisno A, Dajani AS, Durack DT, Gerber MA *et al.* Prevention of bacterial endocarditis. *Am J Dis Child* 1985; **139**: 232–235.

50 Lavie C, Khandheria B, Seward J, Tajik AJ, Taylor CL, Ballard DJ. Factors associated with the recommendation for endocarditis prophylaxis in mitral valve prolapse. *JAMA* 1989; **262**: 3308–3312.

51 Hickey A, MacMahon S, Wilchen D. Mitral valve prolapse and bacterial endocarditis: when is antibiotic prophylaxis necessary? *Am Heart J* 1986; **109**: 431–435.

52 MacMahon S, Hickey A, Wilcken DE, Wittes JT, Feneley MP, Hickie JB. Risk of infective endocarditis in mitral valve prolapse with and without precordial systolic murmurs. *Am J Cardiol* 1986; **58**: 105–108.

53 Scheld W, Sande M. Endocarditis and intravascular infections. In: Mandel R, Douglas R, Bennett J (eds) *Principles and Practice of Infectious Diseases*. John Wiley & Sons, New York, 1985, pp. 504–530.

54 Everett D, Hirschman J. Transient bacteremia and endocarditis prophylaxis: a review. *Medicine* 1977; **56**: 61–77.

55 Von Reyn C, Levy B, Arbeit R, Friedland G, Crumpacker CS. Infective endocarditis: an analysis based on strict case definitions. *Ann Intern Med* 1981; **94**: 505–518.

56 Bayliss R, Clarke C, Oakley C, Somerville W, Whitfield AG, Young SE. The microbiology and pathogenesis of infective endocarditis. *Br Heart J* 1983; **50**: 513–519.

57 Griffin M, Wilson W, Edwards W, O'Fallon WM, Kurland LT. Infective endocarditis— Olmsted County, Minnesota, 1950–1981. *JAMA* 1985; **254**: 1199–1202.

58 Durack D. Prophylaxis of infective endocarditis. In: Mandel R, Douglas R, Bennett J (eds) *Principles and Practice of Infectious Diseases*. John Wiley & Sons, New York, 1985, pp. 539–544.

59 Guntheroth W. How important are dental procedures as a cause of infective

endocarditis? *Am J Cardiol* 1984; **54**: 797–801.

60 Bayliss R, Clarke C, Oakley C, Somerville W, Whitfield AG, Young SE. The bowel, the genitourinary tract and infective endocarditis. *Br Heart J* 1984; **51**: 339–345.

61 Tzukert A, Leviner E, Benollel R, Katz J. Analysis of the American Heart Association's recommendations for the prevention of infective endocarditis. *Oral Surg Oral Med Oral Pathol* 1986; **62**: 276–279.

62 Imperiale T. Does prophylaxis prevent postdental infective endocarditis? *Am J Med* 1990; **88**: 131–136.

63 McGowan D. Nature and prevention of infective endocarditis. In: Cawson R (ed.) *The Medicine Publishing Foundation*. The Medicine Publishing Foundation, Oxford, 1987, pp. 129–142.

64 Pallasch T. A critical appraisal of antibiotic prophylaxis. *Int Dent J* 1989; **39**: 183–194.

65 Kaye D. Prophylaxis for infective endocarditis: an update. *Ann Intern Med* 1986; **104**: 419–423.

66 Tzukert A, Leviner E, Sela M. Prevention of infective endocarditis: not by antibiotics alone. *Oral Surg Oral Med Oral Pathol* 1986; **62**: 383–388.

67 Kaye D. Prophylaxis against bacterial endocarditis: a dilemma. *Am Heart Assoc* 1977; **52**: 67–69.

68 Durack D, Kaplan E, Bisno A. Apparent failures of endocarditis prophylaxis. *JAMA* 1983; **250**: 2318–2322.

69 Richards J. Bacteremia following irritation of foci of infection. *JAMA* 1932; **99**: 1496–1497.

70 Fine B, Sheckman P, Bartlett J. Incision and drainage of soft tissue abscesses and bacteremia. *Ann Intern Med* 1985; **103**: 645–647.

71 Glenchur H, Patel P, Pathmarajah C. Transient bacteremia associated with debridement of decubitus ulcers. *Milit Med* 1981; **146**: 432–433.

72 Sabetta J, Zitelli J. The incidence of bacteremia during skin surgery. *Arch Dermatol* 1987; **123**: 213–215.

73 Wilson W, Van Scoy R, Washington J. Incidence of bacteremia in adults without infection. *J Clin Microbiol* 1975; **2**: 94–95.

74 Zack L, Remlinger K, Thompson K. The incidence of bacteremia following skin surgery. *J Infect Dis* 1989; **159**: 148–150.

75 Halpern A, Leyden J, Dzubow L, McGinley KJ. The incidence of bacteremia in skin surgery of the head and neck. *J Am Acad Dermatol* 1988; **19**: 112–116.

76 Maurice P, Parker S, Azadian B, Cream JJ. Minor skin surgery—are prophylactic antibiotics ever needed for curettage? *Acta Dermatol Venereol (Stockh)* 1991; **71**: 267–268.

77 O'Neill T, Hone R, Blake S. Prosthetic valve endocarditis caused by *Proprionibacterium acnes*. *Br Med J* 1988; **296**: 1444.

78 Spelman D, Weinmann A, Spicer W. Endocarditis following skin procedures. *J Infect* 1993; **26**: 185–189.

79 McGowan D, Hendrey M. Is antibiotic prophylaxis required for dental patients with joint replacements? *Br Dent J* 1985; **158**: 336–338.

80 Fitzgerald R. Infections of hip prostheses and artificial joints. *Infect Dis Clin* 1989; **3**: 329–337.

81 Sanderson P. The choice between prophylactic agents for orthopedic surgery. *J Hosp Infect* 1988; **11**: 57–67.

82 Ainscow D, Denham R. The risk of hematogenous infection in total joint replacements. *J Bone Joint Surg (Br)* 1984; **66**: 580–582.

83 Segreti J, Levin S. The role of prophylactic antibiotics in the prevention of prosthetic device infections. *Infect Dis Clin* 1989; **3**: 357–370.

84 Lattimer G, Keblish P, Dickson TB Jr, Vernick CG, Finnegan WJ. Hematogenous infection in total joint replacement. *JAMA* 1979; **242**: 2213–2214.

Index

Page references in *italics* refer to figures and those in **bold** refer to tables.